PSYCHIATRIC
Words and Phrases

2020 Edition

Mary Ann D'Onofrio
and
Elizabeth D'Onofrio

LITTLE PEBBLE PRESS

Psychiatric Words and Phrases
Copyright © 2020 by Little Pebble Press

www.littlepebblepress.com

ISBN-13: 9798632345361

LEXINGTON, KENTUCKY, UNITED STATES OF AMERICA

All rights reserved. No part of this book may be reproduced or utilized in any form or by any means without the written permission of the author.

PREFACE

Psychiatric Words and Phrases is not a glossary; it is not a coding book. It is a book containing an alphabetical list of terms designed to aid practitioners working in the fields of psychiatry, psychology and learning disabilities, as well as those professionals working with speech, hearing and visually disabled individuals. These doctors, nurses, therapists, even scribes, must work within the parameters proscribed for the electronic health record. Psychiatric and related disorders will be tied to the World Health Organization's International Classification of Diseases (ICD-10) system, modified in the United States as ICD-10-CM. *Psychiatric Words and Phrases* offers both the updated and new terms with selective ICD-10-CM codes for these psychiatric diseases, disorders and other specific conditions.

Under the umbrella category "associations, professsional" we list a wide variety of organizations with their web page addresses. A sample list includes: the American Psychiatric Association, the American Psychological Association, Buros Center for Testing, the Hearing Health Foundation, and the Society for Research in Child Development. We have especially included sources from Australia, Canada, Great Britain, India, and Ireland. Our eBook version of PWP provides a hyperlink to the website of each of the 200+ groups listed.

The *Psychiatric Words and Phrases* entry "test" provides descriptive terms for tests. The entry "tests" lists general tests along with specific spellings of eponymous tests grouped into categories such as Behavior, Development, Education, Neuropsychological, Personality, and Speech and Hearing. We have given added attention to new words and phrases in the areas of hearing, speech, and vision.

In addition to its alphabetical list, *Psychiatric Words and Phrases* offers an Appendix which lists the English names of the muscles of the head and neck with each corresponding Latin name given in parentheses.

This new edition of PWP is also available as an eBook designed for ease of use and quick access to additional information online.

~ Mary Ann D'Onofrio

Psychiatric Words and Phrases 1

A

"A" (street name, LSD; amphetamine)
A+Ox3 (alert and oriented times three)
AAAP (American Academy of Addiction Psychiatry)
AACAP (American Academy of Child and Adolescent Psychiatry)
AACDP (American Association of Chairs of Departments of Psychiatry)
AADPR (American Association of Directors of Psychiatric Residency)
AAFP (American Academy of Family Physicians)
AAGP (American Association for Geriatric Psychiatry)
AAGH (Association for Advancement of Gestalt Therapy)
AAIDD (American Association on Intellectual and Developmental Disabilities)
AAMFT (American Association for Marriage and Family Therapy)
AAMT (*see* Association for Healthcare Documentation Integrity)
AAP (American Academy of Pediatrics)
AAP (Association for Academic Psychiatry)
AAPA (American Association of Psychiatric Administrators)
AAPAA (American Academy of Psychiatrists in Alcoholism and Addictions)
AAPL (American Academy of Psychiatry and the Law)
AAPM&R (American Academy of Physical Medicine and Rehabilitation)
AAS (American Auditory Society)
AASM (American Academy of Sleep Medicine)
AASP (American Association for Social Psychiatry)
AAT (Academic Aptitude Test)
abalienate
   abalienatic mentis
   abalienation
abandoner
abandonment
   fear of
   imagined
   perceived
   real
abandonment concerns
abandominiums (re: abandoned row houses where drugs are sold)
Abbreviated Conners Rating Scale
Abbreviated Conners Teachers Questionnaire
ABC (Aberrant Behavior Checklist)
ABC (Assessment of Basic Competencies)
ABC Inventory—Extended
ABCD (The Arizona Battery for Communication Disorders of Dementia)
ABCT (Association for Behavioral and Cognitive Therapies)
abdominal-diaphragmatic respiration
abdominal distress (a panic attack indicator)
abdominal wall movement

Psychiatric Words and Phrases

abdominis
   musculus obliquus externus
   musculus obliquus internus
abducens (cranial nerve VI)
abducent
abduction
abductor
abductor paralysis
   bilateral
   unilateral
"Abe" (re: drug value)
aberrant behavior
Aberrant Behavior Checklist (ABC)
ABES (Adaptive Behavior Evaluation Scale)
"Abe's cabe" (re: currency)
ABFM (American Board of Family Medicine)
ABFP (American Board of Family Practice)
abilities *(see* ability)
abilities test *(see also* tests)
ability (pl: abilities)
   abstracting
   abstractive
   attention shift
   attentional
   auditory
   cognitive
   communication
   conceptual
   concrete
   constructional
   coping
   disturbance in perceptual motor
   disturbance in word-finding
   drawing
   focal
   general learning
   impaired
   impaired attention
   impaired communication
   impaired focal
   impaired intellectual
   impaired learning
   impaired memory

ability (pl: abilities)
   impaired thinking
   impairment in perceptual-motor
   intellectual
   language
   learning
   mathematical
   memory
   mental
   nonverbal abstraction
   nonverbal synthesizing
   oral sensory
   perceptual
   perceptual motor
   positive
   premorbid
   reality testing (Rorschach)
   reduced attention
   spatial
   thinking
   writing
ability battery (see also *tests*)
ability test *(see also* tests)
Ability-to-Benefit Administration Test
ability to take criticism
ABLL (Alternate Binaural Loudness Balance) test
ABLE (Adult Basic Learning Examination)
ablutomania
abnormal asymmetry
abnormal brain structures
abnormal development
abnormal gait
abnormal involuntary movement scale (AIMS)
abnormal mood
abnormal movements
abnormal pathologic condition
abnormal perceptions due to a psychotic disorder
abnormal perceptions due to drug effect
abnormal perceptions of external reality

abnormal positioning of distal
 limbs
abnormal responsiveness
abnormal sleep-wake schedule
abnormalities in sleep-wake
 timing mechanisms,
 endogenous
abnormality (pl: abnormalities)
 brain
 cranial nerve
 electrolyte
 eye movement
 food intake
 gait
 inherited
 laboratory
 metabolic
 performance
 polysomnographic
 sleep
 sleep-wake
 structural brain
 vocal pitch
abnormality in performance
abnormality of affect
"abolic" (street name, veterinary
 steroid)
"A-bomb" (re: marijuana
 cigarettes with heroin or opium)
"A-boot" (re: under the influence
 of drugs)
abortion
above-average intelligence
ABP (Association for Business
 Psychology)
ABR (auditory brainstem
 response)
ABR audiometry
abrupt onset
abrupt topic shift
abscess, intracranial
absence
absence epilepsy
absence from work, pattern of
 unexplained
absence of feeling
absence of maladaptive behavior

absence seizure (petit mal
 epilepsy)
absence status
absence syndrome
absense seizure
 atonic
 atypical
absent ataxia
absent sexual desire
absentia
absolute agoraphobia
absolute construction of phrases
absolute quantity
absolute scotoma
absolute threshold
absorption of drug
absorption of inhalants,
 pulmonary
abstinence
 alcohol
 drug
 nicotine
 sexual
abstract concept
abstract thinking, excessive use of
abstracting ability
abstraction ladder
abstractive ability
 concrete
 nonverbal
abstractive ability
abulia, cyclic
abulic
abulomania
abuse
 adult physical, by
  nonspouse or nonpartner
 adult psychological, by
  nonspouse or nonpartner
 adult sexual, by nonspouse
  or nonpartner
 child physical (see codes
  under child physical
  abuse)
 child psychological (see
  codes under child
  psychological abuse)

4   Psychiatric Words and Phrases

abuse
   child sexual (see codes
     under child sexual abuse)
   non-parental child
   parental child
   steroid compound drug
     (anabolic steroids)
   stimulant drug
     (amphetamine)
   stimulant drug (cocaine)
   stimulant drug
     (methamphetamine)
abuse and neglect problem
abuse counseling
abuse criteria
abuse or dependence
   adolescent
   adult
   aerosol spray
   alcohol
   amphetamine
   amyl nitrate
   antidepressant type
   anxiolytic
   barbiturate
   caffeine
   cannabis
   chemical
   child
   childhood physical
   childhood sexual
   chronic alcoholic
   club drug
   cocaine
   designer drug
   drug
   elder
   emotional
   hallucinogen
   hashish
   hypnotic (drug)
   inhalant
   laxative
   "laxative habit"
   LSD
   marijuana
   mental

abuse or dependence
   MDMA
   methamphetamine
   mixed drug
   morphine-type
   nonparent
   nonprescription drug
   opioid
   parent
   patent medicinal
   perpetuator of
   phencyclidine/PCP
   physical
   polydrug
   problems related to
   psychoactive substance
   psychological
   ritual
   sadistic
   sedative
   sexual
   spousal
   spouse
   substance
   sympathomimetic
   tobacco
   tranquilizer
   verbal
   victim
   vocal
abused child
abused drugs/substances
   alcohol
   anxiolytic (medications)
   caffeine
   cannabinoids (hashish)
   cannabinoids (marijuana)
   club (ecstasy)
   club (flunitrazepam)
   club (GHB - gamma-
     hydroxybutyrate)
   club (MDMA -
     methylendioxymethamph
     etamine)
   club (Nexus)
   club (Rohypnol)
   compounds (anabolic
     steroids)

Psychiatric Words and Phrases 5

abused drugs/substances
  depressants (medications)
  designer (Alpha-
    ethyltryptamine)
  designer (DMT -
    dimethyltryptamine)
  designer (DXM -
    dextromethorphan)
  designer (fentanyl)
  designer (GHB - gamma-
    hydroxybutyrate)
  designer (ketamine)
  designer (khat)
  designer (methcathinone)
  designer
    (methylendioxymethamph
    etamine)
  designer (4-Bromo-2,5
    dithroxy-phenyl-
    ethylamine)
  designer (2,5-dimethyloxy-
    4-methyl-amphetamine)
  designer (STP)
  hallucinogen (LSD -
    lysergic acid
    diethylamide)
  hallucinogen (mescaline)
  hallucinogen
    (phencyclidine (PCP)
  hallucinogen
    (psilocybin/psilocin)
  hallucinogen (salvia)
  hypnotics (tranquilizers)
  inhalants (nitrites)
  opioid (desomorphine)
  opioid (heroin)
  opioid (methadone)
  opioid (methylmorphine/
    codeine)
  opioid (morphine)
  opioid (opium)
  psychotic (medications)
  sedative (barbiturates)
  stimulant (amphetamine)
  stimulant (cocaine/crack)
  stimulant
    (methamphetamine)
  tobacco (nicotine)
abuser
  adult
  anxious substance
  child
  drug
  non-parent child
  non-spouse adult
  parent
  partner
  spouse
  substance
abusive vocal behavior
abutting consonant(s)
"Abyssinian tea" (street name,
  khat)
AC (air conduction; alternating
  current)
"AC/DC" (street name, codeine
  cough syrup)
"AC/DC" (street name, liquid
  cannabis)
ACA (Affordable Care Act)
Academic Competence
  Evaluation Scale
academic functioning
  marked decline in
  sub-average
Academic Instruction
  Measurement System
academic or educational problems
  (Z55.9)
academic performance
academic problem
academic psychiatry
academically understimulating
  environment
Academy of Integrative Pain
  Management
acalculia
  aphasic
  visual-spatial
"Acapulco gold" (street name,
  cannabis/marijuana from SW
  Mexico)
"Acapulco red" (street name,
  cannabis/marijuana)
accelerated speech
accelerometer

6 Psychiatric Words and Phrases

accent
accent, foreign
acceptable skill, minimum
acceptance of health care, patient
Access Management Survey (AMS)
access to health care services, problems with
accessing cues
accessing cues, eye
accessory nerve, spiral
ACCI (Adult Career Concerns Inventory)
accident-prone behavior
accidents as major childhood stressors
accidents, alcohol-related risk for
accommodation, passive
Accounting Program Admission Test (APAT)
acculturation difficulty (Z60.3)
acculturation problem
acculturation problems with:
    expression of customs
    expression of habits
    expression of political values
    expression of religious values
Accuracy in Children, Test of Listening
accusations, false
accusative case
ACDM (Assessment of Career Decision Making)
ACE (The American Council on Education)
"ace" (street name, cannabis/marijuana; phencyclidine)
ACER Applied Reading Test
ACER Test of Reasoning Ability
ACER Tests of Basic Skills
acetylcholine
ACG (Assessment of Core Goals)
achievement behavior, terminal
achievement quotient (AQ)

achievement
    educational
    exaggerated
aching headache
aching pain
"acid" (street name, LSD)
acid
    drop
    plasma homovanillic (HVA)
acid-base balance
"acid cube" (re: sugar cube with LSD)
acid flashbacks
"acid freak" (re: heavy user of LSD)
"acid head" (re: LSD user)
acidic cannabinoid
"acido" (street name, hallucinogens; LSD)
acidosis
    distal renal tubular
    metabolic
    proximal renal tubular
Ackerman-Schoendorf Scales for Parent Evaluation of Custody
ACNP (American College of Neuropsychopharmacology)
ACO (Assessment of Conceptual Organization)
ACO: Improving Writing, Thinking, and Reading Skills
acouesthesia
acoupedic method
acoupedic method of rehabilitation
acoupedics
acoustic agnosia
acoustic-amnestic aphasia
acoustic analysis
acoustic area
acoustic cell
acoustic contralateral reflex
acoustic crest
acoustic cyst
acoustic energy
acoustic evoked potential
acoustic feedback

acoustic gain
acoustic gain, peak
acoustic gain control
acoustic immittance measurement
   test
acoustic impedance
acoustic impedance, static
acoustic interface
acoustic ipsilateral reflex
acoustic measurement of auditory
   function
acoustic meatus
   external
   internal
acoustic method
acoustic method aural
   rehabilitation
acoustic nerve
acoustic neurilemoma
acoustic neuroma
acoustic noise
acoustic output, maximum
acoustic papilla
acoustic phonetics
acoustic radiation
acoustic ratio, the oral-nasal
   (TONAR)
acoustic reflex
      sensitivity prediction from
         the (SPAR)
      stapedial
acoustic reflex amplitude
acoustic reflex decay
acoustic reflex latency
acoustic reflex pattern
acoustic reflex threshold
acoustic spectrum
acoustic stapedial reflex
acoustic stria
acoustic trauma
acoustic trauma deafness
acoustic tubercle
acoustical
Acoustical Society of America
acousticians
acousticopalpebral reflex
acoustics

ACP (American College of
   Physicians)
ACPA (The American Chronic
   Pain Association)
acquired aphasia
acquired epileptic aphasia
   (Landau-Kleffner syndrome)
acquired fluent aphasia
acquired sexual dysfunction
acquired type dyspareunia
acquired type female orgasmic
   disorder
acquired type female sexual
   arousal disorder
acquired type hypoactive sexual
   desire disorder
acquired type male erectile
   disorder
acquired type male orgasmic
   disorder
acquired type sexual aversion
   disorder
acquired type vaginismus
acrolect
acromania
acrophase
across identity states
act(s)
      biological
      frequency of violence
      instrumental avoidance
      rape
      sadistic rape
      sensorimotor
      serious suicide
      speech
      suicide
      violent
ACT Assessment (Enhanced)
ACT Assessment, The
ACT Evaluation/Survey Service,
   The (ESS)
act of rape, sadistic
ACT Study Power Assessment
   and Inventory (SPA; SPI)
ACT Study Skills Assessment and
   Inventory (SSA; SSI)
act theory, instrumental avoidance

ACTeRS (ADD-H:
  Comprehensive Teacher's
  Rating Scale)
acting out
  asocial
  passive-aggressive
  sexual
acting out potential
acting-out tendencies
action
  amphetamine-like
  brought into
  compulsive
  course of
  duration of drug
  effective
  intensified
  legal
  lengths of
  level of
  modes of
  morphine-like
  plan of
  semiautomatic
  unacceptable
  uncontrolled
Action and Motion, Thinking
  Creatively in
Action Coding System, Facial
  (FACS)
action of lithium
  clinical
  therapeutic
  toxic
action on first messengers,
  lithium's
action on membranes, lithium's
action on second messengers,
  lithium's
action potential
action tremor
action-locative
action-object
active bilingualism
active desire
active displacement of emotive
  energy
active filter

active modification
active phase of schizophrenia
active psychotic symptom
active sleep
active treatment
active voice
active-phase symptoms
active-phase symptoms of
  schizophrenia
activity (pl. activities)
  alpha
  alpha EEG
  anhedonic
  autonomic
  background
  beta
  brain wave
  cross-gender
  decreased
  diminished pleasure in
    everyday
  disturbance in integrating
    tactile information with
    motor
  disturbance in integrating
    visual information with
    motor
  disturbance in integrating
    auditory information with
    motor
  EEG alpha
  EEG delta
  EEG theta
  electromyographic
  electrooculographic
  excessive motor
  fast
  focus of
  frequency of violent
  goal-directed
  hedonistic
  high risk
  impulsive
  limited
  major life
  major point of
  masochistic sexual

activity (pl. activities)
   masturbatory
   motor
   neglect of pleasurable
   nighttime
   nonproductive
   occupational
   organized
   paroxysmal
   peripheral electromyographic
   pharyngeal motor
   phasic REM
   pleasurable
   political
   psychomotor
   random
   rapid change in
   reduced physical
   religious
   repetitious
   role-play
   self-care
   self-initiated
   serious assaultive
   sexual
   slow-frequency (delta) EEG
   slowing
   slow-wave
   solitary
   speech
   stereotyped
   stream of mental
   sweat gland
   take pleasure in few
   voyeuristic
activity in life, everyday
Activity Losses Assessment (ALA)
activity map, brain electrical (BEAM)
activity of daily living, normal
Activity Pattern Indicators (APIs)
activity restriction
actual derailment
Actualizing Assessment Battery I: The Interpersonal Inventories
Actualizing Assessment Battery II: The Interpersonal Inventories
acuity
   auditory
   sensory
acuity level masking technique, sensorineural
acuity level technique, sensorineural
aculturated into a system (e.g. gang)
acute akathisia, neuroleptic-induced
acute amnesia
acute aphonia
acute confusional migraine headache
acute delirium
acute discomfort in close relationships, pattern of
acute dystonia, neuroleptic-induced
acute exacerbation schizophrenia
acute fear
acute intoxication
acute labyrinthine disorder
acute laryngitis
acute mania
acute movement disorder, neuroleptic-induced
acute organic brain syndrome
acute pain
acute phoneme
acute seizure
acute stress disorder (F43.0)
acute toxic effects
"AD" (street name, phencyclidine; drug addict)
AD Scale (Acceptance of Disability Scale)
ADAA (Anxiety and Depression Association of America)
"adam" (re: analog of amphetamine/methamphetamine; MDMA)
Adam's apple, surgical reduction of
adaptability skills, stress

10 Psychiatric Words and Phrases

Adaptability Test
adaptation effect
adaptation effect of stuttering
Adapted Sequenced Inventory of
 Communication Development
adapting, difficulty in
adaption, auditory
adaptive behavior
Adaptive Behavior Evaluation
 Scale (ABES)
Adaptive Behavior Inventory
Adaptive Behavior Scale
adaptive functioning, impairment
 in
adaptive information processing
 (AIP)
adaptive level, high
Adaptive Living Skills
Adaptive Placement Exam
adaptive response
adaptive scale norms
adaptive skill domains
ADARA (American Deafness and
 Rehabilitation Association)
ADAS (Alzheimer's Disease
 Assessment Scale)
ADAS noncognitive subscale
ADC (AIDS dementia complex)
ADC Scale
ADDBRS (Attention Deficit
 Disorder Behavior Rating
 Scales)
added purpose task
ADDES (Attention Deficit
 Disorders Evaluation Scale)
ADD-H: Comprehensive
 Teacher's Rating Scale
addict, drug (DA)
addiction
    absinthe
    alcohol
    biological roots of
    cocaine
    drug
    ethyl alcohol
    heroin
    iatrogenic
    internet

addiction
    methyl alcohol
    methylated spirits
    morphine-type
    nicotine
    opium
    painkiller
    polysurgical
    proneness to
    relation
    relationship
    sex
    social media
    sympathic mimetic
    sympathomimetic
    tobacco
addiction psychiatry
addictive behavior
addictive behavior, sexually
addictive disorders
addictive potential of drug
addictive-related disorders
addition articulation
additional information
adduction
adductor paralysis
    bilateral
    unilateral
adenoid, lateral trim of the
adenoidectomy, lateral
adequate sexual excitement
adequate sexual function
adequate treatment
ADFM (Association of
 Departments of Family
 Medicine)
adhesive otitis media
ADI (Adolescent Diagnostic
 Interview)
ADI (Adolescent Drinking Index)
adjective (parts of speech)
adjective
    derived
    predicate
adjustment
    cultural
    life-cycle
    premorbid

Psychiatric Words and Phrases

adjustment disorder with anxiety (F43.22)
adjustment disorder with depressed mood (F43.21)
adjustment disorder with disturbance of conduct (F43.24)
adjustment disorder with mixed anxiety and depressed mood (F43.23)
adjustment disorder with mixed disturbance of emotions and conduct (F43.25)
adjustment disorder, unspecified (F43.20)
adjustment following migration, cultural
adjustment interface disorder
adjuvant therapy
ADL Index/Scale (see under *Test*)
ADL's, hierarchical scale of
administration
    avenues of
    method of
Administrator Assessment Survey, School
admiration
    excessive
    need for
Admissions Testing program, PAR
admittance
adolescence
    GID of
    late
adolescent abuse
Adolescent Adjustment Profile
Adolescent Alienation Index
adolescent antisocial behavior, child or (Z72.810)
adolescent behavior
adolescent conduct disorder
adolescent cross-gender behavior
Adolescent Diagnostic Interview
Adolescent Drinking Index (ADI)
adolescent group therapies
adolescent guardedness
Adolescent Language Screening Test

Adolescent Multiphasic Personality Inventory
adolescent onset
adolescent personal identity
adolescent psychiatry
adolescent psychology
adolescent risk-taking behavior
Adolescent Separation Anxiety Test
adolescent sexual identity
adolescent suicide
adolescent voice
Adolescent-Coping Orientation for Problem Experiences
Adolescent-Family Inventory of Life Events and Changes
adolescents
    communication with
    evaluation of
    limit-setting for
adoption as major childhood stressor
adoptive family
adrenal hyperplasia, congenital
adrenoleukodystrophy
ADS (American Dialect Society)
adult
    consenting
    nonconsenting
adult abuse
adult antisocial behavior (Z72.811)
Adult Basic Education—Forms 5 and 6, Tests of
Adult Basic Learning Examination
Adult Career Concerns Inventory (ACCI)
adult criminal behavior
adult cross-gender behavior
adult group therapies
adult life
adult maltreatment and neglect problems
Adult Neuropsychological Questionnaire (ANQ)
adult obstructive sleep apnea syndrome

adult-onset fluency disorder
    (F98.5)
Adult Personal Adjustment and
    Role Skills
Adult Personality Inventory (API)
adult physical abuse by nonspouse
    or nonpartner
    confirmed, initial encounter
        (T74.11XA)
    confirmed, subsequent
        encounter (T74.11XD)
    suspected, initial encounter
        (T76.11XA)
    suspected, subsequent
        encounter (T76.11XD)
Adult Protective Services (APS)
adult psychological abuse by
    nonspouse or nonpartner
    confirmed, initial encounter
        (T74.31XA)
    confirmed, subsequent
        encounter (T74.31XD)
    suspected, initial encounter
        (T76.31XA)
    suspected, subsequent
        encounter (T76.31XD)
adult sexual abuse by nonspouse
    or nonpartner
    confirmed, initial encounter
        (T74.21XA)
    confirmed, subsequent
        encounter (T74.21XD)
    suspected, initial encounter
        (T76.21XA)
    suspected, subsequent
        encounter (T76.21XD)
Adult Suicidal Ideation
    Questionnaire (ASIQ)
adult survivor of child abuse
adult survivor of neglect
adulthood psychiatry
adulthood, GID of
adultomorphic behavior role
adult-onset type conduct disorder
advanced dementia
advanced disease
Advanced Measures of Music
    Audiation

Advanced Progressive Matrices
advanced sleep phase pattern
advanced sleep phase syndrome
Advanced Test B90: New Zealand
    Edition, ACER
adventitious deafness
adventitious movement
adverb (parts of speech)
adverse effect of medication,
    other
    initial encounter
        (T50.905.A)
    sequela (T50.905.S)
    subsequent encounter
        (T50.905.D)
adverse effects, potential
adverse effects of medication
advice
    against medical
    excessive need for
aelurophobia
AERA (average evoked response
    audiometry)
aerodynamic analysis
aerodynamics
affair(s)
    accidental
    extramarital
    instrumental
    love
    withdrawal from social
affect (noun)
    abnormalities of
    ambivalent
    angry
    apathetic
    appropriate
    assessment of
    bland
    blunted
    congruent
    constricted
    depressed
    depressive
    diminution of
    dramatic
    dysphoric
    elated

Psychiatric Words and Phrases

affect (noun)
    emptiness of
    euphoric
    flat
    fluctuating
    garrulous
    impaired
    inappropriate
    incongruous
    infantile
    intense
    intense painful
    isolation of
    labile
    labile range of
    modulated
    negative
    normal
    predominant
    preservation of
    removed
    restricted
    restricted range of
    shallow
    short-lived schizophrenic
    silly
    solemn
    superficial
    vacuous
affect modulation, impaired
affect state, opposite
affective arousal
affective disease
affective disorder
    antidepressant use in
    atypical
    atypical bipolar
    electroconvulsive therapy use in
    lithium use in
    major
    organic
    primary (PAD)
affective disorder syndrome
affective dyscontrol
affective experience
affective expression
affective flattening
affective function
affective incontinence
affective lability
affective personality
affective psychosis
    bipolar
    depressive
    involutional
    major depressive
    manic
    manic-depressive
    melancholia
    mixed-type
    mood swings
    senile
affective reactivity
affective responsiveness, mutual
affective set of disturbances
affectivity, flattened
affectivity ratio, high
Affects Balance Scale
afferent (kinesthetic) motor aphasia
afferent feedback
afferent motor aphasia
afferent nerve
affiliation
affirmative care for transgenders
affix
affluenza (affluent neglect)
Affordable Care Act (ACA)
affricate consonant formation
affrication
affricative
Afgani indica" (street name, cannabis/marijuana)
"African" (street name, marijuana/cannabis)
"African black" (street name, cannabis/marijuana)
"African bush" (street name, cannabis/marijuana)
"African salad" (street name, khat)
"African woodbine" (re: cannabis/marijuana cigarette)
aftereffect, figural
aftereffects of drinking

after-glide
afterimage(s)
aftermath of trauma
A. G. Bell Association for the
  Deaf and Hard of Hearing
Agar Score
age
    achievement (AA)
    basal
    Binet
    biologic
    characteristic
    chronological (CA)
    critical
    developmental
    educational (EA)
    emotional
    functional
    individual's
    mental (MA)
    middle
    relation to
    typical
age appropriate education
age appropriate self-help skills
age appropriate societal norms
age appropriate societal norms,
  violation of
age at onset, upper limits
age at onset of schizophrenia,
  pathophysiological significance
  of
age difference
age features
age group
age-matched individual
age mate
age of the child
Age Projection Test (APT)
age range
age-related cognitive decline
age-related cognitive decline
  problems
age-related deterioration
age-related features
age-related physical change
age-specific features aggression

agency (pl. agencies)
    health system
    social service
agenesis
agenitive
agenitive case (parts of speech)
agent(s)
    antianxiety
    antidipsotropic
    antihypertensive
    antimanic
    antipsychotic
    azaspirodecondione
    butyrophenone
    causative
    etiological
    MAOI-serotonergic
    monoamine oxidase
        inhibitor
    monoamine oxidase
        inhibitor-serotonergic
    monoamine oxidase
        inhibitor-tricyclic
    neuroleptic
    offending
    phenothiazine
    possessing
    psychedelic
    psychotomimetic
    sedative-hypnotic
    tranquilizing
    transmissible
agent-action
agent-object
agent of change
Agent Orange
aggression
    child-to-elder parent
    domestic
    husband-to-wife
    parent-to-child
    partner-to-partner
    passive
    physical
    sexual
    spousal
    violent
    wife-to-husband

aggression to animals
aggression to people
aggression without provocation
aggressive behavior
    alleviating
    alleviating violence in
    de-escalating
    management of
    multidisciplinary
      management of
    theories of
aggressive impulses
aggressive type personality disorder
aging
    neuroanatomy of
    neurobiology in
    neuropathology of
aging and PTSD
aging process, normative
agitate
    amentia
    melancholia
agitated behavior
agitated patient
agitation
    emotional
    extreme
    mental
    nightmare
    onset of
    physical
    psychomotor
    purposeless
    unpredictable
    unrelieved
    untriggered
    violent
agitative features
aglossia
AGLP (Association of LGBTQ Psychiatrists)
agnathia
agnosia
    acoustic
    apperceptive visual
    associative visual
    auditory verbal

agnosia
    autotopagnosia
    color
    corporal
    facial
    generalized auditory
    object
    selective auditory
    topographical
    verbal
    verbal auditory
    visual
    visual auditory
agnostic behavior
"agonies" (re: drug withdrawal)
agonist, partial
agonist-antagonist contraction
agonist medication
agonist therapy
agoramania
agoraphobia (F40.00)
    panic disorder with
    panic disorder without
agoraphobia without history of panic disorder
agoraphobic fears
AGP (Archive of General Psychiatry)
AGPA (American Group Psychotherapy Association)
agrammalogia
agrammatic speech
agrammatism agraphia
agraphia
    agrammatism
    alexia with
    alexia without
    aphasic
    apractic
    apraxic
    cerebral
    developmental
    jargon
    lexical
    literal
    mental
    motor
    musical

agraphia
    optic
    phonological
    pure
    spatial
    verbal
agreeableness
agreement
    separation
    subject-verb
AGS Early Screening Profiles
AGT (activity group therapy)
agyiomania
AH (ataxic hemiparesis)
AH5 Group Test of High Grade Intelligence
AH6 Group Tests of High Level Intelligence
AHDI (Association for Healthcare Documentation Integrity)
AHIMA (American Health Information Management Association)
AHPAT (Allied Health Professions Admission Test)
"ah-pen-yen" (street name, opium)
AICPA Orientation Test for Professional Accounting
aid(s)
    air conduction hearing
    binaural hearing
    body hearing
    bone conduction hearing
    canal hearing
    contralateral routing of signals hearing (CROS)
    digital hearing
    external memory
    in-the-ear hearing
    monaural hearing
    pseudobinaural hearing
    vibrotactile
    Y-cord hearing
aid assessment, hearing
aid evaluation, hearing (HAE)
aid selection, hearing
aid systems, hearing
aided augmentative communication
aidoiomania
AIDS (auto-immune deficiency disorder)
AIDS dementia complex (ADC)
AIDS encephalopathy
ailuromania
"aimies" (street name, amphetamine; amyl nitrite)
aimless behavior
AIMS (abnormal involuntary movement scale)
aims, baseline
"AIP" (re: heroin from Afghanistan, Iran and Pakistan)
AIP (adaptive information processing)
air
    complemental
    reserve
    residual
    supplemental
    tidal
air-blade sound
"air blast" (street name, inhalant)
air-bone gap
air conduction (AC)
air conduction, pure tone
air-conduction hearing aid
air-conduction receiver
air-conduction threshold, pure tone
air wastage
"airhead" (re: cannabis/marijuana user)
"airplane" (street name, cannabis/marijuana)
airway dysfunction, lingual
akathisia
    medication-induced, acute (G25.71)
    medication-induced, tardive (G24.01)
    neuroleptic dose-dependent
    neuroleptic-induced acute
akathisia, tardive (G25.71)
akinetic apraxia

akinetic autism
akinetic mania
akinetic seizure
"Al Capone" (street name, heroin)
ALA (Activity Losses
  Assessment)
ala (pl. alae)
alae, nasal
alar flutter
alarm-clock headache
alaryngeal
alaryngeal speech
Alatot
Albrecht syndrome
Alcadd Test
alcohol (ethyl alcohol)
alcohol, toxic effects of
alcohol abuse
alcohol addiction
alcohol amnestic disorder
alcohol amnestic syndrome
alcohol as cause of seizure
Alcohol Assessment and
  Treatment Profile
alcohol drinking
alcohol effect, fetal (FAE)
alcohol habit(s)
alcohol idiosyncratic intoxication
alcohol-induced anxiety
alcohol-induced anxiety disorder
alcohol-induced bipolar disorder
alcohol-induced depressive
  disorder
alcohol-induced major or mild
  neurocognitive disorder
alcohol-induced nighttime sleep
alcohol-induced paranoid state
alcohol-induced persisting
  amnestic disorder
alcohol-induced persisting
  dementia
alcohol-induced psychotic
  disorder
alcohol-induced psychotic
  disorder with delusions
alcohol-induced psychotic
  disorder with hallucinations
alcohol-induced sexual
  dysfunction
alcohol-induced sleep disorder
alcohol intoxication
  acute
  idiosyncratic
  pathological
  signs of
  organic psychosis
alcohol intoxication delirium
alcohol intoxication with mild
  comorbid alcohol use disorder
  (F10.129)
alcohol intoxication with
  moderate/severe comorbid
  alcohol use disorder (F10.229)
alcohol intoxication with no
  comorbidity (F10.929)
alcohol level, blood
alcohol on breath (AOB)
alcohol poisoning
alcohol-precipitated epilepsy
alcohol problem
alcohol-related disorder,
  unspecified (F10.99)
alcohol-related risk for accident
alcohol-related risk for suicide
alcohol-related risk for violence
alcohol seizure
alcohol syndrome, fetal
alcohol therapy agents
  (antidipsotropic agents)
  Antabuse
  calcium carbimide
alcohol therapy agents
  (antidipsotropic agents)
  daidzin
  disulfiram
  Flagyl
  metronidazole
alcohol use disorder, comorbid
  mild (F10.10)
  moderate/severe (F10.20)
alcohol use disorder, comorbid
  mild, with intoxication
  (F10.129)
  moderate/severe, with
  intoxication (F10.229)

alcohol use disorder with alcohol-
induced anxiety disorder with
use disorder
alcohol use disorder with alcohol-
induced bipolar or related
disease
alcohol use disorder with alcohol-
induced brief psychotic disorder
alcohol use disorder with alcohol-
induced delusional disorder
alcohol use disorder with alcohol-
induced major and mild
neurocognitive disorder
alcohol use disorder with alcohol-
induced schizoaffective disorder
alcohol use disorder with alcohol-
induced schizophrenia
alcohol use disorder with alcohol-
induced schizophreniform
disorder
alcohol use disorder with alcohol-
induced schizotypal
(personality) disorder
alcohol use disorder with alcohol-
induced sexual dysfunction
alcohol use disorder with alcohol-
induced sleep disorder
alcohol use disorder without
comorbidity (F10.929)
Alcohol Use Inventory (AUI)
alcohol use questionnaire
alcohol withdrawal
alcohol withdrawal delirium
alcohol withdrawal seizure
alcohol withdrawal syndrome
alcohol withdrawal with
perceptual disturbance
(F10.232)
alcohol withdrawal without
perceptual disturbance
(F10.239)
alcoholic
    child/children of (CoA)
alcoholic
    detoxified
    inactive (IA)
    newly abusive
alcoholic amentia

alcoholic amnesia
alcoholic ataxia
alcoholic brain syndrome, chronic
    (CABS)
alcoholic coma
alcoholic confusional state
alcoholic delirium
    acute
    chronic
alcoholic delirium tremens
alcoholic delirium withdrawal
alcoholic dementia
alcoholic deterioration
alcoholic drunkenness
alcoholic epilepsy
alcoholic hallucination
alcoholic hallucinosis
alcoholic insanity
alcoholic intoxication with
    dependence
alcoholic jealousy
alcoholic liver disease-type
    organic psychosis
alcoholic mania
    acute
    chronic
alcoholic paranoia
alcoholic paranoid psychosis
alcoholic psychosis
    abstinence syndrome
    amnestic confabulatory
    amnestic syndrome
    hallucinosis
    Korsakoff
    paranoid-type
    pathological intoxication
    polyneuritic
    withdrawal delirium
    withdrawal hallucinosis
    withdrawal syndrome
alcoholic wet brain syndrome
Alcoholics Anonymous (AA)
alcoholism
    acute
    chronic
    delirium
    mental disorder due to

alcoholism associated with
  dementia
alcoholism organic psychosis
alcoholism therapy (use of
  dipsotropic agents)
alcoholism with cirrhosis and
  concurrent psychiatric problems
alcoholomania
alcoholophilia
alcoholophobia
ALD (Appraisal of Language
  Disturbances)
alert and oriented times three
  (A+Ox3)
alert and oriented to person, place,
  and time (A+Ox3)
alert awake state
alerting stimulus
alertness
  level of
  state of
Alexander's deafness
alexia (dyslexia)
  anterior
  auditory
  central
  cortical
  incomplete
  motor
  musical
  optical
  posterior
  pure
  sensory
  subcortical
  tactile
  visual
alexia with agraphia
alexia without agraphia
alexic
aliases, use of
"Alice B. Toklas" (street name,
  cannabis/marijuana brownie)
alien obsession
alien thoughts
Alienation Index, Adolescent
alienation, social
alkalosis, metabolic

"all lit up" (re: drug influence)
"all star" (re: multiple drug user)
"all-American drug" (street name,
  cocaine)
allergic encephalopathy
allergy
alleviating aggressive behavior
alleviating violence
alleviating violence in aggressive
  behavior
Allied Health Professions
  Admission Test (AHPAT)
Allied Procedures, The Halstead-
  Reitan Neurological Battery and
alliteration
allomorph
allophone tabulation
allusion (figure of speech)
alogia
alone, living
alopecia
  psychogenic
  trichotillomania-induced
alopecia areata
alpha activity
alpha-adrenergic receptor
alpha EEG activity
alpha-ethyltryptamine (street
  names)
    alpha-ET
    ET
    love pearls
    love pills
    trip
alpha frequency
alpha index
alpha-methyldopa-induced mood
  disorder
alpha-PVP
alpha rhythm
alpha state
alpha wave
alpha wave strains
alphabet
  American Manual
  initial teaching
  International Phonetic
    (IPA)

alphabet
   International Standard
     Manual (ISMA)
   manual
   phonetic
alphabetical index
ALS (amyotrophic lateral
   sclerosis; Lou Gehrig's disease)
alteration in rate of speech
alterations in time perception
alterations, NMDA receptor
altered mental status
altered sensation
altered state
altered vision
altered voice
altering the rate of speech
Alternate Binaural Loudness
   Balance (ABLB)
alternate forms reliability
   coefficient
alternate identity
Alternate Monaural Loudness
   Balance (AMLB)
alternate motion rate (AMR)
alternating current (AC)
alternating pulse
alternative criterion B for
   dysthymic disorder
alternative dimensional
   descriptors for schizophrenia
alternative dimensional
   descriptors of schizophrenia
alveolar angle
alveolar arch
alveolar area
alveolar assimilation
alveolar border of mandible
alveolar canal
alveolar consonant placement
alveolar hypoventilation
   syndrome, central
alveolar nerve
alveolar pattern
alveolar point
alveolar process of maxilla
alveolar ridge
alveolar sac

alveolar septum
alveolar space
alveolar supporting bone
alveolar wall
alveolar yoke
alveolingual
alveolitis
alveolodental canal
alveolodental
alveololabial
alveololingual
alveolopalatal
alveolus (i)
Alzheimer dementia
Alzheimer tangles
Alzheimer type senile dementia
   (SDAT)
Alzheimer's disease (G30.9)
   biology of
   dementia due to
   pathophysiology of
Alzheimer's Disease Assessment
   Scale (ADAS)
Alzheimer's Disease Foundation
AM (amplitude modulation)
AMA (American Medical
   Association)
amaxomania
ambidexterity
ambidextrous
ambient noise
ambiguity
   lexical
   role
   structural
ambiguous genitalia
ambiguous word
ambilaterality
ambisyllabic
amblyopia, toxic
Ambulation Categories,
   Functional
ambulation index
ambulatory care
ambulatory status
amelioration, tendency toward
amenomania

amentia
   nevoid
   phenylpyruvic
   Stern alcoholic
Americamania
American Academy of Addiction Psychiatry (AAAP)
American Academy of Audiology
American Academy of Child and Adolescent Psychiatry (AACAP)
American Academy of Family Physicians (AAFP)
American Academy of Forensic Sciences
American Academy of Otolaryngology
American Academy of Pain Management
American Academy of Pain Medicine
American Academy of Pediatrics (AAP)
American Academy of Physical Medicine and Rehabilitation (AAPM&R)
American Academy of Private Practice in Speech Pathology and Audiology
American Academy of Psychiatrists in Alcoholism and Addictions (AAPAA)
American Academy of Psychiatry and the Law (AAPL)
American Academy of Sleep Medicine (AASM)
American Association of Directors of Psychiatric Residency Training (AADPR)
American Association for Geriatric Psychiatry (AAGP)
American Association for Marriage and Family Therapy (AAMFT)
American Association of Chairs of Departments of Psychiatry
American Association of Psychiatric Administrators
American Association for Social Psychiatry (AASP)
American Association on Intellectual and Developmental Disabilities (AAIDD)
American Auditory Society (AAS)
American Board of Family Medicine (ABFM)
American Board of Forensic Psychology
American Board of Psychiatry and Neurology, Inc.
American Chronic Pain Association, The (ACPA)
American College of Forensic Examiners International
American College of Forensic Psychiatry
American College of Forensic Psychology
American College of Neuropsychiatrists
American College of Neuropsychopharmacology
American College of Osteopathic Neurologists and Psychiatrists
American College of Physicians (ACP)
American Council on Education, The (ACE)
American Deafness and Rehabilitation Association (ADARA)
American Dialect Society (ADS)
American Drug and Alcohol Survey, The
American Group Psychotherapy Association (AGPA)
American Health Information Management Association (AHIMA)
American Hearing Research Foundation
American Hospital Association
American Manual Alphabet
American Medical Association (AMA)

American Music Therapy
  Association (AMTA)
American National Standards
  Institute (ANSI)
American Nurses' Association
  (ANA)
American Occupational Therapy
  Association, Inc.
American Physical Therapy
  Association (APTA)
American Psychiatric Association
  (APA)
American Psychoanalytic
  Association (ApsaA)
American Psychological
  Association (APA)
American Psychology-Law
  Society, Division 41
American Psychopathological
  Association, Inc. (APPA)
American Psychosomatic Society
  (APS)
American Sign Language (ASL)
  (Ameslan)
American Sleep Disorders
  Association
American Society for Adolescent
  Psychiatry (ASAP)
American Society of Addiction
  Medicine (ASAM)
American Society of Clinical
  Hypnosis (ASCH)
American Society of Hospital
  Pharmacists (ASHP)
American Speech-Language-
  Hearing Association (ASLHA)
American Tinnitus Association
Anxiety and Depression
  Association of America
"ames" (street name, amyl nitrite)
Ameslan (American Sign
  Language) (ASL)
amfetyline
AMI (Athletic Motivation
  Inventory)
"Amidone" (street name,
  methadone)

amimia
  amnesic
  ataxic
amimic
amine, biogenic
amine hypothesis, biogenic
amitriptyline-induced mood
  disorder
AMLB (Alternate Monaural
  Loudness Balance)
Ammons Full Range Picture
  Vocabulary Test
amnesia
  acute
  alcoholic
  amnestic state
  antegrade
  anterograde
  asymmetrical
  auditory
  Broca
  childbirth
  chronic
  circumscribed
  complete
  concussion
  continuous
  degree of
  dissociative
  emotional
  episodic
  evidence of
  generalized
  global
  hippocampal
  hysterical
  ictal
  infantile
  Korsakoff
  lacunar
  localized
  nonpathological
  olfactory
  organic
  partial
  patchy
  postconcussive
  posthypnotic

amnesia
    post-traumatic (PTA)
    profound
    psychogenic
    retroactive
    retrograde
    reversible
    selective
    shrinking retrograde
    subsequent
    systematized
    tactile
    toxin-provoked
    transient global
    traumatic
    true
    verbal
    visual
amnesia after trance
amnesiac
amnesia for sleep and dreaming
amnesia for sleep-terror event
amnesia in children
amnesic amimia
amnesic amnesia
amnesic aphasia
amnesic loss of memory
amnesic syndrome
amnestic aphrasia
amnestic apraxia
amnestic confabulatory alcoholic
  psychosis
amnestic confabulatory syndrome
amnestic disorder
    alcohol
    alcohol-induced persisting
    anxiolytic
    substance-induced
      persisting
amnestic psychosis
amnestic state
amnestic syndrome
    alcohol
amnestic syndrome
    drug-induced
    post-traumatic
amobarbital (street names)
    blue angels

amobarbital (street names)
    bluebirds
    blue devils
    Christmas trees
    double trouble
    greenies
    lily
    rainbows
    tooies
"amoeba" (street name,
    phencyclidine)
amotivated behavior
"Amp joint" (re:
  cannabis/marijuana cigarette
  laced with a narcotic)
"amp" (street name,
  amphetamine)
"amped" (re: high on
  amphetamines)
"amped-out" (re: fatigue after
  using amphetamines)
ampere (A)
amphetamine (biphetamine;
  Dexadrine) (street names)
    A
    aimies
    amp
    amped
    amped-out
    back dex
    bam
    bambita
    B-bombs
    beans
    bennies
    bens
    Benz
    benzedrine
    biphetamine
    black and white
    black beauties
    black birds
    black bombers
    black Cadillacs
    blacks
    blue boy
    blue devils
    blue mollies

amphetamine (street names)
- bolt
- bombido
- bombita
- bottles
- brain ticklers
- browns
- bumblebees
- candy
- cartwheels
- chalk
- chicken powder
- chocolate
- Christina
- Christmas tree
- coasts to coasts
- co-pilot
- crank
- crisscross
- crosses
- cross tops
- crossroads
- crystal
- crystal methadrine
- dex
- Dexadrine
- dexies
- diamonds
- diet pills
- dolls
- dominoes
- double cross
- drivers
- elephants
- eye opener
- fasts
- fives
- forwards
- French blue
- gaggler
- glass
- go
- greenies
- hanyak
- head drugs
- hearts
- Hiropon
- horse heads

amphetamine (street names)
- hydro
- iboga
- ice
- in-betweens
- jam
- jam cecil
- jelly baby
- jelly beans
- jolly beans
- jugs
- L.A.
- leapers
- lid poppers
- lightning
- little bomb
- MAO
- marathons
- max
- methedrine
- mini beans
- minibennie
- mollies
- morning shot
- nineteen
- nugget
- oranges
- peaches
- pep pills
- pink hearts
- pixies
- pollutants
- poor man's coke
- powder
- purple hearts
- red phosphorus
- rhythm
- rippers
- road dope
- Rosa
- roses
- slammin'/slamming
- snap
- snot
- snow
- snow pallets
- snow seals
- sparkle plenty

Psychiatric Words and Phrases

amphetamine (street names)
  sparklers
  speed
  speedball
  speedballing
  splash
  splivins
  star
  strawberry shortcake
  sweeties
  sweets
  tens
  The C
  thrusters
  TR-6s
  truck drivers
  turkey
  turnabout
  U.P.S.
  uppers
  uppies
  waffle dust
  wake ups
  West Coast turnarounds
  whiffle dust
  white
  white cross
  whites
  X
amphetamine abuse or dependence
amphetamine challenge test
amphetamine-induced anxiety disorder
amphetamine-induced mood disorder
amphetamine-induced obsessive-compulsive and related disorders
amphetamine-induced psychotic disorder with delusions
amphetamine-induced psychotic disorder with hallucinations
amphetamine-induced sexual dysfunction
amphetamine-induced sleep disorder
amphetamine intoxication
amphetamine intoxication delirium
amphetamine-like action
amphetamine-like substance
amphetamine or other stimulant-related disorder, unspecified (F15.99)
amphetamine or other stimulant withdrawal with perceptual disturbance (F15.23)
amphetamine or other stimulant withdrawal without perceptual disturbance (F15.23)
amphetamine or other stimulant intoxication with perceptual disturbance, with use disorder, mild (F15.122)
amphetamine or other stimulant intoxication with perceptual disturbance, with use disorder, moderate/severe (F15.222)
amphetamine or other stimulant intoxication with perceptual disturbance, without use disorder (F15.922)
amphetamine or other stimulant intoxication without perceptual disturbance, with use disorder, mild (F15.129)
amphetamine or other stimulant intoxication without perceptual disturbance, with use disorder, moderate/ severe (F15.229)
amphetamine or other stimulant intoxication without perceptual disturbance, without use disorder (F15.929)
amphetamine-type substance-related disorders
amphetamine use disorder
amphetamine use disorder with amphetamine-induced anxiety disorder
amphetamine use disorder with amphetamine-induced bipolar or related disease

26 Psychiatric Words and Phrases

amphetamine use disorder with amphetamine-induced brief psychotic disorder
amphetamine use disorder with amphetamine-induced delusional disorder
amphetamine use disorder with amphetamine-induced obsessive-compulsive and related disorders
amphetamine use disorder with amphetamine-induced schizoaffective disorder
amphetamine use disorder with amphetamine-induced schizophrenia
amphetamine use disorder with amphetamine-induced schizophreniform disorder
amphetamine use disorder with amphetamine-induced schizotypal (personality) disorder
amphetamine use disorder with amphetamine-induced sexual dysfunction
amphetamine use disorder with amphetamine-induced sleep disorder
amphetamine withdrawal
amphetamines, manufacturing
amphetaminoethyltheophylline
"amping" (re: accelerated heartbeat)
amplification
    binaural
    compression
    memory
amplifier
amplify
amplitude
    acoustic reflex
    effective
    maximum
    peak
    peak-to-peak
    zero
amplitude asymmetry

amplitude distortion
amplitude gradient
amplitude modulation (AM)
amplitude shimmer
AMR (alternate motion rate)
AMS (Access Management Survey)
"AMT" (street name, amphetamine; dimethyltryptamine)
AMT (Anxiety Management Training)
amt (amount)
AMTA (American Music Therapy Association)
amuck (also amok)
amusia
amyl nitrite (street names)
    aimes
    aimies
    ames
    amys
    boppers
    pearls
    poppers
amyl nitrite abuse
amyl nitrite inhalant
amyloid angiopathy
amyloidosis, metabolic
amyotrophic lateral sclerosis (ALS; Lou Gehrig's disease)
"amys" (street name, amyl nitrite)
ANA (American Nurses Association)
anabolic steroid agents
    Anadrol
    Depo-Testosterone
    Durabolin
    Equipoise
    Oxandrin
anabolic steroids (street names)
    gym candy
    juice
    pumpers
    roids
anacusis
"anadrol" (street name, oral steroid)
anal intercourse

Psychiatric Words and Phrases 27

anal sex
anal stage psychosexual
  development
analog
analog change
analog marking
analysis *(see also* tests)
  aerodynamic
  auditory
  cephalometric
  cerebrospinal fluid (CSF)
  chain
  contrastive
  distal distinctive feature
  Fourier
  gait
  grammatical
  kinesthetic
  kinetic
  morphometric
  neurometric
  perceptual
  phonemic
  phonetic
  phonological
  segmental
  sound
  substitution
  suprasegmental
  task
  task performance and
  toxicological
  traditional phonetic
Analysis of Coping Style
analysis of homonymy
analysis of information
Analysis of Readiness Skills
analytic boundaries
analytic frame
Analytic Learning Disability
  Assessment
analytic method
analytic object
Analytical Reading Inventory
analyze
analyzer
  noise
  Time Use

analyzing information,
  disturbance in rapidity of
anandamide
anaphoric pronoun
anaptyxis (pl. anaptyxes)
anarthria
anatomical site of pain
anatomy, biochemical
"anatrofin" (street name,
  injectable steroid)
"anavar" (street name, oral
  steroid)
anchor
  collapsing
  firing an
  stacking
  stealing an
anchor signs of withdrawal
anchor symptoms
anchors/responses, integrating
androgen
androgen insensitivity syndrome
androgynous individual
andromania
Anglomania
anechoic chamber
anemia, iron deficiency
anemometer, warm-wire
anesthesia
  conversion
  emotional
  first stage of
  halogenated inhalational
  hysterical
  laryngeal
  sensory
  sexual
  stocking-glove
  traumatic
anesthetics, halogenated
  inhalational
aneurysm
  brain
  cerebral
  cranial
  extracerebral
  extracranial
  intracranial

"angel dust" (street name, phencyclidine)
"angel hair" (street name, phencyclidine)
"angel mist" (street name, phencyclidine)
"Angel Poke" (street name, phencyclidine)
"angel" (street name, phencyclidine)
anger
    constant
    difficulty controlling
    fit of
    ineffective
    intense
    marked
    outburst of
anger expression, passivity in
anger mallet
"Angie" (street name, cocaine)
angiopathy, amyloid
angle, alveolar
"Angola" (street name, cannabis/marijuana)
angry behavior
angry reaction
angry reaction to minor stimuli
angular gyrus
anhedonism
aniled sense
aniled sense of self
"animal" (street name, LSD)
"animal trank" (street name, phencyclidine/PCP)
"animal tranq" (street name, phencyclidine/PCP)
"animal tranquilizer" (street name, phencyclidine/PCP)
animal type specific phobia
animals, aggression to
animate
ankyloglossia
ankylosis, cricoarytenoid
Ann Arbor Learning Inventory and Remediation Program
anode
anomalies, craniofacial
anomalous movement
Anomalous Sentences Repetition Test, The (ASRT)
anomaly
anomaly, laryngeal
anomia
    color
    finger
    tactile
anomic aphasia
anomic errors
Anorectic Attitude Questionnaire
anorexia nervosa (AN)
    atypical (F50.8)
    binge-eating/purging type, mild/moderate/ severe/extreme (F50.02)
    restricting type, mild/moderate/severe/extreme (F50.01)
anorexia nervosa and associated disorders (ANAD)
Anorexic Behavior Scale
anorexic fast
anoxia
    cerebral
    dementia due to
anoxic encephalopathy
ANQ (Adult Neuropsychological Questionnaire)
ANSER System, The
ANSI (American National Standards Institute)
answers, syndrome of approximate
antagonism
antagonist
antagonist, beta-adrenergic
antagonist medication
antagonistic muscle strength
antalgic gait
antecedent event
antegrade amnesia
antegrade amnesic
anterior
    alexia
    musculus digastricus
    musculus omohyoideus

Psychiatric Words and Phrases

anterior
    musculus scalenus
    musculus serratus
anterior digastric muscle
anterior feature English phoneme
anterior partial laryngectomy
anterior vertical canal
anterograde amnesia due to
  predatory drug administration
anterograde loss of memory
anthelix
anthomania
anthropological linguistics
anthropomorphic face
anthropophobia
antibulemic agents
    fluoxetine
    Prozac
        anticholinergic delirium
anticipation
anticipatory and struggle behavior
  (theory of stuttering)
anticipatory and struggling
  behavior theories
anticipatory coarticulation
anticonvulsant
anticonvulsant drugs test, blood
  level of
anticonvulsant intoxication
anticonvulsant medication-
  induced postural tremor
antidepressant
    heterocyclic
    monocyclic
antidepressant agents
    Adapin
    Allegron
    amfebutamone HCl
    amitriptyline
    amoxapine
    Asendin
    Aventyl (tricyclic)
    bupropion
    Celexa (SSRI)
    citalopram
    Clomipramine
    Cymbalta (SSRI)
    desipramine

antidepressant agents
    Desyrel
    doxepin
    duloxetine
    Effexor (SSRI)
    Elavil (tricyclic)
    Emsam
    Endep
    escitalopram
    fluoxetine
    fluvoxamine
    imipramine
    imipramine pamoate
    isocarboxazid
    Janimine
    Lexapro (SSRI)
    Ludiomil (tricyclic)
    Luvox (SSRI)
    Manerix
    maprotiline
    Marplan (MAOI)
    mirtazapine
    moclobemide
    Nardil (MAOI)
    nefazodone
    Norpramine (tricyclic)
    nortriptyline
    Pamelor (tricyclic)
    Parnate (MAOI)
    paroxetine
    paroxetine-mesylate
    Paxil (SSRI)
    Pertofrane
    Pexeva (SSRI)
    phenelzine
    Prexa (SSRI)
    protriptyline
    Prozac (SSRI)
    Remeron
    Rhotrimine
    selegiline
    Serafem (SSRI)
    sertraline
    Serzone
    Sinequan (tricyclic)
    sulpiride
    Surmontil (tricyclic)

antidepressant agents
   Symbyax (Prozac and
     Zyprexa combination)
   Tofranil (tricyclic)
   Tofranil-PM (tricyclic)
   tranylcypromine
   trazodone
   trimipramine
   Triptil
   venlafaxine
   Vivactil (tricyclic)
   Wellbutrin
   Zoloft (SSRI)
antidepressant best use via genetic
   testing
antidepressant discontinuation
   syndrome
     initial encounter
       (T43.205A)
     sequela (T43.205S)
     subsequent encounter
       (T43.205D)
antidepressant discontinuation
   syndrome with comorbidity
antidepressant medication-
   induced postural tremor
antidepressant medications,
   serotonin-specific reuptake
   inhibitor
antidepressant treatment
antidepressant use in affective
   disorders
antidipsotropic agents
   Antabuse
   benzodiapin
   benzodiazepines
   calcium carbimide
   carbamazepine
   Carbatrol
   Carbolith
   chlorpromazine
   Cibalith-S
   citalopram
   citalopram hydrobromide
   clomipramine
   clonazepam
   daidzin

antidipsotropic agents
   diazepam
   disulfiram
   Duralith
   Epival
   Flagyl
   fluoxetine
   fluvoxamine
   Lithane
   lithium carbonate
   Lithizine
   Lithobid
   Lithonate
   Lithotabs
   Luvox
   metronidazole
   Prozac
   Tegretol
   Temposil
   trazodone
   tricyclic antidepressants
   Valium
antidote drug
anti-expectancy
"antifreeze" (street name, heroin)
antihelix
antihypertensive agents
antimanic agents
antimongolism
antinociception
antiobsessional agents
antipanic agents
   alprazolam
   Xanax
antiparkinsonism agents
   Amantadine
   anticholinergics
   Aricept (approval pending)
   donepezil (approval
     pending)
   dopamine agonists
   Eldepryl
   Ethopropazine
   Exelon
   galantamine
   L-dopa
   levodopa
   MAO-B inhibitors

antiparkinsonism agents
   memantine (approval
     pending)
   Namenda (approval
     pending)
   profenamine
   Razadyne
   rivastigmine
antipsychotic agents
   Abilify
   aripiprazole
   benzperidol
   buclizine
   butyrophenone
   chlorpromazine
   clozapine
   Clozaril
   Etrafon
   Fanapt
   Fluanxol
   flupenthixol
   fluphenazine decanoate
   Geodon
   Haldol
   haloperidol
   iloperidone
   Largactil
   Loxapac
   loxapine
   Loxitane
   Mellaril
   mesoridazine
   methtrimeprazine
   Moban
   Modecate
   molindone
   Navane
   nozinan
   olanzepine
   Orap
   Permitil
   perphenazine
   phenothiazine
   pimozide
   Piportil
   pipotiazine palmitate
   Prolixin
   quetiapine
antipsychotic agents
   Risperdal
   risperidone
   Serentil
   Seroquel
   Stelazine
   sulpiride
   Symbyax (Prozac and
     Zyprexa combination)
   thioridizine
   thiothixene
   Thixol
   Thorazine
   trifluoperazine
   Trilafon
   ziprasidone
   Zyprexa
antiresonance
antiseizure drug
antisocial behavior
   adult (Z72.811)
   child or adolescent
     (Z72.810)
   pattern of
antisocial personality disorder
   (F60.2)
antitragus
Anton Brenner Developmental
   Gestalt Test of School
   Readiness
antonym
anvil
anxiety
   adjustment disorder with
   alcohol-induced
   amphetamine-induced
   anxiolytic-induced
   caffeine-induced
   cannabis-induced
   clinically significant
   cocaine-induced
   debilitating
   dental
   excessive
   excessive social
   extreme
   feelings of
   focus of

anxiety
    frequency of
    gender differences in
    generalized (GAD)
    hypnotic-induced
    immediate
    intense
    intercurrent
    marked
    neutralized
    nonpathological
    performance
    pervasive
    physical concomitant of
    primary
    prominent
    provoked
    reduction of
    sedative-induced
    severe
    social
    substance-induced
Anxiety and Depression Association of America (ADAA)
anxiety-depressive disorder, mixed
anxiety disorder
    generalized (F41.1)
    other specified (F41.8)
    separation (F93.0)
    social (F40.10)
    unspecified (F41.9)
anxiety disorder, type of:
    agoraphobia (F40.00)
    panic attack (No Code)
    selective mutism (F94.0)
    social phobia (F40.10)
    specific phobia
anxiety disorder, type of (specific phobia):
    animal (F40.218)
    fear of blood (F40.230)
    fear of injections/ transfusions (F40.231)
    fear of injury (F40.233)
    fear of other medical care (F40.232)

anxiety disorder, type of (specific phobia):
    natural environment (F40.228)
    other (e.g. choking) (F40.298)
    situational (e.g. elevators, airplanes) (F40.248)
anxiety disorder due to another medical condition (F06.4)
anxiety disorder due to GMC
anxiety disorder with anxiety disturbance
anxiety due to potential evaluation by others
anxiety illness disorder
anxiety-induced impaired social functioning
anxiety prevention
Anxiety Profile Test
anxiety-related mental disorder
anxiety response
Anxiety Scale
Anxiety Scales for Children and Adults (ASCA)
anxiety symptoms, frequency of
anxiety trends
anxiolytic abuse
anxiolytic agents
    alprazolam
    Ativan
    BuSpar
    buspirone
    Centrax
    chlordiazepoxide
    clonazepam
    clorazepate
    diazepam
    Etrafon
    halazepam
    Klonopin
    Libritabs
    Librium
    lorazepam
    oxazepam
    Paxipam
    perphenazine
    prazepam

Psychiatric Words and Phrases

anxiolytic agents
   Serax
   Stelazine
   T-Quil
   Tranxene
   trifluoperazine
   Trilafon
   Valium
   Valium Injection
   Xanax
anxiolytic-induced anxiety
anxiolytic-induced anxiety disorder
anxiolytic intoxication
anxiolytic intoxication delirium
anxiolytic intoxication with use disorder, mild (F13.129)
anxiolytic intoxication with use disorder, moderate/severe F13.229)
anxiolytic intoxication without use disorder (F13.929)
anxiolytic-related disorder, unspecified (F13.99)
anxiolytic-related disorder with anxiolytic-type withdrawal
anxiolytic substances, long-half-life
anxiolytic use disorder
anxiolytic use disorder in a controlled environment, mild (F13.10)
anxiolytic use disorder in a controlled environment, moderate/ severe (F13.20)
anxiolytic use disorder with anxiolytic-induced anxiety disorder
anxiolytic use disorder with anxiolytic-induced bipolar or related disease
anxiolytic use disorder with anxiolytic-induced brief psychotic disorder
anxiolytic use disorder with anxiolytic-induced delusional disorder
anxiolytic use disorder with anxiolytic-induced major neurocognitive disorder
anxiolytic use disorder with anxiolytic-induced schizoaffective disorder
anxiolytic use disorder with anxiolytic-induced schizophrenia
anxiolytic use disorder with anxiolytic-induced schizophreniform disorder
anxiolytic use disorder with anxiolytic-induced schizotypal (personality) disorder
anxiolytic use disorder with anxiolytic-induced sexual dysfunction
anxiolytic use disorder with anxiolytic-induced sleep disorder
anxiolytic withdrawal delirium
anxiolytic withdrawal with perceptual disturbance (F13.232)
anxiolytic withdrawal without perceptual disturbance (F13.239)
anxious, feeling
anxious clinician
anxious-fearful cluster
anxious mood adjustment
anxious substance abuser
ANZMH (Australian & New Zealand Mental Health Association)
APA (American Psychiatric Association)
APA (American Psychological Association)
APAC (Australian Psychology Accreditation Council)
"Apache" (street name, fentanyl)
APAT (Accounting Program Admission Test)
apathetic type personality disorder
APC (Association of Professional Chaplains)

aperiodic wave
aperta, rhinolalia
aperta voice disorder
aperture apex (pl. apices)
apex of tongue
aphasia *(see also* tests)
    acoustic
    acoustic-amnestic
    acquired
    acquired epileptic
    acquired fluent
    afferent (kinesthetic) motor
    afferent motor
    ageusic
    amnemonic
    amnesic
    anomic
    associative
    ataxic
    auditory
    Broca
    callosal disconnection
      syndrome
    childhood
    combined
    commissural
    complete
    conduction
    contiguity
    contiguity disorder
    cortical
    developmental
    dynamic
    efferent
    efferent (kinetic) motor
    executive
    expressive
    expressive receptive
    fluent
    frontocortical
    frontolenticular
    functional
    gibberish
    global
    graphic
    Grashey
    hypophonic
    idiosyncratic
aphasia
    impressive
    infantile
    intellectual
    isolation
    jargon
    Kussmaul
    lenticular
    Lichtheim
    major motor
    mixed motor
    nominal
    nonfluent
    optic
    parietio-occipital
    partial nominal
    pathomanic
    pictorial
    pragmatic
    psychosensory
    pure
    receptive
    semantic
    sensory
    similarity disorder(s) of
    simple
    speech-reading
    speechreading
    subcortical
    subcortical motor
    syntactic
    tactile
    temporoparietal
    total
    transcortical mixed
    transcortical motor
    transcortical sensory
    true
    verbal
    visual
    Wernicke
Aphasia Clinical Battery
aphasic acalculia
aphasic agraphia
aphasic error(s)
aphasic impairment
aphasic migraine headache
aphasic patient

Psychiatric Words and Phrases 35

aphasic phonological impairment
aphasic seizure
    fluent
    nonfluent
aphasic speech
    fluent
    nonfluent
aphasiologist
aphasiology
aphemia
aphemia, pure
aphonia
    acute
    conversion
    functional
    hysterical
    intermittent
    syllabic
aphonic episode
aphrasia
aphrodisiomania
API (Adult Personality Inventory)
apicalization
apices (sing. apex)
apimania
APIs (Activity Pattern Indicators
aplasia
    cerebral
    cochlear
    labyrinthine
apnea
    central
    central sleep
    idiopathic central sleep
        (G47.31)
    mixed sleep
    obstructive
    obstructive sleep
    sleep
apnea syndrome
    adult obstructive sleep
    central sleep
    obstruction sleep
apneic period
apneic seizure(s)
apneustic breathing
apneustic period
apoplectiform convulsion

apostrophe (figure of speech)
apotemnophilia (fetish to
    amputate healthy limb)
APPA (American
    Psychopathological
    Association, Inc.)
apparent relationship
appearance, body
appendicular ataxia
apperception
apperceptive visual agnosia
appetite
    change in
    loss of
"apple jacks" (street name, crack
    cocaine)
application, ritualized makeup
applied linguistics
applied phonetics
applied psychology
Applied Reading Test, ACER
appositive
APP-R (Assessment of
    Phonological Processes
Appraisal of Language
    Disturbances (ALD)
apprehension test
apprehensiveness, social
approach
    adaptional
    categorical
    checklist
    descriptive
    dimensional
    fundamental
    hear-and-now
    mixture
    nondirect
    psychodynamic
    regressive-reactive
    yawn-sign
approach-avoidance stance
approach-avoidance theory (in
    stuttering)
approaches to dreaming and
    repression, cognitive
appropriate affect

appropriate atmosphere,
    situationally
appropriate avoidant behavior
    culturally
    developmentally
appropriate behavior
appropriate evaluation
appropriate relationship
appropriate self-stimulatory
    behaviors in the young,
    developmentary
appropriate shy behavior
    culturally
    developmentally
appropriate stimulus
appropriate treatment
approval
    excessive need for
    need for
approximate answers, syndrome of
approximation
    successive
    vocal fold
    word
APR (auropalpebral reflex)
apractic agraphia
apractic disorder
apractic dysarthria
apraxia
    akinetic
    buccofacial
    callosal
    cerebral mapping of
    classic
    cortical
    developmental articulatory
    disconnection
    dressing
    ideatory
    ideokinetic
    ideomotor
    innervation
    Liepmann
    magnetic
    motor
    ocular
    oculomotor

apraxia
    oral
    speech
    transcortical
    verbal
Apraxia Battery for Adults (ABA)
apraxic agraphia
apraxic behaviors
apraxic disorder
apraxic dysarthria
aprosody
APS (Adult Protective Services)
APS (American Psychosomatic Society)
APS (Australian Psychological Society)
APsaA (American Psychoanalytic Association)
APSAAR (Asia-Pacific Society for Alcohol and Addiction Research)
APT (Age Projection Test)
APTA (American Physical Therapy Association)
aptitude *(see also* tests)
Aptitude and Achievement Tests
Aptitude Interest Measurement
AQ (achievement quotient)
aquaphobia
arachnephobia
arc
    reflex
    sensorimotor
arch
    alveolar
    dental
    glossopalatine
    pharyngopalatine
architecture, sleep
architecture of brain
Archive of General Psychiatry (AGP)
arcuate fasciculus (AF)
arcuate movement
area(s)
    acoustic
    alveolar
    articulation

Psychiatric Words and Phrases

area(s)
  auditory
  bilabial
  Broca
  Broca's (Brodmann's area 44)
  Brodmann
  Brodmann's, 41
  Brodmann's, 44 (Broca's area)
  callosal (parolfactory nerve)
  culture
  glottal
  health-related
  labiodental
  language
  lingua-alveolar
  linguodental
  motor
  olfactory
  palatal
  parietal association
  parietotemporal
  premotor
  sclerotic
  sclerotome
  septal
  skill
  somesthetic
  velar
  visual
  watershed
  Wernicke
area consonant placement
  bilabial
  glottal
  labiodental
  lingua-alveolar
  linguadental
  palatal
  velar
areas of brain, mapping of language
areata, alopecia
"Are you anywhere?" (re: Do you use marijuana?)
argentophilic Pick inclusion bodies, intraneuronal
argument
"Aries" (street name, heroin)
arithmetic signs
arithmomania
Arizona Articulation Proficiency Scale
Arizona Battery for Communication Disorders of Dementia (ABCD)
Arlin Test of Formal Reasoning
arm swing, decreased
armed services
Armed Services Vocational Aptitude Battery
"Arnolds" (street name, steroids)
"aroma of men" (street name, isobutyl nitrite)
"around the turn" (re: having gone through withdrawal period)
arousal
  affective
  autonomic
  confusional
  erotic
  increased
  intense autonomic
  oxygen-deprived sexual
  problems with sexual
  sense of
  sexual
  sleep
arousal disorder
  acquired type female sexual
  female sexual
  generalized type female sexual
  life-long type female sexual
  male erectile sexual
  situational type female sexual
arousal disorder due to combined factors, female sexual

arousal disorder due to
　psychological factors, female
　sexual
arousal dysfunction
arousal from sleep
　confusional
　increased
arousal problems, sexual
arousing behavior, sexually
arousing fantasy
　sexually
　voyeuristic sexually
arrest of speech
arrest reaction
arresting consonant
arrogant behavior
arson, "communicative"
artery occlusion, cerebral
artery stenosis, carotid
arthropod-borne viral encephalitis
articulate
articulate speech
articulation *(see also* tests)
　addition
　deviant
　distortion
　general oral inaccuracy
　omission
　place of
　point of
　secondary
　substitution
articulation area
articulation curve
articulation disorder
　functional
　organic
articulation error
　phonemic
　phonetic
articulation-gain function
articulation index
articulation programming
articulation-resonance
articulation speech
articulation test
　deep
　diagnostic

articulation test
　screening
　story
articulators
articulatory apraxia,
　developmental
articulatory basis
articulatory disorder
articulatory phonetics
articulatory tic
artificial ear
artificial larynx
　electrical
　electronic
　pneumatic
　reed
artificial mastoid
artificial method
"artillery" (re: drug equipment)
arts, language
aryepiglottic
aryepiglottic folds
aryepiglottic muscle
aryepiglotticus, musculus
arylcyclohexylamine-related
　disorders
arytenoid cartilage(s)
arytenoid muscle
arytenoideus obliquus, musculus
arytenoideus transversus,
　musculus
ASAM (American Society of
　Addiction Medicine)
ASAP (American Society for
　Adolescent Psychiatry)
asapholalia
ASCA (Anxiety Scales for
　Children and Adults)
ascending pitch break
ascending technique
ascending technique audiometry
ascertainment, method of
asceticism
ASCH (American Society of
　Clinical Hypnosis)
asemia
"ashes" (street name,
　cannabis/marijuana)

ASHP (American Society of Hospital Pharmacists)
ASI (Advanced Solutions International) for iMIS online research
Asia-Pacific Society for Alcohol and Addiction Research (APSAAR)
A-SICD (Adapted Sequenced Inventory of Communication Development)
ASIQ (Adult Suicidal Ideation Questionnaire)
ASL (American Sign Language)
ASLHA (American Speech-Language-Hearing Association)
aspect
ASPECT (Ackerman-Schoendorf Scales for Parent Evaluation)
aspects
    linguistic
    speech
aspects of dementia
    ethical
    legal
aspects of schizophrenia
    pharmacological
    psychosocial
Asperger's disorder
Asperger's syndrome
asphyxiophylia
aspirate
aspirate consonant
aspiration
ASPIRE (A Sales Potential Inventory for Real Estate)
"aspirin" (street name, powder cocaine)
ASRT (Anomalous Sentences Repetition Test)
"assassin of youth" (street name, cannabis/marijuana)
assault
    drug facilitated sexual (DFSA)
    sexual
    violent personal
assaulted staff
    post-incident care for the support for the
assaultive acts, serious
assaultive client care
    ethical aspects of
    legal aspects of
    practical aspects of
assay, cocaethylene (CE)
assertive behavior
Assessing Specific Competencies
Assessing Specific Employment Skill Competencies
assessment *(see also* tests)
    behavior-oriented
    comprehensive
    cultural
    disorganized speech
    DSM-5
    endocrine
    environmental
    functional
    global
    hearing aid
    home
    method of
    neurophysiological
    neuropsychological
    personality
    psychiatric diagnosis and quality of life rehabilitation
    quantified cognitive
    specialized language
    standardized cognitive
    written language
assessment and monitoring measures
Assessment and Placement Services for Community Colleges
assessment battery *(see also* tests)
Assessment for Children - Emotional/Behavior Screening
Assessment in Mathematics
assessment inventory *(see also* tests)
Assessment Link Between Phonology and Articulation

assessment methods *(see also* tests)
assessment of affect
Assessment of Career Decision Making (ACDM)
Assessment of Chemical Health Inventory
Assessment of Children's Language Comprehension (ACLC)
Assessment of Conceptual Organization (ACO)
Assessment of Core Goals (ACG)
Assessment of Intelligibility of Dysarthric Speech
Assessment of Phonological Processes (APP)
assessment of recurrent suicidal behavior
Assessment of Suicide Potential
Assessment of Writing
assessment program *(see also* tests)
assessment questionnaire *(see also* tests)
assessment report *(see also* tests)
assessment scale *(see also* tests)
assessment schedule *(see also* tests)
assessment screen *(see also* tests)
assessment survey *(see also* tests)
assessment system *(see also* tests)
assessment techniques *(see also* tests)
assigned responsibility
assigned sex
assimilated nasality
assimilated nasality, voice disorder of
assimilating information
assimilating information, disturbance in rapidity of
assimilation
    alveolar
    double
    labial
    nasal
    progressive

assimilation
    progressive vowel
    reciprocal
    regressive
    velar
assimilation of information
assistant
    physician (PA)
    psychiatric (PA)
assisted suicide
associate learning, paired
associated disability
associated disorder
associated features
associated feelings
associated personality disorder
associated physical examination
association(s) *(see also* associations, professional)
    auditory-vocal
    characteristic
    clang
    direct
    etiological
    free
    frequency encountered
    loose
    loosening of (LOA)
    phoneme/grapheme
    sound-symbol
    tangential
    temporal
    word
Association Adjustment Inventory
association area, parietal
association characteristics, clang
association cortex
Association for Academic Psychiatry (AAP)
Association for Addiction Professionals
Association for Advancement of Gestalt Therapy (AAGH)
Association for Behavioral and Cognitive Therapies (ABCT)
Association for Business Psychology (ABP)

Psychiatric Words and Phrases 41

Association for Healthcare Documentation Integrity (AHDI)
Association for Psychological Science
Association for Research in Nervous and Mental Disease (ARNMD)
Association for Research in Otolaryngology
Association for the Advancement of Gestalt Therapy
Association for the Mentally Challenged
association learning
association mechanism
association neurosis
Association of Departments of Family Medicine (ADFM)
Association of LGBTQ Psychiatrists (AGLP)
Association of Professional Chaplains (APC)
association of sounds and symbols
Association of VA Psychologist Leaders
associations, professional *(see also* academy, board, center, college, conference, consortium, council, foundation, institute, organization, registry, or society)
    Academy of Integrative Pain Management, www.integrativepainmanagement.org
    Acoustical Society of America, acousticalsociety.org
    A. G. Bell Association for the Deaf and Hard of Hearing, www.agbell.org
    Alzheimer's Foundation of America, alzfdn.org
    Alzheimer's Association, www.alz.org

associations, professional
    American Academy of Audiology, www.audiology.org
    American Academy of Child and Adolescent Psychiatry, www.aacap.org
    American Academy of Family Physicians, www.aafp.org
    American Academy of Forensic Psychology, aafpforensic.org
    American Academy of Forensic Sciences, www.aafs.org
    American Academy of Otolaryngology, www.entnet.org
    American Academy of Pain Medicine, www.painmed.org
    American Academy of Pediatrics, www.aap.org
    American Academy of Physical Medicine and Rehabilitation, www.aapmr.org
    American Academy of Private Practice in Speech Pathology and Audiology, www.aappspa.org
    American Academy of Psychiatry and the Law, www.aapl.org
    American Academy of Sleep Medicine, www.aasmnet.org
    American Association of Directors of Psychiatric Residency Training, www.aadprt.org
    American Association for Geriatric Psychiatry, www.aagponline.org

associations, professional
  American Association for
    Marriage and Family
    Therapy, www.aamft.org
  American Association of
    Chairs of Departments of
    Psychiatry,
    www.aacdp.org
  American Association of
    Psychiatric Adminis-
    trators, www.psychiatric
    administrators.org
  American Association for
    Social Psychiatry,
    socialpsychiatry.org
  American Association on
    Intellectual and
    Developmental
    Disabilities,
    www.aaidd.org
  American Auditory
    Society,
    www.amauditorysoc.org
  American Board of Family
    Medicine,
    www.theabfm.org
  American Board of
    Forensic Psychology,
    www.abfp.com
  American Board of
    Psychiatry and
    Neurology, Inc.,
    www.abpn.com
  American Chronic Pain
    Association, The,
    www.theacpa.org
  American College of
    Forensic Examiners
    International,
    www.forensicpsychology
    online.com
  American College of For-
    ensic Psychiatry, www.
    forensicpsychiatry.cc
  American College of
    Forensic Psychology,
    www.forensicpsychology.
    org

associations, professional
  American College of
    Neuropsychiatrists,
    www.acn-aconp.
    webs.com
  American College of
    Neuropsychopharmacol-
    ogy, www.acnp.org
  American College of
    Osteopathic Neurologists
    and Psychiatrists,
    www.acn-aconp.
    webs.com
  American College of
    Physicians,
    www.acponline.org
  American Council on
    Education, The,
    www.acenet.edu
  American Deafness and
    Rehabilitation
    Association,
    www.adara.org
  American Dialect Society,
    www.americandialect.org
  American Group
    Psychotherapy
    Association,
    www.agpa.org
  American Health
    Information Management
    Association,
    www.ahima.org
  American Hearing
    Research Foundation,
    www.american-
    hearing.org
  American Hospital
    Association, www.aha.org
  American Institute of
    Stress, www.stress.org
  American Medical
    Association, www.ama-
    assn.org
  American Music Therapy
    Association,
    www.musictherapy.org

Psychiatric Words and Phrases

associations, professional
American National
Standards Institute,
www.ansi.org
American Nurses
Association,
nursingworld.org
American Occupational
Therapy Association, Inc.,
www.aota.org
American Physical Therapy
Association, www.apta.org
American Psychiatric
Association,
www.psychiatry.org
American Psychoanalytic
Association,
www.apsa.org
American Psychological
Association, www.apa.org
American Psychology-Law
Society,
www.apadivisions.org/
division-41/index
American
Psychopathological
Association, Inc.,
www.appassn.org
American Psychosomatic
Society,
www.psychosomatic.org
American Society for
Adolescent Psychiatry,
www.adolescent-
psychiatry.org
American Society of
Addiction Medicine,
www.asam.org
American Society of
Clinical Hypnosis,
www.asch.net
American Society of
Hospital Pharmacists,
www.ashp.org
American Speech-
Language-Hearing
Association,
wwwasha.org

associations, professional
American Telemedicine
Association, The, www.
americantelemed.org
American Tinnitus
Association, www.ata.org
Anxiety and Depression
Association of America,
www.adaa.org
Asia-Pacific Society for
Alcohol and Addiction
Research,
www.apsaar.org
Association des Sourds du
Canada, www.cad.ca
Association for Academic
Psychiatry, www.
academicpsychiatry.org
Association for Addiction
Professionals,
www.naadac.org
Association for Behavioral
and Cognitive Therapies,
www.abct.org
Association for Business
Psychology,
www.theabp.org.uk
Association for Healthcare
Documentation Integrity,
www.ahdionline.org
Association for Psycho-
logical Science, www.
psychologicalscience.org
Association for Research in
Otolaryngology,
www.aro.org
Association for the
Advancement of Gestalt
Therapy, www.aagt.org
Association for the
Mentally Challenged,
www.amcin.org
Association of Departments
of Family Medicine,
www.adfammed.org
Association of Indian
Psychologists,
aiponline.in

associations, professional
  Association of Indian
    School Counsellors and
    Allied Professionals,
    www.aiscap.com
  Association of LGBTQ
    Psychiatrists, ww.aglp.org
  Association of Professional
    Chaplains, www.
    professionalchaplains.org
  Association of VA
    Psychologist Leaders,
    www.avapl.org
  Australian & New Zealand
    Mental Health
    Association,
    anzmh.asn.au
  Australian Psychological
    Society,
    www.psychology.org.au
  Australian Psychology
    Accreditation Council,
    www.psychologycouncil.
    org.au
  British Association for
    Counselling and
    Psychotherapy,
    www.bacp.co.uk
  British Psychological
    Society, www.bps.org.uk
  British Society of
    Audiology,
    www.thebsa.org.uk
  Buros Center for Testing,
    buros.org
  Canadian Association of
    the Deaf, www.cad.ca
  Center for Medicare and
    Medicaid Services,
    www.cms.gov
  Center for Parent
    Information & Resources,
    www.parentcenterhub.org
  Center for Psychosocial
    Health Research,
    cphr.unt.edu
  Central Institute for the
    Deaf, www.cid.edu

associations, professional
  Certification Board for
    Music Therapists,
    www.cbmt.org
  College of Psychiatrists of
    Ireland,
    www.irishpsychiatry.ie
  Conference of Educational
    Administrators of Schools
    & Programs for the Deaf,
    www.ceasd.org
  Convention of American
    Instructors of the Deaf,
    www.caid.org
  Council for Exceptional
    Children,
    www.cec.sped.org
  Danish Psychological
    Association,
    www.dp.dk/about-the-
    danish-psychological-
    association
  Depression and Bipolar
    Support Alliance,
    www.dbsalliance.org
  Dutch Association of
    Psychologists,
    www.psynip.nl/en
  Educational Audiology
    Association,
    www.edaud.org
  European Association for
    Aviation Psychology,
    www.eaap.net
  European Association for
    Developmental
    Psychology,
    www.eadp.info
  European Association of
    Personality Psychology,
    www.eapp.org
  European Association of
    Work and Organizational
    Psychology,
    www.eawop.org
  European Community
    Psychology Association,
    www.ecpa-online.com

Psychiatric Words and Phrases

associations, professional
European Federation of Psychologists' Associations, www.efpa.eu
European Federation of Sport Psychology, www.fepsac.com
European Society for Biomedical Research on Alcoholism, www.esbra.com
European Society for Traumatic Stress Studies, www.estss.org
Federation of the European Societies of Neuropsychology, www.fesn.eu
Federation of German Psychologists' Associations, www.psychologie.de/en
Gallaudet University Archives and Deaf Collections, www.gallaudet.edu/archives-and-deaf-collections
German Psychological Society, www.dgps.de
Global Alliance for Behavioral Health and Social Justice, www.bhjustice.org
Global Organization for Stress, www.gostress.com
Health Care Compliance Association, www.hcca-info.org
Hearing Health Foundation, hearinghealthfoundation.org
Hearing Industries Association, www.hearing.org
Hearing Loss Association of America, www.hearingloss.org

associations, professional
Helen Keller National Center for Deaf-Blind Youths and Adults, www.hknc.org
Hogan Assessment Systems, www.hoganassessments.com
Indian Academy of Cerebral Palsy, iacp.co.in
Indian Association of Biological Psychiatry, www.iabp.org.in
Indian Association of Clinical Psychologists, iacp.in
Indian Association of Private Psychiatry, www.iapp.co.in
Indian Psychiatric Society, www.indianpsychiatricsociety.org
Indian School Psychology Association, inspa.in
Institute of General Semantics, www.generalsemantics.org
International Association for the Study of Pain, www.iasp-pain.org
International Hearing Society, ihsinfo.org
International Organization for Standardization, www.iso.org
International Phonetic Association, www.internationalphoneticassociation.org
International Society for Biomedical Research on Alcoholism, www.isbra.com
International Society for Mental Health Online, www.ismho.org

associations, professional
- International Society for the Study of Trauma and Dissociation, www.isst-d.org
- International Society for Traumatic Stress Studies, www.istss.org
- International Stress and Behavior Society, www.stressandbehavior.com
- International Stress Management Association, isma.org.uk
- International Union of Psychological Science, www.iupsys.net
- Journal of Interpersonal Violence, journals.sagepub.com/home/jiv
- Korean Psychological Association, www.koreanpsychology.or.kr/eng/index.asp
- Lighthouse Guild, lighthouseguild.org
- Linguistic Society of America, www.lsadc.org
- Medical Journal of Australia, www.mja.com.au
- Mental Health America, www.mentalhealthamerica.net
- Mental Health Association of Central Australia, mhaca.org.au
- Mental Health Australia, mhaustralia.org
- National Academy of Psychology (India), www.naopindia.org
- National Alliance on Mental Illness, www.nami.org

associations, professional
- National Association for Alcoholism & Drug Addiction Counselors, www.naadac.org
- National Association for Behavioral Healthcare, www.nabh.org
- National Association for Special Education Needs, www.nasen.org.uk
- National Association for the Deaf, www.nad.org
- National Association of Academic Psychiatry Administrators, adminpsych.us
- National Association of Forensic Counselors, www.nationalafc.com
- National Association of School Psychologists, www.nasponline.org
- National Association of Social Workers, www.socialworkers.org
- National Association of Special Education Teachers, www.naset.org
- National Bipolar Foundation, www.nationalbipolarfoundation.org
- National Board for Certification in Hearing Instrument Sciences, www.nbc-his.com
- National Captioning Institute, www.ncicap.org
- National Center for Health Statistics, www.cdc.gov/nchs
- National Council for Behavioral Health, www.thenationalcouncil.org

associations, professional
- National Cued Speech Association, www.cuedspeech.org
- National Dissemination Center for Children with Disabilities, nichcy.org
- National Down Syndrome Society, www.ndss.org
- National Drug Intelligence Center, www.justice.gov/archive/ndic
- National Institute of Mental Health, www.nimh.nih.gov
- National Institute of Neurological Disorders and Stroke, www.ninds.nih.gov
- National Institute on Aging, www.nia.nih.gov
- National Institute on Alcohol Abuse and Alcoholism, www.niaaa.nih.gov
- National Institute on Deafness and Other Communication Disorders, www.nidcd.nih.gov
- National Institute on Drug Abuse, www.drugabuse.gov
- National Institutes of Health, www.nih.gov
- National Multiple Sclerosis Society, www.nationalmssociety.org
- National Organization of Forensic Social Work, nofsw.org
- National Sleep Foundation, www.sleepfoundation.org
- National Student Speech Language Hearing Association, www.nsslha.org

associations, professional
- National Survey on Drug Use and Health, nsduhweb.rti.org/respweb/homepage.cfm
- National Technical Institute for the Deaf (Center on Employment), www.ntid.rit.edu
- National Youth Tobacco Survey, www.cdc.gov/tobacco/data_statistics/surveys/nyts/index.htm
- Psychology Today www.psychologytoday.com/us/therapists
- Registry of Interpreters for the Deaf, Inc., www.rid.org
- Research Society on Alcoholism, www.rsoa.org
- Royal College of Psychiatrists, www.rcpsych.ac.uk
- Social Psychiatry and Psychiatric Epidemiology (Journal), link.springer.com/journal/volumesAndIssues/127
- Society for Community Research and Action, www.scra27.org
- Society for Industrial and Organizational Psychology, www.siop.org
- Society for Personality and Social Psychology, www.spsp.org
- Society for Psychotherapy Research, www.psychotherapyresearch.org
- Society for Research in Child Development, www.srcd.org

associations, professional
   Society for the Teaching of
     Psychology,
     teachpsych.org
   Society of Teachers of
     Family Medicine,
     www.stfm.org
   South African Depression
     and Anxiety Group, The,
     www.sadag.org
   Speech-Language &
     Audiology Canada,
     www.sac-oac.ca
   Substance Abuse and
     Mental Health Service
     Administration,
     www.samhsa.gov
   Swedish Psychological
     Association,
     www.saco.se/en/english/o
     ur-22-unions/swedish-
     psychological-association
   Texas Research Society on
     Alcoholism,
     www.trsoa.org
   Voices of Hope,
     www.voicesofhopelex.org
   World Association of
     Social Psychiatry,
     www.waspsocialpsychiatr
     y.com
   World Psychiatric
     Association,
     www.wpanet.org
   Zurinstitute Forensic
     Psychology Resources &
     References, www.
     zurinstitute.com/resources
     /forensic-psychology
associative aphasia
associative visual agnosia
assonance
astasia-abasia, hysterical
astereognosis
asteric seizure
asthenic
asthenic asthenia
astomia
"astroturf" (street name,
   cannabis/marijuana)
astrocytic gliosis
astrophobia
astrotraveling
asymbolia
asymmetrical amnesia
asymmetry
   abnormal
   amplitude
   facial
   interhemispheric
   reflex
   skull
asymptomatic seizure
asynergia
asynergic
asynergy
ATA (American Telemedicine
   Association, The)
atactic ataxia
Ataque de nervios
ataxia
   absent
   alcoholic
   appendicular
   atactic
   autosomal dominant
     cerebellar, deafness, and
     narcolepsy (G47.419)
   Briquet
   Broca
   Bruns
   cerebellar
   crural
   equilibratory
   hysterical
   ipsilateral cerebellar
   kinesigenic
   locomotor
   mild
   moderate
   moral
   psychogenic
   sensory
   severe
ataxia conversion
ataxic cerebral palsy (CP)

Psychiatric Words and Phrases 49

ataxic dysarthria
ataxic gait
ataxiophobia
ataxophobia
atherosclerosis, cerebral
atherosclerotic heart disease
athetoid cerebral palsy (CP)
athetoid movement(s)
athetosis
Athletic Motivation Inventory (AMI)
atmosphere
    situationally appropriate
    situationally optimistic
ATMS (Attitudes Toward Mainstreaming Scale)
"atom bomb" (street name, cannabis and heroin)
atomizer
atonia
atonic absense seizure
atonic cerebral palsy (CP)
atoxic speech
atresia
    aural
    laryngeal
    oral
atrioventricular block
atrophic dementia
atrophy
    brain
    cerebral
    frontotemporal brain
    structural
"atshitshi" (street name, cannabis)
attachment
    Bowlby theory of
    effect of trauma on
    mother-infant
    object
    oscillations of
    selective
    social
    suffocating
    symbiotic
    theory of
    unstable
attachment/commitment, emotional
attachment disorder, reactive
attachment figures
attachment figures, major
attachment –style
    anxious
    avoidant
    secure
attack
    character
    dream anxiety (nightmare)
    full panic
    glottal
    limited-symptom
    motor rage
    nocturnal panic
    panic
    personal
    physical
    psychotic
    rage
    recurrent panic
    refreshing sleep
    road rage
    schizophreniform
    sleep
    terrorist
    transient ischemic
    uncontrollable sleep
    vocal
    word
attacker role
attain power, manipulative behavior to
attempt
    failed suicide
    history of suicide
    risk of suicide
attention
    auditory
    center of
    disturbance in
    fix and focus
    focus of
    focus of clinical
    heightened
    need for constant

attention
    raptus of
    state of heightened
attention ability, impaired
Attention and Adjustment Survey,
    Children's (CAAS)
attention deficit
Attention Deficit Disorder
    Behavior Rating Scales
    (ADDBRS)
Attention Deficit Disorder
    Evaluation Scale (ADDES)
attention-deficit hyperactivity
    disorder
        combined presentation
            (F90.2)
        combined type
        other specified (F90.8)
        predominantly hyperactive
        predominantly hyperactive/
            impulsive presentation
            (F90.1)
        predominantly inattentive
        predominantly inattentive
            presentation (F90.0)
        unspecified (F90.9)
attenuated psychosis syndrome
    (F28)
attention-deficit symptoms
attention to sounds
attention seeking, pattern of
attention shift ability
attention skills, impaired
attentional ability
attentional set of disturbances
attention-deficit
attenuation, interaural
attenuator
attitude
    categorical
    complacent
    cultural
    do-not-care
    gender-based
    hyperdefensive
    inappropriate
    inflexible
    over-dependent

attitude
    primary oppositional
    rigid
    self-centered
    sexual
attitude of health personnel
Attitude Survey Program for
    Business and Industry
attitude to death
attitude to health
Attitudes Toward Mainstreaming
    Scale (ATMS)
attribute-entity
Attributional Style Questionnaire
atypical absense seizure
atypical clefts
atypical clinical course
atypical face pain
atypical features
atypical pain
atypical presentations
audibility threshold
audible blocking in speech
audible field, minimum (MAF)
audible pressure, minimum
    (MAP)
audible range
audible speech blocking
auding
audiogenic seizure
audiogram configurations
    dipper curve
    flat
    gradual falling curve
    gradual rising curve
    marked falling curve
    saddle curve
    saucer curve
    sharply falling curve
    ski slope curve
    steep curve
    sudden drop curve
    trough curve
    U-shaped curve
    waterfall curve
audiologic habilitation
audiological evaluation
audiologist

Psychiatric Words and Phrases

audiology
   clinical
   educational
   experimental
   geriatric
   pediatric
   rehabilitative
audiometer
   automatic
   Bekesy
   crib-o-gram
   group
   limited range
   limited range speech
   narrow range
   pure-tone
   Rudmose
   speech
   wide range
audiometric tests
audiometric zero
audiometry
   ascending technique
   auditory brainstem response (ABR)
   automatic
   average evoked response (AERA)
   behavioral observation (BOA)
   behavioral observational (BOA)
   Bekesy
   brain stem evoked response (BSER)
   brief tone (BTA)
   cardiac evoked response (CERA)
   conditioned orientation reflex (COR)
   delayed feedback (DFA)
   descending technique
   diagnostic
   electric response (ERA)
   electrocochleography (ECoG) (ECochG)
   electrodermal (EDA)

audiometry
   electrodermal response test (EDRA)
   electroencephalic (EEA)
   electroencephalic response (ERA)
   electrophysiologic
   evoked response (ERA)
   galvanic skin response (GSRA)
   group
   high frequency HF
   identification
   industrial
   limited range
   limited range speech
   live voice
   monitored live voice
   monitoring
   narrow range
   neonatal auditory response cradle
   play
   psychogalvanic skin response
   pure-tone (AC)
   pure-tone (BC)
   reduced screening
   screening
   speech
   speech awareness
   speech discrimination
   speech reception
   sweep check test
   tangible reinforcement operant conditioning (TROCA)
   visual reinforcement
   wide range
Audit, Stress
audition
audito-oculogyric reflex
auditory *(see also* tests)
auditory abilities, central
auditory acuity
auditory adaption

auditory agnosia
    generalized
    selective
    verbal
auditory alexia
auditory amnesic
auditory analysis
Auditory Analysis Test
auditory area
auditory attention
auditory blending
auditory brainstem response (ABR)
auditory brainstem response (ABR) audiometry
auditory canal
auditory canal, internal
auditory cortex
auditory cortex, primary
auditory cue
auditory differentiation
auditory discrimination
Auditory Discrimination and Attention Test
Auditory Discrimination Test
auditory disorder
auditory disorder, central
auditory evoked potential, brain stem (BAEP)
auditory evoked response, brain stem (BAER)
auditory fatigue
auditory feedback
    delayed (DAF)
    experimentally delayed
    simultaneous
auditory figure-ground
auditory figure-ground discrimination
auditory flutter
auditory flutter fusion
auditory function
    acoustic measurement of
    central
auditory hallucinations, transient
auditory illusions, transient
auditory imperception
auditory information
auditory information with motor activity, disturbance in integrating
auditory localization
auditory meatus
    external
    internal
auditory memory
auditory memory span
Auditory Memory Span Test/Auditory Sequential Memory Test
auditory method
auditory modality
auditory neglect
auditory nerve (cranial nerve VIII)
auditory pattern
auditory perception
auditory perception, central
auditory phonetics
Auditory Pointing Test
auditory processes
auditory processes, central
auditory processing
auditory processing, temporal
auditory processing disorder
auditory recall
auditory reflex
auditory response cradle audiometry, neonatal
auditory response cradle, neonatal
auditory seizure
auditory selective listening
auditory sensory modality
auditory sequencing
auditory skills
auditory stimulation
auditory stimulus
auditory storage
auditory symptom
auditory synthesis
Auditory Test Lists *(see also* tests)
Auditory Test W-22
auditory tests and procedures
auditory threshold

Psychiatric Words and Phrases 53

auditory trainer
    desk-type
    frequency-modulation
    hard-wire
    loop-induction
auditory training
auditory training units
auditory tube
auditory verbal agnosia
auditory-vocal automaticity
auditory-vocal, association
augmentative communication
    aided
    unaided
augmentative communication system
AUI (Alcohol Use Inventory)
aulophobia
"Aunt Hazel" (street name, heroin)
"Aunt Mary" (street name, cannabis/marijuana)
"Aunt Nora" (street name, cocaine)
"Aunt" (street name, powder cocaine)
"Aunti Emma" (street name, opium)
"Aunti" (street name, opium)
aura
    auditory
    déjà vu
    epigastric
    epileptic
    gustatory
    hysterical
    jamais vu
    kinesthetic
    migraine
    olfactory
    reminiscent
    sensory
    status
    visual
aural *(see also* tests)
aural atresia

aural rehabilitation
    acoustic method
    bimodal method of
    combined
    grammatic method of
    kinesthetic method of
    lipreading
    manual method of
    natural method of
    oral-aural method of
    simultaneous
    speech reading
auricle
auropalpebral reflex (APR)
"aurora borealis" (street name, PCP)
Austin Spanish Articulation Test
Australian Psychological Society (APS)
Australian Psychology Accreditation Council (APAC)
Australian X viral encephalitis
"author" (re: doctor who writes illegal prescriptions)
authoritarianism
autism
    akinetic
    childhood
    infantile
    neuroleptic treatment of childhood
    nonspeaking
    primary
    secondary
    semantics of
Autism Screening Instrument for Educational Planning
autism spectrum disorder (F80.0)
autism spectrum disorder, currently severe (F84.0)
autism spectrum disorder associated with another behavioral disorder (F84.0)
autism spectrum disorder associated with another neurodevelopmental disorder (F84.0)

autism spectrum disorder
  requiring (very) substantial
  support (F84.0)
autism spectrum disorder with a
  known environmental factor
  (F84.0)
autism spectrum disorder with a
  known genetic condition
  (F84.0)
autism spectrum disorder with a
  known medical condition
  (F84.0)
autism spectrum disorder with
  catatonia (F84.0) and (F06.1)
autism spectrum disorder with or
  without accompanying
  intellectual impairment (F84.0)
autism spectrum disorder with or
  without accompanying language
  impairment (F84.0)
Autistic and Other Atypical
  Children - Behavior Rating
Autistic Behavior Composite
  Checklist and Profile
autistic disorder
autistic fantasy
autistic problems
autistic thinking
autobiographical information
autoclitic operant
autoerogenous
autogenic
autogenic training
autogynephilia
automania
Automated Child/Adolescent
  Social History
automatic audiometer
automatic audiometry
automatic gain control
automatic language
automatic line encoding (ALE)
    center placement pop-on
    closed
    closed decoder
    encoder
    encoding
    line-display

automatic line encoding (ALE)
    line 21
    live (ON line)
    master
    open
    pop-on
    real-time dictionary
    reformat
    roll-up
    sub-master
    substitute
    time-code
    timed roll-up
automatic phrase level
automatic psychological process
automatic speech
automatic volume control (AVC)
automaticity, auditory-vocal
automatism
    ambulatory
    chewing
    command
    epileptic
    facial expression
    gestural
    ictal
    mumbling
    swallowing
autonomic activity
autonomic arousal
autonomic arousal, intense
autonomic denervation
autonomic dysfunction
autonomic dysnomia
autonomic hyperactivity
autonomic hyperactivity signs
autonomic hyperarousal
autonomic hyperreflexia
autonomic hyperventilation
autonomic neuropathy, peripheral
autonomic signs
autonomic signs, increased
autophonia
autophonomania
autopsy, brain
autosomal dominant cerebellar
  ataxia, deafness, and narcolepsy
  (G47.419)

Psychiatric Words and Phrases 55

autosomal dominant gene
autosomal dominant narcolepsy, obesity, and type 2 diabetes (G47.419)
autosomal dominant pattern
autotopagnosia agnosia
auxiliary verb
auxiliary verb, modal
available data
AVC (automatic volume control)
Avellis syndrome
avenues of administration
average, pure tone
average evoked response audiometry (AERA)
average full-on gain
    HF
    high-frequency (HF)
average saturation sound pressure level 90, high-frequency
average SSPL 90
    HF
    high-frequency
average SSPL output HF
aversion, occasional sexual
aversion disorder
    acquired type sexual
    generalized type sexual
    life-long type sexual
    sexual
    situational type sexual
aversion disorder due to combined factors, sexual
aversion disorder due to psychological factors, sexual
avoid thinking, to
avoidance
    focus of
    harm
    pain
avoidance act theory, instrumental
avoidance learning
avoidance of an object
avoidance of responsibility
avoidance of situations, phobic
avoidance of speech dysfluencies
avoidance symptoms

avoidance tests (BATs) for OCD, behavioral
avoidant behavior
    culturally appropriate
    developmentally appropriate
avoidant food intake disorder (F50.8)
avoidant personality disorder (F60.6)
avoidant/restrictive food intake disorder (F50.8)
avoiding speech situations
avolition
awake state, alert
awards, potential external
awareness
    conscious
    emotional
    environmental
    heightened
    interoceptive
    lack of
    lack of interoceptive
    lapse of
    leisure
    phonetic
    postural
    sensory (SA)
    state of heightened
    subconscious
awareness audiometry, speech
awareness of the environment
awareness threshold, speech (SAT)
AWOL ideation
axioversion
axioversion of teeth
axon degeneration
axon flare
axon loss
axon terminal
axonal
axonapraxia
axonopathy
Aztec idiocy

B

"B" (re: the marijuana needed to fill a match box)
B12 deficiency
"B-40" (re: cigar laced with marijuana, dipped in malt liquor)
B90: Advanced ACER Test
babbling
    non-reduplicated
    reduplicated
    social
"babe" (re: drug used for detoxification)
Babinski reflex
Babinski sign
"baby" (street name, cannabis/marijuana)
"baby bhang" (street name, cannabis/marijuana)
"baby habit" (re: occasional use of drugs)
"babysit" (re: guidance for first-time drug user)
"babysitter" (street name, cannabis/marijuana)
"Baby T" (street name, crack cocaine)
baby talk
"back breakers" (street name, LSD and strychnine)
"back dex" (street name, amphetamine)
"back door" (re: residue left in a pipe)
back feature English phoneme
"back jack" (re: injecting opium or other drug)
back pain
back pain, low
back phoneme
"back to back" (re: injecting heroin after smoking crack)
"back up" (re: to prepare a vein for injection)
back vowel
background
    educational
    ethnic
    sociocultural
background activity
Background Interference Procedure for Bender Gestalt
background noise
backing to velars
"backtrack" (re: blood flow back into injecting needle)
backward coarticulation
backward masking
"backwards" (street name, barbiturate)
"backwards" (depression)
backwards from 100 test, count
backwards test
    spell
    spell a word
bacterial meningitis
bad behavior
"bad bundle" (re: poor quality heroin)
"bad" (street name, crack; crack cocaine)
"bad go" (re: bad drug reaction)
"bad rock" (street name, crack cocaine)
"bad seed" (street name, mescaline; heroin; cannabis/marijuana)
"bad trip" (re: hallucinogens)
BADGE (Bekesy Ascending-Descending Gap Evaluation)
BAEP (brain stem auditory evoked potential)
BAER (brain stem auditory evoked response)
baffle effect, body (hearing aid)
BaFPE (Bay Area Functional Performance Evaluation

Psychiatric Words and Phrases

"bag" (re: drug container; package of drugs)
"bag bride" (re: crack smoking prostitute)
"bag man" (re: drug dealer)
"bagging" (re: inhalant use)
"bail out" behavior
"baker" (re: marijuana smoker)
balance (pl. balances)
   acid-base
   core body
   dynamic ambulatory
   dynamic standing
   homeostatic
   impaired
   sitting
   spatial
   standing
balance mechanism
balance scale, affects
balance tests *(see also* tests)
balanced words, phonetically (PB words)
"bale" (street name, cannabis/marijuana)
"ball" (street name, crack cocaine; Mexican Black Tar heroin)
"balling" (re: cocaine vaginal concealment)
ballistic movement
ballistomania (missiles)
"balloon" (re: heroin supplier)
"ballot" (street name, heroin)
Balthazar Scales for Adaptive Behavior
"bam" (street name, barbiturate; amphetamine; depressants)
"bamba" (street name, cannabis/marijuana)
"Bambalacha" (street name, cannabis/marijuana)
"bambs" (street name, barbiturate)
"banana split" (re: combination of drugs)
"banano" (re: marijuana cigarettes mixed with cocaine)
band analyzer, octave
band frequency
band-like headache
band-pass filter
band spectrum
"bandits" (street name, methaqualone)
bands, vocal
bandwidth
"bang" (re: drug injection)
"bang" (street name, inhalant)
"banging" (re: under the influence of drugs)
"bank bandit pills" (street name, barbiturate/depressant)
"bank deposit pills" (street name, barbiturate/depressant)
Bankson-Bernthal Test of Phonology (BBTOP)
Bankson Language Test (BLT)
BAP (Behavioral Assessment of Pain Questionnaire)
"bar" (street name, cannabis/marijuana)
"Barb" (street name, barbiturate/depressant)
barbaralalia
Barber Scales of Self-Regard for Preschool Children
"Barbies" (street name, barbiturate/depressant)
barbiturate (street names)
   backwards
   bam
   bambs
   bank bandit pills
   bank deposit pills
   Barb
   Barbies
   beans
   black beauties
   block busters
   blue
   blue bullets
   blue dolls
   blue heavens
   blue tips
   busters
   chorals
   Christmas rolls

barbiturate (street names)
    coral
    courage pills
    disco biscuits
    downie
    drowsy high
    G.B.
    gangster pills
    golf balls
    gorilla pills
    green frog
    idiot pills
    inbetweens
    jellies
    joy juice
    King Kong pills
    lay back
    lib (Librium)
    little bomb
    love drug
    luding out
    luds
    M&M
    marshmallow reds
    Mexican reds
    Mickey Finn
    Mickey's
    Mighty Joe Young
    mother's little helper
    nemmies
    nimbies
    peth
    purple hearts
    Q
    quad
    quas
    red and blue
    red bullets
    red devil
    seggy
    sleeper
    softballs
    sopers
    stoppers
    strawberries
    stumbler
    tooles
    tooties

barbiturate (street names)
    tranq
    tuie
    Uncle Milty
    ups and downs
    yellow
barbiturate-facilitated interview
barbiturate hypnotic drug
"barbs" (street name, cocaine)
bar/cushion/pad/ridge, Passavant's
barotrauma
"barr" (street name, codeine cough syrup)
"barrels" (street name, LSD)
barrenness, inner
Barrett tongue thrust classification
barrier(s)
    blood-brain
    communication
    language
barriers to interventions
Barry Five Slate System
"bars" (street name, heroin mixed with alprazolam)
"Bart Simpson" (street name, heroin)
Barthel ADL Index
BAS (British Ability Scales: Spelling Scale)
BASA (Boston Assessment of Severe Aphasia)
"basa" (street name, crack cocaine)
basal age
basal fluency
basal ganglia
basal ganglia calcification
basal pitch
"base" (street name, cocaine/crack)
base component
"base crazies" (re: crack acquisition)
"base head" (re: a freebaser)
base rule
base structure
base word

Psychiatric Words and Phrases

"baseball" (street name, crack cocaine)
"based" (re: lost control over basing)
baseline aims
baseline symptoms
"bash" (street name, cannabis/marijuana)
basic academic subject specific tests *(see also* tests)
Basic Achievement Skills Individual Screener
Basic Achievement Skills Inventory
Basic Concept Inventory
basic education specific tests *(see also* tests)
Basic Educational Skills Test
basic health, neglect of
Basic Inventory of Natural Language
Basic Language Concepts Test
basic learning skills specific tests *(see also* tests)
Basic Occupational Literacy Test
Basic Personality Inventory (BPI)
Basic Reading Inventory
Basic School Skills Inventory Screen
basic screening specific tests *(see also* tests)
basic skill tests *(see also* tests)
Basic Skills Assessment Program
Basic Skills Inventory
basic skills specific tests *(see also* tests)
Basic Skills Test for Business, Industry, and Government, PSI
basilar insufficiency
basilar membrane
basilar migraine headache
basilect
"basing" (re: crack cocaine)
basis
    articulatory
    biological
"Basson brownies" (street name, MDMA)

"basulco" (street name, cocaine; cigarette laced with cocoa paste)
"basulca" (street name, cocoa paste)
batacas
"batak" (street name, methamphetamine - Philippine term)
Batelle Developmental Inventory
bath, Kwell
"bath salts" (re: narcotics)
bathmophobia
"bathtub crank" (re: poor quality methamphetamine)
"bathtub speed" (street name, methcathinone)
"Batman" (street name, cocaine; heroin)
"Batmans" (street name, MDMA)
bats, encounter
"batt" (re: drug equipment; I.V. needle)
"batted out" (re: apprehended by law)
Battelle Developmental Inventory
batteries of specific tests *(see also* tests)
"battery acid" (street name, LSD)
battery clusters, inner
battery of specific tests *(see also* tests)
battery of tests, neuropsychologic
"batu" (re: smokable methamphetamine)
Bay Area Functional Performance Evaluation
"bazooka" (street name, cocaine; crack; other drug combinations)
"Bazulco" (street name, cocaine)
"B-bombs" (street name, amphetamine; MDMA)
BBTOP (Bankson-Bernthal Test of Phonology)
BC (behavior control; bone conduction)
"BC bud" (re: any high grade marijuana from Canada)

BCAP (British Association for Counselling and Psychotherapy)
BCL (Bekesy comfortable loudness)
BCR (behavior control room)
BCRS (Brief Cognitive Rating Scale)
BD (behavior disorder)
BDAE (Boston Diagnostic Aphasia Examination)
BDIS (Behavior Disorders Identification Scale)
"BDMPEA" (street name, Nexus)
BDRS (Blessed Dementia Rating Scale)
be four-pointed, to (to be restrained)
BEAM (brain electrical activity map)
"beam" (street name, cocaine)
"beam me up Scottie" (street name, crack and phencyclidine)
"beamer" (re: crack user)
"bean" (re: a capsule containing drugs)
"beanies" (street name, methamphetamine)
"beans" (street name, barbiturate; mescaline; crack cocaine)
"beast" (street name, LSD)
"The Beast" (street name, heroin + LSD)
"beat" (street name, crack cocaine)
"beat artist" (re: dealer of bogus drugs)
"beat vials" (re: sham crack)
beating, child
"beautiful boulders" (street name, crack)
beauty, obsession with
"Beavis & Butthead" (street name, LSD; hallucinogen)
"Bebe" (street name, crack)
Beck Depression Inventory
Beck Hopelessness Scale (BHS)
Beck Questionnaire
beclouded dementia

BED (binge-eating disorder) (F50.8)
bed crisis
bed partners
"bedbugs" (re: fellow addict)
Bedside Evaluation and Screening Test of Aphasia
"beedies" (re: cigarettes from India/drug vehicle)
"beemers" (street name, crack)
Beery Picture Vocabulary Test
behavior(s)
    aberrant
    absence of maladaptive
    abusive vocal
    accident prone
    addictive
    adolescent
    adolescent antisocial
    adolescent cross-gender
    adolescent risk-taking
    adult antisocial
    adult antisocial (Z72.811)
    adult criminal
    adult cross-gender
    aggressive
    agitated
    agnostic
    aimless
    alleviating aggressive
    alleviating violence in aggressive
    amotivated
    angry
    apraxic
    arrogant
    assertive
    assessment of recurrent suicidal
    avoidant
    bad
    "bail out"
    "bailout"
    catatonic motor
    child antisocial
    child or adolescent antisocial (Z72.810)
    childhood cross-gender

behavior(s)
- choice
- clinging
- compensatory
- competitive
- complex motor
- compulsive
- compulsive drug-taking
- contractual
- courtship
- crisis management of recurrent suicidal
- cross-dressing
- culturally appropriate avoidant
- culturally appropriate shy
- culturally prescribed ritual
- culturally sanctioned
- cultural-related standards of sexual
- cunning and hiding
- de-escalating aggressive
- delusional
- dementia-related
- developmentally appropriate avoidant
- developmentally appropriate shy
- deviant pattern of inner experience and
- diminution of goal-directed
- disorganized
- disruptive
- disturbance in
- disturbed eating
- dominant-subordinate
- drinking
- driven motor
- driving (automobile)
- drug-seeking
- dysarthric
- empathic
- envious
- eroticized
- exhibitionistic
- exploratory
- explosive
- extramarital

behavior(s)
- feeding
- fidgeting
- flirtatious
- gambling
- goal-directed
- grossly disorganized
- hair-pulling
- haughty
- head-banging
- health
- helping
- help-seeking
- high risk
- homicidal
- hostile
- hyperactive
- hyperactive-impulsive combined
- illness
- imitative
- impulsive
- inappropriate
- inappropriate compensatory
- inappropriate sexual
- inattentive
- incompatible
- infant
- infantile
- initiation of goal-directed
- intense sexual
- interictal
- interpersonal
- intimidating
- irresponsible work
- lawful
- leadership
- learned dysfunctional
- maladaptive
- maladaptive gambling
- maladaptive health
- management of aggressive
- masochistic sexual
- mass
- maternal
- mercurial
- modeled
- motor

behavior(s)
  multidisciplinary
    management of
    aggressive
  negative
  negativistic
  nonfunctional and
    repetitive motor
  nonfunctional motor
  normative
  out-of-control drinking
  pacing
  pain
  paranoid
  paraphiliac
  Parent Rating of Student
  paternal
  pathological
  pattern of antisocial
  pattern(s) of
  persistent pattern of
  pressured
  promiscuous sexual
  psychomotor
  purposeful
  reckless
  regressive
  rehabilitation
  REM sleep
  repetitive
  repetitive pattern of
  repetitive restricted
  repressive
  restless
  risk-taking
  Scales of Independent
  self-damaging
  self-destructive
  self-dramatizing
  self-injurious
  self-stimulation
  self-stimulatory
  semipurposeful
  sensory/motor
  sex-role
  sexual
  sexually addictive

behavior(s)
  sexually arousing
  sexually seductive
  sissyish
  sleepwalking
  social
  social phobic-like
  social stereotypical
  spatial
  speech and language
  speech/language
  stereotyped
  stereotyped restricted
  stereotypic
  stereotypic sex-role
  stereotypical
  Structural Analysis of
    Social
  subliminal
  submissive
  substance-seeking
  substituting
  sucking
  suicidal
  terminal
  terminal achievement
  tests of
  theories of aggressive
  ticlike
  tomboy
  trancelike
  uncued
  unexpected
  unlawful
  unpurposeful
  unusual sexual
  violent
  voyeuristic
  voyeuristic sexual
behavior analyses tests *(see also*
  tests)
Behaviour Assessment Battery
behavior assessment tests *(see*
  also tests)
behavior checklists
behavior control (BC)
behavior control room (BCR)

behavior disorder
 disruptive
 REM sleep
Behavior Disorders Identification Scale (BDIS)
Behavior Evaluation Scale (BES)
behavior for material gratification, manipulative
behavior generator, new
behavior in schizophrenia, disorganized
behavior pattern
behavior patterns, cross-gender
Behavior Problem Checklist
Behavior Rating Instrument for Autistic and Other Atypical Children
Behavior Rating Profile
behavior rating scales
behavior reaction, dangerous
behavior role, adultomorphic
behavior scale tests *(see also* tests)
behavior theories, anticipatory and struggling
behavior theory, operant
behavior to attain power, manipulative
behavior to gain profit, manipulative
Behavioral Academic Self-Esteem
Behavioral Assessment of Pain Questionnaire (BAP; P-BAP)
behavioral avoidance tests *(see also* tests)
behavioral change(s)
behavioral changes, maladaptive
behavioral criterion
Behavioral Deviancy Profile
behavioral disorganization in schizophrenia
behavioral disturbance
behavioral dyscontrol
behavioral dysfunction
 manifestation of
 symptoms of
behavioral flexibility
behavioral genetics
behavioral hearing tests *(see also* tests)
Behavioral Inattention Test (BIT)
behavioral management of dementia
behavioral mapping
behavioral medicine
behavioral monitoring
 distortion of inferential
 exaggeration of inferential
behavioral neurobiology
behavioral neurology
behavioral objective
behavioral observation audiometry (BOA)
Behavioral Observation Scale for Autism
behavioral research orientation
behavioral semantics
behavioral set of disturbances
behavioral syndrome
behavioral training
behavioral undercontrol
Behaviors and Skills for Children Showing Autistic Features
behaviors in sensory deficit individuals, self-stimulatory
behaviors in the young, developmentary appropriate self-stimulatory
"behind the scale" (re: cocaine value)
"beiging" (re: cocaine purity)
being out of control, sense of
being overwhelmed, sense of
being shamed, fear of
being touched, distorted perception of
"Beiruts" (street name, methaqualone)
Bekesy Ascending-Descending Gap Evaluation (BADGE)
Bekesy audiometer
Bekesy audiometry
Bekesy comfortable loudness (BCL)
Bekesy Forward-Reverse Tracings

Bekesy tracing types
bel (logarithmic unit)
belief(s)
    cultural
    culture-bound
    erroneous
    internal world of
    loss of
    odd
    shared delusional
    sustained
    true
    unreasonable
belief in clairvoyance
belief in "sixth sense"
belief in telepathy
belief system, paranoid
Bell mania
Bell Object Relations-Reality Testing Inventory
Bell palsy
Bell paralysis
Bell phenomenon
bell-shaped curve
Bell's Visible Speech
"belladonna" (street name, phencyclidine/PCP)
Bellugi-Klima's Language Comprehension Tests
"belt" (re: intoxication)
"belted" (re: drug intoxication)
"Belushi" (street name, cocaine and heroin)
"Belyando spruce" (street name, cannabis/marijuana)
Bem Sex-Role Inventory
benchmarks
"bender" (re: drug party)
Bender Visual Gestalt drawings
bending, rule
benefit eligibility
benefit remuneration
benefits of the "sick" role, intangible
benign brain neoplasm
benign essential tremor
benign exertional headache
benign habit

benign neonatal familial seizure
"bennie" (street name, amphetamine)
"bens" (street name, amphetamine; MDMA)
Benson-Geschwind classification of aphasia
Benton Revised Visual Retention Test
bent-over neck
"Benz" (street name, amphetamine)
"Benzedrine" (street name, amphetamine; MDMA)
"Benzidrine" (street name, amphetamine)
benzocaine (street names)
    coco snow
    comeback
    flat chunks
    potato chips
benzolecgonine
benzomorphan
bereavement
    biopsychosocial aspects of
    uncomplicated (Z63.4)
bereavement disorder
bereavement disorder, persistent complex
Berko Test
"Bermuda triangles" (re: analog for amphetamine/methamphetamine)
"Bernice" (street name, cocaine)
"Bernie" (street name, cocaine)
"bernie's flakes" (street name, cocaine)
"Bernie's gold dust" (street name, cocaine)
Bernoulli effect
Bernoulli's law
Berry-Talbott Language Test
BES-2 (Behavior Evaluation Scale-2)
best practice decisions using psychiatric tools and algorithms
beta activity
beta-adrenergic antagonist

Psychiatric Words and Phrases 65

beta-adrenergic medication
beta-adrenergic medication-
 induced postural tremor
beta-amyloid protein
beta index
beta pattern on EEG
beta rhythm on EEG
beta wave
beta wave on EEG
"better infamous than invisible"
 (serial killer quote)
better sleep continuity
Bexley-Maudsley Automated
 Psychological Screening
"bhang" (street name, India
 marijuana)
BHS (Beck Hopelessness Scale)
bibliokleptomania (theft of books)
bibliomania (books)
bibliophobia
bibliotherapeutic strategies
bibliotherapy
"bibs" (street name,
 MDMA/methylenedioxymetha
 mphetamine)
BICROS (bilateral contralateral
 routing of signals)
bicuspid teeth
bifid tongue
bifrontal headache
bifurcation
"big 8" (re: 1/8 kilogram of crack)
"big bag" (street name, heroin)
"big bloke" (street name, cocaine)
"big C" (street name, cocaine)
"big D" (street name, LSD)
"big doodig" (street name, heroin)
"big flake" (street name, cocaine)
"big Harry" (street name, heroin)
"big man" (re: drug supplier)
"big O" (street name, opium)
"big rush" (street name, cocaine)
"biker's coffee" (street name,
 methamphetamine and coffee)
bilabial area consonant placement
bilateral abductor paralysis
bilateral adductor paralysis
bilateral cerebral dysfunction

bilateral cleft lip
bilateral cleft palate
bilateral contralateral routing of
 signals (BICROS)
bilateral gaze palsy
bilateral hemisphere dysfunction
bilateral laryngeal paralysis
bilateral migraine headache
bilateral muscle loss
bilateral myoclonic seizure
bilateral scotoma
bilingual
Bilingual Syntax Measure (BSM)
Bilingual Syntax Measure II Test
bilingualism
 active
 passive
"Bill Blass" (street name, crack)
"billie hoke" (street name,
 cocaine)
bimodal aural rehabilitation
bimodal method of aural
 rehabilitation
"Bin Laden" (street name, heroin)
binary principle
binaural CROS (contralateral
 routing of signals)
binaural fusion
binaural hearing aid
binaural integration
binaural resynthesis
binaural separation
binaural summation
binders, breast
"bindle" (re: drug quantity)
Bing Test
"bing" (re: drug quantity for one
 injection)
binge, cocaine
binge-eating behavior
binge-eating disorder (BED)
 (F50.8)
binge-eating disorder in full
 remission (F50.8)
binge-eating disorder in partial
 remission (F50.8)
binge-eating disorder of limited
 duration (F50.8)

binge-eating disorder of low
   frequency (F50.8)
binge-eating pattern
binge-eating/purging behavior
bingeing or binging
"bingers" (re: crack addicts)
"bingo" (re: to inject a drug)
"bings" (street name, crack
   cocaine)
bioacoustics
biooccipital headache
biochemical anatomy
biofeedback feedback
Biographical Inventory Form U
biographical memory, loss of
biolinguistic language theory
biolinguistic theory
biologic age
biologic sign depression
biological act
biological basis
biological causation
biological children
biological dysfunction
   manifestation of
   symptoms of
biological factors
biological orientation
biological parents
biological processes
biological relatives, first-degree
biological research orientation
biological roots of addiction
biological sex
biology-based female traits,
   normal
      emotional sensitivity
      empathetic
      nurturing
biology-based male traits, normal
      aggressiveness
      assertiveness
      competitiveness
      protective vigilance
      stoicism
biology of affective disease
biology of Alzheimer's disease
biology of deceit

biology of major mental disorders
biology of schizophrenia
biopsy, brain
biopsychosocial aspects of
   bereavement
biopsychosocial model
BIP (Background Interference
   Procedure)
biphasic
biphasic potential
"biphetamine" (street name,
   amphetamine; MDMA)
bipolar and related disorder
   other specified (F31.89)
bipolar and related disorder
   substance/medication-
   induced
   unspecified (F31.9)
bipolar and related disorder due to
   another medical condition with
   manic features (F06.33)
bipolar and related disorder due to
   another medical condition with
   manic- or hypomanic-like
   episodes (F06.33)
bipolar and related disorder due to
   another medical condition with
   mixed features (F06.34)
bipolar and related disorder with
   manic or hypomanic-like
   features (F06.33)
bipolar and related disorder with
   mixed features (F06.34)
bipolar I disorder, hypomanic
   episode
      current in full remission
         (F31.74)
      current unspecified (F31.9)
      current in partial remission
         (F31.73)
bipolar I disorder, major
   depressive episode
      current in full remission
         (F31.76)
      current in partial remission
         (F31.75)
      current mild (F31.31)
      current moderate (F31.32)

bipolar I disorder, major
  depressive episode
    current severe (F31.4)
    current unspecified (F31.9)
    current with psychotic
      features (F31.5)
bipolar I disorder, manic episode
    current mild (F31.11)
    current moderate (F31.12)
    current severe (F31.13)
    current with psychotic
      features (F31.2)
    current in full remission
      (F31.74)
    current in partial remission
      (F31.73)
bipolar I disorder, manic episode
    current, unspecified (F31.9)
bipolar I disorder, unspecified
  (F31.9)
Bipolar Psychological Inventory
bipolar II disorder
bipolar II disorder with anxious
  distress (F31.81)
bipolar II disorder with atypical
  features (F31.81)
bipolar II disorder with catatonia
  (F31.81) and (F06.1)
bipolar II disorder with
  melancholic features (F31.81)
bipolar II disorder with mixed
  features (F31.81)
bipolar II disorder with mood-
  congruent (F31.81)
bipolar II disorder with mood-
  incongruent psychotic features
  (F31.81)
bipolar II disorder with
  peripartum onset (F31.81)
bipolar II disorder with psychotic
  features (F31.81)
bipolar II disorder with rapid
  cycling (F31.81)
bipolar II disorder with seasonal
  pattern (F31.81)
"bipping" (re: snorting heroin
  and/or cocaine)
"birdhead" (street name, LSD)

"birdie powder" (street name,
  cocaine; heroin)
birth cry
birth order
Birth to Three Assessment and
  Intervention System
Birth to Three Developmental
  Scale
"biscuit" (re: 50 rocks of crack)
bisensory method
bisexual orientation
bisyllable
BIT (Behavioral Inattention Test)
bite, closed
bite marks
"bite one's lips" (re: to smoke
  marijuana)
bitemporal hemianopsia
biting, nail
biundulant viral encephalitis
"biz" (re: bag/portion of drugs)
bizarre fantasies
bizarre posture
bizarre thought processes
"BJs" (street name, crack cocaine)
"B.J.'s " (street name, crack
  cocaine)
"black" (street name,
  cannabis/marijuana; opium;
  methamphetamine)
"black acid" (street name, LSD;
  LSD & PCP)
"black and white" (street name,
  amphetamine)
"black bart" (street name,
  cannabis/marijuana)
"black beauties" (street name,
  barbiturate; amphetamine)
"black beauty" (street name,
  methamphetamine)
"black birds" (street name,
  amphetamine)
"black bombers" (street name,
  amphetamine)
"black cadillacs" (street name,
  amphetamine)
"black dust" (street name, PCP)

"black eagle" (street name, heroin)
Black English (Ebonics)
"black ganga" (re: cannabis/marijuana resin)
"black gold" (street name, high potency cannabis/marijuana)
"black gungi" (street name, cannabis/marijuana from India)
"black gunion" (street name, cannabis/marijuana)
"black hash" (street name, hashish and opium)
"black hole" (re: feeling a depressant high on ketamine)
"black mo" (street name, high potency cannabis/marijuana)
"black moat" (street name, high potency cannabis/marijuana)
"black mollies" (street name, amphetamine)
"black mote" (street name, cannabis/marijuana and honey)
"black pearl" (street name, heroin)
"black pill" (street name, opium pill)
"black rock" (street name, crack)
"Black Russian" (street name, cannabis/marijuana and opium)
"black star" (street name, LSD)
"black stuff" (street name, heroin)
"black sunshine" (street name, LSD)
"black tabs" (street name, LSD)
"black tar" (street name, heroin)
"black whack" (street name, phencyclidine)
"blacks" (street name, amphetamine)
Blacky Pictures, The
bladder control, loss of
"blade" (street name, crystal methamphetamine)
blade of the tongue
blade of tongue
BLADES (Bristol Language Development Scales)

"blah" feeling
"blahs", the
blame, tendency to externalize
blameworthy
"blanca" (street name, heroin)
"blanco" (street name, heroin plus cocaine)
bland affect
"blank" (re: non-narcotic powder sold as heroin)
blank
 Correctional Officers' Interest
 mind going
 Personnel Reaction
 Rothwell-Miller Interest
 Rotter Incomplete Sentences (RISB)
"blanket" (re: cannabis/marijuana cigarette)
"blanks" (re: low quality drugs)
blasphemous thoughts
"blast" (re: to smoke marijuana or crack cocaine)
"blast a joint" (re: cannabis/marijuana use)
"blast a roach" (re: cannabis/marijuana use)
"blast a stick" (re: cannabis/marijuana use)
"blasted" (re: drug influence)
"blaxing" (re: smoking marijuana)
"blazing" (re: smoking marijuana)
bleeding, self-inflicted rectal
bleeding blast, excessive menstrual
blend, consonant
blended family
blending
 auditory
 sound
blends
Blessed Behavior Scale
Blessed Dementia Rating Scale (BDRS)
Blessed Information-Memory-Concentration Test

BLHI (Brief Life History Inventory)
blind headache
Blind Learning Aptitude Test
blind spot, figurative (scotoma)
blindfolding (sensory bondage)
blindness
    hysterical
    object
"bling bling" (street name, methamphetamine)
blinking, eye
Blissymbolics (ideographs; pictographs)
"blizzard" (re: cocaine smoke)
bloating
"block" (street name, cannabis/marijuana)
block
    atrioventricular
    clonic (in stuttering)
    left bundle branch
    tonic (in stuttering)
"block busters" (street name, barbiturate)
Block Construction Test
block design tests *(see also* tests)
Block Substitution Test
Block Survey and S.L.I.D.E.
blockade, thought
blocking
    audible speech
    emotional
    silent speech
blocking in speech
    audible
    silent
Blom-Singer tracheoesophageal prosthesis
"blonde" (street name, cannabis/marijuana)
blood alcohol level
blood-brain barrier
blood drug screen
blood flow, cerebral (CBF)
blood-injection-injury type
blood level of anti-convulsant drugs test

blood level of illicit drugs test
blood pressure, penile
blood screen for drugs test
Bloods and Crips (street gangs)
Bloom Analogies Test
"blotter" (street name, LSD; crack cocaine)
"blotter acid" (street name, LSD; crack cocaine)
"blotter cube" (street name, LSD; crack cocaine)
"Blou Bulle" (street name, methaqualone)
"blow" (re: inhale cocaine/inject heroin/smoke marijuana)
"blow" (street name, cannabis; cocaine)
"blow a fix" (re: drug injection mishap)
"blow a shot" (re: drug injection mishap)
"blow a stick" (re: to smoke cannabis/marijuana)
"blow blue" (re: to inhale cocaine)
"blow coke" (re: to inhale cocaine)
"blow smoke" (re: to inhale cocaine)
"blow the vein" (re: drug injection)
"blow up" (re: crack cut with lidocaine)
"blow your mind" (re: to get high on hallucinogens)
"blowcaine" (re: crack diluted with cocaine)
blowing, maximum duration of sustained
"blowing one's roof" (re: to smoke marijuana)
"blowing smoke" (street name, marijuana)
"blowout" (street name, crack)
"blows" (street name, heroin)
BLT-2 (Bankson Language Test-2)

"blue" (street name, barbiturate; crack)
"blue acid" (street name, LSD)
"blue barrels" (street name, LSD)
"blue birds" (street name, barbiturate/depressant)
"blue boy" (street name, amphetamine)
"blue bullets" (street name, barbiturate)
"blue caps" (street name, mescaline)
"blue chairs" (street name, LSD)
"blue cheers" (street name, LSD)
"blue clouds" (street name, Amytal)
"blue de hue" (street name, cannabis/marijuana)
"blue devil" (street name, barbiturate/depressants)
"blue devils" (street name, methamphetamine)
"blue dolls" (street name, barbiturate/depressants)
"blue heaven" (street name, LSD)
"blue heavens" (street name, barbiturate/depressants)
"blue kisses" (street name, MDMA)
"blue lips" (street name, MDMA)
"blue madman" (street name, phencyclidine)
"blue meth" (street name, methamphetamine)
"blue microdot" (street name, LSD)
"blue mist" (street name, LSD)
"blue mollies" (street name, amphetamine)
"blue moons" (street name, LSD)
"blue nile" (street name, MDMA)
"blue nile vitality" (re: GBL-containing product)
"blue sage" (street name, cannabis/marijuana)
"blue sky blond" (street name, high potency marijuana)
"blue star" (street name, heroin)
"blue tips" (street name, barbiturate/depressants)
"blue vials" (street name, LSD)
blueness
"blunt" (re: cannabis/marijuana inside a cigar)
blunted
"blunts" (re: street drugs)
blurred vision
blurring, visual
blurring of vision
blushing
BMI (body mass index)
"bo" (street name, cannabis/marijuana)
BOA (Behavioral observation audiometry)
board
    conversation
    direct selection communication
    encoding communication
    scanning communication
"boat" (re: 1000 tabs of MDMA)
"boat" (street name, phencyclidine)
Bobath method
"bo-bo" (street name, cannabis/marijuana)
"bobo" (street name, crack cocaine)
"bobo bush" (street name, cannabis/marijuana)
Boder Test of Reading-Spelling Patterns
bodily disease
bodily illusion
bodily injury, self-inflicted
bodily orifices, nonfunctional and repetitive picking at
bodily signs and symptoms
body (pl. bodies)
    cell
    disease, Lewy
    hitting one's own
    intraneuronal argentophilic Pick inclusion
    loss of control of the

body (pl. bodies)
    material aspects of the
    spiritual aspects of the
body appearance
body baffle effect (hearing aid)
body balances, core
body build
body control, loss of
body dipping
body dissatisfaction
body dysmorphic defect
body dysmorphic disorder
    (F45.22)
body dysmorphic disorder with
    muscle dysmorphia (F42.22)
body dysmorphic-like disorder
    with acute flaws (F42)
body dysmorphic-like disorder
    without repetitive behavior
    (F42)
body dystonia
body fat
body-focused repetitive behavior
    disorder (F42)
body fluids
body functioning
body gestures
body hearing aid
body image
    changed
    distorted
body image distortion
body-image perception
body mass index (BMI)
body mechanics
body memory
body movements
    complex whole
    stereotyped
body of the tongue
body orifices
"body packer" (re: ingestion of
    wrapped cocaine-or-crack)
body parts
    focus on
    "ugly"
body position
body posture

body shape
body size
"body stuffer" (re: crack vials
    ingested for concealment)
body swaying
body temperature
body temperature, core
body temperature measurement,
    core
body tics
body water
body weight
Boehm Test of Basic Concepts
Boehm Test of Basic Concepts-
    Preschool
"Bogart a joint" (re: cannabis use;
    refuse to share)
bogyphobia
"bohd" (street name,
    cannabis/marijuana;
    phencyclidine)
boilermaker's deafness
"bolasterone" (re: injectable
    steroid)
"Bolivian marching powder"
    (street name, cocaine)
"bolo" (re: price of a piece of
    crack)
"bomb" (street name, crack; high
    value heroin; marijuana
    cigarette)
"bomb squad" (re: sellers of
    crack)
"bomber" (street name, marijuana
    cigarette)
"bombido" (street name, heroin;
    injectable amphetamine;
    depressant)
"bombita" (street name, heroin +
    amphetamine; depressants)
"bombs away" (street name,
    heroin)
bond conduction, distortional
bondage
    physical (restraint)
    sensory (blindfolding)
bonding, human-pet

"bone" (street name, cannabis/marijuana; high power crack or heroin)
bone(s)
    alveolar supporting
    deformed
    ethmoid
    fractured
    frontal
    hyoid
    inferior maxillary
    interior turbinated
    lacrimal
    malar
    medial turbinate
    palatine
    sphenoid
    temporal
    zygomatic
bone conduction (BC)
    compression
    inertial
    pure tone
bone-conduction hearing aid
bone-conduction oscillator
bone-conduction receiver
bone-conduction threshold, pure tone
bone-conduction vibrator
bone marrow suppression
bone nasal cavity, nasal
"bonecrusher" (street name, crack)
bonelet
"bones" (street name, crack cocaine)
"bong" (re: cannabis equipment)
"bonita" (street name, heroin)
bony labyrinth
"boo" (street name, cannabis; methamphetamine)
"boo boo bama" (street name, cannabis/marijuana)
"book" (re: 100 unit dosage of LSD)
Booklet Category Test
"boom" (street name, cannabis; marijuana)
"boomers" (street name, psilocybin/psilocin; LSD)
"boost" (re: drug injection; to steal)
"boost" (street name, crack cocaine)
"boost and shoot" (re: to steal to support a habit)
"booster" (re: to inhale cocaine)
"boot" (re: drug injection)
"boot the gong" (re: cannabis/marijuana use)
"booted" (re: drug influence)
"bopper" (street name, crack cocaine)
"boppers" (street name, amyl nitrite)
border, vermillion
border of mandible, alveolar
borderline concept, psychoanalysis and the
borderline intellectual functioning (R41.83)
borderline personality disorder (F60.3)
bore hole
boredom, tendency toward
borrowing, linguistic
Boston Assessment of Severe Aphasia (BASA)
Boston Classification System
Boston Diagnostic Aphasia Examination (BDAE)
Boston Naming Test
Boston University Speech Sound Discrimination Test
Botel Reading Inventory
"botray" (street name, crack)
"bottles" (re: crack vials; amphetamine)
"boubou" (street name, crack)
"boulder" (re: price for a quantity of crack)
"boulder" (street name, crack)
"boulya" (street name, crack)
bounce technique (stuttering)
"bouncing powder" (street name, cocaine)

Psychiatric Words and Phrases

bound
  situationally
  upper
bound (cued) panic attacks,
  situationally
bound morpheme
bound panic attack, situationally
boundaries and gender
boundaries in postanalytic
  supervision
boundaries in psychoanalysis
boundary (pl. boundaries)
  analytic
  ego
  lack of
  language
  little sense of other
    people's
  loss of ego
  posttermination
  role
  subsystem
boundary violations
  nonsexual
  sexual
boundary violations in
  psychoanalysis
bowed vocal folds
bowel control, loss of
Bowen-Chalfant Receptive
  Language
"box labs" (re: small lab
  producing methamphetamine)
"boxcar ventricles" (re: MRI
  finding for Huntington's
  Disease)
"boxed" (re: to be in jail)
"boy" (street name, cocaine;
  heroin)
"boy-girl" (re: heroin mixed with
  cocaine)
"bozo" (street name, heroin)
BPI (Basic Personality Inventory)
BPS (British Psychological
  Society)
Bracken Basic Concept Scale
brackets, square
bradykinesthetic

braggadocio
brain
  architecture of
  concussion of (grades 1-3)
  hemangioma of the
  mapping of language areas of
brain abnormalities
brain abnormalities, structural
brain aneurysm
brain atrophy
brain atrophy, frontotemporal
brain autopsy
brain biopsy
brain cell damage
brain concussion
brain contusion
brain convulsion
brain damage
"brain damage" (street name,
  heroin)
brain death
brain death syndrome
brain degeneration
brain depressant
brain disease
brain disorders, in vivo magnetic
  resonance spectroscopy in
brain dysfunction
  diffuse
  mid
  severe diffuse
brain electrical activity map
  (BEAM)
brain fag
brain function
  integrity of
  semi-autonomous systems
    concept of
brain imaging, functional
brain imaging studies
brain imaging technologies
brain improvement training *(see
  also* tests)
brain injury
  dementia due to traumatic
  traumatic (TBI)
brain injury inventory *(see also*
  tests)

brain involvement, subcortical
brain lesion
brain map
brain neoplasm
    benign
    malignant
brain pathology
"brain pills" (street name, amphetamine)
brain regions
brain spectin
brain structures, abnormal
brain syndrome, acute organic
brain syndrome with psychosis, organic
brain test
    EP (evoked potential)
    ER (evoked response)
    MEP (multimodality evoked potential)
    SEP (somatosensory evoked potential)
    SER (somatosensory evoked response)
    VEP (visual evoked potential)
"brain ticklers" (street name, amphetamine)
brain tiredness
brain trauma
brain tumor
brain tumor, dementia due to
brain washing
brain wave activity
brainstem
brainstem auditory evoked potential (BAEP)
brainstem auditory evoked response (BAER)
brainstem compression
brainstem control
brainstem disease
brainstem displacement
brainstem dysfunction
brainstem evoked potential
brainstem evoked response audiometry (BSER)
brainstem function
brainstem lesion
brainstem reflex
brainstem response, auditory (ABR)
brainstem reticular formation
brainstem signs
brainstem stroke
brainstem symptom
brainstem syndrome
brainstem tumor
brake, descending pitch
branching steps in therapy
branching tree diagram
"bread" (street name, heroin)
break
    ascending pitch
    phonation
    pitch
"break night" (re: pulling a cocaine all-nighter)
break state
"breakdown" (re: break up a crack rock piece for sale)
breakdown theory
breakdown theory of stuttering
breakthrough tearfulness
breast binders
breast rashes
breasts, distorted
breath chewing
breath stream
breathiness
breathing
    apneustic
    crescendo-decrescendo
    daytime mouth
    donkey
    opposition
breathing disorder
breathing method
breathing method of esophageal speech
breathing pauses during sleep
breathing-related sleep disorders
breathing-related sleep disturbances
Brenner Developmental Gestalt Test of School Readiness

"brewery" (re: a drug-making place)
BRI (Basic Reading Inventory
"brick" (street name, crack; 1 kilogram of cannabis/marijuana)
"brick gum" (street name, heroin)
"bridge up" (re: drug injection)
Brief Cognitive Rating Scale (BCRS)
brief depressive disorder, recurrent
Brief Drinker Profile
brief illness anxiety disorder
brief intelligence test *(see also* tests)
Brief Life History Inventory (BLHI)
brief psychotic disorder (F23)
brief psychotic disorder with abnormal psychomotor behavior (F23)
brief psychotic disorder with catatonia (F23) and (F06.1)
brief psychotic disorder with delusions (F23)
brief psychotic disorder with depression (F23)
brief psychotic disorder with disorganized speech (F23)
brief psychotic disorder with hallucinations (F23)
brief psychotic disorder with impaired cognition (F23)
brief psychotic disorder with manic symptoms (F23)
brief psychotic disorder with marked stressor(s) (F23)
brief psychotic disorder with negative symptoms (F23)
brief psychotic disorder with no marked stressor(s) (F23)
brief psychotic disorder with postpartum onset (F23)
brief reactive psychosis
brief somatic symptom disorder
Brief Symptom Inventory
brief tone audiometry (BTA)

BRIGANCE® Diagnostic Assessment of Basic Skills
BRIGANCE® Diagnostic Comprehensive Inventory of Basic Skills
BRIGANCE® Diagnostic Inventory of Basic Skills
BRIGANCE® Diagnostic Inventory of Early Development
BRIGANCE® Diagnostic Inventory of Essential Skills
BRIGANCE® Diagnostic Life Skills Inventory
BRIGANCE® K & 1 Screen for Kindergarten and First Grade Children
"bring up" (re: drug injection)
Brissaud-Marie syndrome
Brissaud syndrome
Bristol Achievement Test
Bristol Language Development Scales (BLADES)
Bristol Social Adjustment Guides
British Ability Scales: Spelling Scale (BAS)
British Association for Counselling and Psychotherapy (BCAP)
British Psychological Society (BPS)
"britton" (street name, mescaline; peyote)
broad phonemic transcription
broad transcription
Broca's aphasia
Broca's area (Brodmann's area 44)
"broccoli" (street name, cannabis/marijuana)
Brodmann's area 44 (Broca's area)
"broja" (street name, heroin)
broken words
"broker" (re: a go-between in a drug deal)
bromine compound
bromism (due to bromide intoxication)

"bromo" (street name, Nexus)
bronchial respiration
bronchus (pl. bronchi)
brooding about the past
brought into action
"brown" (street name, heroin; cannabis/marijuana; methamphetamine)
"brown bombers" (street name, LSD)
"brown crystal" (street name, heroin)
"brown dots" (street name, LSD)
"brown rhine" (street name, heroin)
"brown sugar" (street name, heroin)
"brown tape" (street name, heroin)
brownian motion
brownian movement
"brownies" (street name, amphetamine)
"browns" (street name, amphetamine)
Bruhn method
Bruininks-Oseretsky Standardized Test
Bruininks-Oseretsky Test of Motor Proficiency
bruises
Bruns ataxia
bruxomania (grinding of teeth)
Bryngelson-Glaspey Test of Articulation
BSER (Brain-stem evoked response audiometry)
BTA (brief tone audiometry)
"bubble gum" (street name, cocaine; crack; cannabis/marijuana)
buccal cavity
buccal speech
buccal whisper
buccofacial apraxia
buccolabial
buccoversion
buccoversion of teeth

"buck" (re: to shoot someone in the head)
"bud" (street name, cannabis/marijuana)
"buda" (street name, crack-laced cannabis cigarette)
"Buddha" (street name, opium-laced high-grade cannabis)
"buffer" (re: a crack prostitute or user)
"bugged" (re: drug user with sores from injections)
"bugged" (re: to be annoyed)
build, body
building restrictions
bulbar paralysis
bulimia nervosa (F50.2)
    in full remission (F50.2)
    in partial remission (F50.2)
bulimia nervosa of limited duration (F50.8)
bulimia nervosa of low frequency (F50.8)
"bull" (re: a narcotics agent or police officer)
"bull dog" (street name, heroin)
"bullet" (street name, inhalant; isobutyl nitrite)
"bullet bolt" (street name, inhalant)
"bullia capital" (street name, crack; fake crack)
"bullion" (street name, crack)
"bullyon" (street name, cannabis/marijuana)
"bumblebees" (street name, amphetamine)
"bummer trip" (re: a bad PCP experience)
"bump" (re: drug intoxication; fake crack; the price for ketamine)
"bump up" (re: bolstering MDMA with cocaine or crack)
"bumper" (street name, crack cocaine)
"bumping up" (re: combining MDMA with powder cocaine)

Psychiatric Words and Phrases

Bunavail (buprenorphine/naloxone)
"bundle" (street name, heroin)
"bunk" (re: fake cocaine; crack cocaine)
buprenorphine *(see also* medications)
buprenorphine/naloxone
bupropion/naloxone
Burks' Behavior Rating Scale
"burn one" (re: cannabis/marijuana use)
"burn the main line" (re: drug injection)
"burned" (re: to purchase fake drugs)
"burned out" (re: drug use/injection)
"Burnese" (street name, cocaine)
"burnie" (street name, cannabis/marijuana)
burning pain
burnout, professional
"burnout" (re: a drug user)
burnout inventory *(see also* tests)
Burnout Scale for Health Professionals and Staff
Burns Depression/Anxiety Checklists
Burns/Roe Informal Reading Inventory
Buros Center for Testing
"bush" (street name, cocaine; cannabis; PCP)
"bushman tea" (street name, khat)
Business and Industry Attitude Survey
Business, Industry, and Government PSI Basic Skills Test
"businessman's LSD" (street name, dimethyltryptamine)
"businessman's special" (street name, dimethyltryptamine)
"businessman's trip" (street name, dimethyltryptamine)
"busted" (re: to be arrested)

"busters" (street name, barbiturate)
"busy bee" (street name, phencyclidine)
"butler" (street name, cannabis/marijuana; crack)
"butt naked" (street name, phencyclidine)
"butter" (street name, cannabis/marijuana; crack)
"butter flower" (street name, cannabis/marijuana)
button, stoma
"buttons" (street name, mescaline)
"butu" (street name, heroin)
butyl nitrate inhalant
butyrophenone-based neuroleptics
butyrophenone-based tranquilizer
"buzz" (re: drug influence)
"buzz bomb" (street name, nitrous oxide)
buzzing sensation
Bzoch-League Receptive-Expressive Emergent Language Scale

"C" (street name, cocaine)
"C, the" (street name, methcathinone)
"C & M" (street name, cocaine and morphine)
"C.J." (street name, PCP)
"C joint" (re: cocaine-buying place)
"C.S." (street name, cannabis/marijuana)
CAAS (Children's Attention and Adjustment Survey)
"cabello" (street name, cocaine; heroin)
"caca" (street name, heroin)
cacodemonomania (possession by evil spirits)
"cactus" (street name, mescaline)
"cactus buttons" (street name, mescaline)
"cactus head" (street name, mescaline)
"cad/Cadillac" (re:1 ounce)
CADeT (Communication Abilities Diagnostic Test)
"Cadillac express" (street name, methamphetamine)
"Cadillac" (street name, PCP)
cafard
caffeine
    dietary
    powdered
caffeine abuse
caffeine intoxication (F15.929)
caffeine-induced anxiety disorder without use disorder (F15.980)
caffeine-induced disorders, other
caffeine-induced excitement
caffeine-induced postural tremor
caffeine-induced sleep disorder (no use disorder (F15.982)
caffeine-induced sleep disorder, insomnia type
caffeine-related disorder, unspecified (F15.99)
caffeine supplements
caffeine toxicity
caffeine use disorder with mild caffeine-induced anxiety disorder (F15.180)
caffeine use disorder with m/s caffeine-induced anxiety disorder (F15.280)
caffeine use disorder with mild caffeine-induced sleep disorder (F15.182)
caffeine use disorder with m/s caffeine-induced sleep disorder (F15.282)
caffeine withdrawal disorder (F15.93)
CAGE alcohol use questionnaire
CAID (Convention of American Instructors of the Deaf)
CAIN (Computer Anxiety Index)
"caine" (street name, cocaine; crack)
Cain-Levine Social Competency Scale
cainophobia
cainotophobia
"cakes" (re: round discs of crack)
calcification, basal ganglia
calculation skills
calculations test
calibrate
calibrated loop
California Achievement Tests (CAT/5)
California Child Q-Set
California Consonant Test
California cornflakes"(cocaine)
California Critical Thinking Dispositions Inventory (CCTDI)

Psychiatric Words and Phrases

California Critical Thinking Skills Test (CCTST)
California Life Goals Evaluation Schedules
California Marriage Readiness Evaluation (CMRE)
California Motor Accuracy Test, Southern
California Phonics Survey
California Q-Sort
"California sunshine" (street name, LSD)
California Verbal Learning Test
California viral encephalitis
Callier-Azusa Scale
calling, word
callomania (beauty)
callosal apraxia
callosal area (parolfactory nerve)
callosal commissurotomy
callosal disconnection syndrome
callosal disconnection syndrome aphasia
callosal gyrus
callosal lesion
callosal sulcus
callosum, corpus
Caloric Stimulation Test for Vestibular Function
Caloric Test
CALS (Checklist of Adaptive Living Skills)
"cam red" (street name, cannabis/marijuana)
"cam trip" (street name, high potency cannabis/marijuana)
"Cambodian red" (street name, cannabis/marijuana)
Cambridge battery
"came" (street name, cocaine)
CAML (Coarticulation Assessment in Meaningful Language)
camouflage the defect
camp counselor
Campbell Leadership Index (CLI)
Campbell Organizational Survey (COS)

"can" (re: 1 oz. of cannabis/marijuana)
Canadian Association of Speech-Language Pathologists and Audiologists (see Speech-Language & Audiology Canada)
"Canadian black" (street name, cannabis/marijuana)
Canadian Cognitive Abilities Test (CCAT)
Canadian Comprehensive Assessment Program: Achievement Series
Canadian Comprehensive Assessment Program: Developing Cognitive
Canadian Comprehensive Assessment Program: School Attitude Measure
Canadian Neurological Scale
canal
   alveolar
   alveolodental
   anterior vertical
   auditory
   cochlear
   craniopharyngeal
   ear
   Guyon
   horizontal
   internal auditory
   intramedullary
   lateral
   medullary
   posterior vertical
   semicircular
   vestibular
canal caps
canal caps hearing protection device
canal hearing aid
"canamo" (street name, cannabis/marijuana)
"canappa" (street name, cannabis/marijuana)
cancellation test, letter

"cancelled stick" (street name, cannabis/marijuana cigarette)
cancer and concurrent psychiatric problems
Cancer, Imagery of
Candidate Profile Record, The
candor, radical
"candy" (street name, crack cocaine; depressant; amphetamine)
"candy C" (street name, cocaine)
"candy flipping" (re: mixing LSD and MDMA)
"candy flipping on a string" (re: sequencing LSD, MDMA, and cocaine on a string)
"candy rave" (street name, club drug)
"candy ravers" (re: rave attendees wearing candy necklaces)
Canfield Instructional Styles Inventory
canine teeth
cannabichromene (CBC)
cannabidiol (CBD)
cannabidiolic acid (CBDA)
cannabidivarin (CBDV)
cannabigerol (CBG)
cannabigerolic acid (CBGA)
cannabinoid(s)
    acidic
    cross-reacting (CRC)
    non-acidic
cannabinoid hyperemesis syndrome (CHS)
"cannabinol" (street name, CBN)
cannabis (marijuana) (street names)
    3750
    420
    51
    A-bomb
    Acapulco gold
    Acapulco red
    AC/DC (liquid)
    ace
    Afgani indica
    African

cannabis (street names)
    African black
    African bush
    African woodbine
    airhead
    airplane
    Alice B. Toklas
    amp
    amp joint
    Angola
    Are you anywhere?
    ashes
    assassin of youth
    astroturf
    atom bomb
    atshitshi
    Aunt Mary
    B
    B-40
    baby
    baby bhang
    babysitter
    bad seed
    bag
    bale
    Bambalacha
    bammies
    bammy
    banano
    bar
    bash
    basuco (Spanish)
    bazooka
    BC bud
    beedies
    Belyando spruce
    bhang
    bite one's lips
    black
    black bart
    black ganga
    black gold
    black gungi
    black gunion
    black mo
    black moat
    black mote
    blanket

cannabis (street names)
- blast
- blast a joint
- blast a roach
- blast a stick
- blaxing
- blazing
- block
- blonde
- blow
- blowing smoke
- blue de hue
- blue sage
- blue sky blond
- blunt
- BO
- bo-bo
- bobo bush
- Bogart a joint
- bohd
- bomb
- bomber
- bone
- bong
- boo
- boo boo bama
- boom
- boot the gong
- brick
- broccoli
- brown
- bubble gum
- bud
- buda
- Buddha
- bullyon
- burn one
- burnie
- bush
- butter
- butter flower
- C.S.
- Cam red
- Cam trip
- Cambodian red
- can
- Canada
- Canadian black

cannabis (street names)
- canamo
- canappa
- cancelled stick
- candy blunt
- candy stick
- cannabis tea
- cartucho (Spanish)
- catnip
- caviar
- Cavite all star
- cest
- champagne
- charas
- Charge/Charge+
- Charlotte's Web (liquid)
- chase
- cheeba
- cheeo
- chemo
- chiba chiba
- Chicago black
- Chicago green
- chiefing
- chillum
- chips
- chira
- chocolate
- chocolate Thai
- Christmas bud
- Christmas tree
- chronic
- chunky
- churus
- Cid
- citrol
- clam bake
- clicker
- clickums
- cochornis
- cocoa puff
- colas
- coli
- coliflor tostao
- Colombian
- Colorado cocktail
- Columbus black
- cosa (Spanish)

cannabis (street names)
- crack back
- crazy weed
- cripple
- crying week
- cryppie
- cryptonic
- cubes
- culican
- dagga
- dank
- dawamesk
- dew
- Diablo (Spanish)
- diambista
- dimba
- ding
- dinkie dow
- dipped joints
- dips
- dirt grass
- dirties
- dirty joints
- ditch dirty joints
- ditch weed
- djamba
- dody
- don jem
- Don Juan (Spanish)
- Dona Juana (Spanish)
- Dona Juanita (Spanish)
- donk
- doob
- doobee
- doobie/dubbe/duby
- dope
- dope smoke
- doradilla
- draf
- draf weed
- drag weed
- dry high
- dube
- duby
- Durog
- Duros (Spanish)
- dust
- dust blunt

cannabis (street names)
- dusting
- earth
- El Diablito (Spanish)
- El Diablo (Spanish)
- El Gallo ("Rooster")
- elephant
- endo
- Esra
- Fallbrook red hair
- fatty
- feed bag
- feeling
- fiend
- fine stuff
- finger
- fir
- firewood
- flower
- flower tops
- Fly Mexican Airlines
- fraho/frajo
- frios (Spanish)
- fry
- fry daddy
- fry sticks
- fu
- fuel
- fuma D'Angola (Portuguese)
- gage/gauge
- gange
- gangster
- ganja
- ganoobies
- garbage
- gash
- Gasper
- Gasper stick
- gauge butt
- geek
- geek-joints
- get a gage up
- Ghana
- giggle smoke
- giggle weed
- gimmie
- gold

cannabis (street names)
   gold star
   golden
   golden leaf
   gong
   gonj
   good butt
   good giggles
   good stuff
   goody-goody
   goof butt
   gorge
   grass
   grass brownies
   grass hopper
   grata
   Greek
   green
   green buds
   green goddess
   greens
   greeter
   gremmies
   Greta
   griefo
   griefs
   grifa (Spanish)
   griff
   griffa
   griffo
   grows
   G-shot
   gunga
   gungeon
   gungun
   gunja
   gyve
   haircut
   hanhich
   happy cigarette
   Harlequin (liquid)
   Hawaiian
   Hawaiian black
   Hawaiian homegrown hay
   hay
   hay butt
   hemp
   herb

cannabis (street names)
   Herb and Al
   herba
   hit
   hit the hay
   hocus
   homegrown hay
   honey blunts
   hooch
   hooter
   hot stick
   hydro
   hydrogrows
   illies
   illing
   illy
   Indian boy
   Indian hay
   Indian hemp
   Indica
   Indo
   Indonesian bud
   instaga
   instagu
   J
   Jamaican gold
   Jamaican red hair
   Jane
   jay
   jay smoke
   Jim Jones
   jive
   jive stick
   joint
   jolly green
   joy smoke
   joy stick
   Juan Valdez (Spanish)
   Juanita (Spanish)
   juice joint
   juja
   ju-ju
   jumbos
   K2/Spice
   kabak
   kaff
   kalakit
   Kali

cannabis (street names)
    Kansas grass
    Kate bush
    Kawaii electric
    Kay
    kaya
    KB
    kee
    Kentucky blue
    KGB (killer green bud)
    khayl
    Ki
    kick stick
    kief
    kiff
    killer
    killer weed
    kilter
    kind
    kind bud
    king bud
    Kona gold
    krippy
    Kryptonite
    Kumba
    kush
    L.L.
    lace
    lakbay diva
    laughing grass
    laughing weed
    leaf
    leak
    Leno (Spanish)
    LG (lime green)
    lid
    light stuff
    Lima
    liprimo
    little smoke
    llesca
    loaf
    lobo
    loco (Spanish)
    locoweed
    log
    loose shank
    love boat

cannabis (street names)
    love leaf
    love weed
    loveboat
    lovelies
    lubage
    M
    M.J.
    M.O.
    M.U.
    macaroni
    macaroni and cheese
    machinery
    Macon
    Maconha
    mafu (Spanish)
    magic smoke
    Manhattan silver
    Mari
    marijuana
    marimba (Spanish)
    Mary
    Mary and Johnny
    Mary Ann
    Mary Jane
    Mary Jonas
    Mary Warner
    Mary Weaver
    matchbox
    Maui wauie
    Maui-wowie
    Meg
    Megg
    Meggie
    messorole
    Mexican brown
    Mexican green
    Mexican locoweed
    Mexican red
    mighty mezz
    Mo
    modams
    mohasky
    mohasty
    monte
    mooca/moocah
    mooster
    moota/mutah

cannabis (street names)
- mooters
- mootie
- mootos
- mor a grifa
- mota/moto (Spanish)
- mother
- mow the grass
- Mu
- muggie
- muggle/muggles
- muta
- mutha
- nail
- Nigra
- Northern lights
- number
- O.J.
- oolies
- Ozone
- P.R. (Panama Red)
- pack
- pack a bowl
- pack of rocks
- pakaloco
- Pakistani black
- Panama cut
- Panama gold
- Panama red
- panatella
- paper blunts
- parsley
- pasto (Spanish)
- Pat
- P-dogs
- Philly blunts
- pin
- pipe
- pocket rocket
- pod
- poke
- pot
- potlikker
- potten bush
- premos
- prescription
- pretendica
- pretendo

cannabis (street names)
- primo
- primo square
- primo turbo
- Puff the dragon
- purple haze
- Queen Ann's lace
- ragweed
- railroad
- rainy day woman
- Rangood
- rasta weed
- red but
- red cross
- red dirt
- reefer
- righteous bush
- righteous weed
- rip
- roach
- roacha
- roasting
- rockets
- rompums
- root
- rope
- Rose Marie
- rough stuff
- ruderalis
- salt and pepper
- sandwich bag
- Santa Marta (Spanish)
- sasfras
- sativa
- schwagg
- scissors
- scrub
- seeds
- sen
- sess
- sezz
- shake
- Sherman stick
- shotgun
- Siddi
- sinse (Spanish)
- sinsemilla
- skunk

cannabis (street names)
- skunkweed
- smoke
- smoke a bowl
- smoke Canada
- snop
- spark it up
- speedboat
- Spice/K2
- spliff
- splim
- splitting
- square mackerel
- squirrel
- stack
- stems
- stick
- sticky icky
- stink weed
- stoney weed
- straw
- sugar weed
- super pot
- supergrass
- swag
- Sweet Lucy
- swishers
- synthetic
- syrup
- T
- taima
- Takkouri
- tea
- tea party
- Texas pot
- Texas tea
- Tex-Mex
- Thai sticks
- thirteen
- thirty-eight
- thumb
- tin
- tio
- toke
- torc
- torch
- torch up
- torpedo

cannabis (street names)
- trauma
- tray
- trees
- triple A
- trupence bag
- twist
- twistum
- unotque
- vega
- viper
- viper's weed
- wac
- wacky weed
- wake and bake
- water
- water-water
- weed
- weed tea
- wet
- wet daddies
- wet sticks
- whack
- whackatabacky
- wheat
- white-haired lady
- White Russian
- white tiger
- wicky
- wicky stick
- wollie
- woolah
- woolas
- woolies
- wooly blunts
- X
- yeh
- yellow submarine
- yen pop
- yerba (Spanish)
- yerba mala (Spanish)
- yerhia
- yesca
- yesco
- Zacatecas purple
- zambi
- zay
- zig zag man

cannabis (street names)
   zol
   zooie
   zoom
cannabis abuse, long-term
cannabis/alcohol, "Herb and Al"
cannabis/cocaine/heroin, "el diablo"
cannabis/cocaine/heroin/PCP, "el diablito"
cannabis cocktail
cannabis grown domestically
cannabis/heroin, "atom bomb"
cannabis intoxication
cannabis intoxication delirium
cannabis intoxication (perceptual disturbance) with mild use disorder (F12.122)
cannabis intoxication (perceptual disturbance) with m/s use disorder (F12.222)
cannabis intoxication (perceptual disturbance) wit no use disorder (F12.922)
cannabis intoxication (no perceptual disturbance) with mild use disorder (F12.129)
cannabis intoxication (no perceptual disturbance) with m/s use disorder (F12.229)
cannabis intoxication (no perceptual disturbance) with no use disorder (F12.929)
cannabis-induced anxiety disorder
cannabis-induced disorder
cannabis-induced psychotic disorder with delusions
cannabis-induced psychotic disorder with hallucinations
cannabis/marijuana, synthetic (street names)
   Black Mamba
   Joker
   Kronic
   K2
   Kush
   Spice

cannabis/opium (street names)
   black hash
   Black Russian
cannabis/PCP, "killer weed"
cannabis/PCP/crack "speed boat"
cannabis-related disorder, unspecified (F12.99)
cannabis use disorder
   mild (F12.10)
   m/s (F12.20)
cannabis use disorder with cannabis-induced anxiety disorder
cannabis use disorder with cannabis-induced delirium
cannabis use disorder with cannabis-induced obsessive-compulsive disorder and related disorders
cannabis use disorder with cannabis-induced psychotic disorder
cannabis use disorder with cannabis-induced sexual disorder
cannabis use disorder with cannabis-induced sleep disorder
cannabis use, recreational
cannabis withdrawal with use disorder, m/s (F12.288)
cannula
Canter Background Interference Procedure for the Bender
CAP Assessment of Writing
"cap" (street name, crack; LSD)
"cap up" (re: drug containers; transfer bulk drugs to capsules)
Capabilities Test, Minimum Auditory (MAC)
capacitance
Capacities Battery, Rand Physical
capacitor
capacity
   carcinoma
   dissociative
   functional
   functional residual (FRC)
   hedonic

capacity
- inspiratory (IC)
- intellectual
- lung
- measured
- mental
- nonverbal intellectual
- orgasmic
- oxygen-carrying
- respiratory
- self-regulatory
- speaking
- vital (VT)

capacity for independent living
Capacity Questionnaire, Toronto Functional (TFCQ)
Capgras syndrome
"capital H" (street name, heroin)
"caps" (street name, crack; heroin; psilocybin/psilocin)
caps, canal
Captagon (brand name, amphetamine; psychostimulant)
caption file
caption(s) (for the hearing impaired)
captioning (for the hearing impaired)
- live (ON line)
- prerecorded (OFF line)
- real-time

captive, indoctrination while
carbamazepine for mood disorders
carbon dioxide intoxication
carbon monoxide intoxication
carbonyl modification
"carburetor" (re: crack equipment)
Card, Mother
cardiac evoked response audiometry (CERA)
cardinal ocular movement
cardinal vowel(s)
cardiovascular disease and concurrent psychiatric problems
cardiovascular seizure

care
- ambulatory
- clinical
- continuum of
- excessive need for
- foster
- grossly pathogenic
- health
- inappropriate dependent
- individual
- medical
- need for
- pastoral
- pathogenic
- pathological
- personal
- primary

care organization
Care Questionnaire, Health
care seekers
care services, health
career analysis *(see also* tests)
Career Assessment Inventories for the Learning Disabled
career assessment inventory *(see also* tests)
Career Beliefs Inventory (CBI)
career change problem
Career Concerns Inventory
career course planning *(see also* tests)
career decision making assessment *(see also* tests)
Career Decision Scale
Career Decision-Making System
Career Development Inventory
Career Problem Check List
career problem, new
Career Quest
Caregiver Strain Index
caregiver, adoptive
Caregiver's School Readiness Inventory (CSRI)
"carga" (street name, heroin)
Cargot ear
Carhart notch
caries, dental
caring, quality of

"carmabis" (street name, cannabis)
"carne" (street name, heroin)
"carnie" (street name, cocaine)
carotid artery stenosis
"carpet patrol" (re: crack search and acquisition)
Carrell Discrimination Test
"Carrie Nation" (street name, cocaine)
carrier phrase
Carrow Auditory-Visual Abilities Test
carryover coarticulation
cartilage
    arytenoid
    corniculate
    cricoid
    cuneiform
    thyroid
cartilage shaving, thyroid
"cartucho" (re: package of marijuana/cannabis cigarettes)
"cartwheels" (street name, amphetamine)
case
    accusative
    genitive
    grammar
    nominative
    objective
    possessive
    primary
    prototypical
    subjective
    unusual
case grammar
case management of recurrent suicidal behavior
case relations
case series
case study
CASH (Comprehensive Assessment of Symptoms and History)
"Casper the Ghost" (street name, crack)
Cassipa (buprenorphine/naloxone)
CAST (Children's Apperceptive Story-Telling Test)
CAT (California Achievement Tests)
CAT (Children's Articulation Test)
CAT (computer axial tomography)
"cat" (street name, methcathinone)
cat cry syndrome (cri du chat)
"Cat in the Hats" (street name, ecstasy; MDMA)
"cat valium" (street name, ketamine)
catabolism
cataclysmic headache
cataplexy
cataplexy, episode of
cataplexy syndrome, narcolepsy
cataracts, traumatic
catarrh
catarrhal deafness
catastrophic reaction
catastrophic response
catatonia
    lethal
    unspecified (R29.8) and (F06.1)
catatonia associated with another medical condition (F06.1)
catatonia disorder due to another medical condition (F06.1)
catatonic behavior
catatonic disorder
catatonic disorder due to GMC
catatonic features
catatonic features, mood disorders with
catatonic motor behavior(s)
catatonic mutism
catatonic negativism
catatonic presentation
catatonic rigidity
catatonic schizophrenia
catatonic symptom
catatonic type
catatonic type schizophrenia

catch, glossal
categorical approach
categorical classification
categorical definition
categorical model
categorical name
categorical perspective
categorical system(s)
categories
    checklist of problem
    grammatical
    lexical
category tests *(see also* tests)
catenative
cathard
cathisophobia
cathode (C or Ca)
"catnip" (street name, cannabis/marijuana cigarette)
catoptrophobia
Cattell Scales
Cattell Personality Factor Questionnaire
caudal
causal component
causal factor
causal link
causal relationship
causalgic pain
causality
    direct
    presumed
causation
    biological
    epidemiological
causative agent(s)
causative pathophysiological mechanism, direct
cause and effect, laws of
cause of death
cause of seizure
    alcohol as
    emotion as
cause of seizure
    fatigue as
causes, substance-related
caution, special

cavernosography
"caviar" (street name, crack)
"Cavite all star" (street name, cannabis/marijuana)
cavity
    buccal
    oral
CAVLT (Children's Auditory Verbal Learning Test
CBC (cannabichromene)
CBD (cannabidiol)
CBD e-juice
CBD e-liquid
CBD full-spectrum vape oil
CBD isolate vape oil
CBD oil
CBD oil milligram catch
CBD tincture
CBD vape cartridge
CBD vape juice
CBD vape oil
CBD vape pen
CBDA (cannabidiolic acid)
CBDV (cannabidivarin)
CBF (cerebral blood flow)
CBG (cannabigerol)
CBG oil
CBGA (cannabigerolic acid)
CBI (Career Beliefs Inventory)
CBMT (Certification Board for Music Therapists)
CBS (culture-bound syndrome)
CCAE (Checklist for Child Abuse Evaluation)
CCAT (Canadian Cognitive Abilities Test
CCQ (Chronicle Career Quest)
CCSEQ (Community College Student Experiences Questionnaire)
CCTDI (The California Critical Thinking Dispositions Inventory)
CCTST (California Critical Thinking Skills Test)
CDC–NCHS (Center for Disease Control – National Center for Health Statistics)

CDMS (The Harrington-O'Shea Career Decision-Making System)
CDR (Clinical Dementia Rating Scale)
CDS (Children's Depression Scale)
"C-dust" (street name, cocaine)
CE (cocaethylene assay)
CEASD (Conference of Educational Administrators of Schools & Programs for the Deaf)
CEC (Council for Exceptional Children)
"Cecil" (street name, cocaine)
cecocentral scotoma
CEHRT (Certified Electronic Health Record Technology)
cell(s)
    acoustic
    hair
    nerve
cell body
cellular effects of lithium
cellulitis
Celtophobia
center(s)
    hearing
    language
    motor
    speech
    visual
Center for Disease Control – National Center for Health Statistics (CDC–NCHS)
Center for Epidemiological Studies
Center for Medicare and Medicaid Services (CMS)
center of attention
center of facial paresis
center of gravity (CG)
center of gray matter
centeredness
central alexia
central alveolar hypoventilation, congenital (G47.35)

central alveolar hypoventilation syndrome
central apnea
central auditory abilities
central auditory abilities *(see also* tests)
central auditory disorder
central auditory function
central auditory perception
central auditory processes
central auditory tests *(see also* tests)
central convulsion
central deafness
central drive for respiration
Central European viral encephalitis
central excitatory state
central hearing
central incisor teeth
Central Institute for the Deaf (CID)
Central Institute for the Deaf Preschool Performance Scale
central language deficit
central language disorder (CLD)
central language imbalance
central masking
central motor pathways disease
central nervous system effect
central nervous system pathology
central neurogenic hyperventilation
central scotoma
central sensory deficit
central sensory loss
central sleep apnea, idiopathic (G47.21)
central sleep apnea comorbid with opioid use (G47.37)
central sleep apnea disorder
central sleep apnea syndrome
central speech range
central sulcus
central vowel
centration
centrencephalic seizure
centrotemporal epilepsy

cephalic seizure
cephalometric analysis
cephalometry
CERA (cardiac evoked response audiometry)
CERAD (Consortium to Establish a Registry for Alzheimer's Disease)
CERAD Assessment Battery
ceraunophobia
cerebellar ataxia
cerebellar ataxia, ipsilateral
cerebellar cortex
cerebellar degeneration
cerebellar disease
cerebellar disease, tremor from
cerebellar fits (seizure)
cerebellar mass
cerebellar pathway
cerebellar scanning quality speech
cerebellar scanning type speech
cerebellar signs
cerebellar syndrome
cerebellar tremor
    essential
    progressive
cerebellum (pl. cerebella)
cerebral aneurysm
cerebral anoxia
cerebral aplasia
cerebral artery occlusion
cerebral atherosclerosis
cerebral atrophy
cerebral blood flow (CBF)
cerebral brain death
cerebral contusion
cerebral convulsion
cerebral cortex
cerebral death
cerebral disorder
cerebral dominance
cerebral dominance and handedness theory of stuttering
cerebral dominance, mixed
cerebral dysfunction
    bilateral
    higher (HCD)
cerebral edema

cerebral fissure, longitudinal
cerebral gait
cerebral lipidosis
cerebral localization
cerebral mapping of apraxia
cerebral outflow tremor
cerebral palsy (CP)
    ataxic
    athetoid
    atonic
    choreoathetoid
    clonic
    dyskinetic
    dystonic
    extrapyramidal
    flaccid
    hypotonic
    pyramidal
    rigid
    spastic
    tremulous
cerebral palsy tests for children (*see also* tests)
cerebral paraplegia
cerebral potential
cerebral seizure
cerebral signs
cerebral syndrome, posttraumatic
cerebral thumb
cerebral trauma
cerebral tremor, essential
cerebral zero
cerebri, pseudotumor
cerebrospinal convulsion
cerebrospinal fluid (CSF) analysis
cerebrovascular disease
cerebrovascular insufficiency
cerebrum
ceremonial behavior
Certified Electronic Health Record Technology (CEHRT)
ceruloplasmin
cerumen, impacted
cervical
cessation
cessation, smoking
cessation of a medication
cessation of seizure

"cest" (street name,
   cannabis/marijuana)
CF (Coalition for the Family)
CFBRS (Cooper-Farran
   Behavioral Rating Scales)
CFQ (Cognitive Failure
   Questionnaire)
CFSEI (Culture-Free Self-Esteem
   Inventories)
CG (center of gravity)
"C-game" (street name, cocaine)
CGIC (Clinical Global Impression
   of Change)
chain, ossicular
chain analysis
chaining
chaining responses
"chalk" (street name, methamphetamine; amphetamine)
"chalked up" (re: cocaine
   influence)
"chalking" (re: chemically
   whitening cocaine)
challenge, neuroendocrine
challenge test, tyramine
chamber
   anechoic
   echo
   no-echo
chance, pure
"chandoo/chandu" (street name,
   opium)
change
   agent
   agent of
   age-related physical
   analog
   behavioral
   digital
   life
   life-cycle
   maladaptive behavioral
   maladaptive psychological
   mental
   mental status
   personality
   psychomotor
   psychophysiological
change
   reflex
   time-zone
   transitional
   unpredictable mood
Change, Clinical Global
   Impression of (CGIC)
changed body image
change events, life
change in activity, rapid
change in adolescent/family life
   events
change in level of consciousness
change in mentation
change in mood
change in personality
   characteristics
change in treatment
change of consciousness, episodic
change problem, career
changing response set, difficulty
   in
changing sleep-wake pattern
"channel" (re: drug injection)
channel, membrane ion
"channel swimmer" (re: heroin
   injection user)
chaotic
character
   abusive
   costumed
   dependent
   histrionic
   oral
   out of
   perceived attack on one's
character attack
character disorder, psychoanalysis
   and
character of a substance
character pathology
characteristic age
characteristic association
characteristic durations of
   intoxication
characteristic features
characteristic paraphiliac focus
characteristic pattern

characteristic sex ratio
characteristic sign of
   schizophrenia
characteristic symptoms of
   schizophrenia
characteristic syndrome
characteristic withdrawal
   syndrome
characteristics
     change in personality
     clang association
     primary sex
     psychometric performance
     secondary sex
     sex
characteristics of cleft palate,
   language and speech
characteristics of pain, temporal
characteristics of stuttering
     primary
     secondary
"charas" (street name, cannabis;
   marijuana from India)
"Charge" (street name, cannabis;
   cocaine; club drug)
"Charge+" (re: powdery
   substance with ecstasy effect)
"charged up" (re: drug influence)
"Charley" (street name, heroin)
"Charlie" (street name, cocaine)
"Charlotte's Web" (street name,
   liquid cannabis)
charm superficial
Charteris Reading Test
charts
     developmental evaluation
     Northampton
chase (gambling), long-term
"chase" (re: cannabis or cocaine
   use)
"chaser" (re: compulsive crack
   user)
"chasing" one's losses
"chasing the dragon" (re: crack
   and heroin use)
"chasing the tiger" (re: smoking
   heroin)
"chasm of insanity"

"cheap basing" (street name,
   crack)
"check" (re: personal drug supply)
check test, audiometry sweep
checklist (or check list)
checklist approach
Checklist for Child Abuse
   Evaluation (CCAE)
Checklist of Adaptive Living
   Skills (CALS)
checklist of problem categories
   (see also tests)
"cheeba" (street name,
   cannabis/marijuana)
cheeking medication
"cheeo" (street name,
   cannabis/marijuana)
cheerlessness
cheiloschisis
chemical health assessment (see
   also tests)
chemical messengers
"chemical" (street name, crack)
chemotherapeutic
cheromania (heavenly desire)
cherophobia
chest discomfort (a panic attack
   indicator)
chest pain (a panic attack
   indicator)
chest pulse
chest voice
"chewies" (street name, crack)
chewing, breath
chewing automatism
chewing method
Cheyne-Stokes breathing (R06.3)
Cheyne-Stokes respiration
CHI (closed head injury)
"chiba chiba" (street name,
   cannabis/marijuana from
   Columbia)
"Chicago black" (street name,
   cannabis/marijuana
"Chicago green" (street name,
   cannabis/marijuana)
"chicken powder" (street name,
   amphetamine)

"chicken scratch" (re: crack acquisition)
"chicle" (street name, heroin)
"chief" (street name, mescaline)
"chieva" (street name, heroin)
child
    age of the
    exceptional
    gifted
    middle
    only
child abuse
    adult survivor of
    non-parental
    perpetrator of non-parental
    perpetrator of parental
child abuse evaluation *(see also* tests)
Child Abuse Potential Inventory
Child/Adolescent Social History (automated)
child affected by parental relationship distress (Z62.898)
Child and Adolescent Adjustment Profile
Child Anxiety Scale
Child Assessment Schedule
Child "At Risk" for Drug Abuse Rating Scale (DARS)
child behavior *(see also* tests)
Child Behavior Checklist
Child Behavior Rating Scale
child care and guidance competency *(see also* tests)
Child Care Inventory
child counselor
Child Depression Scale
child development *(see also* tests)
Child Development Age Scale
Child Development Inventory
child exploitation
child group therapies
child guidance
child issues, inner
child language development *(see also* tests)
child maltreatment and neglect problems
child neglect
    (Confirmed/Initial) encounter (T74.02XA)
    (Confirmed/Subsequent) encounters (T74.02XD)
    (Suspected/Initial) encounter (T76.02XA)
    (Suspected/Subsequent) encounters (T76.02XD)
    victim of
Child Neuropsychological Questionnaire (CNQ)
child or adolescent antisocial behavior (Z72.810)
child physical abuse
    circumstances related to
    (Confirmed/Initial) encounter (T74.12XA)
    (Confirmed/Subsequent) encounters (T74.12XD)
    (Suspected/Initial) encounter (T76.12XA)
    (Suspected/Subsequent) encounters (T76.12XD)
child psychiatry, psychopharmacology in
child psychological abuse
    circumstanced related to
    (Confirmed/Initial) encounter (T74.32XA)
    (Confirmed/Subsequent) encounter (T74.32XD)
    (Suspected/Initial) encounter (T76.32XA)
    (Suspected/Subsequent) encounter (T76.32XD)
child rearing
child sexual abuse
    circumstances related to
    (Confirmed/Initial) encounter (T74.22XA)
    (Confirmed/Subsequent) encounters (T74.22XD)
    (Suspected/Initial) encounter (T76.22XA)
    (Suspected/Subsequent) encounters (T76.22XD)
child support

childbirth amnesia
childhood
    cross dressing in
    developmental
      experimentation in
    GID of
    physical abuse in
    psychological abuse in
    sexual abuse in
childhood phasia *(see also* tests)
childhood autism, neuroleptic
  treatment of
childhood conduct disorders,
  neuroleptic treatment of
childhood cross-gender behavior
childhood disintegrative disorder
childhood disorders *(see also*
  tests)
childhood encephalopathy
childhood epilepsy
childhood-onset fluency disorder
  (stuttering) (F80.81)
childhood-onset type conduct
  disorder
childhood physical abuse
childhood psychological affliction
childhood psychosis
childhood schizophrenia,
  neuroleptic treatment of
childhood services systems
childhood sexual abuse
childhood stressors
    accidents as major
    adoption as major
    divorce as major
    natural disasters as major
    sexual abuse as major
    violence as major
childhood Tourette's syndrome,
  neuroleptic treatment of
childhood trauma symptom
  checklist *(see also* tests)
childlike silliness
children
    amnesia in
    biological
    emotional maltreatment of
    mental disturbance in
    neurological dysfunctions
      of
    school-age
    severe stress in
children and adults anxiety scales
  (see also tests)
children and adults depression
  inventories *(see also* tests)
children and adults intelligence
  tests *(see also* tests)
Children and Emotional/Behavior
  Screening Program
Children's Academic Intrinsic
  Motivation Inventory
Children's Adaptive Behavior
  Scale
children's apperception tests *(see*
  also tests)
Children's Apperceptive Story-
  Telling Test (CAST)
Children's Articulation Test
  (CAT)
Children's Attention and
  Adjustment Survey (CAAS)
Children's Auditory Verbal
  Learning Test (CAVLT)
Children's Coma Score
Children's Depression Inventory
Children's Depression Scale
  (CDS)
Children's early communication
  skills *(see also* tests)
children's fear survey *(see also*
  tests)
Children's Hypnotic
  Susceptibility Scale
children's intelligence tests *(see*
  also tests)
Children's Inventory of Self-
  Esteem (CISE)
Children's Language Assessment
  Test
Children's Language Battery
Children's language competence
  tests *(see also* tests)
Children's Language Processes

Psychiatric Words and Phrases

children's life event scale *(see also* tests)
Children's listening accuracy tests *(see also* tests)
Children's Manifest Anxiety Scale (CMAS)
Children's Perception of Speech Test
children's personality inventory *(see also* tests)
Children's self-perception profile *(see also* tests)
children's temperament assessment *(see also* tests)
Children's Version Family Environment Scale
Children with Specific Language Disability
Children with Suspected Learning and Behavioral Disabilities
chills (a panic attack indicator)
"China cat" (street name, heroin)
"China girl" (street name, fentanyl)
"China town" (street name, fentanyl)
"China white" (street name, heroin analog of fentanyl)
Chinamania (China/things; Chinese)
"Chinese molasses" (street name, opium)
"Chinese red" (street name, heroin)
"Chinese tobacco" (street name, opium)
chink, glottal
chionomania (snow)
"chip" (street name, heroin)
"chipper" (re: occasional Hispanic drug user)
"chipping" (re: occasional drug se)u
"chippy" (street name, cocaine)
"chira" (street name, cannabis/marijuana)
"chiva" (street name, heroin)
chlamydia
chloral hydrate
chloride, methylene
chlorthiazides
"chocolate chips" (street name, LSD)
"chocolate ecstasy" (re: chocolate milk added to crack processing)
"chocolate" (street name, opium; amphetamine)
"choe" (street name, cocaine)
choice behavior *(see also* tests)
choice reaction time test, visual
choking during sleep
choking, feeling of
cholecystitis
cholera
cholesteatoma
cholesterol
cholinergic neurons
"cholly" (street name, cocaine)
choral reading
choral speaking
"chorals" (street name, barbiturate)
chorditis nodosa
chorditis tuberosa
chorea
    senile
    Sydenham's
choreiform movement(s)
choreoathetoid cerebral palsy (CP)
choreoathetosis
choreomania (dance)
"Christina" (street name, amphetamine)
"Christmas rolls" (street name, barbiturate)
"Christmas trees" (street name, barbiturate/depressant; amphetamine; cannabis/marijuana)
chromosomal
chromosome 21-trisomy syndrome
chromosomes, sex
chronaxie

"chronic" (street name, cannabis/marijuana mixed with crack)
chronic amnesia
chronic disability, posttraumatic
chronic epilepsy
Chronic Family Invalid - Depressed (MMPI)
chronic fatigue
chronic feelings
chronic feelings of emptiness
chronic forms of pain
chronic headache
chronic insomnia
chronic intoxication
chronic irritable dysphoria
chronic laryngitis
chronic mania
chronic motor or vocal tic disorder
chronic motor tic disorder
chronic phase of stable sleep difficulty
chronic psychosis
chronic pulmonary heart disease
chronic renal failure
chronic sedative-hypnotic use
chronic sleep disturbance
chronic subglottic laryngitis
chronic suppurative otitis media
chronic tiredness
chronic tissue damage
chronic toxic effects
chronic vocal tic disorder
Chronicle Career Quest (CCQ)
chronobiological disorder
chronobiological disturbances
chronological relationship
chronology
CHS (cannabinoid hyperemesis syndrome)
"chucks" (re: heroin withdrawal)
chunk size
chunking
"churus" (street name, cannabis/marijuana)
(C/I) confirmed/initial episode

"Cid" (street name, cannabis/marijuana cigarette; LSD)
CID (Central Institute for the Deaf)
CID Preschool Performance Scale
"cigarette paper" (re: packet of heroin)
cigarette tobacco
cigarette-related pathology
cigarettes, electronic
"cigarrode cristal" (street name, PCP)
cinefluorography
cinefluoroscopy
cineradiography
cineroentgenography
cipher method, numerical
circadian pacemaker, endogenous
circadian period, endogenous
circadian phase of sleep
circadian rhythm phase, endogenous
circadian rhythm sleep disorder
circadian rhythm sleep-wake disorder (G47.22)
    irregular type (G47.23)
    non-24-hour type (G47.24)
    overlapping non-24-hour type (G47.21)
    shift work type (G54.26)
    unspecified (G54.20)
    voyeuristic type disorder (F65.3)
circadian system
circle of thoughts, wide
circuit
    convergence
    divergence
    neuronal
circular thinking
circumaural hearing protection device(s)
circumflex
circumlocution
circumlocution of speech
circumlocutory
circumscribed delusion

Psychiatric Words and Phrases 99

circumstances
    difficult life
    living
    real-life
circumstances related to adult abuse by nonspouse or nonpartner
circumstances related to spousal or partner abuse, psychological
circumstances related to spousal or partner violence
    physical
    sexual
circumstantial migraine headache
CIRCUS
CISE (Children's Inventory of Self-Esteem)
"citrol" (street name, high potency cannabis/marijuana from Nepal)
city and state tests *(see also* tests)
clairvoyance, belief in
clammy hands, cold
clang association
clang association characteristics
"clarity" (street name, MDMA)
clarity of language
Clark-Madison Test of Oral Language
Clark Picture Phonetic Inventory
Clarke Reading Self-Assessment Survey
clasp knife" phenomenon
class, closed
Class Activities Questionnaire
class word
classes, word
classic apraxia
classical migraine
classical migraine headache
classification
    Barrett tongue thrust
    categorical
    Garliner tongue thrust
    sentence
classification of aphasia, Benson-Geschwind
classification system

classification tests
classifications of the cleft palate
Classroom Environment Index
classroom performance, decline in
claudication, neurogenic
clausa, rhinolalia
clause
    constituent
    dependent
    embedded
    independent
    main
    principal
    subordinate
    terminal
clause voice disorder, rhinolalia
clavicular respiration
Claybury Selection Battery
CLCS (Comprehensive Level of Consciousness Scale)
CLD (central language disorder)
clear sensorium
clear up"(re: stop drug use)
clearing, throat
clearly demarcated relationships
CLEF (Clinical Evaluation of Language Functions)
cleft(s)
    atypical
    labial
    nose
    rare
cleft lip
    bilateral
    median
    unilateral
cleft palate
    bilateral
    classifications of the
    complete
    incomplete
    language and speech characteristics of
    occult
    partial
    prosthetic management of
    speech and language characteristics of

cleft palate
    submucous
    subtotal
    total
    unilateral
cleft palate fistula
clenching, fist
CLEP (College-Level Examination Program General Examination)
cleptophobia
clerical assessment tests *(see also* tests)
clerical response (Q)
CLI (Campbell Leadership Index)
click, glottal
"clicker" (street name, crack and PCP)
client care
    ethical aspects of assaultive
    legal aspects of assaultive
    practical aspects of assaultive
"cliff of sanity"
"cliffhanger" (street name, PCP)
"climate", emotional
"climax" (street name, crack cocaine; isobutyl nitrite; heroin)
"climb" (street name, cannabis/marijuana cigarette)
clinging behavior, pattern of
clinic patient populations
clinical action of lithium
clinical attention, focus of
clinical audiology
Clinical Battery, Aphasia
clinical course, atypical
Clinical Dementia Rating Scale (CDR)
clinical evaluation
Clinical Evaluation of Language Functions (CLEF)
clinical evaluation, process of
clinical experience
clinical features
Clinical Global Impression of Change (CGIC)
clinical information
clinical judgment
clinical management
Clinical Multiaxial Inventory-II, Obsessive-Compulsive}
Clinical Probes of Articulation Consistency (C-PAC)
clinical psychobiology
clinical psychopharmacology
Clinical Rating Scale (CRS)
clinical scales *(see also* tests)
Clinical Scales (MMPI)
clinical setting
clinical status
Clinical Support System Battery
clinical training
clinical utility
clinically significant anxiety
clinically significant distress
clinically significant impairment
clinician
    anxious
    language
    speech and language
    voice
clinics, maternal addiction
clinomania (bending)
clipped word
clipping, peak
"clips" (re: drug vials)
"clocking paper" (re: drug profits)
clonic block (in stuttering)
clonic cerebral palsy (CP)
clonic convulsion
clonic movement
clonic seizure
clonic-tonic-clonic seizure
clonus
close phonetic transcription
close relationship
close relationships, pattern of discomfort in
close transcription
close vowel
close watch restrictions
closed bite
closed bite malposition of teeth
closed class
closed head injury (CHI)

Psychiatric Words and Phrases

closed head trauma
closed juncture
closed syllable
closed to experience
"closet baser" (re: crack user)
closure processes
closure
    grammatic
    perceptual
    velopharyngeal
closure task, sentence
clothing, feminine
"cloud nine" (street name, crack)
"cloud" (street name, crack)
clozapine for mood disorders
club drug (dance club drug use and users) (street names)
    007s
    2CB
    banana split
    Batman
    bean
    Bermuda triangles
    bibs
    blue Nile
    BOMPEA
    boomers
    bromo
    bump up
    bumping up
    candy rave
    caps
    Care Bears
    Cat in the Hats
    cat killer
    Charge+
    charity
    circles
    clarity
    cloud nine
    dead road
    easy lay
    E-bombs
    Egyptians
    elephant flipping
    elephants
    E-puddle
    E-tard

club drug (street names)
    exiticity
    fantasy
    flatliners
    flipping
    forget-me pill
    four leaf clover
    Georgia home boy
    golden eagle
    goop
    green triangles
    gum
    GWM
    hammerheading
    happy drug
    happy pill
    H-bomb
    herbal bliss
    hawkers
    hippieflip
    hugs and kisses
    igloo
    ivory wave
    jellies
    Jerry Garcias
    kitty flipping
    K-lots
    letter biscuits
    liquid ecstasy
    liquid X
    love flipping
    love pill
    lovers' special
    Mercedes
    MFT
    Mitsubishi
    Molly
    moonstone
    Nexus
    Nexus flipping
    NOX
    ocean burst
    on the ball
    orange bandits
    P and P
    party pack
    peace
    peeper(s)

club drug (street names)
    piggybacking
    Pikachu
    pink partners
    Playboy bunnies
    playboys
    pure ivory
    purple wave
    rave energy
    red devils
    rib
    ritual spirit
    roach-2
    Rolls Royce
    scoop
    sextasy
    sleep
    sleep-500
    smurfs
    snackies
    soap
    Somatomax
    Spectrum
    stacking
    stacks
    stars
    Superman
    super-X
    swans
    tabs
    tachas
    Tom and Jerries
    toonies
    triple crowns
    triple Rolexes
    triple stacks
    troll
    tutus
    twenty birds
    ultimate xphoria
    vanilla sky
    Venus
    Vita-G
    wafers
    waffle dust
    water
    ya ba
"cluck" (re: crack user)
clucking, tongue
Clunis inquiry forensic psychiatry
cluster
    anxious-fearful
    consonant
    dramatic-emotional
    odd-eccentric
Cluster A Personality Disorder - Paranoid
Cluster A Personality Disorder - Schizoid
Cluster A Personality Disorder - Schizotypal
Cluster B Personality Disorder - Antisocial
Cluster B Personality Disorder - Borderline
Cluster B Personality Disorder - Histrionic
Cluster B Personality Disorder - Narcissistic
Cluster C Personality Disorder - Avoidant
Cluster C Personality Disorder - Dependent
Cluster C Personality Disorder - Obsessive/Compulsive
cluster consonant
cluster headache
cluster migraine headache
cluster of situations
cluster reduction
clusters, reduction of
"cluttering"
Clymer-Barrett Readiness Test
CMA (Conflict Management Appraisal)
CMAS (Children's Manifest Anxiety Scale)
CMEE (Content Mastery Examinations for Educators)
CMII (College Major Interest Inventory)
CMRE (California Marriage Readiness Evaluation)
CMS (Center for Medicare and Medicaid Services)

CNQ (Child Neuropsychological
  Questionnaire)
CNS disease group
CNT ("could not test")
coalescence
Coalition for the Family (CF)
coalitions
coarctated personality
coarse tremor
coarticulation
  anticipatory
  backward
  carryover
  forward
Coarticulation Assessment in
  Meaningful Language (CAML)
"coasting" (re: drug influence)
"coasts to coasts" (street name,
  amphetamine)
"coca" (street name, cocaine)
cocaethylene (CE) assay
cocaine (street names)
  51
  All-American drug
  Angie
  aspirin
  Aunt
  Aunt Nora
  balling
  banano
  barbs
  basa
  base
  base crazies
  base head
  based out
  basing
  basuco
  Batman
  bazooka
  Bazulco
  beam
  beam me up Scottie
  behind the scale
  beiging or beigeing
  Belushi
  Bernice
  Bernie

cocaine (street names)
  Bernie's flakes
  Bernie's gold dust
  big bloke
  big C
  big flake
  big rush
  billie hoke
  black rock
  Blanca
  Blanco
  Blast
  blizzard
  blotter
  blow
  blow blue
  blow coke
  blow smoke
  blunt
  body packer
  Bolivian marching powder
  booster
  bopper
  bouncing powder
  boy
  boy-girl
  break night
  brick
  bubble gum
  bump
  bump up
  bumper
  bumping up
  bunk
  Burese
  Burnese
  bush
  C
  C & M
  C joint
  caine
  California cornflakes
  came
  candy C
  candy flipping on a string
  candy sticks
  candy sugar
  caps

cocaine (street names)
- Carnie
- Carrie Nation
- Caviar
- CDs
- Cecil
- chalked up
- chalking
- champagne
- Charge/Charge+
- Charlie
- chase
- chicken scratch
- chippy
- choe
- cholly
- cigamos
- coca
- cocktail
- coconut
- cola
- combol
- comeback
- Connie
- cooking up
- coolie
- cork the air
- Corrinne
- cotton brothers
- crack
- crack bash
- crisscrossing
- croak
- crystal
- Dama Blanca
- Devil's dandruff
- dirties
- do a line
- double breasted dealing
- double bubble
- draf
- dream
- duct
- DUST
- dynamite
- El diablito
- El diablo
- El Perico

cocaine (street names)
- Electric Kool Aid
- five-way
- flake
- flame cooking
- flamethrowers
- flash
- flave
- fleece
- flex
- Florida snow
- foo-foo
- foo-foo dust
- foo-foo stuff
- foolish powder
- freebase
- freeze
- Frisco special
- Frisco speedball
- friskie powder
- frontloading
- gaffel
- Geek-joints
- geeze
- ghost busting
- gift-of-the-sun
- gift-of-the-sun-god
- gin
- girl
- girlfriend
- glad stuff
- go on a sleigh ride
- gold dust
- goofball
- green gold
- G-rock
- half piece
- handlebars
- happy dust
- happy powder
- happy trails
- have a dust
- heaven
- heaven dust
- Henry VIII
- her
- he-she
- hitch up the reindeers

cocaine (street names)
- hooter
- horn
- horning
- hunter
- ice
- icing
- Inca message
- ivory wave
- jam
- jejo
- jelly
- Jim Jones
- joy powder
- junk
- king
- king's habit
- lace
- lady caine
- lady snow
- late night
- leaf
- line
- love affair
- Ma'a
- macaroni and cheese
- mama coca
- marching dust
- mayo
- Merck
- merk
- mighty white
- mix
- mo
- Mojo
- mon
- monkey
- monos (Spanish)
- monster
- mosquitos
- movie star drug
- mujer
- murder one
- nieve
- nose
- nose powder
- nose stuff
- number 3

cocaine (street names)
- ocean burst
- one and one
- one bomb
- one on one house
- one plus one sales
- onion
- oyster stew
- paradise
- paradise white
- pearl
- percia
- percio
- perico
- Peruvia
- Peruvian
- Peruvian flake
- Peruvian lady
- picking
- piece
- pimp
- polvo blanco
- pop
- powder
- powder diamonds
- premos
- press
- primo(s)
- primo turbo
- pseudocaine
- pure ivory
- purple caps
- purple haze
- purple wave
- quill
- Racehorse Charlie
- rane
- raw
- ready rock
- real tops
- recompress
- rider
- rocks
- Roxanne
- rush
- sandwich
- schmeck
- schoolboy

cocaine (street names)
- scorpion
- Scottie
- Scotty
- scramble
- seconds
- serial speedballing
- Serpico 21
- Seven-up
- shabu
- shaker/baker/water
- she
- shebanging
- Sherman stick
- shot
- shrile
- sleigh ride
- smoke houses
- smoking gun
- sniff
- snort
- snow
- snow bird
- snow cones
- snow seals
- Snow White
- society high
- soda
- soft
- soup
- space
- spaceball
- speedball
- speedballing
- speedballs – nose style
- splitting
- sporting
- squirrel
- stacks
- star
- stardust
- star-spangled powder
- studio fuel
- sugar
- sugar boogers
- sweet stuff
- T
- talco

cocaine (street names)
- tardust
- teenager
- teeth
- The five way
- thing
- tio
- toke
- toot
- trey
- turkey
- tutti-frutti
- Twinkie
- uptown
- vanilla sky
- white boy
- white dragon
- white girl
- white horse
- white lady
- white mosquito
- white powder
- whiz bang
- wicky
- wild cat
- window pane
- wings
- wired on
- witch
- woo blunts
- woolas
- woolie
- woolie blunt
- wooties
- working bags
- yao
- yarn
- yay
- yeyo
- zip

cocaine, toxic effects of
cocaine/amphetamine, "snow seals"
"cocaine blues" (re: cocaine use)
"cocaine crash" (re: cocaine use)
cocaine craving, cue-elicited
cocaine dependence, long-term

cocaine/heroin (street names)
    Belushi
    flamethrower (cigarette)
    number 3
    snowball
    whiz bang
cocaine intoxication
    no perceptual disturbance, no use disorder (F14.929)
    no perceptual disturbance, with mild use disorder (F14.129)
    no perceptual disturbance, with m/s use disorder (F14.229)
    perceptual disturbance, no use disorder (F14.922)
    perceptual disturbance, with mild use disorder (F14.122)
    perceptual disturbance, with m/s use disorder (F14.222)
cocaine intoxication delirium
cocaine-induced anxiety disorder
cocaine-induced disorder
cocaine-induced disorder with obsessive-compulsive and related disorders
cocaine-induced mood disorder
cocaine-induced psychotic disorder with delusions
cocaine-induced psychotic disorder with hallucinations
cocaine-induced sexual dysfunction
cocaine-induced sleep disorder
cocaine-laced cigarette (street names)
    cocktail
    coolie
    monkey
    monos
    primos
    wild cat
cocaine/PCP, "stardust"
cocaine problem
cocaine-produced insomnia
cocaine-related disorder, unspecified (F14.99)
cocaine-related headache
cocaine run
cocaine use disorder with cocaine-induced anxiety disorder
cocaine use disorder with cocaine-induced bipolar or related disease
cocaine use disorder with cocaine-induced brief psychotic disorder
cocaine use disorder with cocaine-induced delirium
cocaine use disorder with cocaine-induced delusional disorder
cocaine use disorder with cocaine-induced depressive disorder
cocaine use disorder with cocaine-induced obsessive-compulsive and related disorders
cocaine use disorder with cocaine-induced psychotic disorder
cocaine use disorder with cocaine-induced schizoaffective disorder
cocaine use disorder with cocaine-induced schizophrenia
cocaine use disorder with cocaine-induced schizophreniform disorder
cocaine use disorder with cocaine-induced schizotypal (personality) disorder
cocaine use disorder with cocaine-induced sexual disorder
cocaine use disorder with cocaine-induced sleep disorder
cocaine withdrawal
    no perceptual disturbance (F14.23)
    perceptual disturbance (F14.23)
cocaine withdrawal disorder
cochlea
cochlea, fenestra
cochlear aplasia
cochlear canal
cochlear duct
cochlear implant

cochlear microphonia
cochlear nerve
cochlear nucleus
    dorsal
    ventral
cochlear reflex
cochlear window
cochleo-orbicular reflex
cochleopalpebral reflex (CPR)
"cochornis" (street name, cannabis/marijuana)
"cocktail" (street name, cocaine/crack-laced cigarette; marijuana cigarette inside a regular cigarette)
"coco rocks" (street name, crack made with chocolate pudding)
"coco snow" (street name, benzocaine cutting agent for crack)
"cocoa puff" (re: smoking cocaine and marijuana)
"coconut" (street name, cocaine)
"cod" (re: currency)
code 1
codeine, "schoolboy" (street name, opioid)
coefficient
    alternate forms reliability
    comparable forms reliability
    odd-even method reliability
    split half reliability
    test-retest reliability
coefficient of correlation (product moment)
coefficient of correlation (rank order)
coefficient of correlation, Pearson product-moment
coercion, sexual
coercive communication
"coffee" (street name, LSD)
COG (Cognitive Observation Guide)
cognate confusion
cognate(s)
cognition

cognition, empiric
cognition scale, need for
Cognitive Abilities Test
cognitive approaches to dreaming and repression
cognitive assessment technique(s), standardized
cognitive assessment, quantified
Cognitive Behavior Rating Scales
cognitive-behavioral technique
cognitive-behavioral treatments
Cognitive Control Battery
cognitive decline problems, age-related
cognitive decline
    age-related
    communication in
cognitive deficit
cognitive deficit(s)
    global
    multiple
cognitive development stages (Period I-IV)
cognitive development stages, Piaget's
Cognitive Diagnostic Battery
cognitive disorder
cognitive distancing
cognitive distortion
cognitive distortions, pattern of
cognitive dysfunction
Cognitive Failures Questionnaire (CFQ)
cognitive function
    higher level
    impairment of
cognitive functioning
    impaired
    impairment in
cognitive impairment
cognitive impairment, level of
cognitive limitations
cognitive mapping
Cognitive Observation Guide (COG)
cognitive personality traits
cognitive processes
Cognitive Rating Scale

cognitive research orientation
cognitive restructuring
cognitive science
cognitive self-hypnosis training
cognitive set of disturbances
Cognitive Skills Assessment Battery
cognitive status, current
cognitive structures tests *(see also* tests)
cognitive style
Cognitive Style in Mathematics Test
cognitive tests for the elderly *(see also* tests)
cognitive variables, preexisting
cogwheel rigidity
coherent stream of thought
cohesion evaluation scales *(see also* tests)
cohesive devices
coil, induction
coital orgasm
"coke" (street name, cocaine; crack)
"coke bar" (re: cocaine use)
"coke bugs" (street name, cocaine)
"cola" (street name, cocaine)
cold clammy hands
cold-running speech
Cold-Running Speech Test
"cold turkey" (re: sudden drug withdrawal)
coldness, emotional
"coli" (street name, cannabis/marijuana)
"coliflor tostao" (street name, cannabis) (Spanish)
collapsing anchors
collar, shower
collateral sources
collected data
collection, complete data
collective monologue
College Admission Test
College Basic Academic Subjects Examination

college-level examinations *(see also* tests)
College Major Interest Inventory (CMII)
College of Psychiatrists of Ireland
college questionnaires *(see also* tests)
colloquial
colloquialism
color
    flashes of
    sound-produced sensation of
color agnosia
color and word tests *(see also* tests)
color anomia
color perception
color responses
color therapy
"Colorado cocktail" (street name, cannabis/marijuana)
Colorado Educational Interest Inventory
Coloured Progressive Matrices
"Columbian" (street name, cannabis/marijuana)
"Columbo" (street name, phencyclidine)
"Columbus black" (street name, cannabis/marijuana)
columella (pl. columellae)
coma-like state, hysteric
Coma Scale
    Edinburgh-2
    Glasgow (GCS)
Coma Score, Children's
comatose patient
combat
    military
    trauma effects on soldiers in
combat tension
combative patient
combination headache
combinative thinking
combined aural rehabilitation
combined behavior, hyperactive-impulsive

combined factors
    dyspareunia due to
    female orgasmic disorder
        due to
    female sexual arousal
        disorder due to
    hypoactive sexual desire
        disorder due to
    male erectile disorder due
        to
    male orgasmic disorder due
        to
    sexual aversion disorder
        due to
    sexual dysfunction due to
    vaginismus due to
combined method
combined type attention-deficit/hyperactivity disorder
combined type personality disorder
"come home" (re: ending an LSD "trip")
"comeback" (re: adulterated cocaine used in crack conversion)
comfortable loudness
    Bekesy (BCL)
    most (MCL)
comfortable loudness range, most (MCLR)
command
    embedded
    negative
command test, three-stage
commentary
commissural aphasia
commissure
commissurotomy, callosal
commitment of mentally ill
common experience
common language
common migraine
common migraine headache
common objects test, naming
common precipitant exposure
common sense
common shared features

Communicating Empathy
communicating hydrocephalus
communicating with adolescents
communication
    aided augmentative
    coercive
    distortion of language and
    exaggeration of language and
    impaired
    impaired effective
    language and
    limited verbal
    manual
    non-oral
    nonvocal
    persuasive
    problem-solving
    qualitative impairment in
    short-phrase
    total
    unaided augmentative
Communication Abilities Diagnostic Test (CADeT)
Communication Abilities Diagnostic Test and Screen
communication ability, impaired
communication barriers
communication board
    direct selection
    encoding
    scanning
communication/cognition treatment
communication disorder
    social (pragmatic) (F80.89)
    unspecified (F80.9)
communication disorders battery (*see also* tests)
communication evaluation and rating scales (*see also* tests)
communication failure theory
communication failure theory of stuttering
communication in schizophrenia
    distorted
    exaggerated
communication sciences

communication sciences and
   disorders (CSD)
Communication Screen
Communication Sensitivity
   Inventory
communication skills
communication skills evaluation
   (see also tests)
communication system,
   augmentative
"communicative" arson
communicative competence
communicative competence
   evaluation (see also tests)
communicative disorder
communicative interaction
communicative technique
communicatively impaired
community
      dialect speech
      speech
community-based survey
community college-level
   screening (see also tests)
Community College Student
   Experiences Questionnaire
   (CCSEQ)
community-institutional relations
community mental health services
Community-Oriented Programs
   Environment Scale (COPES)
community populations
community setting
community study
comorbid sleep-related
   hypoventilation (G47.36)
compact phoneme
comparable forms reliability
   coefficient
comparative, superlative
comparative linguistics
comparative research
comparison
      comparative
      positive
compartmentalize
compensatory behavior,
   inappropriate

compensatory movement
compensatory technique
competence
      communicative
      linguistic
      velopharyngeal
competency, mental
competency scales and tests (see
   also tests)
competent relational functioning
competing messages integration
Competing Sentence Test
competitive behavior
complaining, help-rejecting
complaints
      pain
      sleep
      somatic
complaints of insomnia
complaints of pain
complement, objective
complemental air
complementary distribution
complete amnesia
complete cleft palate
complete cross-dressing
complete data collection
complete predicate
complete recruitment
complete subject
complete unawareness of
   environment
complete visual loss
completed suicide
completion, task
complex, AIDS dementia (ADC)
complex adaptation, symptoms of
complex equivalence
Complex Figure Test
complex motor behavior
complex motor tics
complex multistep task
complex noise
complex partial seizure (CPS)
complex seizure, partial
complex sentence
Complex Speech-Sound
   Discrimination Test

complex syllabics
complex thematic pictures test
complex tone
complex vocal tics
complex wave
complex whole body movements
complex word
complexes, K
compliance, patient
compliance masking covert resistance, overt
complicated migraine headache
complications, psychosocial
complications of pregnancy
complications of treatment
component
    base
    grammatical
    morphological linguistic
    morphophonemic
    phonological linguistic
    pragmatic linguistic
    semantic linguistic
    syntactic linguistic
component of evaluation
compound
    bromine
    methaqualone
    nominal
compound-complex sentence
compound consonant
compound sentence
compound word
comprehension
comprehension deficit
comprehension impairment, reading
comprehension skills
comprehension span
comprehension tests *(see also* tests)
Comprehensive Articulation Test
comprehensive assessment
Comprehensive Assessment of Symptoms and History (CASH)
Comprehensive Assessment Program
Comprehensive Developmental Evaluation Chart
Comprehensive Drinker Profile
comprehensive evaluation
Comprehensive Level of Consciousness Scale (CLCS)
comprehensive review
Comprehensive Teacher's Rating Scale
Comprehensive Test of Adaptive Behavior
Comprehensive Test of Basic Skills
Comprehensive Test of Visual Functioning (CTVF)
compressed speech
Compressed Speech Test
compression, brain stem
compression amplification
compression bone conduction
compromise formation
Compton Speech and Language Screening Evaluation
Compton-Hutton Phonological Assessment
compulsion
compulsive action
compulsive behavior
compulsive drug-taking behavior
compulsive mania
compulsive substance use
    pattern of
    signs of
compulsive thoughts
computed tomography (CT)
Computer Anxiety Index
Computer Aptitude, Literacy and Interest Profile
computer language
computer literacy test *(see also* tests)
Comrey Personality Scales
con-artists
concatenation
concentrating
    difficulty in
    subjective sense of difficulty

concentration
    disturbance in
    poor
concentration ability, impaired
concept
    abstract
    concrete
    critical band
    grandiose
    object
    self-role
    self-derogatory
concept formation tests *(see also tests)*
concept in medicine
concept of brain function, semi-autonomous systems
conceptual ability
conceptual disorder
Conceptual Series Completion Mental Status Test
conceptualization
concerns
    focus on
    health
    lack of abandonment
concerns about contracting an illness
concha (pl. conchae)
concha
    inferior nasal
    medial nasal
    nasal
concomitant of anxiety, physical
concrete concept
concrete operations period
concrete thought process(es)
concreteness
concurrent psychiatric problems
    alcoholism with cirrhosis and
    cancer and
    cardiovascular disease and
    gastrointestinal conditions and
    HIV infection and
    kidney disease and
    pulmonary disease and

concussion
    amnesic
    brain
concussion amnesia
concussion of brain (grades 1-3)
concussion syndrome, post
condenser
condescending evaluation
condition(s)
    abnormal pathologic
    dementia due to endocrine
    dementia due to hepatic
    dementia due to metabolic
    dementia due to neurological
    dermatological
    etiological neurological
    impaired
    living
    metabolic
    victim's
conditioned disintegration theory
conditioned disintegration theory of stuttering
conditioned orientation reflex audiometry (COR)
conditioned reinforcer
conditioned response
conditioned stimulus
conditioning
    counter
    eyelid
    phonological
    tangible reinforcement of operant (TROCA)
conditioning audiometry, tangible reinforcement operant (TROCA)
conditioning for sleep, negative
conduct and emotional problems testing *(see also tests)*
conduct disorder(s)
    adolescent onset type (F91.2)
    childhood-onset type (F91.1)
    disruptive impulse-control

conduct disorder(s)
    neuroleptic treatment of childhood
    undersocialized
    unspecified onset (F91.9)
    unspecified onset, with limited prosocial emotions (F91.9)
conductance
conduction
    air (AC)
    bone (BC)
    compression bone
    distortional bond
    ephaptic
    inertial bone
    motor nerve
    pure tone air
    pure tone bone
conduction studies, nerve
conduction test for hearing loss *(see also* tests)
conductive deafness
conductivity
"conductor" (street name, LSD)
cone of light
confabulate
confabulation of speech
confabulator
Conference, Hearing Aid Industry (HAIC)
confessions, false
confident, feeling
confident status
configuration(s)
    confused language
    dipper curve audiogram
    flat audiogram
    gradual falling curve audiogram
    gradual rising curve audiogram
    language
    marked falling curve audiogram
    saddle curve audiogram
    saucer curve audiogram

configuration(s)
    sharply falling curve audiogram
    ski slope curve audiogram
    steep curve audiogram
    sudden drop curve audiogram
    trough curve audiogram
    U-shaped curve audiogram
    waterfall curve audiogram
    word
confirmed/initial episode (C/I)
confirmed/subsequent episode (C/S)
conflict, emotional
Conflict Management Appraisal (CMA)
conflict resolution, internalizing style of
conflict-resolution strategies
conflict-resolving skills
Conflict Tactics Scale
conflict with the law
conflicting motives
conflicts, increased interpersonal
conflictual situation
conformity, social
confrontation naming test
confused language
confused language configuration
confusion
    cognate
    episodic
    gender
    nocturnal
    postictal
confusional arousal(s)
confusional arousals from sleep
confusional episode
confusional migraine headache
confusional seizure, ictal
congenital adrenal hyperplasia
congenital central alveolar hypoventilation (G47.35)
congenital deafness
congenital hydrocephalus
congenital hypertrophic pyloric stenosis

congenital intersex condition
congruent, mood
congruent affect
conjoiner (parts of speech)
conjunction (parts of speech)
"connect" (re: drug buyer or
    supplier)
connected speech
connectedness, family
Conners Hyperkinesis Index –
    Parent Form
Conners Hyperkinesis Index –
    Teacher Form
Conners Parent Rating Scale
Conners Rating Scale
Conners Teacher Rating Scale
connotation
conscientiousness
conscious awareness
conscious state, parasomniac
consciousness
    change in level of
    crude
    declining
    depression of
    discrimination
    disturbance in
    effect of trauma on
    episodic changes of
    impaired
    impairment of
    loss of
consequated
consequence(s)
    health-related
    high potential for painful
consequences of illness
consequences of stroke,
    psychiatric
consequences of suicidal behavior
consequences of suicidal thinking
conservation
    hearing
    speech
considered thought
consistency, perceptual
consistency effect
consistency effect of stuttering

consistent failure to speak
consistent irresponsibility
consolidated sleep
consonance
consonant(s)
    abutting
    arresting
    aspirate
    blend
    cluster
    compound
    deletion of final
    deletion of initial
    devoicing of final
    double
    flap
    flat
    fortis
    lax
    lenis
    nasal
    prevocalic voicing of
    releasing
    velarized
    vibrant
    voiced
    voiceless
consonantal feature English
    phoneme
consonantal sound
consonant blend
consonant cluster
consonant formation
    affricate
    continuant
    dark lateral
    frictionless
    fricative
    glide
    groove fricative
    implosive
    light lateral
    liquid
    nasal
    nonsonorant
    obstruent
    plosive
    retroflex

consonant formation
    semi-vowel
    sibilant
    slit fricative
    sonant
    sonorant
    spirant
    stop
    trill
consonant-injection method
consonant placement
    alveolar
    bilabial area
    glottal area
    labiodental area
    lingua-alveolar area
    linguadental area
    palatal area
    velar area
consonant position
    final
    initial
    intervocalic
    medial
    postvocalic
    prevocalic
consonant tests *(see also* tests)
consonant voicing
consonant-vowel (C-V)
consonant-vowel-consonant (C-V-C)
consonant-vowel-consonant syllable
consonant-vowel preference
consonant-vowel syllable
Consonant-Vowel Test (Dichotic
consort
constancy
constant anger
constant attention, need for
constant worry
constantly threatened, feeling
constellation of signs and symptoms
constellation of symptoms
constituent clause
constituent sentence

constituents
    immediate sentence
    sentence
constraint
constraints, semantic
constricted affect
constricted vocal production
constriction
    nares
    vocal
constriction of affect
constrictor
    inferior pharyngeal
    middle pharyngeal
constrictor muscle of pharynx
    inferior
    middle
    superior
constrictor pharyngis inferior, musculus
constrictor pharyngis medius, musculus
constrictor pharyngis superior, musculus
construct theory, personal
construction
    endocentric
    exocentric
    visual field
construction of femininity
construction of phrases
    absolute
    endocentric
    exocentric
Construction Test, Three-Dimensional Block (3DBCT)
consultation/liaison patient populations
consultation/liaison service, hospital
contact, genital sexual
contacts, hard
"contact lens" (street name, LSD)
contact ulcer
contact with reality, inconsistent
contamination

content
    dream
    grandiose
    language
    paucity of speech
    poverty of
    self-derogatory
    speech
    thought
Content Mastery Examinations for Educators (CMEE)
content scale
Content Scales (MMPI)
content speech, serial
content word
contentive word
context, phonetic
context reframing
contextual therapy
contiguity aphasia
contiguity disorder
contiguity disorder aphasia
continence, fecal
contingency management
continua seizure, epilepsia partialis
continuant
continuant consonant formation
continuant feature English phoneme
continued drinking
continued drinking pattern
continued evaluation, need for
continuing petit mal seizure
continuing sign of schizophrenia
continuity
    better sleep
    sleep
    specific sleep
    worse sleep
continuity disturbance, sleep
continuous course
continuous observation
continuous pain
continuous performance tetanic facilitation test
continuous period of illness

continuous reinforcement schedule
Continuous Visual Memory Test (CVMT)
continuum of care
contour(s)
    equal loudness
    intonation
contract
    formal
    group
    informal
    legal
    quasi
contracting an illness, concerns about
contraction, rhythmic
contraction headache, muscle
contractual behavior
contradictory information
contralateral neglect syndrome
contralateral reflex, acoustic
contralateral routing of signals (CROS)
    bilateral (BICROS)
    focal (FOCALCROS)
contralateral routing of signals hearing aid (CROS)
contrast sensitivity
contrastive analysis
contrastive distribution
contrastive linguistics
contrasts
    maximal
    minimal
contrasts processes, feature
Contrave (bupropion/naloxone)
contributing role
control
    acoustic gain
    automatic gain
    automatic volume (AVC)
    brain stem
    degree of
    diminished
    external
    feeling out of
    image

control
    impaired
    internal-external
    interpersonal
    island of
    lack of
    losing
    loss of
    manual volume
    mind
    need to
    neurological
    not in
    one's own
    outside
    rate
    sensation of lack of
    sense of being out of
    superego
    swing phase
    taking
    tone
    unable to
    ventilatory
control of the body, loss of
control of the mind, loss of
control others, need to
control problem, leaving parental
controlled drinking
controlled emotion
controlled environment
controlled release drug (CR)
controlling anger, difficulty
controlling external entities
controlling external spirits
controlling identity
controls, psycho-optical reflex
contusion
    brain
    cerebral
convergence circuit
conversation board
conversational postulates
conversion anesthesia
conversion aphonia
conversion deafness
conversion problem, faith
conversion seizure

conversion symptoms
Conversion V (MMPI)
conviction, delusional
conviction in civil or criminal
    court proceedings without
    imprisonment (Z65.0)
convolution
convulsion
    apoplectiform
    brain
    central
    cerebral
    cerebrospinal
    clonic
    coordinate
    eclamptic
    epileptic
    essential
    febrile
    generalized
    generalized tonic/clonic
    infantile
    local
    myoclonic
    paroxysmal
    puerperal
    recurrent
    reflex
    repetitive
    salaam
    spasmodic
    spontaneous
    tetanic
    tonic/clonic
    uncinate
    uremic
convulsive seizure
convulsive status epilepticus
co-occurrence of depression
co-occurring mental disorders
cooing
"cook" (re: heating heroin to
    prepare for injection)
"cook down" (re: liquefy heroin
    to prepare for injection)
"cooker" (re: drug injection)
"cookies" (street name, crack)

"cooler" (street name, drug-laced cigarette)
"coolie" (street name, cocaine-laced cigarette)
Cooperation Preschool Inventory—Revised
Cooper-Farran Behavioral Rating Scales (CFBRS)
Cooper-MacGuire Diagnostic Word Analysis Test
Coopersmith Self-Esteem Inventories
coordinate convulsion
coordination
    impaired
    subaverage motor
    visual-motor
coordination disorder, developmental
"cop" (re: to obtain drugs)
COPES (Community-Oriented Programs Environment Scale)
"co-pilot" (street name, amphetamine)
coping, rational/cognitive
coping ability
coping assessments (see also tests)
Coping Resources Inventory (CRI)
coping strategies
coping style
coping style, extratensive
Coping with Stress
Coping with Tests
"copping zone" (re: drug-buying area)
coprolalomania (foul language)
COPSystem Interest Inventory
copula
copy geometric designs test
copy intersecting pentagons test
coquetting, flirting and
COR (conditioned orientation reflex audiometry)
"coral" (street name, barbiturate)
cordectomy
cords, vocal
core body temperature
core body temperature measurement
core vocabulary
"coriander seeds" (re: currency)
"cork the air" (re: cocaine use)
Cornell Critical Thinking Tests
Cornell Scale for Depression/Dementia (CSDD)
corniculate cartilage(s)
coronal feature English phoneme
coronal orientation
coronal plane
Coronavirus Disease 2019 (COVID-19)
coronavirus pandemic
corporal agnosia
corpus (pl. corpora)
corpus callosum
correction, speech
Correctional Institutions Environment Scale
Correctional Officers' Interest Blank
correctionist, speech
corrective feedback
correlates, psycho-physiologic
correlation
    negative
    Pearson product-moment coefficient of
    positive
"Corrinne" (street name, cocaine)
cortex (pl. cortices)
    association
    auditory
    cerebellar
    cerebral
    deep
    motor
    primary auditory
    sensory
cortical aphasia
cortical apraxia
cortical deafness
cortical dysfunction
    higher
    posttraumatic

cortical epilepsy
cortical evoked potential
cortical function, mapping of
cortical gray matter
cortical lateralization
cortical mapping
cortical respiration
cortical sensory loss
cortical testing
cortical thumb position
cortices
corticoadrenal insufficiency
cortisol secretion
COS (Campbell Organizational Survey)
"cosa" (street name, cannabis/marijuana)
cosine wave
costarum, musculi levatores
Costen's syndrome
costumed character
Cotard delusion
"cotics" (street name, heroin)
"coties" (street name, codeine)
cotinine
"cotton" (re: currency)
"cotton brothers" (street name, cocaine, heroin and morphine)
coulomb (Q)
counseling, sex (Z70.9)
counseling and development inventories *see also* tests)
counseling (consultation), other (Z71.9)
counselor
    camp
    child
    couples
    disability
    drug
    family
    genetic
    grief
    individual
    legal
    marital
    marriage
    pastoral

counselor
    personal
    professional
    rehabilitation
    school
    spiritual
    substance abuse
    youth
count, word
count backwards from 100 test
counter conditioning
counting-money tremor
coup de glotte
coupler
couples counselor
Couple's Pre-Counseling Inventory
coupling
coupling, nasal
"courage pills" (street name, heroin; barbiturate)
course
    atypical clinical
    continuous
    episodic
    rapid-cycling
"course note" (re: currency)
course of abuse, long-term
course of action
course of illness
course of treatment
course patterns, prototypical
courtship behavior
covert feelings
covert resistance, overt compliance masking
covert response
COVID-19 (Coronavirus Disease 2019)
COVID-19 Peritraumatic Distress Index (CPDI)
"Cozmo's" (street name, phencyclidine)
C-PAC (Clinical Probes of Articulation Consistency)
CPDI (COVID-19 Peritraumatic Distress Index)
CPDI score

Psychiatric Words and Phrases

CPRS (Conners Parent Rating Scale)
CPS (complex partial seizure)
cps (cycle per second) tremor
CPS (cycles per second)
CR (controlled release)
crack (processed cocaine) (street names)
   151
   24-7
   2-for-1 sale
   3750
   51
   apple jack(s)
   B.J.s or BJs
   Baby T
   back-to-back
   bad
   bag bride
   ball
   basa
   base
   base crazies
   base head
   baseball
   basing
   Batman
   bazooka
   Beam me up Scottie
   beamer(s)
   beans
   beat
   beat vials
   beautiful boulders
   Bebe
   bedrock
   beemers
   Bill Blass
   bings
   biscuit
   black rock
   blast
   blotter
   blowcaine
   blowout
   blowup
   blue
   bobo
crack (street names)
   body packer
   body stuffer
   bollo
   bolo
   bomb
   bomb squad
   bone
   bonecrusher
   bones
   boost
   bopper
   botray
   bottles
   boubou
   boulder
   boulya
   breakdown
   brick
   bubble gum
   buda
   buffer
   bullia capital
   bullion
   bump
   bumper
   bunk
   butler
   butter
   caine
   cakes
   candy
   cap(s)
   capsula (Spanish)
   carburetor
   carpet patrol
   Casper
   Casper the ghost
   caviar
   CDs
   chalk
   chaser
   chasing the dragon
   cheap basing
   chemical
   chewies
   chicken scratch
   chocolate ecstasy

crack (street names)
- chocolate rock
- chronic
- cigamos
- clicker
- climax
- clocker
- cloud
- cloud nine
- cluck
- cock snow
- cocktail
- coco rocks
- coke
- comeback
- cookies
- cooking up
- crack attack
- crack back
- crack bash
- crack cooler
- crack gallery
- crack house
- crack spot
- cracker jack(s)
- crank
- credit card
- crib
- crimmie
- croak
- crumbs
- crunch and munch
- cubes
- demo
- demolish
- devil drug
- devil's dandruff
- devilsmoke
- dime
- dime special
- dip
- dipping out
- dirty basing
- dirty joints
- DOA
- dope fiend
- doub
- double rock

crack (street names)
- double up
- double u-s
- double yoke
- dove
- dragon roc
- dub
- Eastside player
- egg
- eightball
- Electric Kool Aid
- eye opener
- famous dimes
- fat bags
- feenin
- fifty-one
- fire
- fish scales
- flat chunks
- fleece
- flex
- freebase
- freebasing
- French fries
- fries
- fry
- fry daddy
- gank
- garbage heads
- garbage rock
- geek
- geek joints
- geeker
- ghostbusting
- gick monster
- gimmie
- girl
- glo
- gold
- golf ball
- gone
- gravel
- grit
- groceries
- hail
- half a football field
- half track
- hamburger helper

crack (street names)
    handlebars
    hand-to-hand man
    hard ball
    hard line
    hard rock
    hell
    henpecking
    hit
    hotcakes
    house fee
    house piece
    How do you like me now?
    hubba
    hubba pigeon
    Hubba, I am back
    hubbas
    I am back
    ice
    ice cube
    interplanetary mission
    issues
    jelly beans
    Johnson
    juice joint
    jum
    jumbos
    kabuki
    kangaroo
    kibbles and bits
    kissing
    Klingons
    Kokomo
    Kryptonite
    Lamborghini
    liprimo
    love
    Ma'a
    Masarati
    mission
    mist
    mixed jive
    moonrock
    morning wakeup
    nickelodians
    nontoucher
    nuggets
    on a mission

crack (street names)
    one bomb
    one tissue box
    one-fifty-one
    onion
    outer limits
    ozone
    parachute
    parlay
    paste
    patico
    P-dogs
    pebbles
    Pee Wee
    perp
    P-funk
    pianoing
    picking
    piece
    piedras
    piles
    pimp your pipe
    pipe
    pony
    potato chips
    power puffer
    premos
    press
    prime time
    primo
    primo square
    primo turbo
    product
    pseudocaine
    puffer
    pullers
    pumping
    purple caps
    purple haze
    pusher
    raspberry
    raw
    ready rock
    real tops
    red caps
    regular P
    res
    rest in peace

crack (street names)
- ringer
- roca (Spanish)
- rock attack
- rock house
- rock star
- rocks of hell
- Rocky III
- rooster
- rox
- Roxanne
- Roz
- schoolcraft
- Scotty
- scramble
- scrape and snort
- scruples
- seconds
- server
- Seven-up
- shabu
- sheet rocking
- Sherman stick
- sherms
- shot to the curb
- sixty-two
- skeegers/skeezers
- slab
- sleet
- smoke
- smoke house
- snow coke
- soap
- soup
- space
- space base
- spaceball
- speed
- speedball
- speedboat
- square time Bob
- squirrel
- stacks
- steerer
- stem
- stones
- strawberry
- sugar

crack (street names)
- sugar block
- swell up
- tar
- taxing
- teardrops
- teeth
- tension
- the devil
- thing
- thirst monster(s)
- thirty-eight
- tissue
- top gun
- torpedo
- toss up(s)
- toucher
- tragic magic
- trey
- troop
- turbo
- tweak mission
- tweaker
- tweaking
- tweaks
- twenties
- two for nine
- ultimate
- uzi
- wave
- weightless
- whack
- white ball
- white cloud
- white ghost
- white stick
- white sugar
- white tornado
- window pane
- wollie
- woolah
- woolas
- woolie blunt
- woolies
- wooly blunts
- wooties
- working
- working bags

crack (street names)
   working fifty
   working half
   wrecking crew
   yahoo/yeaho
   Yale
   yam
   yay
   yayoo
   yeah-O
   yeo
   yeola
   yimyom
   zoomer
   zulu
"crack attack" (re: crack craving)
"crack back" (street name, crack and cannabis)
crack/benzocaine (street names)
   flat chunks
   potato chips
crack/cannabis (street names)
   crack back
   fry daddy
   geek
   gimmie
   torpedo
   turbo
crack/cocaine, "blowcaine"
"crack cooler" (street name, crack soaked in wine cooler)
"cracker jack" (street name, crack cocaine)
"cracker jacks" (re: crack users)
"crackers" (street name, LSD)
"crack gallery" (re: crack-buying place)
crack/heroin (street names)
   casing the dragon
   lightball
   moonrock
"crack kits" (re: glace pipes and copper mesh)
crack-laced cigarette (street names)
   cocktail
   crimmie
   fry daddy

crack/lidocaine, "blow up"
crack/LSD (street names)
   outer limits
   sheet rocking
crack/methamphetamine (street names)
   croak
   fire
crack/PCP (street names)
   beam me up Scottie
   double rock
   missile basing
   parachute
   P-funk
   space base
   space cadet
   space dust
   tragic magic
"crack spot" (re: crack-buying place)
cradle audiometry, neonatal auditory response
cradle, neonatal auditory response
cramp, writer's
cramping pain
cranial aneurysm
cranial nerve abnormalities
cranial nerve deficit
cranial nerve I (olfactory)
cranial nerve II (optic)
cranial nerve III (oculomotor)
cranial nerve IV (trochlear)
cranial nerve V (trigeminal)
cranial nerve VI (abducens)
cranial nerve VII (facial)
cranial nerve VIII (auditory)
cranial nerve IX (glossopharyngeal)
cranial nerve X (vagus)
cranial nerve XI (spinal accessory)
cranial nerve XII (hypoglossal)
cranial nerve involvement
cranial nerve palsy
craniocerebral trauma
craniofacial anomalies
craniopharyngeal canal

"crank" (street name, methamphetamine; amphetamine; methcathinone)
"cranking up" (re: drug injection)
"crankster" (re: user or maker of methamphetamine)
cranky mood
"crap/crop" (re: low quality heroin)
"crash" (re: sleep off effect of drugs)
"crash" (street name, cocaine)
craving
    cue-elicited cocaine
    drug
"crazy coke" (street name, phencyclidine)
"Crazy Eddie" (street name, phencyclidine)
"crazy weed" (street name, cannabis/marijuana)
CRC (cross-reacting cannabinoids)
Creative Perception Inventory, Khatena-Torrance
Creative Talent, Group Inventory for Finding
Creatively in Action and Motion, Thinking
creativeness
Creativity Assessment Packet
Creativity Checklist
"credit card" (re: crack equipment)
creeping-crawling sensation
cremnomania (precipices)
crepuscular state
crescendo-decrescendo breathing
cresomania (dramatic buildup/climax)
crest, acoustic
Creutzfeldt-Jakob disease
CRI (Coping Resources Inventory)
cri du chat syndrome
"crib" (street name, crack)
crib-o-gram
crib-o-gram audiometer

cricoarytenoid ankylosis
cricoarytenoid joint
cricoarytenoid muscle
    lateral
    posterior
cricoarytenoideus lateralis, musculus
cricoarytenoideus posterior, musculus
cricoid cartilage
cricothyroid muscle
cricothyroid paralysis
cricothyroideus, musculus
cri-du-chat syndrome
crime
    multiple personality
    victim of
crime-ridden neighborhood, living in a
criminal behavior, adult
Criminal Responsibility Scale, Rogers
criminal sex acts
"crimmie" (street name, crack-laced cigarette)
"crink" (street name, methamphetamine)
"cripple" (street name, cannabis/marijuana cigarette)
"cris" (street name, methamphetamine)
cris-CROS (contralateral routing of signals)
crisis
    bed
    oculogyric
    parkinsonian
crisis management of recurrent suicidal behavior
"crisscross" (street name, amphetamine)
criss-crossing (re: parallel lines of cocaine and heroin to snort)
"Cristal" (street name, ecstasy/MDMA)
"Cristina" (street name, methamphetamine)

Psychiatric Words and Phrases

"Cristy" (street name, smokable methamphetamine)
criteria
    abuse
    equivalent
    equivalent intoxication
    equivalent withdrawal
    full symptom
    method of defining
    relevant diagnostic
criteria set, single
criterion
    behavioral
    evaluation of
    impairment
criterion-referenced test
criterion B for dysthymic disorder, alternative
criterion related validity
Criterion Test of Basic Skills
critical band concept
critical period of learning
Critical Reasoning Tests (CRT)
critical submodalities
critical thinking tests *(see also* tests*)*
criticism, fear of
Crk protein
"croak" (street name, crack and methamphetamine)
CROS (contralateral routing of signals)
    binaural
    high (HICROS) frequency
CROS hearing aid
cross-bite
cross-bite malposition of teeth
cross-consonant injection method
cross-dress
cross-dressing
    complete
    forced
    motivation for
    partial
cross-dressing behavior
cross dressing in childhood
cross-dressing skill
cross-gender activity

cross-gender behavior
    adolescent
    adult
    childhood
cross-gender behavior patterns
cross-gender identification
cross-gender interests
cross-gender wishes
cross hearing
cross-modality perception
cross-over mirroring
cross-sex roles
cross-talk
"cross tops" (street name, amphetamine)
crossed laterality
"crossroads" (street name, amphetamine)
croup
    inflammatory
    spasmodic
croupous laryngitis
crowding
"crown crap" (street name, heroin)
CRS (Clinical Rating Scale)
CRT (Critical Reasoning Tests)
crude consciousness
"crumbs" (re: tiny pieces of crack)
"crunch and munch" (street name, crack)
crural ataxia
crus (pl. crura)
"Cruz" (street name, opium from Veracruz, Mexico)
cry, birth
"crying weed" (street name, cannabis/marijuana)
cryomania (cold)
"crypto" (street name, methamphetamine)
cryptococcal meningitis
cryptogenic seizure
"crystal" (street name, methamphetamine; PCP; amphetamine; cocaine)

"crystal joint" (street name, phencyclidine)
"crystal meth" (street name, methamphetamine)
"crystal methadrine" (street name, methamphetamine; MDMA)
"crystal T" (street name, phencyclidine)
"crystal tea" (street name, LSD)
(C/S) confirmed/subsequent episode
CSDD (Cornell Scale of for Depression, Dementia)
CSRI (Caregiver's School Readiness Inventory)
CT (computed tomography)
CT (corrective therapy)
CTRS (Conners Teacher Rating Scale)
CTVF (Comprehensive Test of Visual Functioning)
"cube" (re: 1 ounce LSD)
"cubes" (street name, cannabis/marijuana tablets)
cue(s)
    accessing
    auditory
    eye accessing
    learning
    kinesthetic
    visual
cue-elicited cocaine craving
cued by an object
cued speech
cul-de-sac
cul de sac voice disorder
"culican" (street name, cannabis/marijuana)
cult of manhood
cults, killer
cultural adjustment
cultural adjustment following migration
cultural assessment
cultural attitudes
cultural background, evaluation of
cultural belief
cultural content of evaluation
cultural differences
cultural elements
cultural experience
cultural explanations for illness
cultural factors
cultural features
cultural formulation
cultural identity
cultural information
Cultural Literacy Test
cultural norm(s)
cultural reference group
cultural-related standards of sexual behavior
cultural setting
cultural training
culturally appropriate avoidant behavior
culturally appropriate shy behavior
culturally bound syndromes
culturally prescribed ritual behavior
culturally sanctioned behavior
culturally sanctioned experience
culturally sanctioned response
culturally unsanctioned response
culture
    host
    individual's
    industrialized
    person's
    street-drug
culture area
culture-bound belief
culture-bound syndrome (CBS)
culture features, specific
Culture-Free Self-Esteem Inventories for Children and Adults
culture of candor
culture of origin
culture-related features
Culture Shock Inventory
culture-specific features
cuneiform cartilage(s)
cunning and hiding behavior
"cupcakes" (street name, LSD)

"cura" (street name, heroin)
current
    alternating (AC)
    direct (DC)
current cognitive status
current defense level
current drug toxicity
current episode
current state
current tics
Curriculum Achievement Levels Test Scaled (SCALE)
cursing
Curtis Completion Form
Curtis Interest Scale
curve
    articulation
    bell-shaped
    dipper
    discrimination
    falling
    frequency response
    gaussian
    gradual falling
    gradual rising
    marked falling
    normal
    normal probability
    probability
    saddle
    saucer
    shadow
    sharply falling
    ski slope
    steep
    steep drop
    sudden drop
    trough
    U-shaped
    waterfall
curve audiogram configurations
    dipper
    gradual falling
    gradual rising
    marked falling
    saddle
    saucer
    sharply falling

curve audiogram configurations
    ski slope
    steep
    sudden drop
    trough
    U-shaped
    waterfall
curve discrimination
"cushion" (re: drug injection)
cuspid teeth
Custody Quotient
"cut" (re: adulterate drugs)
cut, visual field
"cut-deck" (street name, heroin mixed with powdered milk)
cuts
cutting
CV (consonant-vowel)
C-V (consonant-vowel)
CVA (stroke)
CVC (consonant-vowel-consonant)
C-V-C (consonant-vowel-consonant)
CVMT (Continuous Visual Memory Test)
cyanosis
cybermotion sickness
cybernetic theory of stuttering
cycle(s)
    desire phase of sexual response
    duration duty
    excitement phase of sexual response
    glottal
    menstrual
    orgasmic phase of sexual response
    phase shift of sleep-wake
    resolution phase of sexual response
    sexual response
    short
    sleep
    sleep-wake
    sleep-wakefulness
    sleep-waking

cycle(s)
    vibratory
    vicious
cycle and occurrence of seizure, sleep-waking
cycle change, life
cycle noise hum, sixth
cycle per second (cps) tremor
cycles per second (CPS)
cyclical pattern of symptoms
"cycline" (street name, PCP/phencyclidine)
cycling
    mood disorder with rapid
    rapid
"cyclones" (street name, PCP/phencyclidine)
cyclothymic disorder (F34.0)
cynomania (dogs)
cyst, acoustic
cystic fibrosis
cytoskeleton
Czechoslovakian viral encephalitis

D

"D" (street name, LSD)
DAB-2 (Diagnostic Achievement Battery, Second Edition)
"dabble" (re: drug use)
Daberon Screening for School Readiness
dactyl speech
dactylology
Daily Coping Assessment, Stone and Neale
daily living
Daily Living, Communicative Abilities in (CADL)
daily symptom ratings
daily treatment
dam, dental
"dama blanca" (street name, cocaine)
damage
    brain
    brain cell
damaged, feeling permanently
damaged hair follicles
damped wave
damping
"dance fever" (street name, fentanyl)
danger, feelings of
dangerous behavior reaction
dancing mania
Dantomania (writings of Dante)
DAP (Diversity Awareness Profile)
DAP:SPED (Draw A Person: Screening Procedure for Emotional Disturbance)
DAR (Diagnostic Assessments of Reading)
dark environment
dark lateral consonant formation
darkening of vision
DARS (The Child "At Risk" for Drug Abuse Rating Scale)
DART Phonics Testing Program (Diagnostic and Achievement Tests)
DAT (Differential Aptitude Tests)
data
    available
    collected
    empirical
    epidemiological
    field
    insufficient
    laboratory
    long-term
    NIMH
    normative
    reanalyzed
    recent
    survey
data collection, complete
data reanalysis strategy
data sets
date test, name the
dative case (parts of speech)
"dawa mesk" (street name, cannabis/marijuana)
day of month test
daytime fatigue
daytime functioning, impaired
daytime mouth breathing
daytime sedation
daytime sleep episodes
daytime sleep episodes, unintentional
daytime sleepiness
dB (decibel)
DBD (Dementia Behavior Disturbance Scale)
DBSA (Depression and Bipolar Support Alliance)
DBT (dialectical behavior therapy)
DBT distress tolerance skill
DBT group therapy/skills training
DBT individual therapy
DBT phone coaching

DBT therapist consultation team
DC (direct current)
de Lange syndrome
"dead on arrival" (street name, heroin)
dead room (no-echo chamber)
deadness, emotional
Deaf
    Central Institute for the (CID)
    National Association for the
    telephone device for the (TDD)
deaf mute
Deaf Preschool Performance Scale
deaf speech
deafferentiation
deafness
    acoustic trauma
    adventitious
    Alexander's
    autosomal dominant cerebellar ataxia, and narcolepsy (G47.419)
    boilermaker's
    catarrhal
    central
    conductive
    congenital
    conversion
    cortical
    functional
    HF
    high frequency
    industrial
    labyrinthine
    low tone
    midbrain
    mixed
    Mondini
    nerve
    noise-induced
    nonorganic
    occupational
    organic
    perceptive

deafness
    postlingual
    prelingual
    prevocational
    psychogenic
    pure word
    retrocochlear
    Scheibe
    sensorineural
    tone
    toxic
dealing, drug
death
    attitude to
    brain
    cause of
    cerebral
    cerebral brain
    expectation of
    fear of
    hypoxyphilia-caused
    impending
    nerve cell
    news of
    premature
    preoccupation with
    reaction to
    sudden sniffing
    suffering
    survivors of
    thoughts of
    threat of
    unexpected
    violent
death from suicide
death rate
death syndrome, brain
death wish, Klein's
debilitating anxiety
"decadence" (street name, methylenedioxy-methamphetamine)
"deca-duabolin" (re: injectable steroid)
decay
    acoustic reflex
    tone
decay period

decay rate
Decay Test, Tone
"decadence" (street name,
   amphetamine/
   methamphetamine)
deceit
   biology of
   detection of
   determinants of
   technological detection of
deceitfulness, therapeutic
   approaches for
decentration
deception, effects of
decibel (dB)
deciduous molar
   first
   second
deciduous teeth
Decision, Tarasoff
decision making assessments
Decision Making Inventory
Decision-Making Organizer
decision-making process
Decision-Making System
decision scale *(see also* tests)
decision theory
decision trees
"deck" (re: 1 to 15 grams of
   heroin; a packet of drugs)
declarative sentence
decline
   age-related cognitive
   Rating Scale of
     Communication in
     Cognitive (RSCCD)
decline in academic functioning,
   marked
decline in classroom performance
decline in occupational
   functioning, marked
decline in performance
decline problems, age-related
   cognitive
declining consciousness
decoder
Decoding Skills Test
deconditioning

decreased activity
decreased arm swing
decreased effectiveness
decreased energy
decreased fluency of speech
decreased frequency
decreased interest
decreased interest in usual
   activities
decreased motivation
decreased need for sleep
decreased peripheral sensation
decreased productivity
decreased productivity of speech
decreased reactivity to
   environment
decreased sleep
decussation
deduction
"deeda" (street name, LSD)
deep articulation test
deep cortex
deep emptiness, feelings of
deep sensation
deep sleep
deep structure
deep tendon reflexes,
   exaggeration of
Deep Test of Articulation:
   Screening
deep trance identification
de-escalating aggressive behavior
defect
   body dysmorphic
   camouflage the
   developmental
   exaggerated
   excessive concern for
   imagined
   physical
   preoccupation with
   slight
   speech
   visual field
defenestrated
defense level, current
defensive dysregulation, level of
defensive functioning axis

Defensive Functioning Scale
   (DFS)
deficiency (pl. deficiencies)
      dementia due to vitamin
      environmental
      hearing
      hypocretin
      nutritional
      vitamin
      vitamin B12
deficiency anemia, iron
deficient sexual desire
deficit
      attention
      central language
      central sensory
      cognitive
      comprehension
      cranial nerve
      emotional
      gaze
      global cognitive
      gross neurologic
      language
      linguistic
      mental
      motor
      multiple cognitive
      neural
      neurologic
      sensory
      speech perception
      speech-motor
deficit of symptoms
deficit symptoms
defining criteria, method of
definition, categorical
deformed bones
degeneration
      axon
      brain
      cerebellar
      granulovascular
      olivopontocerebellar
degeneration of the true folds,
   polypoid
degenerative dementia, primary

degenerative disease
      inherited progressive
      progressive
deglutition
degree of amnesia
degree of control
degree of disability
Degrees of Reading Power (DRP)
deictic
deity or famous person, themes of
   special relationship to a
deixis
      person
      place
      time
déjà vu aura
dejected mood
dejection, feeling of
Dejerine syndrome
Del Rio Language Screening Test:
   English/Spanish
"delatestryl" (re: injectable
   steroid)
delay, developmental
delayed auditory feedback (DAF)
delayed auditory feedback,
   experimentally
delayed development
delayed ejaculation (lifetime,
   acquired, generalized,
   situational; F52.32)
delayed feedback audiometry
   (DFA)
delayed language
delayed reflex
delayed reinforcer
delayed response
delayed sleep phase syndrome
delayed sleep phase type
   dyssomnia
delayed speech
delayed toilet training
deletion
      stridency
      syllable
      unstressed syllable
      weak syllable

Psychiatric Words and Phrases

deletion of final consonant
deletion of initial consonant
deletion of unstressed syllables
deliberate fire setting
deliberate therapy
Delineator, Gregorc Style
delirious mania
delirium *(see also* intoxication
   delirium)
        alcohol intoxication
        amphetamine intoxication
        anticholinergic
        anxiolytic intoxication
        anxiolytic withdrawal
        cannabis intoxication
        cocaine intoxication
        digitalis-induced
        full-blown
        hallucinogen intoxication
        hypnotic intoxication
        hypnotic withdrawal
        hypoglycemic
        inhalant intoxication
        medication-induced
        opioid intoxication
        other specified (R41.0)
        phencyclidine intoxication
        sedative intoxication
        sedative withdrawal
        substance intoxication
        substance withdrawal
        substance-induced
        superimposed
        trauma-induced
        unspecified (R41.0)
delirium and concurrent
  psychiatric problems
delirium due to another medical
  condition
        acute or persistent
          hyperactive (F05)
        acute or persistent mixed
          level of activity (F05)
delirium due to GMC
delirium due to hepatic
  encephalopathy
delirium due to multiple etiologies
    acute or persistent
      hyperactive (F05)
    acute or persistent
      hypoactive (F05)
delirium due to multiple etiologies
    acute or persistent mixed
      level of activity (F05)
delirium-like state
delirium-related disorder
delirium-related mental disorder
delta activity, EEG
delta index
delta 9 THC
delta opiate receptors
delta receptors
delta rhythm
delta wave(s)
delusion(s)
    alcohol-induced psychotic
      disorder with
    amphetamine-induced
      psychotic disorder with
    cannabis-induced psychotic
      disorder with
    circumscribed
    cocaine-induced psychotic
      disorder with
    Cotard
    erotomanic type
    established
    expressive
    fist rank symptoms of
    focus of the
    Fregoli
    grandiose type
    jealous type
    mixed type
    monothematic
    mood-incongruent
    non-bizarre
    object of a
    persecutory type
    referential
    somatic type
    unspecified type

delusional behavior
delusional belief
    dominant
    shared
delusional conviction
delusional disorder (F22)
    continuous (F22)
    erotomanic type of (F22)
    first episode currently acute (F22)
    first episode in full remission (F22)
    first episode in partial remission (F22)
    grandiose type of (F22)
    jealous type of (F22)
    mixed type of (F22)
    multiple episodes of (F22)
    persecutory type of (F22)
    somatic type of (F22)
    unspecified type of (F22)
delusional disorder with abnormal psychomotor behavior (F22)
delusional disorder with bizarre content (F22)
delusional disorder with delusions (F22)
delusional disorder with depression (F22)
delusional disorder with disorganized speech (F22)
delusional disorder with hallucinations (F22)
delusional disorder with impaired cognition (F22)
delusional disorder with manic symptoms (F22)
delusional disorder with negative symptoms (F22)
delusional equivalent
delusional interpretation of a perceptual disturbance
delusional jealousy
delusional misidentification syndromes (DMS)
delusional network
delusional projection
delusional proportions
delusional system, focus of
delusional thinking
delusional thoughts
delusions in schizophrenia, fragmentary
delusions of control
demands of society
demarcated relationships, clearly
demarcation in sensory testing, level of
dementia
    advanced
    alcohol-induced persisting
    Alzheimer's type senile (SDAT)
    atrophic
    beclouded
    behavioral management of
    early
    ethical aspects of
    evaluation of
    familial
    frontal lobe
    global
    HIV-based
    impairments of
    lacunar
    language disorder in
    legal aspects of
    neuropsychological evaluation of
    onset of
dementia, persisting
    pharmacological management of
    pharmacological treatment of
    Pike
    preexisting
    primary degenerative
    psychobiological process of
    psychological management of
    remitting
    severe
    stages of
    static
    subcortical

dementia
   substance-induced
      persisting
   traumatic
   vascular
Dementia Behavior Disturbance
  Scale (DBD)
dementia complex, AIDS (ADC)
dementia due to:
   Alzheimer's disease
   anoxia
   brain tumor
   endocrine conditions
   hepatic conditions
   Huntington's disease
   immune disorders
   infectious disorders
   metabolic conditions
   neurological conditions
   normal-pressure
    hydrocephalus
   Parkinson's disease
   Pick's disease
   prion diseases
   traumatic brain injury
   vitamin deficiencies
Dementia Mood Assessment
  Scale (DMAS)
Dementia Rating Scale (DRS)
dementia-related behavior
dementia-related disorder
dementia-related mental disorder
dementing illness, progressive
dementing processes
"demo" (re: sample quantity of
  crack; crack equipment)
"demolish" (street name, crack)
demomania (people)
demonomania (demons)
demonstrative-entity
demyelinating encephalopathy
denasality voice disorder
denasalization
dendrite
dendrophobia
denervation
    autonomic
    level of

denial, psychotic
denigrated self-esteem
denotation
dense scotoma
dense sensory loss
density
dental anxiety
dental arch
dental caries
dental dam
dental erosion
dental lisp
dentition
denuding, hair
Denver Prescreening
  Development Questionnaire
Depade (naltrexone)
depalatalization
Department of Health and Human
  Services (U.S.)
dependence
   analgesic drug
   cannabis
   emotional
   GBH (amino acid
    concoction)
   inhalant
   long-term
   reward
   substance
   substance dependence with
    physiological
   substance dependence
    without physiological
   tendency for
dependence-independence, field
dependency needs, unmet
dependent care, inappropriate
dependent character
dependent clause
dependent personality disorder
  (F60.7)
depersonalization
depersonalization experience
depersonalization/derealization
  disorder (F48.1)
depletion, metabolic volume
depolarizing muscle relaxants

depreciated subsystem
depressant, brain
depressants (street names)
    backwards
    bam
    bambs
    Barb
    Barbies
    beans
    black bandit pills
    black beauties
    block busters
    blue
    blue angels
    blue birds
    blue bullets
    blue clouds
    blue devil
    blue dolls
    blue heavens
    blue tips
    bombido
    bombita
    busters
    candy
    chorals
    Christmas rolls
    Christmas tree
    coral
    courage pills
    disco biscuit(s)
    dolls
    double trouble
    gangster pills
    golf balls
    goofers
    gorilla pills
    green dragons
    green frog
    idiot pills
    in betweens
    jellies
    jelly bean
    joy juice
    King Kong pills
    lay back
    lib (Librium)
    little bomb

depressants (street names)
    love drug
    ludes
    luding out
    luds
    M&M
    marshmallow reds
    Mexican reds
    Mickey Finn
    Mickey's
    Mighty Joe Young
    Mother's little helper
    nebbies
    nemmies
    nimbies
    no worries
    on the nod
    pancakes and syrup
    peanut
    Peter
    purple hearts
    Q
    quads
    quas
    rainbows
    red and blue
    red bullets
    red devil
    red rock opium
    red rum
    red stuff
    reds
    schoolboy
    seccy
    seggy
    sleeper
    sleeper and red devil
    slumber
    softballs
    sopers
    speedballing
    stoppers
    strawberries
    tooles
    tooties
    tranq
    tuie
    Uncle Milty

depressants (street names)
    ups and downs
    V
    yellow
    yellow bullets
    yellows
depressed
    economically
    feeling
depressed mood
    adjustment disorder with
    adjustment disorder with mixed anxiety and
    markedly
depressed reflex
depressiform
depression
    biologic sign
    co-occurrence of
    double
    episodes of
    exogenous
    history of
    marked
    moderate
    opticochiasmatic
    periods of
    post partum major
    post psychotic
    postictal
    postpsychotic
    psychoanalysis and
    risk for
    severe
    somatic treatment for
    symptoms of
    unipolar
depression disorder of schizophrenia, postpsychotic
depression episode, single major
depression in epilepsy
depression inventories *(see also* tests)
depression of consciousness
depression phase of seizure, past ictal
depression questionnaires *(see also* tests)
depression rating scales *(see also* tests)
depression-related disorder
depression-related mental disorder
depression scale
    adolescent
    children's
    geriatric
    hospital anxiety and
depressive affect
depressive disorder *(see also* major depressive disorder; persistent depressive disorder)
    medication/substance-induced
    minor
    other specified (F32.8)
    postpsychotic
    recurrent brief
    unspecified (F32.9)
depressive disorder due to another medical condition with depressive features (F06.31)
depressive disorder due to another medical condition with major depressive-like episode (F06.32)
depressive disorder due to another medical condition with mixed features (F06.34)
depressive disorder of schizophrenia, postpsychotic
depressive episode
depressive episode, pattern of major
depressive experience
depressive feelings
depressive personality disorder
depressive phase
depressive symptoms, frequency of
depressive symptoms in schizophrenia
depressors
deprivation
    environmental
    food
    paternal

deprivation
    psychosocial
    severe environmental
    sleep
    water
"dep-testosterone" (re: injectable steroid)
depth of sleep
depth perception
derailment
    actual
    frequent
    speech
derangements, metabolic
derealization (a panic attack indicator)
derealization, feelings of
derealization/depersonalization disorder (F48.1)
derivation, sentence
derivation of a sentence
derived adjective
derived sentence
dermatological conditions
dermatophobia
DES (Dissociative Experiences Scale)
descending pitch brake
descending technique
descending technique audiometry
descent through non-REM to REM
Description of Body Scale
descriptive approach
descriptive features
descriptive linguistics
descriptive phonetics
descriptive validity
descriptor for preschool and kindergarten interests *see* test
descriptors for schizophrenia, alternative dimensional
desensitization
desensitization, psychologic
deserved punishment
design
    human
    Kohs Block

design
    study
design tests (*see also* tests)
designer drugs (street names)
    45 minute psychosis
    Adam
    alpha-ET
    AMT
    apache
    banana split
    bath salts
    bathtub speed
    B-bombs
    BDMPEA
    bean
    bens
    Benzedrine
    biphetamine
    black hole
    blue kisses
    blue lips
    bromo
    bump
    businessman's LSD
    businessman's special
    businessman's trip
    Cadillac express
    candy raver
    cat
    cat valium
    change
    clarity
    cloud nine
    crank
    cristal (Spanish)
    dance fever
    dead road
    debs
    decadence
    DET
    dex
    Dexedrine
    diamonds
    disco biscuit(s)
    DMT
    doctor
    dolls
    domex

Psychiatric Words and Phrases

designer drugs (street names)
- drivers
- ecstasy
- ephedrone
- essence
- exiticity
- fantasia
- fastin
- forget me drug
- forget pill
- friend
- gagers
- gaggers
- gaggier
- Georgia home boy
- GHB
- Go
- Go-fast
- goob
- goodfellas
- gravel
- great bear
- green
- greenies
- grievous bodily harm
- gum
- GWM
- happy drug
- happy pill
- hawkers
- he-man
- herbal bliss
- iboga
- ice
- ivory wave
- jackpot
- jet
- K2
- ket
- K-hole
- king ivory
- kit kat
- Kleenex
- La Rocha
- liquid ecstasy
- love drug
- love pearls
- love pills

designer drugs (street names)
- love trip
- lunch money drug
- MAD
- Max
- MDM
- MDMA
- methedrine
- Mexican valium
- MFT
- mini beans
- murder 8
- Nexus
- Nexus flipping
- nineteen
- ocean burst
- party pack
- Pikachu
- pingus
- pink
- poison
- pollutants
- pure ivory
- purple
- purple wave
- Qat
- R-2
- rave energy
- Reynolds
- rip
- ritual spirit
- roaches
- roachies
- roapies
- Robutal
- roca (Spanish)
- rochas dos
- roche
- rophy
- ropies
- roples
- row-shay
- ruffles
- running
- scoop
- Shabu
- slammin/slamming
- slick superspeed

designer drugs (street names)
    sniff
    Somali tea
    Somatomax
    Special "K"
    special la coke
    spectrum
    speed for lovers
    speedballing
    spice
    spivias
    star
    stat
    strawberry shortcake
    super acid
    super C
    sweeties
    TNT
    toonies
    totally spent
    trip
    tweeker
    U-4
    U.S.P.
    ultimate xphoria
    vanilla sky
    Venus
    vitamin K
    waters
    West Coast turnarounds
    wheels
    whiffledust
    wild cat
    wolfies
    wonder star
    X
    X-ing
    XTC
designs test, copy geometric
desirability, social desire, "low"
desire
    absent sexual
    active
    deficient sexual
    disturbance in sexual
    hyperactive sexual
    hypoactive sexual
    impaired

desire
    intense
    lack of
    levels of
    loss of
    loss of sexual
    low sexual
    problems with sexual
    sexual
    stated
desire disorder
    hypoactive sexual
    sexual
desire for personal gain
desire for revenge
desire phase of sexual response cycle
desired effect
desk-type auditory trainer
desomorphine, krokodil (synthetic morphine; opioid)
despair, feelings of
Destrezas en Desarrollo, Lista de (La Lista)
destruction, nerve cell
destructive tendencies
"DET" (street name, dimethyltryptamine)
detached, feeling
detachment
    feeling of
    pattern of
    sense of
    social
detachment from social relationships, pattern of
detail, minimization of emotional
detailed dream
detailed history
detailed plan, meticulously
details, preoccupation with
detectability threshold
detectability threshold, speech (SDT)
detection
    lie
    signal
detection of deceit, technological

detection threshold
    noise (NDT)
    speech (SDT)
deterioration
    functioning
    grooming
    hygiene
    language function
    mood
    motivation
    social skills
    status
deteriorative disorder, simple
determinants of deceit
determination, forensic
Determination in Exploration and Assessment System
Determination Test for Dyslexia
determiner, regular
Determining Needs in Your Youth Ministry
determining risk
determinism, linguistic
"Detroit pink" (street name, PCP/phencyclidine)
Detroit Test of Learning Aptitude—Adult (DTLA-A)
Detroit Test of Learning Aptitude—Primary (DTLA-P)
"deuce" (re: $2 worth of drugs)
"deuce" (street name, heroin)
Deutsche Gesellschaft für Psychologie (DGPs)
devaluation
Developing Skills Checklist (DSC)
development
    abnormal
    anal stage psychosexual
    child
    child language
    delayed
    expressive language
    gender identity psychosexual
    human
    impaired
    intellectual

development
    language
    late speech
    latency period psychosexual
    motor
    normal
    optimal
    oral stage psychosexual
    perinatal
    pervasive impairment of
    phallic stage psychosexual
    psychomotor
    receptive
    receptive language
    slow rate of language
    speech sound
    subsequent
development stages
    cognitive (Period I-IV)
    Piaget's cognitive
Developmental Articulation Test (DAT)
developmental articulatory apraxia
Developmental Assessment of Life Experiences
developmental coordination disorder (F82)
developmental defect
developmental delay
developmental delay, global (F88)
developmental disorder
    disinhibited type of passive pervasive
    pervasive disinhibited type of
    specific (SDD)
developmental experimentation in childhood
Developmental Gestalt Test of School Readiness (Anton Brenner)
developmental imbalance
Developmental Indicators for the Assessment of Learning
developmental inventories *(see also* tests)

developmental period
developmental phase
developmental phonological
  processes
Developmental Profiles, S.E.E.D.
developmental scale *(see also*
  tests)
developmental screening *(see also*
  tests)
Developmental Sentence Scoring
developmental skills inventory
  (see also tests)
developmental stage
Developmental Test of Visual
  Perception
Developmental Test of Visual-
  Motor Integration
developmentally appropriate
  avoidant behavior
developmentally appropriate shy
  behavior
developmentally expected speech
  sounds
developmentally inappropriate
  social relatedness
developmentary appropriate self-
  stimulatory behaviors in the
  young
Devereux Adolescent Behavior
  Rating Scale
Devereux Child Behavior Rating
  Scale
deviance disorder, sexual
deviant articulation
deviant language
deviant pattern of inner
  experience and behavior
deviant speech
deviant swallowing
deviated septum
deviation, statistical
deviation from physiological
  norm
device
    canal caps hearing
      protection
    circumaural hearing
      protection

device
    cohesive
    earmuffs hearing protection
    earplugs hearing protection
    hearing protection (HPD)
    insert hearing protection
    interrupter
    protection device, insert
    semiaural hearing
      protection
    presyntactic
device for the deaf, telephone
  (TDD)
"devil, the" (street name, crack)
"devil's dandruff" (street name,
  crack)
"devil's dick" (re: crack
  equipment)
"devil's dust" (street name,
  phencyclidine)
"devil smoke" (street name,
  crack)
Devine Inventory
devious manner
devoicing of final consonants
"dew" (street name,
  cannabis/marijuana)
"dews" (re: $10 worth of drugs)
dexamethasone non-suppression
dexamethasone suppression test
dexterity
dextral
dextrality
DFA (Delayed Feedback
  Audiometry)
DFS (Defensive Functioning
  Scale)
DFSA (drug-facilitated sexual
  assault)
DFSA (drugs facilitating sexual
  assault: alcohol; GHB;
  Rohypnol)
DFTT (Digital Finger Tapping
  Test)
DGPs (Deutsche Gesellschaft für
  Psychologie, German
  Psychological Society)

DHHS (U.S. Department of
  Health and Human Services)
diabetes (type 2), autosomal
  dominant narcolepsy, obesity,
  and (G47.419)
Diabetes Opinion Survey and
  Parent Diabetes Opinion Survey
diabetic ketoacidosis
diacetylmorphine (heroin; opioid)
diachronic linguistics
diacritic
diadochokinesis
diagnoses associated with caffeine
diagnosis
        differential
        equivalent
        focus of
        principal
        psychiatric
        rule in a
        rule out a
diagnosis and assessment,
  psychiatric
diagnosogenic theory of stuttering
Diagnostic Achievement Battery
Diagnostic Achievement Test for
  Adolescents
Diagnostic Analysis of Reading
  Errors
diagnostic articulation test
Diagnostic Assessments of
  Reading (DAR)
diagnostic audiometry
Diagnostic Checklist for
  Behavior-Disturbed Children
  Form
diagnostic criteria, relevant
Diagnostic Employability Profile
diagnostic features
diagnostic information
Diagnostic Inventory of Early
  Development (BRIGANCE)
diagnostic judgment
Diagnostic Mathematics Profiles
diagnostic questionnaires *(see
  also* tests)
Diagnostic Reading Aptitude and
  Achievement Tests
Diagnostic Reading Scales
Diagnostic Reading Test of Word
  Analysis Skills
Diagnostic Reading Test of Word
  Recognition Skills
Diagnostic Screening Batteries:
  Adolescent, Adult, and Child
Diagnostic Skills Battery
diagnostic subtypes
diagnostic teaching
Diagnostic Tests and Self-Helps
  in Arithmetic
diagnostic therapy
diagnostic use of hypnosis
Diagnostic Word Analysis Test
diagram, branching tree
dialect, regional
dialect speech community
dialectical behavior therapy
  (DBT)
"diambista" (street name,
  cannabis/marijuana)
"dianabol" (re: veterinary steroid)
diaphragm
diaphragmatic-abdominal
  respiration
diarrhea
diary, symptom
diathesis
dichotic
Dichotic Consonant-Vowel Test
Dichotic Digits Test
dichotic listening
dichotic listening tasks
dichotic messages
dichotomy
diction
dielectric
diencephalic seizure
diencephalon
diet
        improper
        limited
        low-tyramine
        restricted
diet foods, low-calorie
"diet pills" (street name,
  amphetamine)

difference
    age
    cultural
    just noticeable (JND)
    language
    masking level
    qualitative
difference limen (DL)
difference tone
differences in interpretation
different foods, intolerance to
differential, semantic
differential diagnosis
differential function
differential reinforcement
differential relaxation
differential response
differential threshold
differentiation, auditory
difficult life circumstances
difficulties in speech or language
difficulties with problem solving
difficulties with the law
difficulty (pl. difficulties)
    emotional
    interpersonal
    language
    learning
    level of
    memory
    multiple life
    speech
    word-finding
difficulty concentrating, subjective sense of
difficulty controlling anger
difficulty in adapting
difficulty in changing response set
difficulty in concentrating
difficulty in initiating sleep
difficulty in maintaining sleep
difficulty maintaining sleep
difficulty sleeping
difficulty swallowing
difficulty thinking
diffidence (culturally appropriate)
diffracted wave
diffuse brain dysfunction
diffuse encephalopathy
diffuse Lewy body disease
diffuse pain
diffuse phoneme
diffuse traumatic brain injury with LOC of unspecified duration
    sequela with behavioral disturbance (S06.2X9S) and (F02.81)
    sequela without behavioral disturbance (S06.2X9S) and (F02.80)
digastric muscle
    anterior
    posterior
digastricus anterior, musculus
digastricus posterior, musculus
digit repetition test
digit reversal test
digit span recall test, reverse
digit span test
digit symbol test
digital change
Digital Finger Tapping Test (DFTT)
digital hearing aid
digital manipulation
digital motion sickness
digital span recall test, forward
digitalis-induced delirium
digits test
    dichotic
    memory for
diglossia
digraph diminutive
digressive speech
"dihydrolone" (re: injectable steroid)
"dimba" (street name, cannabis/marijuana)
"dime" (street name, crack)
"dime bag" (re: $10 worth of drugs)
"dime bag" (street name, cocaine)
dimension of positive schizophrenic symptoms
    disorganization
    psychotic

Psychiatric Words and Phrases 147

dimension of schizophrenia
    disorganization
    psychotic
dimension scale, social-emotional
dimensional approach
dimensional descriptors for
  schizophrenia, alternative
dimensional model of
  schizophrenia, 3-factor
"dime's worth" (re: amount of
  heroin to cause death)
dimethyltryptamine (DMT) (street
  names)
    45 minute psychosis
    AMT
    businessman's LSD
    businessman's special
    businessman's trip
    DET
    DMT
    DPT
    Fantasia
diminished control
diminished effect
diminished feeling of emotion
diminished libido
diminished pleasure in everyday
  activities
diminished reality testing
diminished reflex
diminished response to pain
diminished responsiveness
diminished sensation
diminished sexual interest
diminution of affect
diminution of goal-directed
  behavior
diminution of thought(s)
diminutive, digraph
DIMS (disorder of initiating and
  maintaining sleep)
"ding" (street name,
  cannabis/marijuana)
"dinkie dow" (street name,
  cannabis/marijuana)
dinomania (terror/fright)
dinophobia
diode

diotic listening
diotic messages
"dip" (street name, crack)
diphasic meningoencephalitis
  viral encephalitis
diphasic spike
diphthong
diplegia
diplophonia
"dipper" (street name,
  phencyclidine/PCP)
dipper curve audiogram
  configurations
dipping, body
"dipping out" (re: crack dealing)
dipsomania (alcohol
  consumption)
dipsomaniac
direct association
direct causality
direct causative
  pathophysiological mechanism
direct current (DC)
direct laryngoscopy
direct motor system
direct object
direct observation
direct physiological effect
direct selection communication
  board
direction profile, neurotic
directional microphone
directionality
Directionality and Lateral
  Awareness Test
directivity
"dirt" (street name, heroin)
"dirt grass" (street name,
  cannabis/marijuana)
dirtiness, feelings of
"dirty" (re: drug-injecting
  equipment)
"dirty basing" (street name, crack)
Disabilities Basic Screening and
  Referral Form (for Children)
disability
  associated
  degree of

disability
    functional
    global measures of
    intellectual, mild (F70)
    intellectual, moderate (F71)
    intellectual, profound (F73)
    intellectual, severe (F72)
    level of
    manifested
    measures of
    mental
    mild
    mobility
    neurologic
    observable
    partial permanent
    permanent
    posttraumatic chronic
    progressive
    severe
    social
    work
disability assessments *(see also tests)*
disability counselor
Disability Factor Scales—General
Disability Screening Questionnaire
disabled, learning (LD)
disabling headache
disaccharide malabsorption
disadvantage
disapproval, fear of
disassimilation
disassociation
disasters
    man-made
    natural
disavowal level
discharge, recent hospital
discipline
    harsh
    inadequate
    inconsistent parental
discipline problem, school
disclosure
    prevention of
    truth

"disco biscuits" (street name, barbiturate)
discomfort
    threshold of
    tolerance level of
discomfort in close relationships, pattern of
discomfort threshold
discomfort with emotion
discomfort with gender role, persistent
disconnection apraxia
disconnection syndrome aphasia, callosal
disconnection syndrome, callosal
discord with landlord (Z59.2)
discord with lodger (Z59.2)
discord with neighbor (Z59.2)
discord with social service provider – case manager (Z64.4)
discord with social service provider – probation officer (Z64.4)
discord with social service provider – social service worker (Z64.4)
discourse, disorganization in
discrepant intellectual function
discrepant intellectual functioning
discriminate validity
discrimination audiometry, speech
discrimination consciousness
discrimination curve
discrimination learning
discrimination loss
discrimination of sounds
discrimination score
discrimination score, word
discrimination training
discrimination audiometry, speech
discrimination consciousness
discrimination curve
discrimination learning
discrimination loss
discrimination of sounds
discrimination score
discrimination score, word

discrimination training
"disease" (re: drug of choice)
disease
    advanced
    Alzheimer's (G30.9)
    atherosclerotic heart
    biology of affective
    bodily
    brain
    brain stem
    central motor pathways
    cerebellar
    cerebrovascular
    chronic pulmonary heart
    Creutzfeldt-Jakob
    degenerative
    dementia due to
      Alzheimer's
    dementia due to
      Huntington's
    dementia due to
      Parkinson's
    dementia due to Pick's
    dementia due to prion
    diffuse Lewy body
    end-stage renal
    feared
    Gaucher's
    Hirshprung
    HIV (infection; B20)
    Huntington (G10)
    hypertensive heart
    hypertensive renal
    inherited
    inherited progressive
      degenerative
    Krabbe's
    Kufs'
    Lewy body (G31.83)
    life-threatening
    Lou Gehrig's (ALS;
      amyotrophic lateral
      sclerosis)
    Meniere's
    multiple sclerosis (G35)
    neurodegenerative
    parathyroid
    Parkinson's (G20)
disease
    pathophysiology of
      Alzheimer's
    peripheral vascular
    primary Parkinson's
    prion (A81.9)
    progressive degenerative
    rheumatic pulmonary valve
    serious
    severe
    sexually transmitted (STD)
    suspected
    Tay-Sachs
    tremor from cerebellar
    tricuspid valve
    white matter
disease process
disequilibrium state
disfluency dyskinesia
disgust, feeling
disinhibited social engagement
    disorder (F94.2)
disinhibited type
disinhibited type of
    developmental disorder,
    pervasive
disinhibited type of pervasive
    developmental disorder
disinhibited type personality
    disorder
disinhibited type reactive
    attachment disorder
disinhibition, emotional
disintegration theory, conditioned
disintegrative disorder, childhood
disorder(s)
    abnormal perceptions due
      to a psychotic
    acquired type female
      orgasmic
    acquired type female
      sexual arousal
    acquired type hypoactive
      sexual desire
    acquired type male erectile
    acquired type male
      orgasmic

disorder(s)
    acquired type sexual aversion
    acute labyrinthine
    acute stress (F43.0)
    addictive
    addictive-related
    adjustment interface
    adolescent conduct
    adult-onset fluency (F98.5)
    adult-onset type conduct
    aggressive type personality
    agoraphobia without history of panic
    alcohol-induced anxiety
    alcohol-induced bipolar
    alcohol-induced depressive
    alcohol-induced major or mild neurocognitive
    alcohol-induced persisting amnestic
    alcohol-induced psychotic
    alcohol-induced sleep
    alcohol-related
    alcohol-related, unspecified (F10.99)
    alcohol use, mild (F10.10)
    alcohol use, moderate/severe (F10.20)
    alcohol use, with alcohol-induced anxiety
    alpha-methyldopa-induced mood
    alternative criterion B for dysthymic
    amitriptyline-induced mood
    amphetamine-induced anxiety
    amphetamine-induced mood
    amphetamine-induced, with obsessive-compulsive and related
    amphetamine-type substance-related
    amphetamine use

disorder(s)
    amphetamine use, with amphetamine-induced anxiety
    amphetamine use, with amphetamine-induced obsessive-compulsive and related
    antidepressant use in affective
    antisocial personality (F60.2)
    anxiety, (agoraphobia; F40.00)
    anxiety, due to another medical condition (F06.4)
    anxiety, generalized (F41.1)
    anxiety, other specified (F41.8)
    anxiety, panic attack (not coded)
    anxiety, selective mutism (F94.0)
    anxiety, social phobia (F40.10)
    anxiety, specific phobia (animal) (F40.218)
    anxiety, specific phobia (fear of blood) (F40.230)
    anxiety, (specific phobia, fear of injections/ transfusions; F40.231)
    anxiety, specific phobia (fear of injury; F40.233)
    anxiety, specific phobia (fear of other medical care; F40.232)
    anxiety, specific phobia (natural environment (F40.228)
    anxiety, specific phobia (other e.g. choking; F40.298)
    anxiety, specific phobia (situational e.g. elevators, airplanes; F40.248)

disorder(s)
  anxiety, unspecified
    (F41.9)
  anxiety illness
  anxiety-related mental
  anxiolytic-induced anxiety
  anxiolytic-related
  anxiolytic use
  anxiolytic use, with
    anxiolytic-induced
    anxiety
  apathetic type personality
  apractic
  apraxic
  articulatory
  arylcyclohexylamine-
    related
  arylcyclohexylamine use
  Asperger's
  Asperger-type autistic
  associated personality
  attention
    deficit/hyperactivity,
    combined presentation
    (F90.2)
  attention
    deficit/hyperactivity,
    other specified (F90.8)
  attention
    deficit/hyperactivity,
    predominantly
    hyperactive/impulsive
    presentation (F90.1)
  attention
    deficit/hyperactivity,
    predominantly inattentive
    presentation (F90.0)
  attention
    deficit/hyperactivity,
    unspecified (F90.9)
  auditory processing
  avoidant food intake
    (F50.8)
  avoidant personality
    (F60.6)
  avoidant/restrictive food
    intake (F50.8)
  bereavement

disorder(s)
  bereavement, persistent
    complex (F44.0)
  binge-eating (BED) (F50.8)
  binge-eating, in full
    remission (F50.8)
  binge-eating, in partial
    remission (F50.8)
  binge-eating, of limited
    duration (F50.8)
  binge-eating, of low
    frequency (F50.8)
  bipolar and related
  bipolar I
  bipolar II
  body dysmorphic (F45.22)
  body dysmorphic, with
    muscle dysmorphia
    (F42.22)
  body dysmorphic-like, with
    acute flaws (F42)
  body dysmorphic-like,
    without repetitive
    behavior (F42)
  body-focused repetitive
    behavior (F42)
  borderline personality
    (F60.3)
  breathing
  breathing-related sleep
  brief illness anxiety
  brief psychotic
  brief somatic symptom
  caffeine use, with caffeine-
    induced anxiety
  caffeine-induced anxiety
  caffeine-induced sleep
  caffeine-related
  caffeine-related,
    unspecified (F15.99)
  caffeine withdrawal
    (F15.93)
  cannabis-induced anxiety
  cannabis-related
  cannabis use
  cannabis use, with
    cannabis-induced anxiety

disorder(s)
- cannabis withdrawal (F12.288)
- catatonic
- central auditory
- central language (CLD)
- central sleep apnea, idiopathic (G47.31)
- cerebral
- childhood
- childhood disintegrative
- chronic motor tic
- childhood-onset fluency (stuttering; F80.81)
- childhood-onset type conduct
- chronic vocal tic
- chronobiological
- circadian rhythm sleep
- cocaine-induced anxiety
- cocaine-induced mood
- cocaine-induced sleep
- cocaine-induced, with obsessive-compulsive and related
- cocaine-related
- cocaine use
- cocaine use, with cocaine-induced anxiety
- cocaine use, with cocaine-induced obsessive-compulsive and related
- cognitive
- combined type personality
- communication
- communication, unspecified (F80.9)
- communicative
- conceptual
- conduct
- contiguity
- co-occurring mental
- cul de sac voice
- delirium-related
- delirium-related mental
- delusional (F22)
- dementia due to immune
- dementia due to infectious

disorder(s)
- dementia-related
- dementia-related mental
- denasality voice
- dependent personality (F60.7)
- depression-related
- depression-related mental
- depressive, other specified (F32.8)
- depressive, unspecified (F32.9)
- depressive personality
- developmental coordination
- disinhibited social engagement, persistent (F94.2)
- disinhibited social engagement, severe (F94.2)
- disinhibited type personality
- disruptive behavior
- disruptive mood dysregulation (F34.8)
- dissociative identity
- dissociative interface
- dissociative trance
- dream anxiety
- drug-related
- dyssocial personality
- electroconvulsive therapy-induced mood
- elimination (encopresis; F98.1)
- elimination (enuresis; F98.0)
- evidence of dissociation
- evolution of the
- exacerbated symptoms of a preexisting mental
- excoriation (skin-picking; L98.1)
- expressive language
- factitious interface
- false role
- feeding and eating

disorder(s)
    female orgasmic
    female sexual arousal
    fluency
    functional articulation
    gait
    gambling-related
    gaming
    gender identity (GID)
    generalized anxiety (GAD)
    generalized type female
      orgasmic
    generalized type female
      sexual arousal
    generalized type
      hypoactive sexual desire
    generalized type male
      erectile
    generalized type male
      orgasmic
    generalized type sexual
      aversion
    group of
    hallucinogen persisting
      perception
    hallucinogen-related
    hallucinogen use
    hearing
    histrionic personality
    hoarding, excessive (F42)
    hyperactivity
    hypernasality voice
    hyperrhinolalia voice
    hyperrhinophonia voice
    hypersomnia related to
      another mental
    hypnotic use
    hypnotic-related
    hypoactive sexual desire
    impulse-control interface
    in-vivo magnetic resonance
      spectroscopy in
    inhalant use
    inhalant-related
    insomnia related to another
      mental
    insomnia type caffeine-
      induced sleep

disorder(s)
    insomnia type substance-
      induced sleep
    intermittent explosive
    labile type personality
    labyrinthine
    language
    late luteal phase dysphoric
    learning
    lifelong type female
      orgasmic
    lifelong type female sexual
      arousal
    lifelong type hypoactive
      sexual desire
    lifelong type male erectile
    lifelong type male
      orgasmic
    lifelong type sexual
      aversion
    light therapy-induced mood
    limbic system
    lithium use in affective
    male erectile
    male erectile arousal
    male hypoactive sexual
      desire
    male orgasmic
    malingering
    mathematics
    medical/neurological
    medical/psychiatric sleep
    medication-induced
      movement
    mild neurocognitive
    minor depressive
    mixed anxiety-depressive
    mixed nasality voice
    mixed receptive-expressive
      language
    moderate substance use
    motor
    motor or vocal tic,
      persistent (chronic; F95.1)
    motor or vocal tic,
      persistent (chronic), with
      motor tics only (F95.1)

disorder(s)
    motor or vocal tic, persistent (chronic), with vocal tics only (F95.1)
    motor skills
    multiple personality (PD)
    narcissistic personality (F60.81)
    negativistic personality
    neurocognitive, unspecified (R41.9)
    neurocognitive, with Lewy body disease (G31.83)
    neurodevelopmental
    neuroleptic-induced acute movement
    neuropsychiatric
    neuropsychiatric movement
    nicotine-related
    nicotine use
    night-eating (F50.8)
    nightmare
    non-substance-induced mental
    non-substance-related
    obsessive-compulsive (F42)
    obsessive-compulsive and related, due to another medical condition (F06.8)
    obsessive-compulsive and related, other specified (F42)
    obsessive-compulsive and related, unspecified (F42)
    obsessive-compulsive, due to another medical condition with appearance preoccupations (F06.8)
    obsessive-compulsive, due to another medical condition with hair-pulling symptoms (F06.8)
    obsessive-compulsive, due to another medical condition with hoarding symptoms (F06.8)

disorder(s)
    obsessive-compulsive, due to another medical condition with obsessive-compulsive disorder-like symptoms (F06.8)
    obsessive-compulsive, due to another medical condition with skin-picking symptoms (F06.8)
    obsessive-compulsive personality (F60.5)
    obsessive-compulsive, tic related (F42)
    opioid-induced anxiety
    opioid-related
    opioid use
    opioid use, with opioid-induced anxiety
    oppositional-defiant (F91.3)
    organic articulation
    orgasmic
    other (or unknown) caffeine-induced
    other (or unknown) hallucinogen-related
    other (or unknown) substance-induced, with obsessive-compulsive and related
    other (or unknown) substance/medication-related
    other (or unknown) substance use, with other (or unknown) substance-induced
    other stimulant-induced, with obsessive-compulsive and related
    other stimulant use, with other stimulant-induced obsessive-compulsive and related
    other type personality
    over-the-counter drug-related

disorder(s)
- pain
- paranoid personality (F60.0)
- paraphilic
- parasomnia type substance-induced sleep
- passive-aggressive personality
- "patient" role in factitious
- PCP use
- pedophilia (F65.4)
- perceptual
- personality, other specified (F60.89)
- personality, unspecified (F60.9)
- pervasive
- pervasive disinhibited type of developmental
- phencyclidine-induced anxiety
- phencyclidine-related
- phencyclidine use
- phencyclidine use, with phencyclidine-induced anxiety
- phonatory
- phonological
- pica
- polysubstance-related
- postconcussional
- postpsychotic depressive
- post-traumatic stress (PTSD; F42.10)
- post-traumatic stress (children 6 YO and younger; F42.10)
- post-traumatic stress, with delayed expression (F42.10)
- post-traumatic stress, with dissociative symptoms (F42.10)
- premenstrual dysphoria (N94.3)
- prescription drug-related
- primary anxiety

disorder(s)
- primary mental
- primary psychotic
- primary sleep
- psychiatric
- psychiatric system(s) interface
- psychoactive substance-induced organic mental
- psychoactive substance use
- psychotic
- purging (50.8)
- rapid eye movement sleep behavior (G47.52)
- reactive attachment
- reading
- receptive language
- recurrent brief depressive
- related sleep
- REM sleep behavior
- resonance
- respiratory
- restrictive food intake (F50.8)
- Rett
- rhinolalia aperta voice
- rhinolalia clause voice
- rumination (F98.21)
- schizoid personality (F60.1)
- schizophrenia spectrum and other related psychotic
- schizophrenic speech and language
- schizotypal personality (F21)
- sedative-induced anxiety
- sedative-related
- sedative use
- sedative use, with sedative-induced anxiety
- separation anxiety (F93.0)
- severe substance use
- sexual and gender identity
- sexual arousal
- sexual aversion
- sexual desire
- sexual deviance

disorder(s)
- sexual identity
- sexual pain
- sexual sadism (F65.52)
- shared psychotic
- simple deteriorative
- situational type female orgasmic
- situational type female sexual arousal
- situational type hypoactive sexual desire
- situational type male erectile
- situational type male orgasmic
- situational type sexual aversion
- sleep-related, idiopathic, hypoventilation (G47.34)
- sleep-wake
- social anxiety (F40.10)
- social (pragmatic) communication (F80.89)
- somatic symptoms and related
- somatoform
- somatoform interface
- specific developmental (SDD)
- speech
- speech and language
- speech-sound (F80.0)
- stereotypic movement
- stereotypy/habit
- stimulant-induced
- stimulant-induced anxiety
- stimulant-related
- stimulant use
- stimulant use, with stimulant-induced anxiety
- substance use
- substance-related
- substance/medication-induced anxiety
- substance/medication-induced depressive, with onset during intoxication

disorder(s)
- substance/medication-induced depressive, with onset during withdrawal
- substance/medication-induced mental
- substance/medication-induced mood
- substance/medication-induced obsessive-compulsive and related
- substance/medication-induced persisting
- substance/medication-induced persisting amnestic
- substance/medication-induced psychotic
- substance/medication-induced sleep
- substance/medication-related
- substance/medication-related and addiction
- substance/medication use
- tic
- tobacco-related
- tobacco use
- transient tic
- transvestic (F65.1)
- trauma- and stress-related
- trauma- and stress-related, other specified (F43.8)
- trauma- and stress-related, unspecified (F43.9)
- trichotillomania (hair-pulling; F63.3)
- unconscious processing of dissociative states and
- unknown substance/medication-induced
- unspecified bipolar I
- unspecified caffeine-related
- unspecified type personality
- visual
- visuospatial

Psychiatric Words and Phrases 157

disorder(s)
    vocal tic
    voice
    voyeuristic, in a controlled
      environment (F65.3)
    voyeuristic, in full
      remission (F65.3)
disorder affecting GMC
    mental
    psychological
disorder aphasia, contiguity
disorder by proxy, factitious
disorder due to combined factors
    female orgasmic
    female sexual arousal
    hypoactive sexual desire
    male erectile
    male orgasmic
    sexual aversion
disorder due to epilepsy,
  parasomnia type sleep
disorder due to GMC
    anxiety
    parasomnia type sleep
    sleep
disorder due to psychological
  factors
    female orgasmic
    female sexual arousal
    hypoactive sexual desire
    male erectile
    male orgasmic
    sexual aversion
disorder in dementia, language
disorder of assimilated nasality,
  voice
disorder of initiating and
  maintaining sleep (DIMS)
disorder of schizophrenia
disorder of schizophrenia,
  postpsychotic depressive
disorder of sex development
disorder of written expression
disorder syndrome, reversible
  affective
disorder with agoraphobia, panic
disorder with delusions,
  amphetamine-induced psychotic
disorder with hallucinations
    alcohol-induced psychotic
    amphetamine-induced
      psychotic
    cannabis-induced psychotic
    cocaine-induced psychotic
disorder with psychotic features,
  primary mood
disorder with rapid cycling, mood
disorder with seasonal pattern,
  mood
disorder without agoraphobia,
  panic
disordered mental status
disordered sleep
disorders in psychiatry, speech
  and language
disorders of aphasia, similarity
disorders of phonation, voice
disorders of resonance, voice
disorders of sexual response
disorders with catatonic features,
  mood
disorganization
    linguistic
    psychotic
    spatial
disorganization dimension of
  positive schizophrenic
  symptoms
disorganization dimension of
  schizophrenia
disorganization in discourse
Disorganization in Dyspraxic
  Children
disorganization in schizophrenia
    behavioral
    linguistic
    psychotic
disorganized behavior
disorganized behavior in
  schizophrenia
disorganized behavior, grossly
disorganized factor
disorganized factor in
  schizophrenia
disorganized speech
disorganized speech assessment

disorganized speech in
  schizophrenia
disorganized thinking
disorganized type schizophrenia
disorientation
  graphic
  right-left
  spatial
  visuospatial
disoriented patient
disparity, vision
displaced speech
displacement, brain stem
displacement of emotive energy,
  active
display of emotion, public
disproportionate impairment
disregard for the rights of others
disrupt sleep organization
disrupted relational functioning
disrupted sleep
disruption
  increased sleep
  marital
  sleep
disruption of family by separation
  or divorce (Z63.5)
disruptive behavior
disruptive behavior disorder
disruptive emotion
disruptive impulse-control and
  conduct disorder, other
  specified (F91.8)
disruptive impulse-control and
  conduct disorder, unspecified
  (F91.9)
disruptive mood dysregulation
  disorder (F34.8)
disruptive of family functioning
dissatisfaction
  body
  marital
dissociated sensory loss
dissociation, syndrome of sensory
dissociation disorder, evidence of
dissociative amnesia (F44.0)
dissociative amnesia with
  dissociative fugue (F44.11)

dissociative capacity
dissociative disorder
  other specified (F44.89)
  unspecified (F44.9)
dissociative episode, experience
  of
Dissociative Experiences Scale
  (DES)
dissociative fugue
dissociative identify disorder
  (F44.81)
dissociative interface disorder
dissociative phenomenon
dissociative states and disorders,
  unconscious processing of
dissociative symptoms
dissociative trance
dissociative trance disorder
distal distinctive feature analysis
distal limbs, abnormal positioning
  of
distal renal tubular acidosis
distance, social
distance perception
distancing, cognitive
distinct identities, multiple
distinctive feature analysis, distal
distoclusion of teeth
distorted body image
distorted breasts
distorted communication in
  schizophrenia
distorted inferential thinking in
  schizophrenia
distorted language in
  schizophrenia
distorted perception in
  schizophrenia
distorted perception of being
  touched
distorted perception of odor
distorted perception of physical
  sensations
distorted perception of sound
distorted perception of taste
distorted perception of the
  environment

distorted perception of visual
 sensations
distortion
 amplitude
 body image
 cognitive
 figure-ground
 harmonic
 intermodulary
 nonlinear
 perceptual
 psychotic
 speech
 transient
 visual-spatial
 waveform
distortion articulation
distortion of inferential behavioral
 monitoring
distortion of inferential perception
distortion of inferential thinking
distortion of language and
 communication
distortional bond conduction
distoversion of teeth
distractibility
distress
 clinically significant
 emotional
 intense psychological
 significant subjective
distress questionnaires *(see also*
 tests)
distressing thoughts
distribution
 complementary
 contrastive
 gaussian
 noncontrastive
 normal
 parallel
distribution of power
distrust
 interpersonal
 malevolent
 pervasive
distrust of others' motives

disturbance
 affective
 anxiety
 attentional
 behavioral
 breathing-related sleep
 chronic sleep
 chronobiological
 cognitive
 electrolyte
 fluctuating mood
 fluid
 focal neurologic
 global assessment of
  sensory
 high level perceptual
 identity
 infancy and early
  childhood
 language
 linguistic
 metabolic
 mixed symptom picture
  with perceptual
 motor skill
 oculomotor
 overall severity of
  psychiatric
 perceptual
 predominant mood
 psychiatric
 psychic
 psychotic
 sleep continuity
 stress-related
 visual
 visual field
disturbance in attention
disturbance in behavior
disturbance in children, mental
disturbance in concentration
disturbance in consciousness
disturbance in excitement
disturbance in executive
 functioning
disturbance in feeding and eating,
 infancy and early childhood
disturbance in fluency

disturbance in integrating auditory information with motor activity
disturbance in integrating tactile information with motor activity
disturbance in integrating visual information with motor activity
disturbance in language
disturbance in learning new information
disturbance in memory
disturbance in perception
disturbance in perceptual motor abilities
disturbance in planning
disturbance in rapidity of analyzing information
disturbance in rapidity of assimilating information
disturbance in rate of fluency
disturbance in reasoning
disturbance in recalling new information
disturbance in sexual desire
disturbance in sleep
disturbance in social relatedness
disturbance in speech
disturbance in speed of information processing
disturbance in the normal fluency of speech
disturbance in the time patterning of speech
disturbance in word-finding ability
disturbance of conduct
disturbance of conduct, adjustment disorder with
disturbance of emotions
disturbance of emotions and conduct, adjustment disorder with
disturbance of gait
disturbed eating behavior
disturbed orientation
disturbed sleep, easily
disturbed sleep pattern
disturbed social relatedness
disturbing experiences
disturbing feelings
disturbing problems
disturbing thoughts
disturbing wishes
disyllabic
disyllable
"ditch" (street name, cannabis/marijuana)
"ditch weed" (street name, cannabis/marijuana)
diurnal enuresis
diurnal epilepsy
divergence circuit
diverse group
diversity, group
Diversity Awareness Profile (DAP)
divorce as major childhood stressor
divorce problem
dizziness (a panic attack indicator)
dizziness, feelings of
dizzy, feeling
"djamba" (street name, cannabis/marijuana)
DL (difference limen)
DMAS (Dementia Mood Assessment Scale)
DMI Mathematics Systems Instructional Objectives Inventory
DMS (delusional misidentification syndromes)
"DMT" (street name, dimethyltryptamine; hallucinogen)
"do a joint" (re: cannabis/marijuana use)
"do a line" (re: cocaine use)
"do it Jack" (street name, phencyclidine)
"DOA" (street name, phencyclidine; crack)
"doctor" (street name, analog of amphetamine/methamphetamine; MDMA)
doctrine, usage

Dodd Test of Time Estimation
Doerfler-Stewart Test
"dog" (re: good friend)
"dog food" (street name, heroin)
"dogie" (street name, heroin)
Dole Vocational Sentence Completion Blank
"dollar" (re: $100 worth of drugs)
doll's eye reaction
doll's eye reflex
domain of information
domains, adaptive skill
"domes" (street name, LSD; phencyclidine and amphetamine/ methamphetamine)
"domestic" (re: locally grown cannabis)
domestic environment
domestic violence (D-V)
"domex" (re: methylenedioxy-methamphetamine and phencyclidine)
domiciliary, VA
dominance
    cerebral
    lateral
    left hemisphere
    left/right hemisphere
    mixed cerebral
    right hemisphere
    social
dominance-subordination
dominant delusional belief
dominant features
dominant gene, autosomal
dominant language
dominant pattern, autosomal
dominant person
dominant-subordinate behavior
dominant trait
dominant waking frequency
"dominoes" (street name, amphetamine)
"don jem" (street name, cannabis)
"Dona Juana" (street name, cannabis)
"Dona Juanita" (street name, cannabis)
donkey breathing
do-not-care attitude
"doobie/dubbe/duby" (street name, cannabis/marijuana)
"doogie/doojee/dugie" (street name, heroin)
"dooley" (street name, heroin)
dopamine metabolite
dopaminergic medication-induced postural tremor
"dope fiend" (street name, crack addict)
"dope smoke" (re: cannabis use)
"dopium" (street name, opium)
Doppler effect
Doppler phenomenon
Doppler shift
"doradilla" (street name, cannabis/marijuana)
doramania (animal skin/fur)
Doren Diagnostic Reading Test of Word Recognition Skills
dorsal cochlear nucleus
dorsal dorsum (pl. dorsa)
dorsal gray matter
dorsi
    musculus iliocostalis
    musculus latissimus
dorsi muscle, latissimus
dorsum of tongue
Dos Amigos Verbal Language Scales
dosage, equivalent
dosage reduction, trial of
dose-dependent effect
dosing, need for frequent drug
"dots" (street name, LSD)
"doub" (re: fixed worth of rock cocaine)
double assimilation
double bind theory
"double bubble" (street name, cocaine)
double consonant
double depression
"double dome" (street name, LSD)

"double rock" (re: crack diluted with procaine)
"double ups" (re: drug value)
double vision
"double yoke" (street name, morphine)
doubling
doubting mania
doubts of loyalty, unjustified
doubts of trustworthiness, unjustified
dovetail
"downie" (street name, barbiturate)
"downward drift"
DPP (Dropout Prediction & Prevention)
"draf" (re: ecstasy with cocaine)
"draf weed" (street name, cannabis/marijuana)
"drag weed" (street name, cannabis/marijuana)
dramatic affect
dramatic-emotional cluster
dramatic interpersonal style
drapetomania (running away from home)
Dravet syndrome
draw a clock face test
draw a house test
"Draw-A-Man" test
Draw A Person: Screening Procedure for Emotional Disturbance
draw a picture from memory test
drawings tests *(see also* tests)
dread of insanity
dreaded situation
"dream" (street name, cocaine)
dream
    detailed
    erotic
dream anxiety disorder
dream content
dream experience
"dream gum" (street name, opium)
dream image
    fragmentary
    vivid
dream recall, vivid
dream sequence
    elaborate
    story-like
dream state
"dream stick" (street name, opium)
"dreamer" (street name, morphine)
dreaming and repression, cognitive approaches to
dreamless sleep
dreamlike hallucination
"dreams" (street name, opium)
dreams, erotic
"dreck" (street name, heroin)
dressing apraxia
DRI (Driver Risk Inventory)
"drink" (street name, phencyclidine)
Drinker Profile
    Brief
    Comprehensive
    Follow-up
drinkers
    first-time
    persistent heavy
    repeated heavy
drinking
    aftereffects of
    alcohol
    continued
    controlled
    early-onset
    non-problematic
    social
    state markers of heavy (GGT)
    volitional
drinking behavior, out-of-control
drinking history
drinking pattern
    continued
    moderate
    to moderate one's

drinking period
drinking syndrome, nocturnal
drive
    failure to resist a
    hedonic
    hunger
    lack of
    sex
    subjective
    thirst
drive for thinness
driven motor behavior
Driver Risk Inventory (DRI)
driving (automobile) behavior
driving habits, reckless
dromomania (wander or travel)
"drop acid" (re: LSD use)
drop curve audiogram configurations, sudden
Dropout Prediction & Prevention (DPP)
dropouts, student
"dropper" (re: drug injection)
drowsiness, marked
"drowsy high" (street name, barbiturate)
DRP (Degrees of Reading Power)
drug
    absorpti narcotic
    absorption of
    addictive potential of
    amphetamine
    antidote
    antiseizure
    anxiolytic
    barbiturate
    barbiturate hypnotic
    benzodiazepine
    bromine compound
    butyrophenone-based tranquilizer
    chloral hydrate
    controlled release (CR)
    designer
    glutethimide group
    hallucinogen
    heterocyclic antidepressant
    high-dose
drug
    hypnotic
    inhalation of
    intranasal
    intravenous
    long-acting (LA)
    methaqualone compound
    mixed sedative
    monoamine oxidase inhibitor (MAOI)
    monocyclic antidepressant
    narcotic agonist
    negative effect of
    paraldehyde
    phenothiazine-based tranquilizer
    psychiatric
    psychodysleptic
    psychostimulant
    psychotic
    psychotropic (PTD)
    sedative
    sedative/hypnotic/ anxiolytic (S-H-A)
    slow release (SR)
    sublingual (SL)
    toxic effect of
    tranquilizer
    tricyclic antidepressant
drug abuse
    dissociative (DMT – dimethyltryptamine)
    dissociative (DXM - dextromethorphan)
    dissociative (ketamine)
    dissociative (PCP - phencyclidine)
    dissociative (salvia)
drug action, duration of
drug categories, major
    alcohol (F10.xxx)
    amphetamine/stimulants (F15.xxx)
    caffeine (F15.xxx)
    cannabis (F12.xxx)
    cocaine (F14.xxx)
    hallucinogens, other (F16.xxx)

drug categories, major
    inhalants (F18.xxx)
    opioids (F11.xxx)
    other (or unknown)
      substances (F19.xxx)
    phencyclidine/PCP;
      F16.xxx)
    sedatives/hypnotics/
      anxiolytics (S-H-A;
      F13.xxx)
    tobacco (F17.xxx)
drug counselor
drug craving
drug dealing
drug dosing, need for frequent
drug effect
drug effect, abnormal perceptions due to
drug facilitated sexual assault (DFSA)
drug-facilitated sexual assault using alcohol
drug-facilitated sexual assault using GHB
drug-facilitated sexual assault using Rohypnol
drug holiday, therapeutic
drug-induced floating sensation
drug-induced seizure
drug-injecting equipment
    "dirty"
    used
drug intolerance
drug paraphernalia, shared
drug possession
drug problem
drug-related disorder
    over-the-counter
    prescription
drug-related violence
drug screen
    blood
    urine
drug screening test
drug-seeking behavior
drug supplies
drug-taking behavior, compulsive
drug toxicity, current

drug treatment for personality disorders
drug treatment for sexual disorders
drug treatment for the elderly
drug types, abused (listed by type)
    amobarbital (sodium)
    amphetamine
    amyl nitrite
    alcohol
    anabolic steroids
    barbiturates
    cannabis
    club drugs
    cocaine
    crack cocaine
    depressants
    desomorphine
    designer drugs
    dimethyltryptamine
    ecstasy/MDMA
    fentanyl
    GBL (gamma butyrolactone)
    GHB (gamma hydroxybutyrate)
    hallucinogens
    hashish
    heroin
    inhalants
    ketamine
    khat
    LSD/lysergic acid diethylamide
    mescaline
    methadone
    methamphetamine
    methcathinone
    methylendioxy-methamphetamine/MDMA
    methylmorphine (codeine)
    methylphenidate
    Nexus (2-CB)
    nicotine
    opioids
    peyote
    phencyclidine/PCP

drug types, abused (listed by type)
    psilocybin/psilocin
    Rohypnol (flunitrazepam)
    Ritalin (methylphenidate)
    Sedative-Hypnotic-
      Anxiolytic (S-H-A)
    steroid compounds
    stimulants
    strychnine
    STP (pseudo-
      phencyclidine)
    Sudafed
    Talwin (pentazocine HCl)
    tobacco
drug use
    high frequency of
    low frequency of
drug users, injection
drug withdrawal
drug-withdrawal seizure
drugs
    frequency of self-
      administration of
    sex for
    wearing-off effect of
drugs, street names (*See also street drug names in the following categories:* alcohol, amobarbital, amphetamine, amyl nitrite, anabolic steroids, barbiturates, cannabis, club drugs, cocaine, crack cocaine, depressants, desomorphine, designer drugs, dimethyltryptamine, ecstasy/MDMA), fentanyl, GBL (gamma butyrolactone), GHB (gamma hydroxybutyrate), hallucinogens, hashish, heroin, inhalants, ketamine, khat, LSD (lysergic acid diethylamide), mescaline, methadone, methamphetamine, methcathinone, methylendioxy-methamphetamine (MDMA), methylmorphine (codeine), methylphenidate, Nexus (2-CB), nicotine, opioids, peyote, phencyclidine(PCP), psilocybin/psilocin, Rohypnol/flunitrazepam, Ritalin (methylphenidate), Sedative-Hypnotic-Anxiolytic (S-H-A), steroid compounds, stimulants, strychnine, STP (2,5-dimethyl-oxy-4-methylamphetamine), Sudafed, Talwin (pentazocine), and tobacco)
    007s (club drug; ecstasy/MDMA; stimulant)
    100s (LSD; hallucinogen)
    151 (crack cocaine; stimulant)
    24-7 (crack cocaine; stimulant)
    25s (LSD; hallucinogen)
    2C1 (ecstasy/MDMA; stimulant)
    2CB (club drug; Nexus; hallucinogen)
    2CE (ecstasy/MDMA; stimulant)
    2-CT-7 (Nexus; hallucinogen)
    2-for-1 sale (crack cocaine; stimulant)
    3750 (cannabis; crack cocaine; stimulant)
    4 Dot (ecstasy/MDMA; stimulant)
    40 (OxyContin; opioid)
    40-bar (OxyContin; opioid)
    420 (cannabis)
    45 minute psychosis (designer drug; dimethyltryptamine; hallucinogen)
    51 (cannabis; crack cocaine with marijuana or tobacco)
    69s (ecstasy/MDMA; stimulant)
    714 (depressant)
    7-up (Nexus; hallucinogen)
    80 (OxyContin; opioid)
    A (amphetamine; stimulant; LSD; hallucinogen)

drugs (street names)
  abolic (steroid compound)
  A-bomb (re: marijuana cigarette with heroin or cocaine)
  Abyssinian tea (khat; stimulant)
  AC/DC (cocaine)
  Acapulco gold (cannabis)
  Acapulco red (cannabis)
  ace (cannabis; phencyclidine/PCP; hallucinogen)
  acid (LSD; hallucinogen)
  acid cube (sugar cube with LSD; hallucinogen)
  acid freak (re: user of LSD; hallucinogen)
  acid head (re: user of LSD; hallucinogen)
  acido (LSD; hallucinogen)
  AD (phencyclidine/PCP; hallucinogen)
  Adam (designer drug; ecstasy/MDMA; stimulant)
  aeon flux (LSD; hallucinogen)
  Afgani indica (cannabis)
  African (cannabis)
  African black (cannabis)
  African bush (cannabis)
  African salad (khat; stimulant)
  African woodbine (cannabis)
  Ah-pen-yen (heroin; opium; opioid)
  aimies (amphetamine; stimulant; amyl nitrite; inhalant)
  AIP (re: heroin from Afghanistan, Iran, or Pakistan)
  air blast (inhalant)
  airhead (cannabis)
  airplane (cannabis)
  Al Capone (heroin; opioid)
  Alice B. Toklas (cannabis)
  All-American drug (cocaine)

drugs (street names)
  alpha-ET (designer drug)
  ames (amyl nitrite; inhalant)
  amidone (methadone; hallucinogen)
  amoeba (phencyclidine/PCP; hallucinogen)
  amp (amphetamine; stimulant; cannabis; phencyclidine/PCP; hallucinogen)
  amp head (LSD; hallucinogen)
  amp joint (cannabis)
  amped (amphetamine; stimulant)
  amped-out (re: amphetamine use; stimulant)
  ampL (stimulant)
  AMT (designer drug; dimethyltryptamine; hallucinogen)
  amyl nitrate (inhalant)
  amys (amyl nitrite; inhalant)
  Anadrol (steroid compound)
  anatrofin (steroid compound)
  anavar (steroid compound)
  angel (phencyclidine/PCP; hallucinogen)
  angel dust (phencyclidine/PCP; hallucinogen)
  angel hair (phencyclidine/PCP; hallucinogen)
  angel mist (phencyclidine/PCP; hallucinogen)
  Angel Poke (phencyclidine/PCP; hallucinogen)
  Angie (cocaine)
  Angola (cannabis)
  animal (LSD; hallucinogen)
  animal trank (phencyclidine/PCP; hallucinogen)

drugs (street names)
  animal tranq
    (phencyclidine/PCP;
    hallucinogen)
  animal tranquilizer
    (phencyclidine/PCP;
    hallucinogen)
  antifreeze (heroin; opioid)
  Apache (designer drug;
    fentanyl; opioid)
  apple jack (crack cocaine)
  Are you anywhere?
    (cannabis)
  Aries (heroin; opioid)
  Arnolds (steroid compound)
  aroma of men (inhalant)
  ashes (cannabis)
  aspirin (cocaine)
  assassin of youth (cannabis)
  astroturf (cannabis)
  atom bomb (cannabis; heroin;
    opioid)
  atom bomb (re: marijuana
    mixed with heroin)
  atshitshi (cannabis)
  Aunt (cocaine)
  Aunt Emma (opium; heroin;
    opioid)
  Aunt Hazel (heroin; opioid)
  Aunt Mary (cannabis)
  Aunt Nora (cocaine)
  Aunti (opium; opioid)
  aurora borealis
    (phencyclidine/PCP;
    hallucinogen)
  B (cannabis)
  B's (Nexus; hallucinogen)
  B-40 (cannabis; nicotine;
    tobacco)
  B.J.s or BJs (crack cocaine)
  baby (cannabis)
  baby bhang (cannabis)
  Baby T (crack cocaine)
  babysitter (cannabis)
  back breakers (LSD and
    strychnine; hallucinogen)
  back dex (amphetamine;
    stimulant)

drugs (street names)
  back to back (re: smoking
    crack after injecting heroin)
  backwards (barbiturate;
    depressant; S-H-A)
  bad (crack cocaine)
  bad bundle (re: inferior
    heroin)
  bad seed (cannabis; heroin;
    opioid; marijuana with
    mescaline/peyote;
    hallucinogen)
  bag (cannabis)
  bag (re: a package of drugs,
    usually marijuana or heroin)
  bag bride (crack cocaine)
  bag man (re: drug pusher)
  bagging (re: using inhalants)
  bain (stimulants
  bale (cannabis)
  ball (crack cocaine; Mexican
    Black Tar heroin; opioid)
  balling (re: cocaine use)
  balloon (re: a penny balloon
    containing heroin; re: heroin
    supplier)
  ballot (heroin; opioid)
  bam (amphetamine;
    stimulant; barbiturate;
    depressant; S-H-A)
  Bambalacha (cannabis)
  bambita (amphetamine;
    stimulant)
  bambs (barbiturate;
    depressant; S-H-A)
  bammies (cannabis)
  bammy (cannabis)
  banana split (club drug;
    designer drug; Nexus with
    LSD; hallucinogen)
  banano (cannabis; cocaine;
    nicotine; tobacco)
  bandits (depressant)
  bang (inhalant)
  banimal (LSD; hallucinogen)
  bank bandit pills (barbiturate;
    S-H-A)

drugs (street names)
  bank deposit pills
    (barbiturate; S-H-A)
  bar (cannabis)
  Barb (barbiturate; depressant;
    S-H-A)
  Barbies (barbiturate;
    depressant; S-H-A)
  barbs (cocaine)
  barr (codeine cough syrup;
    depressant; S-H-A)
  barrels (LSD; hallucinogen)
  bars (re: heroin mixed with
    alprazolam/Xanax; opioid)
  Bart Simpson (heroin;
    opioid)
  basa (cocaine; crack cocaine)
  base (cocaine; crack cocaine)
  base crazies (cocaine; crack
    cocaine)
  base head (cocaine; crack
    cocaine)
  baseball (crack cocaine)
  based out (re: cocaine use)
  bash (cannabis)
  basing (cocaine; crack
    cocaine)
  basuco (cannabis; cocaine;
    nicotine; tobacco)
  batak (methamphetamine;
    stimulant)
  bath salts (designer drug;
    synthetic cannabinoids;
    hallucinogen)
  bathtub crank
    (methamphetamine;
    stimulant)
  bathtub speed (designer drug;
    methcathinone; stimulant)
  Batman (club drug;
    ecstasy/MDMA; stimulant;
    crack cocaine; cocaine;
    heroin; opioid)
  battery acid (LSD;
    hallucinogen)
  batu (methamphetamine;
    stimulant)

drugs (street names)
  bazooka (cannabis; crack
    cocaine; cocaine; nicotine;
    tobacco)
  Bazulco (cocaine)
  B-bombs (designer drug;
    amphetamine;
    ecstasy/MDMA; stimulant)
  BC bud (cannabis)
  BDMPEA (designer drug;
    Nexus; hallucinogen)
  beam (cocaine;
    MDMA/ecstasy; stimulant)
  Beam me up Scotty (cocaine;
    crack cocaine;
    phencyclidine/PCP;
    hallucinogen)
  beamer(s) (crack cocaine)
  bean (club drug; designer
    drug; ecstasy/MDMA;
    stimulant)
  beanies (methamphetamine;
    stimulant)
  beans (amphetamine;
    stimulant; barbiturate;
    depressant; S-H-A; crack
    cocaine; mescaline;
    hallucinogen)
  beast (LSD; hallucinogen;
    heroin; opioid)
  beat (crack cocaine)
  beat vials (re: crack cocaine
    use)
  beautiful boulders (crack
    cocaine)
  Beavis & Butthead (LSD;
    hallucinogen)
  Bebe (crack cocaine)
  bedrock (crack cocaine)
  beedies (cannabis; nicotine;
    tobacco)
  beemers (crack cocaine)
  bees (designer drug; Nexus;
    hallucinogen)
  behind the scale (cocaine)
  beiging or beigeing (re:
    cocaine use)
  Beiruts (depressant)

drugs (street names)
  belladonna
    (phencyclidine/PCP;
    hallucinogen)
  Belushi (cocaine plus heroin;
    opioid)
  Belyando spruce (cannabis)
  bennies (amphetamine;
    stimulant)
  bens (designer drug; re:
    ecstasy mixed with
    ketamine)
  benz (amphetamine;
    stimulant)
  benzedrine (designer drug;
    amphetamine; ecstasy;
    stimulant)
  Bermuda triangles (club
    drug; ecstasy/MDMA;
    stimulant)
  Bernice (cocaine)
  Bernie (cocaine)
  Bernie's flakes (cocaine)
  Bernie's gold dust (cocaine)
  bhang (cannabis)
  bibs (club drug;
    ecstasy/MDMA; stimulant)
  big bag (heroin; opioid)
  big bloke (cocaine)
  big C (cocaine)
  Big D (LSD; hallucinogen)
  big doodig (heroin; opioid)
  big flak (cocaine)
  Big H (heroin; opioid)
  Big Harry (heroin; opioid)
  Big Henry (heroin; opioid)
  Big O (opium; opioid)
  big rush (cocaine)
  biker coffee
    (methamphetamine mixed
    with coffee; stimulant)
  Bill Blass (crack cocaine)
  billie hoke (cocaine)
  bin Laden (re: heroin after
    9/11 event)
  bindle (heroin; opioid; re:
    heroin; small packet)
  bings (crack cocaine)

drugs (street names)
  biphetamine (designer drug;
    amphetamine;
    ecstasy/MDMA)
  bipping (re: snorting heroin
    & cocaine – separately or
    together)
  birdhead (LSD;
    hallucinogen)
  birdie powder (cocaine;
    heroin; opioid)
  biscuit (crack cocaine)
  bite one's lips (cannabis)
  black (cannabis;
    methamphetamine;
    stimulant; opium; opioid)
  black acid (LSD;
    phencyclidine/PCP;
    hallucinogen)
  black and white
    (amphetamine; stimulant)
  black bandit pills (depressant;
    S-H-A)
  black bart (cannabis)
  black beauties (amphetamine;
    stimulant; barbiturate;
    depressant; S-H-A)
  Black Beauty
    (methamphetamine;
    stimulant)
  black birds (amphetamine;
    stimulant)
  black bombers
    (amphetamine; stimulant)
  black Cadillacs
    (amphetamine; stimulant)
  black dust
    (phencyclidine/PCP;
    hallucinogen)
  black eagle (heroin; opioid)
  black ganga (cannabis)
  black gold (cannabis)
  black gungi (cannabis)
  black gunion (cannabis)
  black hash (hashish and
    opium; hallucinogen;
    opioid)

drugs (street names)
    black hole (designer drug; re: depressant high associated with ketamine)
    black jack (re: injecting opium)
    black mo (cannabis)
    black moat (cannabis)
    black mollies (amphetamine; stimulant)
    black mote (cannabis)
    black pearl (heroin; opioid)
    black pill (opium; opioid)
    black rock (cocaine; crack cocaine)
    black Russian (hashish; hallucinogen; opium; opioid)
    black star (LSD; hallucinogen)
    black stuff (heroin; opium)
    black sunshine (LSD; hallucinogen)
    black tabs (LSD; hallucinogen)
    black tar (heroin; opioid)
    black whack (phencyclidine/PCP; hallucinogen)
    blacks (amphetamine; stimulant)
    blade (crystal methamphetamine; stimulant)
    Blanca (cocaine)
    Blanco (cocaine; heroin; opioid)
    blanket (cannabis)
    blast (cannabis; cocaine; crack cocaine)
    blast a joint (cannabis)
    blast a roach (cannabis)
    blast a stick (cannabis)
    blaxing (cannabis)
    blazing (cannabis)
    bling bling (methamphetamine; stimulant)

drugs (street names)
    blizzard (cocaine)
    block (cannabis)
    block busters (barbiturate; depressant; S-H-A)
    blonde (cannabis)
    blotter (cocaine; crack cocaine; LSD; hallucinogen)
    blotter acid (LSD; hallucinogen; phencyclidine/PCP)
    blotter cube (LSD; hallucinogen)
    Blou Bulle (depressant)
    blow (cannabis; cocaine)
    blow blue (cocaine)
    blow coke (cocaine)
    blow smoke (cocaine)
    blow up (re: crack cut with lidocaine to increase size, weight, or value)
    blow your mind (re: get high on hallucinogens)
    blowcaine (crack cocaine)
    blowing smoke (cannabis)
    blowout (crack cocaine)
    blowup (crack cocaine)
    blue (barbiturate; depressant; S-H-A; crack cocaine; OxyContin; opioid)
    blue acid (LSD; hallucinogen)
    blue angels (amobarbital; depressant; S-H-A)
    blue barrels (LSD; hallucinogen)
    blue birds (amobarbital; depressant; S-H-A)
    blue boy (amphetamine; stimulant)
    blue bullets (barbiturate; depressant; S-H-A)
    blue caps (LSD; mescaline; hallucinogen)
    blue chairs (LSD; hallucinogen)

drugs (street names)
- blue cheers (LSD; hallucinogen)
- blue clouds (depressant; S-H-A)
- blue de hue (cannabis)
- blue devils (amphetamine; methamphetamine; stimulant; amobarbital; depressant; S-H-A)
- blue dolls (barbiturate; depressant; S-H-A)
- blue heaven (LSD; hallucinogen)
- blue heavens (barbiturate (depressant; S-H-A)
- blue kisses (designer drug; ecstasy/MDMA; stimulant)
- blue lips (designer drug; ecstasy/MDMA; stimulant)
- blue madman (phencyclidine/PCP; hallucinogen)
- blue meth (methamphetamine; stimulant)
- blue microdot (LSD; hallucinogen)
- blue mist (LSD; hallucinogen)
- blue mollies (amphetamine; stimulant)
- blue moons (LSD; hallucinogen)
- blue Nile (club drug; ecstasy/MDMA; stimulant)
- blue nitrate vitality (contains GBL; depressant; S-H-A)
- blue sage (cannabis)
- blue sky blond (cannabis)
- blue star (heroin; opioid)
- blue tips (barbiturate; depressant; S-H-A)
- blue vials (LSD; hallucinogen)
- blunt (cocaine; cannabis)
- BO (cannabis)
- boat (phencyclidine/PCP; hallucinogen)

drugs (street names)
- boat (re: 1000 tabs of MDMA or ecstasy; stimulant)
- bo-bo (cannabis)
- bobo (crack cocaine)
- bobo bush (cannabis)
- body packer (cocaine; crack cocaine)
- body stuffer (crack cocaine)
- Bogart a joint (cannabis)
- bohd (cannabis; phencyclidine/PCP; hallucinogen)
- bolasterone (steroid compound)
- Bolivian marching powder (cocaine)
- bollo (crack cocaine)
- bolo (crack cocaine)
- bolt (amphetamine; stimulant)
- bolt (inhalant)
- bomb (cannabis; crack cocaine; heroin; opioid)
- bomb squad (crack cocaine)
- bomber (cannabis)
- bombido (depressant; S-H-A; amphetamine; stimulant; heroin; opioid)
- bombita (depressant; S-H-A; amphetamine; stimulant; heroin + amphetamine; Spanish depressant)
- bombs away (heroin; opioid)
- BOMPEA (club drug)
- bone (cannabis; crack cocaine; re: high purity heroin)
- bonecrusher (crack cocaine)
- bones (crack cocaine)
- bong (cannabis)
- Bonita (heroin; opioid)
- boo (cannabis; methamphetamine; stimulant)
- boo boo bama (cannabis)
- book (re: 100 dosage units of LSD)

drugs (street names)
    boom (cannabis)
    boomers (club drug; psilocybin/psilocin; hallucinogen)
    boost (crack cocaine)
    booster (cocaine)
    boot the gong (cannabis)
    bopper (cocaine; crack cocaine)
    boppers (amyl nitrite; inhalant)
    botray (crack cocaine)
    bottles (crack cocaine; amphetamine; stimulant)
    boubou (crack cocaine; stimulants)
    boulder (crack cocaine)
    boulya (crack cocaine)
    bouncing powder (cocaine)
    box labs (re: small labs used to produce methamphetamine)
    boy (cocaine; heroin; opioid)
    boy-girl (heroin mixed with cocaine)
    Bozo (heroin; opioid)
    brain damage (heroin; opioid)
    brain ticklers (amphetamine; stimulant)
    Brea (heroin; opioid)
    break night (cocaine)
    breakdown (crack cocaine)
    brick (cannabis; cocaine; crack cocaine)
    brick gum (heroin; opioid)
    britton (mescaline/peyote; hallucinogen)
    broccoli (cannabis)
    broja (heroin; opioid)
    broma mescaline (club drug; Nexus; hallucinogen)
    bromo (designer drug; Nexus; hallucinogen)
    brown (cannabis; heroin; opioid; methamphetamine; stimulant)

drugs (street names)
    brown bombers (LSD; hallucinogen)
    brown crystal (heroin; opioid)
    brown dots (LSD; hallucinogen)
    brown rhine (heroin; opioid)
    brown sugar (heroin; opioid)
    brown tape (heroin; opioid)
    brownies (stimulant)
    browns (amphetamine; stimulants)
    bubble gum (cannabis; cocaine; crack cocaine)
    bud (cannabis)
    buda (cannabis; crack cocaine)
    Budda (opium; opioid)
    Buddha (cannabis)
    buffer (crack cocaine)
    bull dog (heroin; opioid)
    bullet (inhalant)
    bullet bolt (inhalant)
    bullia capital (crack cocaine)
    bullion (cannabis; crack cocaine)
    bumblebees (amphetamine; stimulant)
    bummer trip (re: unsettling trip from PCP intoxication)
    bump (cocaine; crack cocaine)
    bump (re: hit of ketamine - $20)
    bump up (cocaine; club drug)
    bump up (re: bolstering MDMA with cocaine; stimulant)
    bumper (cocaine; crack cocaine)
    bumping up (cocaine; club drug; re: combining MDMA with powder cocaine; stimulant)
    bundle (heroin; opioid)
    bunk (cocaine; crack cocaine)
    burn one (cannabis)

drugs (street names)
  Burnese (cocaine)
  burnie (cannabis)
  bush (cannabis; cocaine; phencyclidine/PCP; hallucinogen)
  bushman's tea (khat; stimulant)
  businessman's LSD (designer drug; dimethyltryptamine; hallucinogen)
  businessman's special (designer drug; dimethyltryptamine; hallucinogen)
  businessman's trip (designer drug; dimethyltryptamine; hallucinogen)
  busters (barbiturate; depressant; S-H-A)
  busy bee (phencyclidine/PCP; hallucinogen)
  butler (crack cocaine)
  butt naked (phencyclidine/PCP; hallucinogen)
  butter (cannabis; crack cocaine)
  butter flower (cannabis)
  buttons (mescaline; hallucinogen)
  Butu (heroin; opioid)
  butyl nitrate (inhalant)
  buzz bomb (nitrous oxide; inhalant)
  C (cocaine)
  C & M (cocaine and morphine)
  C joint (cocaine)
  C.S. (cannabis)
  caballo (heroin; opioid)
  caca (heroin; opioid)
  cactus (mescaline; hallucinogen)
  cactus buttons (mescaline; hallucinogen)

drugs (street names)
  cactus head (mescaline; hallucinogen)
  Cadillac (phencyclidine/PCP; hallucinogen)
  Cadillac express (designer drug; methcathinone; stimulant)
  caine (cocaine; crack cocaine)
  cakes (crack cocaine)
  calbo (heroin; opioid)
  California cornflakes (cocaine)
  California sunshine (LSD; hallucinogen)
  Cam red (cannabis)
  Cam trip (cannabis)
  Cambodian red (cannabis)
  came (cocaine)
  can (cannabis)
  Canada (cannabis)
  canade (heroin + marijuana)
  Canadian black (cannabis)
  canamo (cannabis)
  canappa (cannabis)
  cancelled stick (cannabis)
  candy (depressant; S-H-A; amphetamine; crack cocaine)
  candy blunt (cannabis)
  candy C (cocaine)
  candy flipping (LSD and ecstasy)
  candy flipping on a string (LSD/MDMA/cocaine)
  candy rave (designer drug; GHB; depressant)
  candy ravers (re: rave club attendees wearing candy necklaces)
  candy stick (cannabis; cocaine)
  candy sugar (cocaine)
  cannabis tea (cannabis)
  cap(s) (club drug; cocaine; GHB; heroin; LSD; psilocybin/psilocin)

drugs (street names)
    Capital H (heroin; opioid)
    capsula (crack cocaine)
    carburetor (crack cocaine)
    Care Bears (club drug; ecstasy/MDMA; stimulant)
    carga (heroin; opioid)
    carne (heroin; opioid)
    Carnie (cocaine)
    carpet patrol (crack cocaine)
    Carrie Nation (cocaine)
    cartucho (cannabis)
    cartwheels (amphetamine; stimulant
    Casper (crack cocaine)
    Casper the ghost (crack cocaine)
    cat (designer drug; methcathinone; stimulant)
    Cat in the Hats (club drug; ecstasy/MDMA; stimulant)
    cat killer (club drug; ketamine; dissociative hallucinogen)
    cat Valium (designer drug; ketamine; dissociative hallucinogen)
    catnip (cannabis)
    caviar (cannabis; cocaine; crack cocaine)
    Cavite all star (cannabis)
    CB's (Nexus; hallucinogen)
    CDs (cocaine; crack cocaine)
    Cecil (cocaine)
    cest (cannabis)
    cha (methamphetamine; stimulant)
    chalk (amphetamine; crack cocaine; stimulant)
    chalked up (cocaine)
    chalking (cocaine)
    champagne (cannabis; cocaine)
    chandoo/chandu (opium)
    change (designer drug)
    channel swimmer (re: a heroin injector)
    chapopote (heroin; opioid)

drugs (street names)
    charas (cannabis)
    Charge (cannabis; club drug; cocaine)
    Charge+ (re: powdery substance with effects like ecstasy)
    charity (club drug; ecstasy/MDMA; stimulant)
    Charley (heroin; opioid)
    Charlie (cocaine)
    Charlotte's Web (liquid cannabis)
    chase (cannabis; cocaine)
    chaser (crack cocaine)
    chasing the dragon (crack and heroin mix)
    chasing the tiger (re: smoking heroin)
    chatarra (heroin; opioid)
    cheap basing (crack cocaine)
    cheeba (cannabis)
    cheeo (cannabis)
    chemical (crack cocaine)
    chemo (cannabis)
    cherry mein (GHB; depressant; S-H-A)
    chewies (crack cocaine)
    chiba (heroin; opioid)
    chiba chiba (cannabis)
    Chicago black (cannabis)
    Chicago green (cannabis)
    chicken feed (methamphetamine; stimulant)
    chicken powder (amphetamine; stimulant)
    chicken scratch (cocaine; crack cocaine)
    chicle (heroin; opioid)
    chief (LSD; mescaline; hallucinogen)
    chiefing (cannabis)
    chieva (heroin; opioid)
    chillum (cannabis; hashish; opium)
    China cat (re: high potency heroin)

drugs (street names)
    China girl (fentanyl; opioid)
    China town (fentanyl; opioid)
    China white (heroin + fentanyl; synthetic heroin; opioid)
    Chinese molasses (opium)
    Chinese red (heroin; opioid)
    Chinese tobacco (opium)
    chip (heroin; opioid)
    chipper (re: occasional heroin user)
    chippy (cocaine)
    chips (cannabis; nicotine/tobacco; phencyclidine/PCP)
    chira (cannabis)
    chiva (heroin; opioid)
    choco-fan (heroin; opioid)
    chocolate (amphetamine; cannabis; opium)
    chocolate chip cookies (re: MDMA with heroin or methadone)
    chocolate chips (LSD; hallucinogen)
    chocolate ecstasy (crack cocaine)
    chocolate rock (re: crack smoked with heroin)
    chocolate Thai (cannabis)
    choe (cocaine)
    cholly (cocaine)
    chorals (barbiturate; depressant; S-H-A)
    Christina (amphetamine; stimulant)
    Christmas bud (cannabis)
    Christmas rolls (barbiturate; depressant; S-H-A)
    Christmas tree (amphetamine; cannabis; methamphetamine)
    Christmas tree meth (green-tinted methamphetamine using Drano)
    Christmas trees (amobarbital; depressant; S-H-A)

drugs (street names)
    chrome (crystal methamphetamine; stimulant)
    chronic (cannabis; crack cocaine)
    chucks (re: hunger after heroin withdrawal)
    chunky (cannabis)
    churus (cannabis)
    Cid (cannabis; LSD)
    cigamos (cocaine; crack cocaine)
    cigarette paper (re: packet of heroin)
    cigarrode cristal (phencyclidine/PCP; hallucinogen)
    cinnamon (methamphetamine; stimulant)
    circles (club drug; Rohypnol/flunitrazepam; S-H-A)
    citrol (cannabis)
    CJ (phencyclidine/PCP; hallucinogen)
    clam bake (cannabis)
    clarity (designer drug; ecstasy/MDMA; stimulant)
    clear (methamphetamine; stimulant)
    clicker (cannabis; crack cocaine; phencyclidine/PCP)
    clickum (cannabis)
    climax (crack cocaine; heroin; isobutyl inhalant)
    clocker (crack cocaine)
    cloud (crack cocaine)
    cloud nine (club drug; designer drug; crack cocaine; ecstasy/MDMA)
    cluck (crack cocaine)
    coasts to coasts (amphetamine; stimulant)
    coca (cocaine)
    cochornis (cannabis)

drugs (street names)
- cock snow (crack cocaine)
- cocktail (cocaine; crack cocaine; nicotine/tobacco)
- coco-fan (brown tar heroin; opioid)
- coco rocks (crack cocaine)
- cocoa puff (cannabis)
- coconut (cocaine)
- coffee (LSD; hallucinogen)
- coke (crack cocaine)
- cola (cocaine)
- colas (cannabis)
- coli (cannabis)
- coliflor tostao (cannabis)
- Colombian (cannabis)
- Colorado cocktail (cannabis)
- Columbo (phencyclidine/PCP; hallucinogen)
- Columbus black (cannabis)
- combol (cocaine)
- come home (LSD; re: end a "trip" from LSD)
- comeback (cocaine; crack cocaine)
- comic book (LSD; hallucinogen)
- conductor (LSD; hallucinogen)
- Connie (cocaine)
- contact lens (LSD; hallucinogen)
- cook (re: heroin prep for injection)
- cook down (re: heating heroin to liquefy before inhaling it)
- cook/cooker (re: drug manufacturer of methamphetamine)
- cookies (crack cocaine)
- cooking up (cocaine; crack cocaine)
- cooler (nicotine/tobacco)
- coolie (cocaine; nicotine/tobacco)
- co-pilot (amphetamine)

drugs (street names)
- coral (barbiturate; depressant; S-H-A)
- cork the air (cocaine)
- Corrinne (cocaine)
- cosa (cannabis)
- cotica (heroin; opioid)
- coties (cocaine; heroin)
- cotton (OxyContin) opioid)
- cotton brothers (cocaine + heroin + morphine)
- courage pills (barbiturate; depressant; heroin)
- Cozmo's (phencyclidine/PCP; hallucinogen)
- CR (methamphetamine; stimulant)
- crack (chemically processed cocaine)
- crack attack (crack cocaine)
- crack back (cannabis; crack cocaine)
- crack cooler (crack cocaine)
- crack gallery (re: crack cocaine use)
- crack house (re: crack cocaine site)
- crack spot (re: crack cocaine place)
- cracker jack (crack cocaine)
- cracker jacks (re: crack users)
- crackers (LSD; Talwin/Ritalin mix simulating heroin/cocaine effect)
- crank (designer drug; amphetamine; crack cocaine; heroin; methamphetamine)
- crankster (re: user or manufacturer of methamphetamine)
- crap (re: low quality heroin)
- crazy coke (phencyclidine/PCP; hallucinogen)
- Crazy Eddie (phencyclidine/PCP; hallucinogen)

drugs (street names)
    crazy weed (cannabis)
    credit card (crack cocaine)
    crib (crack cocaine)
    crimmie (crack cocaine; nicotine/tobacco)
    crink (methamphetamine; stimulant)
    cripple (cannabis)
    cris (methamphetamine; stimulant)
    crisscross (amphetamine; stimulant)
    crisscrossing (re: cross snorting cocaine and heroin)
    cristal (designer drug; ecstasy/MDMA; stimulant)
    Cristina (methamphetamine; stimulant)
    Cristy (stimulant)
    croak (cocaine; crack cocaine; methamphetamine; stimulant)
    crop (re: low quality heroin)
    cross tops (amphetamine; stimulant)
    crosses (amphetamine)
    crossies (stimulant)
    crossroads (amphetamine; stimulant)
    crown crap (heroin; opioid)
    crumbs (crack cocaine)
    crunch and munch (crack cocaine)
    crush and rush (re: starch not removed from ephedrine or pseudo-ephedrine tablets in manufacture)
    Cruz (opium from Vera Cruz, Mexico)
    crying week (cannabis)
    cryppie (cannabis)
    crypto (methamphetamine; stimulant)
    cryptonic (cannabis)
    crystal (cocaine; amphetamine; methamphetamine; phencyclidine/PCP)

drugs (street names)
    crystal glass (crystal shards of methamphetamine; stimulant)
    crystal joint (phencyclidine/PCP; hallucinogen)
    crystal meth (methamphetamine; stimulant)
    crystal methadrine (amphetamine; ecstasy/MDMA; stimulant)
    crystal T (phencyclidine/PCP; hallucinogen)
    crystal tea (LSD; hallucinogen)
    cube (LSD – 1 ounce; hallucinogen)
    cubes (cannabis; crack cocaine)
    culican (cannabis)
    cupcakes (LSD; hallucinogen)
    cura (heroin; opioid)
    cut-deck (re: heroin mixed with powdered milk)
    cycline (phencyclidine/PCP; hallucinogen)
    cyclones (phencyclidine/PCP; hallucinogen)
    D (LSD; phencyclidine/PCP; hallucinogen)
    dagga (cannabis)
    Dama Blanca (cocaine)
    dance fever (designer drug; fentanyl; opioid)
    dank (cannabis; nicotine/tobacco)
    dawamesk (cannabis)
    dead on arrival (heroin; opioid)
    dead president (heroin; opioid)
    dead road (club drug; designer drug; ecstasy/MDMA; stimulant)

drugs (street names)
  debs (designer drug; ecstasy/MDMA; stimulant)
  decadence (designer drug; ecstasy/MDMA; stimulant)
  deca-duabolin (steroid compound)
  deck (re: 1 to 15 grams of heroin)
  deeds (LSD; hallucinogen)
  delatestryl (steroid compound)
  Demerol (meperidine; opioid)
  demo (crack cocaine)
  demolish (crack cocaine;
  dep-testosterone (steroid compound)
  desocsins (methamphetamine; stimulant)
  desogtion (methamphetamine; stimulant)
  DET (designer drug; dimethyltryptamine; hallucinogen)
  Detroit pink (phencyclidine/PCP; hallucinogen)
  deuce (heroin; opioid; re: $2 of drugs)
  devil drug (crack cocaine)
  devil's dandruff (cocaine; crack cocaine)
  devil's dust (phencyclidine/PCP; hallucinogen)
  devilsmoke (crack cocaine)
  dew (cannabis)
  dex (designer drug; amphetamine; ecstasy/MDMA; stimulant)
  Dexadrine (amphetamine; designer drug; ecstasy/MDMA; stimulant)
  dexies (amphetamine; stimulant)

drugs (street names)
  diablo (cannabis)
  diambista (cannabis)
  diamonds (designer drug; amphetamine; ecstasy/MDMA; stimulant)
  dianabol (steroid compound)
  diet pills (amphetamine; stimulant)
  dihydrolone (steroid compound)
  dimba (cannabis)
  dime (crack cocaine)
  dime special (crack cocaine)
  ding (cannabis)
  dinkie dow (cannabis)
  dinosaurs (re: older population of heroin users)
  dip (crack cocaine)
  dip sticks (re: cigarettes dipped in PCP oil)
  dipped joints (re: marijuana, PCP, and formaldehyde)
  dipper (phencyclidine/PCP; hallucinogen)
  dipping out (crack cocaine)
  dips (cannabis)
  dirt (heroin; opioid)
  dirt grass (cannabis)
  dirties (cannabis; cocaine)
  dirty basing (crack cocaine)
  dirty joints (cannabis; crack cocaine)
  disco biscuit(s) (barbiturate; depressant; designer drug; ecstasy/MDMA)
  disco pellets (stimulant)
  discorama (inhalant)
  ditch dirty joints (cannabis)
  ditch weed (cannabis)
  diviner's sage (salvia divinorum; hallucinogen)
  djamba (cannabis)
  DMT (designer drug; dimethyltryptamine; phencyclidine/PCP; hallucinogen)
  do a line (cocaine)

drugs (street names)
  do it Jack
    (phencyclidine/PCP;
    hallucinogen)
  DOA (crack cocaine; heroin;
    PCP)
  doctor (designer drug;
    ecstasy/MDMA; stimulant)
  doctor shopping (re: using
    doctors to obtain meds)
  dody (cannabis)
  dog food (heroin; opioid)
  doggie (heroin; opioid)
  dogs (heroin; opioid)
  dolls (amphetamine;
    depressant; designer drug;
    ecstasy/MDMA)
  domes (LSD; hallucinogen;
    methamphetamine;
    stimulant)
  domex (designer drug;
    ecstasy/MDMA and PCP
    mix)
  dominoes (amphetamine;
    stimulant)
  don jem (cannabis)
  Don Juan (cannabis)
  Dona Juana (cannabis)
  Dona Juanita (cannabis)
  donk (re: marijuana and PCP
    mix)
  doob (cannabis)
  doobee (cannabis)
  doobie/dubbe/duby
    (cannabis)
  doogie/doojee/dugie (heroin;
    opioid)
  dooley (heroin; opioid)
  doosey (heroin; opioid)
  dope (marijuana; heroin;
    other drugs)
  dope fiend (crack cocaine)
  dope smoke (cannabis)
  dopium (opium)
  doradilla (cannabis)
  dors and 4s (Doriden and
    Tylenol #4 combo)
  doses (LSD; hallucinogen)

drugs (street names)
  dosure (LSD; hallucinogen)
  dots (LSD; hallucinogen)
  doub (crack cocaine)
  double breasted dealing (re:
    dealing cocaine/heroin
    together)
  double bubble (cocaine)
  double cross (amphetamine;
    stimulant)
  double dome (LSD;
    hallucinogen)
  double rock (crack cocaine)
  double trouble (amobarbital;
    depressant; S-H-A)
  double up (crack cocaine)
  double u-s (crack cocaine)
  double yoke (crack cocaine;
    morphine)
  dove (crack cocaine)
  Dover's deck (opium)
  Dover's powder (opium)
  downie (barbiturate; S-H-A)
  DPT (dimethyltryptamine;
    hallucinogen)
  Dr. Feelgood (heroin; opioid)
  draf (cannabis; cocaine;
    ecstasy with cocaine)
  draf weed (cannabis)
  drag weed (cannabis)
  dragon roc (crack cocaine)
  dragon rock (mixture of
    heroin & crack)
  dream (cocaine)
  dream gun (opium)
  dream stick (opium)
  dreamer (morphine; opioid)
  dreams (opium)
  dreck (heroin; opioid)
  drink (phencyclidine/PCP;
    hallucinogen)
  drivers (amphetamine;
    designer drug; ecstasy/
    MDMA; stimulant)
  drop dean (fentanyl; opioid)
  dropping (re: wrapping
    methamphetamine in bread
    and eating it)

drugs (street names)
> drowsy high (barbiturate; S-H-A)
> dry high (cannabis)
> dub (crack cocaine)
> dube (cannabis)
> duby (cannabis)
> duct (cocaine)
> duji (heroin; opioid)
> dujra (heroin; opioid)
> dujre (heroin; opioid)
> dummy dust (phencyclidine/PCP; hallucinogen)
> durabolin (steroid compound)
> Durog (cannabis)
> dust (marijuana; cocaine; heroin; phencyclidine/PCP)
> dust blunt (cannabis; phencyclidine/PCP)
> dust joint (phencyclidine/PCP; hallucinogen)
> dust of angels (phencyclidine/PCP; hallucinogen)
> dusted parsley (phencyclidine/PCP; hallucinogen)
> dusting (re: adding heroin, PCP, or another drug to marijuana)
> dusting (re: using inhalants)
> dymethzine (steroid compound)
> dynamite (cocaine; cocaine mixed with heroin)
> dyno (heroin; opioid)
> dyno-pure (heroin; opioid)
> E (ecstasy; MDMA; stimulant)
> earth (cannabis; phencyclidine/PCP; hallucinogen)
> easing powder (opium)
> Eastside player (crack cocaine)
> easy lay (club drug)

drugs (street names)
> E-bombs (club drug; MDMA/ecstasy; stimulant)
> ecstasy (designer drug; MDMA; stimulant)
> egg (crack cocaine)
> Egyptians (club drug; ecstasy/MDMA; stimulant)
> eightball (crack cocaine; crack mixed with heroin)
> eighth (heroin; opioid)
> el diablito (cannabis; cocaine; heroin; PCP)
> el diablo (cocaine; marijuana; heroin)
> El Gallo ("Rooster"; cannabis)
> El Perico ("Parrot"; cocaine)
> elbows (re: one pound of methamphetamine)
> Electric Kool Aid (cocaine; crack cocaine; LSD; hallucinogen)
> elephant (cannabis; phencyclidine/PCP; hallucinogen)
> elephant flipping (club drug; re: use of PCP and MDMA)
> elephant trank (phencyclidine/PCP; hallucinogen)
> elephant tranquilizer (phencyclidine/PCP; hallucinogen)
> elephants (club drug; ecstasy/MDMA; stimulant)
> Elvis (LSD; hallucinogen)
> embalming fluid (phencyclidine/PCP; hallucinogen)
> emsel (morphine; opioid)
> endo (cannabis)
> energizer (phencyclidine/PCP; hallucinogen)
> enoltestovis (steroid compound)
> ephedrine (designer drug)

drugs (street names)
 ephedrone (methcathinone; stimulant)
 E-puddle (club drug; re: sleeping after MDMA/ecstasy use)
 equipoise (steroid compound)
 Esra (cannabis)
 essence (designer drug; ecstasy/MDMA; stimulant)
 estuffa (heroin; opioid)
 E-tard (club drug; re: under the influence of MDMA or ecstasy)
 Eve (ecstasy/MDMA; stimulant)
 everclear (GHB; depressant; S-H-A)
 Ewings (depressant)
 exiticity (club drug; designer drug; ecstasy/MDMA; stimulant)
 Explorers Club (re: group of LSD users)
 eye opener (amphetamine; crack cocaine; stimulant)
 fake STP (phencyclidine/PCP; hallucinogen)
 Fallbrook red hair (cannabis)
 famous dimes (crack cocaine)
 fantasia (designer drug; dimethyltryptamine; hallucinogen)
 fantasy (club drug; GHB; depressant; S-H-A)
 fast (methamphetamine; stimulant)
 fastin (designer drug; ecstasy/(MDMA; stimulant)
 fasts (amphetamine)
 Fat Albert (fentanyl; opioid)
 fat bags (crack cocaine)
 fatty (cannabis)
 feed bag (cannabis)
 feeling (cannabis)
 feenin (crack cocaine)
 Felix the Cat (LSD; hallucinogen)

drugs (street names)
 ferry dust (heroin; opioid)
 fi-do-nie (opium)
 fields (LSD; hallucinogen)
 fiend (cannabis)
 fifty-one (crack cocaine)
 finajet/finaject (steroid compound)
 fine stuff (cannabis)
 finger (cannabis)
 fir (cannabis)
 fire (crack and methamphetamine; stimulant)
 firewater (contains GBL; depressant; S-H-A)
 firewood (cannabis)
 first line (morphine; opioid)
 fish scales (crack cocaine)
 five-way (re: snorting heroin/cocaine/methamphetamine/ crushed flunitrazepam pills, and drinking alcohol)
 fizzies (methadone; hallucinogen)
 flake (cocaine)
 flakes (phencyclidine/PCP; hallucinogen)
 flame cooking (re: cocaine use)
 flamethrowers (cocaine, heroin, and tobacco combined)
 flamingos (depressant)
 flash (cocaine; LSD; hallucinogen)
 flat blues (LSD; hallucinogen)
 flat chunks (crack cocaine)
 flatliners (club drug)
 flave (cocaine)
 flea powder (re: low purity heroin)
 fleece (cocaine; crack cocaine)
 flex (cocaine; crack cocaine)
 flipping (club drug; ecstasy/MDMA; stimulant)

drugs (street names)
    Florida snow (cocaine; heroin; opioid)
    flower (cannabis)
    flower flipping (ecstasy/MDMA mixed with mushrooms; psilocybin/psilocin; hallucinogen)
    flower tops (cannabis)
    flowers (depressant)
    Fly Mexican Airlines (cannabis)
    foil (heroin; opioid)
    foo-foo (cocaine)
    foo-foo dust (cocaine)
    foo-foo stuff (cocaine; heroin)
    foolish powder (cocaine; heroin)
    forget me drug (designer drug; Rohypnol/flunitrazepam; S-H-A)
    forget pill (designer drug; Rohypnol/flunitrazepam; S-H-A)
    forget-me pill (club drug; Rohypnol/flunitrazepam; S-H-A)
    forwards (amphetamine)
    four leaf clover (club drug; ecstasy/MDMA; stimulant)
    fraho/frajo (cannabis)
    freebase (cocaine; crack cocaine)
    freebasing (crack cocaine)
    freeze (cocaine)
    French blue (amphetamine)
    French fries (crack cocaine)
    fresh (phencyclidine/PCP; hallucinogen)
    friend (designer drug; fentanyl; opioid)
    fries (crack cocaine)
    frios (cannabis; phencyclidine/PCP; hallucinogen)

drugs (street names)
    Frisco special (cocaine/heroin/LSD)
    Frisco speedball (cocaine/heroin/ a dash of LSD)
    friskie powder (cocaine)
    frontloading (cocaine)
    fry (cannabis; crack cocaine; phencyclidine/PCP)
    fry daddy (cannabis; crack cocaine)
    fry sticks (cannabis; phencyclidine/PCP; tobacco)
    fu (cannabis)
    fuel (cannabis; phencyclidine/PCP; hallucinogen)
    fuel fuma D'Angola (Portuguese cannabis)
    furra (heroin)
    G (GHB; depressant; S-H-A)
    G.B. (barbiturate; S-H-A)
    gaffel (cocaine)
    gage/gauge (cannabis)
    gaggers (designer drug; methcathinone; stimulant)
    gaggler (designer drug; amphetamine; MDMA; stimulant)
    gallop (heroin; opioid)
    galloping horse (heroin; opioid)
    gallup (heroin; opioid)
    gamut (heroin; opioid)
    gange (synthetic cannabis)
    gangster (cannabis)
    gangster (re: user or manufacturer of methamphetamine)
    gangster pills (barbiturate; depressant; S-H-A)
    ganja (cannabis)
    gank (crack cocaine)
    ganoobies (cannabis)
    garbage (re: low quality marijuana or heroin)

Psychiatric Words and Phrases

drugs (street names)
  garbage heads (crack cocaine)
  garbage rock (crack cocaine)
  gash (cannabis)
  Gasper (cannabis)
  Gasper stick (cannabis)
  gato (heroin; opioid)
  gauge butt (cannabis)
  GB (gamma hydroxybutyrate; depressant; S-H-A)
  GBH (gamma hydroxybutyrate)
  GBL (gamma butyrolactone is used to make GHB)
  gee (opium)
  geek (cannabis; crack cocaine)
  geek joints
  geeker (crack cocaine)
  geek-joints (cannabis; cocaine; crack cocaine; tobacco)
  geep (methamphetamine; stimulant)
  geeter (methamphetamine; stimulant)
  geeze (cocaine)
  geigo (stimulants
  genuines (depressant)
  George (heroin; opioid)
  George smack (heroin; opioid)
  Georgia home boy (club drug; designer drug; GHB; depressant; S-H-A)
  get a gage up (cannabis)
  get high (cannabis)
  get-off houses (re: places drug users buy/use heroin for a fee)
  get the wind (cannabis)
  get-go (methamphetamine; stimulant)
  getting glassed (re: snorting methamphetamine)
  getting roached (re: using Rohypnol)

drugs (street names)
  getting snotty (heroin; opioid)
  GGT (gamma-glutamyltransferase)
  Ghana (cannabis)
  GHB (designer drug; gamma hydroxybutyrate; depressant; S-H-A)
  ghost (LSD; hallucinogen)
  ghost busting (cocaine; crack cocaine)
  gick monster (crack cocaine)
  gift-of-the-sun (cocaine)
  gift-of-the-sun-god (cocaine)
  giggle smoke (cannabis)
  giggle weed (cannabis)
  gimmie (cannabis; crack cocaine)
  gin (cocaine)
  girl (cocaine; crack cocaine; heroin)
  girlfriend (cocaine)
  give wings (re: injecting or teaching someone to inject heroin)
  glacines (heroin; opioid)
  glad stuff (cocaine)
  glading (re: using inhalants)
  glass (amphetamine)
  glass (heroin; opioid)
  glass (heroin; amphetamine; meth; re: hypoderm. needle)
  glo (crack cocaine)
  gluey (re: glue sniffer or inhaler)
  Go (designer drug; amphetamine; ecstasy/MDMA; stimulant)
  go on a sleigh ride (cocaine)
  goat (heroin; opioid)
  God's drug (morphine; opioid)
  God's flesh (psilocybin/psilocin; hallucinogen)
  God's medicine (opium)

Psychiatric Words and Phrases

drugs (street names)
Go-fast (designer drug; methamphetamine; stimulant)
gofers (depressant; S-H-A)
gold (cannabis; crack cocaine; heroin)
gold dust (cocaine)
gold star (cannabis)
golden (cannabis)
golden dragon (LSD; hallucinogen)
golden eagle (club drug)
golden girl (heroin; opioid)
golden leaf (cannabis)
golf ball (crack cocaine)
golf balls (barbiturate; depressant; S-H-A)
golpe (heroin; opioid)
goma (black tar heroin + opium; opioid)
gondola (opium)
gone (crack cocaine)
gong (cannabis; opium)
gonj (cannabis)
goob (designer drug; methcathinone; stimulant)
Good (phencyclidine/PCP; hallucinogen)
Good and Plenty (heroin; opioid)
good butt (cannabis)
good giggles (cannabis)
good H (heroin; opioid)
good horse (heroin; opioid)
good stuff (cannabis)
goodfelas (designer drug; fentanyl; opioid)
goody-goody (cannabis)
goof butt (cannabis)
goofball (cocaine; cocaine mixed with heroin)
goofy's (LSD; hallucinogen)
goon (phencyclidine/PCP; hallucinogen)
goon dust (phencyclidine/PCP; hallucinogen)

drugs (street names)
goop (club drug; GHB; depressant; S-H-A)
gorge (cannabis)
goric (opium; opioid)
gorilla biscuits (phencyclidine/PCP; hallucinogen)
gorilla pills (barbiturate; depressant; S-H-A)
gorilla tab (phencyclidine/PCP; hallucinogen)
gram (hashish; hallucinogen)
granulated orange (methamphetamine; stimulant)
grape parfait (LSD; hallucinogen)
grass (cannabis)
grass brownies (cannabis)
grass hopper (cannabis)
grata (cannabis)
gravel (crack cocaine)
gravy (heroin; opioid; re: to inject a drug)
great bear (designer drug; fentanyl; opioid)
great hormones at bedtime (GHB; depressant; S-H-A)
great tobacco (opium)
Greek (cannabis)
green (designer drug; phencyclidine/PCP; hallucinogen; cannabis; re: inferior quality of ketamine)
green buds (cannabis)
green double domes (LSD; hallucinogen)
green dragons (depressant; S-H-A)
green frog (barbiturate; depressant; S-H-A)
green goddess (cannabis)
green gold (cocaine)
green leaves (phencyclidine/PCP; hallucinogen)

Psychiatric Words and Phrases

drugs (street names)
  green single dome (LSD; hallucinogen)
  green triangles (club drug; ecstasy/MDMA; stimulant)
  green wedge (LSD; hallucinogen)
  greenies (designer drug; amphetamine; ecstasy/MDMA)
  greens (cannabis)
  greeter (cannabis)
  gremmies (cannabis)
  Greta (cannabis)
  grey shields (LSD; hallucinogen)
  griefo (cannabis)
  griefs (cannabis)
  grievous bodily harm (designer drug; GHB; depressant; S-H-A)
  grifa (cannabis)
  griff (cannabis)
  griffa (cannabis)
  G-riffic (GHB; depressant; S-H-A)
  griffo (cannabis)
  grit (crack cocaine)
  groceries (crack cocaine)
  G-rock (cocaine)
  ground control (re: guide during a hallucinogenic "trip")
  grows (cannabis)
  G-shot (cannabis)
  gum (club drug; designer drug; ecstasy/MDMA; stimulant)
  guma (opium; opioid)
  gunga (cannabis)
  gungeon (cannabis)
  gungun (cannabis)
  gunja (cannabis)
  GWM (club drug; designer drug; ecstasy/MDMA; stimulant)
  gym candy (anabolic steroid compound)

drugs (street names)
  gyve (cannabis)
  H & C (heroin and cocaine)
  H (heroin; opioid)
  H caps (heroin; opioid)
  hache (heroin; opioid)
  hail (crack cocaine)
  haircut (cannabis)
  hairy (heroin; opioid)
  half a football field (crack cocaine)
  half elbows (re: 1/2 pound of methamphetamine)
  half load (re: 15 bags/decks of heroin)
  half moon (mescaline/peyote; hallucinogen)
  half piece (re: 1/2 ounce of heroin or cocaine)
  half track (crack cocaine)
  hamburger helper (crack cocaine)
  hammerheading (club drug; re: MDMA or ecstasy with Viagra)
  handlebars (cocaine; crack cocaine)
  hand-to-hand man (crack cocaine)
  hanhich (cannabis)
  hanyak (amphetamine; smokable methamphetamine; stimulant)
  happy cigarette (cannabis)
  happy drug (club drug; designer drug; ecstasy/MDMA; stimulant)
  happy dust (cocaine)
  happy pill (club drug; designer drug; ecstasy/MDMA; stimulant)
  happy powder (cocaine)
  happy stick (re: marijuana & PCP combination)
  happy trails (cocaine)
  hard ball (crack cocaine)
  hard candy (heroin; opioid)

drugs (street names)
- hard line (crack cocaine)
- hard rock (crack cocaine)
- hard stuff (heroin; opioid)
- hardware (inhalant)
- Harry (heroin; opioid)
- hats (LSD; hallucinogen)
- have a dust (cocaine)
- Hawaiian (cannabis)
- Hawaiian black (cannabis)
- Hawaiian homegrown hay (cannabis)
- Hawaiian sunshine (LSD; hallucinogen)
- hawk (LSD; hallucinogen)
- hawkers (re: sellers of drugs at a club)
- hay (cannabis)
- hay butt (cannabis)
- Hayron (heroin; opioid)
- haze (LSD; hallucinogen)
- Hazel (heroin; opioid)
- H-bomb (club drug; ecstasy/MDMA mixed with heroin)
- HCP (phencyclidine/PCP; hallucinogen)
- head drugs (amphetamine; stimulants)
- head light (LSD; hallucinogen)
- heart-on (inhalant)
- hearts (amphetamine; stimulants)
- heaven (cocaine; heroin)
- heaven and hell (phencyclidine/PCP; hallucinogen)
- heaven dust (cocaine; heroin)
- heavenly blue (LSD; hallucinogen)
- Helen (heroin; opioid)
- hell (crack cocaine)
- hell dust (heroin; opioid)
- he-man (designer drug; fentanyl; opioid)
- hemp (cannabis)
- henpecking (crack cocaine)

drugs (street names)
- Henry (heroin; opioid)
- Henry VIII (cocaine)
- her (cocaine)
- Hera (heroin; opioid)
- herb (cannabis)
- Herb and Al (cannabis and alcohol)
- herba (cannabis)
- herbal bliss (club drug; designer drug; ecstasy/MDMA; stimulant)
- herms (phencyclidine/PCP; hallucinogen)
- hero (heroin; opioid)
- hero of the underworld (heroin; opioid)
- heroin (diacetylmorphine)
- heroina (heroin; opioid)
- herone (heroin; opioid)
- he-she (cocaine)
- hessle (heroin; opioid)
- hiagra in a bottle (inhalant)
- highball (inhalant)
- hikori (mescaline/peyote; hallucinogen)
- hikuli (mescaline/peyote; hallucinogen)
- hillbilly heroin (OxyContin; opioid)
- him (heroin; opioid)
- Hinkley (phencyclidine/PCP; hallucinogen)
- hippie crack (inhalant)
- hippieflip (re: use of MDMA or ecstasy with mushrooms)
- hironpon (smokable methamphetamine; stimulant)
- hit (cannabis; crack cocaine)
- hit the hay (cannabis)
- hitch up the reindeers (cocaine)
- hitters (re: people who inject others in exchange for drugs)
- hocus (cannabis; opium)
- hog (phencyclidine/PCP; hallucinogen)

Psychiatric Words and Phrases

drugs (street names)
holiday meth (re: green methamphetamine using Draino)
holly terror (heroin; opioid)
hombre (heroin; opioid)
hombrecitos (psilocybin/psilocin; hallucinogen)
homegrown hay (cannabis)
homicide (re: heroin cut with scopolamine or strychnine)
honey blunts (cannabis)
honey oil (ketamine; dissociative hallucinogen; inhalant)
hong-yen (re: heroin in pill form; opioid)
hooch (cannabis)
hooter (cannabis; cocaine)
hop/hops (opium)
horn (cocaine)
horning (cocaine; heroin)
horse (heroin; opioid)
horse heads (amphetamine; stimulant)
horse tracks (phencyclidine/PCP; hallucinogen)
horse tranquilizer (phencyclidine/PCP; hallucinogen)
horsebite (heroin; opioid)
hospital heroin (re: Dilaudid)
hot dope (heroin; opioid)
hot heroin (re: poisoned heroin for informant)
hot ice (smokable methamphetamine; stimulant)
hot rolling (re: liquefying methamphetamine; inhaling it)
hot stick (cannabis)
hotcakes (crack cocaine)
hotrailing (re: heat methamphetamine; inhale through nose)

drugs (street names)
house fee (re: crack cocaine use)
house piece (re: crack cocaine use)
How do you like me now? (crack cocaine)
hows (morphine; opioid)
HRN (heroin; opioid)
hubba (crack cocaine)
Hubba, I am back (crack cocaine)
hubba pigeon (crack cocaine)
hubbas (crack cocaine)
huff (inhalant)
huffer (re: inhalant drug abuser)
huffing (re: sniffing an inhalant)
hug (ecstasy; stimulant)
hug drug (MDMA/ecstasy; stimulant)
hugs and kisses (club drug; methamphetamine with MDMA; stimulant)
hunter (cocaine)
hyatari (mescaline/peyote; hallucinogen)
hydro (amphetamine; cannabis; ecstasy/MDMA)
hydrogrows (cannabis)
hype (heroin; opioid)
hype (re: MDMA or ecstasy addict)
I am back (crack cocaine)
iboga (designer drug; amphetamine; ecstasy/MDMA; stimulant)
ice (amphetamine; cocaine; crack cocaine; ecstasy/MDMA; PCP; smokable methamphetamine; stimulant)
ice cube (crack cocaine)
icing (cocaine)
idiot pills (barbiturate; depressant; S-H-A)

drugs (street names)
    igloo (club drug;
      ecstasy/MDMA; stimulant)
    ill (phencyclidine/PCP;
      hallucinogen)
    illies (re: marijuana dipped in
      PCP)
    illing (re: marijuana dipped
      in PCP)
    illy (cannabis)
    illy momo
      (phencyclidine/PCP;
      hallucinogen)
    in-betweens (amphetamine;
      barbiturate; depressant;
      LSD)
    Inca message (cocaine)
    incredible hulk (fentanyl;
      opioid)
    Indian boy (cannabis)
    Indian hay (cannabis)
    Indian hemp (cannabis)
    Indica (cannabis)
    Indo (cannabis)
    Indonesian bud (cannabis;
      opium)
    instaga (cannabis)
    instagu (cannabis)
    instant zen (LSD;
      hallucinogen)
    interplanetary mission (crack
      cocaine)
    Isda (heroin; opioid)
    issues (crack cocaine)
    ivory wave (club drug;
      cocaine; ecstasy/MDMA;
      stimulant)
    J (cannabis)
    jackpot (designer drug;
      fentanyl; opioid)
    jam (amphetamine; cocaine)
    jam cecil (amphetamine;
      stimulants
    Jamaican gold (cannabis)
    Jamaican red hair (cannabis)
    Jane (cannabis)
    jay (re: to smoke cannabis)
    je gee (heroin; opioid)

drugs (street names)
    jejo (cocaine)
    jellies (club drug; re:
      combination of MDMA and
      depressants in gel form)
    jelly (cocaine)
    jelly baby (amphetamine;
      stimulants
    jelly bean (depressant; S-H-
      A)
    jelly beans (amphetamine;
      crack cocaine; stimulants
    Jerry Garcias (club drug;
      ecstasy/MDMA; stimulant)
    Jerry Springer (heroin;
      opioid)
    jet (designer drug; ketamine;
      dissociative hallucinogen)
    jet fuel (methamphetamine
      combined with PCP)
    Jib (GHB; depressant; S-H-
      A)
    Jim Jones (cannabis; cocaine;
      phencyclidine/PCP)
    Jim Jones jive (cannabis)
    jive (marijuana; heroin)
    jive doo jee (heroin; opioid)
    jive stick (cannabis)
    joharito (heroin; opioid)
    Johnson (crack cocaine)
    joint (cannabis)
    jojee (heroin; opioid)
    jolly beans (amphetamine;
      stimulant)
    jolly green (cannabis)
    jolly pop (re: casual heroin
      user)
    Jones (heroin; opioid)
    joy (heroin; opioid)
    joy flakes (heroin; opioid)
    joy juice (barbiturate;
      depressant; S-H-A)
    joy plant (opium)
    joy powder (cocaine; heroin)
    joy smoke (cannabis)
    joy stick (cannabis;
      phencyclidine/PCP;
      hallucinogen)

drugs (street names)
  Juan Valdez (cannabis)
  Juanita (cannabis)
  jugs (amphetamine; stimulants)
  juice (phencyclidine/PCP; hallucinogen)
  juice (anabolic steroid compound)
  juice joint (cannabis; crack cocaine)
  juja (cannabis)
  ju-ju (cannabis)
  jum (crack cocaine)
  jumbos (cannabis; crack cocaine)
  junk (cocaine; heroin)
  K (phencyclidine/PCP; hallucinogen)
  K2 (designer drug; synthetic cannabis; hallucinogen)
  kabak (cannabis)
  kabayo (heroin; opioid)
  kabuki (crack cocaine)
  kaff (cannabis)
  Kaksonjae (methamphetamine; stimulant)
  kalakit (cannabis)
  Kali (cannabis)
  kangaroo (crack cocaine)
  Kansas grass (cannabis)
  Karachi (heroin; phenobarbital, and methaqualone)
  Karo (cocaine cough syrup)
  Kate bush (cannabis)
  Kawaii electric (cannabis)
  Kay (cannabis)
  kaya (cannabis)
  KB (cannabis)
  K-blast (phencyclidine/PCP; hallucinogen)
  kee (cannabis)
  keel (re: heroin (other narcotics) laced with fentanyl; opioid)
  Kentucky blue (cannabis)

drugs (street names)
  ket (designer drug; ketamine; dissociative hallucinogen)
  KGB (killer green bud; cannabis)
  khayl (cannabis)
  K-hole (designer drug; re: depressant high associated with ketamine)
  Ki (cannabis)
  kibbles and bits (crack cocaine)
  kick (inhalant)
  kick stick (cannabis)
  kicker OxyContin; opioid)
  kief (cannabis)
  kiff (cannabis)
  kill (re: heroin (other narcotics) laced with fentanyl)
  killer (cannabis; phencyclidine/PCP; hallucinogen)
  killer weed (cannabis) (phencyclidine/PCP; hallucinogen)
  kilter (cannabis)
  kind (cannabis)
  kind bud (cannabis)
  king (cocaine)
  king bud (cannabis)
  king ivory (designer drug; fentanyl; opioid)
  King Kong pills (barbiturate; depressant; S-H-A)
  king's habit (cocaine)
  kissing (crack cocaine)
  kit kat (designer drug; ketamine; dissociative hallucinogen)
  kitty flipping (club drug; re: ketamine and MDMA/ecstasy use)
  KJ (phencyclidine/PCP; hallucinogen)
  Kleenex (designer drug; ecstasy (MDMA; stimulant)
  Klingons (crack cocaine)

drugs (street names)
K-lots (club drug; re: bags of 1000 MDMA or ecstasy pills)
Kokomo (crack cocaine)
koller joints (phencyclidine/PCP; hallucinogen)
kona gold (cannabis)
kools (phencyclidine/PCP; hallucinogen)
krippy (cannabis)
krokodil (desomorphine; synthetic morphine (opioid)
Kryptonite (cannabis; crack cocaine)
krystal (phencyclidine/PCP; hallucinogen)
krystal joint (phencyclidine/PCP; hallucinogen)
Kumba (cannabis)
kush (cannabis)
KW (phencyclidine/PCP; hallucinogen)
L (LSD; hallucinogen)
L.A. (amphetamine)
L.A. glass (smokable methamphetamine; stimulant)
L.A. ice (smokable methamphetamine; stimulant)
L.L. (cannabis)
la buena (heroin; opioid)
la chiva (heroin; opioid)
la rocha (designer drug; Rohypnol/flunitrazepam; S-H-A)
lace (cannabis; cocaine)
lactone (GBL/gamma butyrolactone; depressant; S-H-A)
lady (heroin; opioid)
lady caine (cocaine)
lady snow (cocaine)
lakbay diva (cannabis)
Lamborghini (crack cocaine)

drugs (street names)
las mujercitas (psilocybin/psilocin; hallucinogen)
lason sa daga (LSD; hallucinogen)
late night (cocaine)
laughing gas (nitrous oxide; inhalant)
laughing grass (cannabis)
laughing weed (cannabis)
lay back (barbiturate; depressant; S-H-A)
laze (LSD; hallucinogen)
LBJ (heroin + LSD + PCP)
leaf (cannabis; cocaine)
leak (cannabis; re: Marijuana/PCP combination)
leaky bolla (phencyclidine/PCP; hallucinogen)
leaky leak (phencyclidine/PCP; hallucinogen)
lean (cocaine cough syrup)
leapers (amphetamine; stimulants
lemon 714 (phencyclidine/PCP; hallucinogen)
lemon drop (yellow tinged methamphetamine; stimulant)
lemons (depressant)
lemonade (heroin; re: poor quality drugs; re: blunts mixed with marijuana & heroin)
Lennons (depressant)
Leno (cannabis)
lenos (phencyclidine/PCP; hallucinogen)
lens (LSD; hallucinogen)
lethal injection (fentanyl; opioid)
lethal weapon (phencyclidine/PCP; hallucinogen)

drugs (street names)
    letter biscuits (club drug; ecstasy/MDMA; stimulant)
    LG (lime green; cannabis)
    lib (Librium (barbiturate; depressant; S-H-A)
    lid (cannabis)
    lid poppers (amphetamine; stimulants
    light stuff (cannabis)
    lightning (amphetamine; stimulants
    lily (amobarbital; S-H-A)
    Lima (cannabis)
    lime acid (LSD; hallucinogen)
    line (cocaine)
    liprimo (cannabis; crack cocaine)
    liquid E (GHB; depressant; S-H-A)
    liquid ecstasy (club drug; designer drug; GHB; depressant; S-H-A)
    liquid G (GHB; depressant; S-H-A)
    liquid X (club drug; GHB; depressant; S-H-A)
    lithium (re: better grade of methamphetamine; re: skin lesions due to meth abuse)
    little bomb (amphetamine; barbiturate; depressant; heroin)
    little boy (heroin; opioid)
    little ones (phencyclidine/PCP; hallucinogen)
    little smoke (cannabis; LSD; psilocybin/psilocin; hallucinogen)
    live ones (phencyclidine/PCP; hallucinogen)
    llesca (cannabis)
    load (re: 25 bags of heroin)
    load of laundry (methamphetamine; stimulant)

drugs (street names)
    loaf (cannabis)
    lobo (cannabis)
    locker room (inhalant)
    loco (cannabis)
    locoweed (cannabis)
    log (cannabis; phencyclidine/PCP; hallucinogen)
    logor (LSD; hallucinogen)
    Looney Toons (LSD; hallucinogen)
    loose shank (cannabis)
    love (crack cocaine)
    love affair (cocaine)
    love boat (cannabis; heroin)
    love boat (re: marijuana/PCP combination)
    love drug (barbiturate; depressant; designer drug; ecstasy/MDMA; stimulant)
    love flipping (club drug; mescaline & MDMA)
    love leaf (cannabis; phencyclidine/PCP; hallucinogen)
    love pearls (designer drug)
    love pill (club drug; designer drug; ecstasy/MDMA; stimulant)
    love trip (designer drug; ecstasy/MDMA and mescaline)
    love weed (cannabis)
    lovelies (cannabis; re: marijuana laced with PCP)
    lovely (phencyclidine/PCP; hallucinogen)
    lovers (depressant)
    lovers' special (club drug; ecstasy/MDMA; stimulant)
    lovers' speed (ecstasy (MDMA; stimulant)
    LSD (lysergic acid diethylamide)
    lubage (cannabis)
    Lucy in the sky with diamonds (LSD; hallucinogen)

drugs (street names)
   ludes (depressant; S-H-A)
   luding out (barbiturate; depressant; S-H-A)
   luds (barbiturate; depressant; S-H-A)
   lunch money drug (designer drug; Rohypnol/flunitrazepam; S-H-A)
   M (cannabis; morphine)
   M&M (barbiturate; depressant; S-H-A)
   M.J. (cannabis)
   M.O. (cannabis)
   M.S. (morphine; opioid)
   M.U. (cannabis)
   Ma'a (cocaine; crack cocaine)
   mac (heroin; opioid)
   macaroni (cannabis)
   macaroni and cheese (cannabis; cocaine)
   machinery (cannabis)
   Macon (cannabis)
   Maconha (cannabis)
   MAD (designer drug)
   mad dog (phencyclidine/PCP; hallucinogen)
   madman (phencyclidine/PCP; hallucinogen)
   mafu (cannabis)
   magic (phencyclidine/PCP; hallucinogen)
   magic dust (phencyclidine/PCP; hallucinogen)
   magic mink (salvia divinorum; hallucinogen)
   magic mushroom (psilocybin/psilocin; hallucinogen)
   magic smoke (cannabis)
   mama coca (cocaine)
   Mandies (depressant)
   Manhattan silver (cannabis)
   mansakow (heroin)
   manteca (heroin; opioid)
   MAO (amphetamine; ecstasy (MDMA; stimulant)

drugs (street names)
   Mapergan (meperidine; opioid)
   marathons (amphetamine)
   marching dust (cocaine)
   Mari (cannabis)
   Maria Pastora (salvia divinorum; hallucinogen)
   marimba (cannabis)
   marshmallow reds (barbiturate; depressant; S-H-A)
   Mary (cannabis)
   Mary and Johnny (cannabis)
   Mary Ann (cannabis)
   Mary Jane (cannabis)
   Mary Jonas (cannabis)
   Mary Warner (cannabis)
   Mary Weaver (cannabis)
   Masarati (crack cocaine)
   matchbox (cannabis)
   Matsakow (heroin; opioid)
   Maui wauie (cannabis)
   Maui-wowie (cannabis; methamphetamine)
   max (designer drug; re: water-diluted GHB/amphetamine mixture)
   maxibolin (steroid compound)
   mayo (cocaine; heroin)
   M-cat (stimulants)
   MDM (designer drug; MDMA/ecstasy; stimulant)
   MDMA (designer drug; methylendioxymethamphetamine; stimulant)
   mean green (phencyclidine/PCP; hallucinogen)
   Medusa (inhalant)
   Meg (cannabis)
   Megg (cannabis)
   Meggie (cannabis)
   mellow yellow (LSD; hallucinogen)
   Mercedes (club drug)
   Merck (cocaine)

drugs (street names)
  merk (cocaine)
  mesc (mescaline; hallucinogen)
  mescal (mescaline; hallucinogen)
  mese (mescaline; hallucinogen)
  messorole (cannabis)
  meth (methamphetamine; stimulant)
  meth head (re: regular methamphetamine user; stimulant)
  meth monster (re: a violent reaction to methamphetamine; stimulant)
  meth speedball (methamphetamine and heroin)
  methatriol (steroid compound)
  methedrine (amphetamine; designer drug; ecstasy/MDMA; stimulant)
  methlies quik (methamphetamine; stimulant)
  methnecks (re: methamphetamine addicts)
  methyltestosterone (steroid compound)
  Mexican brown (cannabis; heroin)
  Mexican crack (methamphetamine; stimulant)
  Mexican horse (heroin; opioid)
  Mexican locoweed (cannabis)
  Mexican mud (heroin; opioid)
  Mexican mushroom (psilocybin/psilocin; hallucinogen)
  Mexican red (cannabis)
  Mexican reds (barbiturate; depressant; S-H-A)

drugs (street names)
  Mexican speedballs (crack and methamphetamine; stimulant)
  Mexican Valium (designer drug; Rohypnol/flunitrazepam)S-H-A)
  mezc (mescaline; hallucinogen)
  MFT (club drug; designer drug; Nexus; hallucinogen)
  miaow (stimulant)
  Mickey Finn (barbiturate; depressant; S-H-A)
  Mickey's (barbiturate; depressant; LSD)
  microdot (LSD; hallucinogen)
  midnight oil (opium)
  Mighty Joe Young (barbiturate; depressant; S-H-A)
  mighty mezz (cannabis)
  Mighty Quinn (LSD; hallucinogen)
  mighty white (cocaine)
  mind detergent (LSD; hallucinogen)
  mini beans (amphetamine; designer drug; ecstasy/MDMA; stimulant)
  mini bennie (amphetamine; stimulant)
  mint leaf (phencyclidine/PCP; hallucinogen)
  mint weed (phencyclidine/PCP; hallucinogen)
  mira (opium; opioid)
  Mirra (khat; stimulant)
  Miss Emma (morphine; opioid)
  missile basing (phencyclidine/PCP; hallucinogen)
  mission (crack cocaine)
  mist (crack cocaine)

drugs (street names)
    Mister Blue (morphine; opioid)
    Mitsubishi (club drug; ecstasy/MDMA; stimulant)
    mix (cocaine)
    mixed jive (crack cocaine)
    Mo (cannabis; cocaine)
    modams (cannabis)
    mohasky (cannabis)
    Mojo (cocaine; heroin)
    Molly (club drug; purest form of MDMA; stimulant)
    mon (cocaine)
    mone (heroin; opioid)
    money talks (heroin; opioid)
    monkey (cocaine; heroin)
    monkey dust (phencyclidine/PCP; hallucinogen)
    monkey tranquilizer (phencyclidine/PCP; hallucinogen)
    monoamine oxidase (MAO; MDMA/ecstasy; stimulant)
    monos (cocaine; nicotine/tobacco)
    monster (cocaine)
    monte (cannabis)
    mooca/moocah (cannabis)
    moon (mescaline; hallucinogen)
    mon gas (inhalant)
    moonrock (crack cocaine; crack mixed with heroin)
    moonstone (club drug; re: dealer shaves MDMA into a bag of heroin)
    mooster (cannabis)
    moota/mutah (cannabis)
    mooters (cannabis)
    mootie (cannabis)
    mootos (cannabis)
    mor a grifa (cannabis)
    more (phencyclidine/PCP; hallucinogen)
    morf (morphine; opioid)
    morning shot (amphetamine; ecstasy/MDMA; stimulant)

drugs (street names)
    morning wakeup (crack cocaine)
    Morotgara (heroin; opioid)
    morpho (morphine; opioid)
    mortal combat (re: high potency heroin)
    mosquitos (cocaine)
    mota/moto (cannabis)
    mother (cannabis)
    mother's little helper (barbiturate; depressant; S-H-A)
    movie star drug (cocaine)
    mow the grass (cannabis)
    Mu (cannabis)
    mud (heroin + opium; opioid)
    muggie (cannabis)
    muggle/muggles (cannabis)
    mujer (cocaine)
    murder 8 (designer drug; fentanyl; opioid)
    murder one (heroin and cocaine)
    murotugora (heroin; opioid)
    mushrooms (psilocybin/psilocin; hallucinogen)
    musk (psilocybin/psilocin; hallucinogen)
    muta (cannabis)
    mutha (cannabis)
    muzzle (heroin; opioid)
    nail (cannabis)
    nanoo (heroin; opioid)
    Nazimeth (methamphetamine; stimulant)
    nebbies (depressant; S-H-A)
    nemmies (barbiturate; depressant; S-H-A)
    new acid (phencyclidine/PCP; hallucinogen)
    New Jack Swing (heroin and morphine; opioid)
    new magic (phencyclidine/PCP; hallucinogen)

drugs (street names)
- Nexus (club drug; designer drug; 2-CB; hallucinogen)
- Nexus flipping (club drug; designer drug; re: use of 2CB and MDMA)
- nice and easy (heroin; opioid)
- nickel bag (re: $5 worth of heroin)
- nickel deck (heroin; opioid)
- nickelodians (crack cocaine)
- niebla (phencyclidine/PCP; hallucinogen)
- nieve (cocaine)
- Nigra (cannabis)
- nimbies (S-H-A; barbiturate; depressant; S-H-A)
- nineteen (amphetamine; designer drug; MDMA/ecstasy; stimulant)
- nitrite (an inhalant)
- no worries (depressant; S-H-A)
- nod (re: effect of heroin)
- nods (codeine cough syrup; opioid)
- noise (heroin; opioid)
- nontoucher (crack cocaine)
- Northern lights (cannabis)
- nose (cocaine; heroin)
- nose drops (liquid heroin; opioid)
- nose powder (cocaine)
- nose stuff (cocaine)
- NOX (club drug; re: use of nitrous oxide and MDMA)
- nubs (mescaline/peyote; hallucinogen)
- nugget (amphetamine; stimulant)
- nuggets (crack cocaine)
- number 1 (cocaine and heroin)
- number 3 (cocaine and heroin)
- number 4 (heroin; opioid)
- number 6 (heroin; opioid)
- number 8 (heroin; opioid)

drugs (street names)
- nurse (heroin; opioid)
- O (opium; opioid)
- O.J. (cannabis)
- O.P. (opium; opioid)
- O.P.P. (phencyclidine/PCP; hallucinogen)
- ocean burst (club drug; cocaine; designer drug; re: powdery substance mimics effect of ecstasy)
- OCs (OxyContin) opioid)
- octane (phencyclidine/PCP; hallucinogen)
- ogoy (heroin; opioid)
- oil (heroin; phencyclidine/PCP)
- old garbage (heroin; opioid)
- old navy (heroin; opioid)
- Old Steve (heroin; opioid)
- on a mission (crack cocaine)
- on the ball (club drug; re: dealer shaving MDMA into a bag of heroin)
- on the nod (re: under the influence of depressants/narcotics)
- one and one (cocaine and heroin mix)
- one and ones (Talwin & Ritalin combined injection simulates effect of heroin mixed with cocaine)
- one bomb (cocaine; crack cocaine)
- one on one house (re: place to purchase cocaine and heroin)
- one plus one sales (re: selling cocaine and heroin together)
- one tissue box (crack cocaine)
- one way (heroin; opioid; LSD; hallucinogen)
- one-fifty-one (crack cocaine)
- onion (cocaine; crack cocaine)
- oolies (cannabis)

drugs (street names)
  OP (opium; opioid)
  ope (opium; opioid)
  optical illusions (LSD; hallucinogen)
  orange bandits (club drug; ecstasy/MDMA; stimulant)
  orange barrels (LSD; hallucinogen)
  orange crystal (phencyclidine/PCP; hallucinogen)
  orange cubes (LSD; hallucinogen)
  orange haze (LSD; hallucinogen)
  orange line (heroin; opioid)
  orange micro (LSD; hallucinogen)
  orange wedges (LSD; hallucinogen)
  oranges (amphetamine; stimulant)
  organic Quaalude (GHB; depressant; S-H-A)
  Os (OxyContin) opioid)
  outer limits (crack cocaine and LSD)
  Owsley (LSD; hallucinogen)
  Owsley's acid (LSD; hallucinogen)
  Ox (OxyContin; semi-synthetic opiate)
  Oxicotton (OxyContin; semi-synthetic opiate)
  Oxy 80s (OxyContin; semi-synthetic opiate)
  Oxycet (OxyContin; semi-synthetic opiate)
  oyster stew (cocaine)
  Oz (inhalant)
  ozone (cannabis; crack cocaine)
  ozone (phencyclidine/PCP; hallucinogen)
  OZs (methamphetamine; stimulant)
  P (phencyclidine/PCP; hallucinogen)

drugs (street names)
  P (peyote; hallucinogen)
  P and P (club drug) (re: combing of MDMA/ecstasy & Viagra)
  P.R. (Panama Red; cannabis)
  pack (cannabis; heroin)
  pack a bowl (cannabis)
  pack of rocks (cannabis)
  pakaloco (cannabis)
  Pakistani black (cannabis)
  Panama cut (cannabis)
  Panama gold (cannabis)
  Panama red (cannabis)
  panatela (cannabis)
  pancakes and syrup (depressant; S-H-A)
  pane (LSD; hallucinogen)
  Pangonadalot (heroin; opioid)
  paper (re: 1/10 of gram of heroin; methamphetamine)
  paper acid (LSD; hallucinogen)
  paper blunts (cannabis)
  paper boy (re: heroin peddler)
  parabolin (steroid compound)
  parachute (crack cocaine)
  parachute (phencyclidine/PCP; hallucinogen; smoked heroin)
  parachute down (re : use of MDMA after heroin)
  paradise (cocaine)
  paradise white (cocaine)
  parlay (crack cocaine; phencyclidine/PCP)
  parsley (cannabis)
  party and play (re: MDMA or ecstasy combined with Viagra)
  party pack (club drug; designer drug; re: combing Nexus with ecstasy or other drug)
  paste (crack cocaine)

Psychiatric Words and Phrases

drugs (street names)
  pasto (cannabis)
  Pat (cannabis)
  patico (crack cocaine)
  paz (phencyclidine/PCP; hallucinogen)
  PCPA (phencyclidine/PCP; hallucinogen)
  P-dogs (cannabis; crack cocaine)
  P-dope (re: 20-30% pure heroin)
  peace (club drug; phencyclidine/PCP; LSD; MDMA)
  peace pill (phencyclidine/PCP; hallucinogen)
  peace tablets (LSD; hallucinogen)
  peace weed (phencyclidine/PCP; hallucinogen)
  peaches (amphetamine; stimulant)
  peanut (depressant; S-H-A)
  peanut butter (methamphetamine; phencyclidine/PCP)
  pearl (cocaine)
  pearls (amyl nitrite; inhalant)
  pearly gates (LSD; hallucinogen)
  pebbles (crack cocaine)
  Pee Wee (crack cocaine)
  peep (phencyclidine/PCP; hallucinogen)
  peeper(s) (club drug; ecstasy/MDMA; stimulant)
  Peg (heroin; opioid)
  pellets (LSD; hallucinogen)
  pen yan (opium; opioid)
  pep pills (amphetamine; stimulant)
  perc-a-pop (re: fentanyl lozenge for cancer pts. – diverted)
  Percia (cocaine)
  Percio (cocaine)

drugs (street names)
  Perfect High (heroin; opioid)
  perias (re: street dealers of heroin)
  Perico (cocaine)
  perp (crack cocaine)
  Peruvian (cocaine)
  Peruvian flake (cocaine)
  Peruvian lady (cocaine)
  Peter (depressant; S-H-A)
  Peter Pan (phencyclidine/PCP; hallucinogen)
  peth (barbiturate; S-H-A)
  Pethidine (meperidine; opioid)
  peyote (mescaline; hallucinogen)
  P-funk (crack with PCP; heroin)
  pharming (re: taking a mixture of prescription medication)
  Philly blunts (cannabis)
  pianoing (crack cocaine)
  picking (cocaine; crack cocaine)
  piece (cocaine; crack cocaine)
  piedras (crack cocaine)
  Pig Killer (phencyclidine/PCP; hallucinogen)
  piggybacking (club drug; re: injecting two drugs together)
  Pikachu (club drug; designer drug; re: pills containing PCP and ecstasy)
  piles (crack cocaine)
  pill ladies (re: female senior citizens selling OxyContin)
  pills (OxyContin) opioid)
  pimp (cocaine)
  pimp your pipe (crack cocaine)
  pin (cannabis)
  pin gon (opium; opioid)
  pin yen (opium; opioid)

drugs (street names)
pingus (designer drug; Rohypnol/flunitrazepam; S-H-A)
Pink (methamphetamine; stimulant)
pink blotters (LSD; hallucinogen)
pink elephants (amphetamine; methamphetamine; stimulant)
pink hearts (amphetamine; methamphetamine; stimulant)
Pink Panther (LSD; hallucinogen)
Pink Panthers (ecstasy/MDMA; stimulant)
pink partners (club drug)
pink robots (LSD; hallucinogen)
pink wedges (LSD; hallucinogen)
pink witches (LSD; hallucinogen)
pipe (cannabis; crack cocaine)
pit (phencyclidine/PCP; hallucinogen)
pixies (amphetamine; stimulant)
Playboy bunnies (club drug; ecstasy/MDMA; stimulant)
playboys (club drug; ecstasy/MDMA; stimulant)
Pluto (heroin; opioid)
pocket rocket (cannabis)
pod (cannabis)
poison (designer drug; fentanyl; heroin; opioid)
poke (cannabis)
pollutants (designer drug; amphetamine; ecstasy/MDMA; stimulant)
polo (mixture of heroin and motion sickness drugs)
polvo (phencyclidine/PCP; heroin)

drugs (street names)
polvo blanco (cocaine)
polvo de angel (phencyclidine/PCP; hallucinogen)
polvo de estrellas (phencyclidine/PCP; hallucinogen)
pony (crack cocaine)
poor man's coke (amphetamine)
poor man's heroin (Talwin/Ritalin injections together)
poor man's pot (inhalant)
pop (cocaine)
poppers (amyl nitrite; inhalant)
poppy (heroin; opioid)
poro (heroin + PCP)
pot (cannabis)
potato (LSD; hallucinogen)
potato chips (crack cocaine)
potlikker (cannabis)
potten bush (cannabis)
powder (cocaine; heroin; amphetamine)
powder diamonds (cocaine)
power puffer (crack cocaine)
pox (opium)
predator (heroin)
premos (cannabis; cocaine; crack cocaine)
prescription (cannabis)
press (cocaine; crack cocaine)
pretendica (cannabis)
pretendo (cannabis)
primbolin (steroid compound)
prime time (crack cocaine)
primo (re: mix of cannabis/heroin/cocaine/crack/tobacco)
primo square (cannabis; crack cocaine)
primo turbo (cannabis; crack cocaine; cocaine)

Psychiatric Words and Phrases

drugs (street names)
primobolan (steroid compound)
primos (nicotine/tobacco)
product (crack cocaine)
proviron (steroid compound)
pseudocaine (cocaine; crack cocaine)
Puff the dragon (cannabis)
puffer (crack cocaine)
puffy (phencyclidine/PCP; hallucinogen)
pulborn (heroin; opioid)
pullers (crack cocaine)
pumpers (anabolic steroid compound)
pumping (crack cocaine)
pure (heroin; opioid)
pure ivory (club drug; cocaine; designer drug)
pure ivory (re: drug effects similar to ecstasy)
pure love (LSD; hallucinogen)
purple (designer drug)
purple (ketamine; dissociative hallucinogen)
purple barrels (LSD; hallucinogen)
purple caps (cocaine; crack cocaine)
purple drank (re: mixture: promethazine/cocaine syrup)
purple flats (LSD; hallucinogen)
purple gel tabs (LSD; hallucinogen)
purple haze (cannabis; LSD; cocaine; crack cocaine)
purple hearts (amphetamine; barbiturate; depressant; LSD)
purple ozoline (LSD; hallucinogen)
purple rain (phencyclidine/PCP; hallucinogen)

drugs (street names)
purple wave (club drug; designer drug; re:drug effects similar to ecstasy)
purple wave (cocaine)
pusher (crack cocaine)
Q (barbiturate; depressant; S-H-A)
Qaat (methcathinone; stimulant)
Qat (designer drug)
Qua (depressant)
Quaaludes (depressant)
quack (depressant)
quads (barbiturate; depressant; S-H-A)
quarter moon (hashish; hallucinogen)
quartz (smokable methamphetamine; stimulant)
quas (barbiturate; depressant; S-H-A)
Queen Ann's lace (cannabis)
quill (cocaine; heroin; methamphetamine)
quinolone (steroid compound)
R-2 (designer drug; Rohypnol/flunitrazepam; S-H-A)
Racehorse Charlie (cocaine; heroin)
ragweed (re: inferior marijuana or heroin)
railroad (cannabis)
rainbows (amobarbital; depressant; LSD)
rainy day woman (cannabis)
Rambo (heroin; opioid)
Randy Mandies (depressant)
rane (cocaine; heroin)
rangood (cannabis)
raspberry (crack cocaine)
rasta weed (cannabis)
rave energy (club drug; designer drug; ecstasy/MDMA; stimulant)

drugs (street names)
    raw (cocaine; crack cocaine)
    raw (re: high purity heroin)
    raw fusion (heroin; opioid)
    raw hide (heroin; opioid)
    ready rock (cocaine; crack cocaine; heroin)
    real tops (cocaine; crack cocaine)
    recompress (cocaine)
    recycle (LSD; hallucinogen)
    red (methamphetamine; stimulant)
    red and blue (barbiturate; depressant; S-H-A)
    red bullets (barbiturate; depressant; S-H-A)
    red but (cannabis)
    red caps (crack cocaine)
    red chicken (heroin; opioid)
    red cross (cannabis)
    red devil (barbiturate; depressant; S-H-A; heroin; opioid; phencyclidine/PCP; hallucinogen)
    red devils (club drug; ecstasy/MDMA; stimulant)
    red dirt (cannabis)
    red eagle (heroin; opioid)
    red lips (LSD; hallucinogen)
    red phosphorus (amphetamine) stimulant)
    red rock (heroin; opioid)
    red rock opium (re: heroin/barbital/strychnine/caffeine combo)
    red rum (re: heroin/barbital/strychnine/caffeine combo use)
    red stuff (re: heroin/barbital/strychnine/ caffeine combo use)
    redneck cocaine (methamphetamine; stimulant)
    reds (depressant; S-H-A)
    reefer (cannabis)
    regular P (crack cocaine)

drugs (street names)
    reindeer dust (heroin; opioid)
    RenewTrient (contains GBL; depressant; S-H-A)
    rest in peace (crack cocaine)
    revivarant (GBL product; depressant; S-H-A)
    revivarant-G (GBL product; depressant; S-H-A)
    Reynolds (designer drug; Rohypnol/flunitrazepam; S-H-A)
    Rhine (heroin; opioid)
    rhythm (amphetamine; stimulant)
    rib (club drug; ecstasy/MDMA; stimulant; Rohypnol/flunitrazepam; S-H-A)
    rider (re: 5k heroin given with 100 kilos cocaine purchase)
    righteous bush (cannabis)
    righteous weed (cannabis)
    ringer (crack cocaine)
    rip (designer drug; cannabis)
    rippers (amphetamine; stimulant)
    Ritalin and coffee (methylphenidate and caffeine; stimulant)
    ritual spirit (club drug; designer drug; ecstasy/MDMA; stimulant)
    roach (cannabis)
    roach clip (re: cannabis cigarette holder)
    roach-2 (club drug; Rohypnol/flunitrazepam; S-H-A)
    roacha (cannabis)
    roachas dos (Rohypnol/flunitrazepam; S-H-A)
    roaches (designer drug; Rohypnol/flunitrazepam; S-H-A)

drugs (street names)
  roachies (designer drug; Rohypnol/flunitrazepam; S-H-A)
  road dope (amphetamine) (stimulant)
  roapies (designer drug; Rohypnol/flunitrazepam; S-H-A)
  roasting (cannabis)
  robin's egg (stimulant)
  robotripping (re: under the influence of Sudafed and DXM-dextromethorphan)
  Robutal (designer drug; Rohypnol/flunitrazepam; S-H-A
  roca (designer drug; crack cocaine; ecstasy/MDMA; stimulant)
  rochas dos (designer drug; Rohypnol/flunitrazepam; S-H-A)
  roche (designer drug; Rohypnol/flunitrazepam; S-H-A)
  Rock (methamphetamine; stimulant)
  rock attack (crack cocaine)
  rock house (crack cocaine)
  rock star (crack cocaine)
  rocket fuel (phencyclidine/PCP; hallucinogen)
  rockets (cannabis)
  rocks (cocaine)
  rocks of hell (crack cocaine)
  Rocky III (crack cocaine)
  roid rage (steroid compound)
  roids (anabolic steroids)
  rolling (MDMA/ecstasy; stimulant)
  Rolls Royce (club drug; ecstasy/MDMA; stimulant)
  rompums (cannabis)
  roofies (Rohypnol/flunitrazepam; S-H-A)
  rooster (crack cocaine)
  root (cannabis)

drugs (street names)
  rope (cannabis; Rohypnol/flunitrazepam)
  rophies (Rohypnol/flunitrazepam; S-H-A)
  rophy (designer drug; Rohypnol/flunitrazepam; S-H-A)
  ropies (designer drug; Rohypnol/flunitrazepam; S-H-A)
  Rosa (amphetamine; stimulants
  Rose Marie (cannabis)
  roses (amphetamine; stimulant)
  rough stuff (cannabis)
  row-shay (designer drug; Rohypnol/flunitrazepam; S-H-A)
  rox (crack cocaine)
  Roxanne (cocaine; crack cocaine)
  royal blues (LSD; hallucinogen)
  Roz (crack cocaine)
  ruderalis (cannabis)
  ruffies (Rohypnol/flunitrazepam; S-H-A)
  ruffles (designer drug; Rohypnol/flunitrazepam; S-H-A)
  running (designer drug; ecstasy/MDMA; stimulant)
  rush (cocaine)
  rush hour (heroin; opioid)
  Rusko (Nexus; hallucinogen)
  Russian sickles (LSD; hallucinogen)
  sack (heroin; heroin; opioid)
  sacrament (LSD; hallucinogen)
  sacred mushroom (psilocybin/psilocin; hallucinogen)
  sage of the seers (salvia divinorum; hallucinogen)

drugs (street names)
- Sally D (salvia divinorum; hallucinogen)
- salt (heroin; opioid) salt and pepper (cannabis)
- salty water (GHB; depressant; S-H-A)
- salvia (salvia divinorum; hallucinogen)
- sandoz (LSD; hallucinogen)
- sandwich (cocaine/heroin/ cocaine layers)
- sandwich (re: outer layers of cocaine; inner layer of heroin)
- sandwich bag (cannabis)
- Santa Marta (cannabis)
- sasfras (cannabis)
- satan's secret (inhalant)
- sativa (cannabis)
- scaffle (phencyclidine/PCP; hallucinogen)
- scag (heroin; opioid)
- scat (heroin; opioid)
- scate (heroin; opioid)
- schmeck (cocaine)
- Schmiz (methamphetamine; stimulant)
- schoolboy (cocaine; depresssant; methylmorphine/(codeine)
- schoolcraft (crack cocaine)
- schwagg (cannabis)
- scissors (cannabis)
- Scooby snacks (MDMA/ecstasy; stimulant)
- scoop (club drug; designer drug; GHB; depressant; S-H-A)
- Scootie (methamphetamine; stimulant)
- scorpion (cocaine)
- Scott (heroin; opioid)
- Scottie (cocaine; crack cocaine)
- Scotty (cocaine; crack cocaine)

drugs (street names)
- scramble (re: low quality heroin plus crack cocaine)
- scrape and snort (crack cocaine)
- scrub (cannabis)
- scruples (crack cocaine)
- scuffle (phencyclidine/PCP; hallucinogen)
- seccy (depressant; S-H-A)
- second to none (heroin; opioid)
- seconds (cocaine; crack cocaine)
- seeds (cannabis)
- seggy (barbiturate; depressant; S-H-A)
- sen (cannabis)
- seni (mescaline/peyote; hallucinogen)
- serial speedballing (re: sequencing cocaine/cough syrup/heroin)
- sernyl (phencyclidine/PCP; hallucinogen)
- Serpico 21 (cocaine)
- server (crack cocaine)
- sess (cannabis)
- set (Talwin/Ritalin injection simulates heroin/cocaine effect)
- set (re: place where drugs are sold)
- Seven-up (cocaine; crack cocaine)
- sextasy (club drug; re: ecstasy used with Viagra)
- sezz (cannabis)
- Shabu (designer drug; powder cocaine and methamphetamine; MDMA; stimulant)
- shake (cannabis)
- shaker/baker/water (cocaine)
- she (cocaine)
- shebanging (cocaine)
- sheet rocking (crack cocaine)

drugs (street names)
  sheet rocking (LSD; hallucinogen)
  sheets (phencyclidine/PCP; hallucinogen)
  sherms (phencyclidine/PCP; psychedelic mushrooms; hallucinogen)
  sherman stick (cannabis; cocaine; crack cocaine)
  shermans (phencyclidine/PCP; hallucinogen)
  sherms (crack cocaine)
  shit (heroin; opioid)
  shmeck/schmeek (heroin; opioid)
  shoot (heroin) opioid)
  shoot the breeze (nitrous oxide; inhalant)
  shot (cocaine)
  shot to the curb (crack cocaine)
  shotgun (cannabis)
  shrile (cocaine)
  shrooms (psilocybin/psilocin; hallucinogen)
  Siddi (cannabis)
  Silly Putty (psilocybin/psilocin; hallucinogen)
  Simple Simon (psilocybin/psilocin; hallucinogen)
  sinse (cannabis)
  sinsemilla (cannabis)
  sixty-two (crack cocaine)
  skag (heroin; opioid)
  skee (opium)
  skeegers/skeezers (re: crack use)
  Sketch (methamphetamine; stimulant)
  skid (heroin; opioid)
  skittle-ing (re: under the influence of Sudafed and DXM-dextromethorphan)
  skuffle (phencyclidine/PCP; hallucinogen)

drugs (street names)
  skunk (cannabis; heroin)
  skunkweed (cannabis)
  slab (crack cocaine)
  slammin/slamming (designer drug; amphetamine; ecstasy/MDMA; stimulant)
  sleep (club drug; GHB; depressant; S-H-A)
  sleep-500 (club drug; GHB (depressant; S-H-A)
  sleeper (barbiturate; depressant; heroin)
  sleeper & red devil (heroin and a depressant)
  sleet (crack cocaine)
  sleigh ride (cocaine)
  slick superspeed (designer drug; methcathinone; stimulant)
  slime (heroin; opioid)
  slum (phencyclidine/PCP; hallucinogen)
  slumber (depressant; S-H-A)
  smack (heroin; opioid)
  smears (LSD; hallucinogen)
  smoke (cannabis; heroin and crack cocaine)
  smoke a bowl (cannabis)
  smoke Canada (cannabis)
  smoke houses (re: cocaine/crack cocaine use)
  smoking (phencyclidine/PCP; hallucinogen)
  smoking gun (heroin and cocaine)
  Smurf (nicotine/tobacco)
  Smurfs (club drug; MDMA/ecstasy; stimulant)
  snackies (club drug; re: MDMA adulterated with mescaline)
  snap (amphetamine; inhalant)
  sniff (cocaine)
  sniff (re: inhaling methcathinone or other designer drugs)

drugs (street names)
    sniffer bag (re: $5 bag of heroin – for inspection)
    snop (cannabis)
    snort (cocaine)
    snort (re: to use inhalants)
    snorting (re: using inhalants)
    snorts (phencyclidine/PCP; hallucinogen)
    snot (amphetamine; stimulant)
    snotballs (re: inhaling fumes from burned rubber cement)
    snotty (heroin; opioid)
    snow (cocaine; heroin; amphetamine)
    snow bird (cocaine)
    snow coke (crack cocaine)
    snow cones (cocaine)
    snow pallets (amphetamine; stimulant)
    snow seals (cocaine; amphetamine; stimulant)
    Snow White (cocaine)
    snowball (cocaine and heroin)
    snowmen (LSD; hallucinogen)
    soap (crack cocaine; methamphetamine; stimulant)
    soap (club drug; GHB; depressant)
    soap dope (pink tinted methamphetamine; stimulant)
    soaper (depressant)
    society high (cocaine)
    soda (cocaine)
    soft (cocaine)
    softballs (barbiturate; depressant; S-H-A)
    soles (hashish; hallucinogen)
    soma (phencyclidine/PCP; hallucinogen)
    Somali tea (designer drug; khat; methcathinone; stimulant)

drugs (street names)
    Somatomax (club drug; designer drug; GHB; depressant; S-H-A)
    sopers (barbiturate; depressant; S-H-A)
    sopes (depressant)
    soup (cocaine; crack cocaine)
    South Parks (LSD; hallucinogen)
    space (cocaine; crack cocaine)
    space base (crack cocaine; phencyclidine/PCP; hallucinogen)
    space cadet (phencyclidine/PCP; hallucinogen)
    space dust (phencyclidine/PCP; hallucinogen)
    spaceball (cocaine/crack; phencyclidine/PCP)
    spackle (methamphetamine; stimulant)
    spark it up (cannabis)
    Sparkle (methamphetamine with a shiny appearance; stimulant)
    sparkle plenty (amphetamine; stimulant)
    sparklers (amphetamine; stimulant)
    Special "K" (designer drug; ketamine; dissociative hallucinogen)
    special la coke (designer drug; ketamine; dissociative hallucinogen)
    Speckled birds (methamphetamine; stimulant)
    Spectrum (club drug; designer drug; Nexus; hallucinogen)
    speed (amphetamine; crack cocaine; methamphetamine; stimulant)

drugs (street names)
- speed for lovers (designer drug; ecstasy/MDMA; stimulant)
- speed freak (re: habitual user of methamphetamine)
- speedball (amphetamine) (crack/heroin mix) (Ritalin/heroin mix)
- speedballing (re: ecstasy/MDMA mixed with ketamine; cocaine & heroin smoked together)
- speedballs – nose style (cocaine)
- speedboat (cannabis; crack cocaine; phencyclidine/PCP; hallucinogen)
- speedies (re: MDMA adulterated with amphetamine; stimulant)
- spice (designer drug; synthetic cannabinoids; hallucinogen)
- Spice/K2 (synthetic cannabis)
- spider (heroin; opioid)
- spider blue (heroin; opioid)
- spike (re: heroin cut with strychnine or scopolamine)
- spivias (designer drug; ecstasy/MDMA; stimulant)
- splash (amphetamine; stimulant)
- spliff (cannabis)
- splim (cannabis)
- splitting (cannabis; cocaine)
- splivins (amphetamine; stimulant)
- spoon (re: 1/16 oz of heroin)
- spoosh (methamphetamine; stimulant)
- spores (phencyclidine/PCP; hallucinogen)
- sporting (cocaine)
- spray (inhalant)
- square mackerel (cannabis)

drugs (street names)
- square time Bob (crack cocaine)
- squirrel (cannabis; cocaine; crack)
- swuirrel (LSD; phencyclidine/PCP; hallucinogen)
- stack (cannabis)
- stackers/stacking (steroid compound)
- stacking (club drug; re: use of 3 or more MDMA tablets in combination)
- stacks (club drug; crack cocaine; re: adulterated MDMA with heroin or crack)
- star (amphetamine; cocaine; designer drug; methamphetamine; stimulant)
- stardust (cocaine; phencyclidine/PCP; hallucinogen)
- stars (club drug; ecstasy/MDMA; stimulant)
- star-spangled powder (cocaine)
- stat (designer drug; methcathinone; stimulant)
- steerer (crack cocaine)
- stem (crack cocaine)
- stems (cannabis)
- stick (cannabis; phencyclidine/PCP)
- sticky icky (cannabis)
- stink weed (cannabis)
- stones (crack cocaine)
- stoney weed (cannabis)
- stoppers (barbiturate; depressant; S-H-A)
- stove top (crystal methamphetamine; stimulant)
- STP (re: fake PCP)
- straw (cannabis)
- strawberries (barbiturate; depressant; S-H-A)

drugs (street names)
- strawberry (crack cocaine; LSD)
- strawberry fields (LSD; hallucinogen)
- Strawberry Quik (re: strawberry-flavored methamphetamine; stimulant)
- strawberry shortcake (amphetamine; designer drug; ecstasy/MDMA; stimulant)
- street rocking (crack and LSD)
- studio fuel (cocaine)
- stuff (heroin; opioid; re: heroin injection paraphernalia)
- stumbler (barbiturate; S-H-A)
- sugar (cocaine; crack cocaine; heroin; LSD)
- sugar block (crack cocaine)
- sugar boogers (cocaine)
- sugar cubes (LSD; hallucinogen)
- sugar lumps (LSD; hallucinogen)
- sugar weed (cannabis)
- sunshine (LSD; hallucinogen)
- super (phencyclidine/PCP; hallucinogen)
- super acid (designer drug; ketamine; dissociative hallucinogen)
- super C (designer drug; ketamine; dissociative hallucinogen)
- super grass (phencyclidine/PCP; hallucinogen)
- super ice (smokable methamphetamine; stimulant)
- super joint (phencyclidine/PCP; hallucinogen)

drugs (street names)
- super kools (phencyclidine/PCP; hallucinogen)
- super pot (cannabis)
- super weed (phencyclidine/PCP; hallucinogen)
- super X (re: mix MDMA and methamphetamine; stimulant)
- supergrass (cannabis)
- Superlab (re: clandestine lab able to produce 10 lbs. of meth in 24 hours)
- Superman (club drug; ecstasy/MDMA; LSD)
- super-X (club drug)
- surfer (phencyclidine/PCP; hallucinogen)
- sustanon 250 (steroid compound)
- swag (cannabis)
- swans (club drug; ecstasy/MDMA; stimulant)
- Sweet Lucy (cannabis)
- sweet dreams (heroin; opioid)
- Sweet Jesus (heroin; opioid)
- sweet stuff (cocaine; heroin/opioid)
- sweeties (amphetamine; designer drug; ecstasy/MDMA)
- sweets (amphetamine; stimulant)
- swell up (crack cocaine)
- swishers (cannabis)
- synthetic (cannabis)
- synthetic cocaine (phencyclidine/PCP)
- synthetic THT (phencyclidine/PCP; hallucinogen)
- syrup (cannabis)
- T (cannabis; cocaine)
- T.N.T. (heroin; Fentanyl)
- T-7 (Nexus; hallucinogen)
- tabs (club drug; ecstasy/MDMA; LSD)

drugs (street names)
    TAC (phencyclidine/PCP; hallucinogen)
    tachas (club drug; ecstasy/MDMA; stimulant)
    tail lights (LSD; hallucinogen)
    taima (cannabis)
    taking a cruise (phencyclidine/PCP; hallucinogen)
    Takkouri (cannabis)
    talco (cocaine)
    Tango and Cash (fentanyl; opioid)
    tar (crack/heroin smoked together; opium; opioid)
    tar dust (cocaine)
    taste (heroin; opioid; re: small sample of drugs)
    taxing (crack cocaine)
    T-buzz (phencyclidine/PCP; hallucinogen)
    tea (cannabis; phencyclidine/PCP; hallucinogen)
    tea party (cannabis)
    teardrops (crack cocaine)
    tecate (heroin; opioid)
    tecatos (re: Hispanic heroin addict)
    teenager (cocaine)
    teeth (cocaine; crack cocaine)
    ten pack (re: 1,000 dosage units of LSD)
    tens (amphetamine; ecstasy/MDMA; stimulant)
    tension (crack cocaine)
    Tex-Mex (cannabis)
    Texas pot (cannabis)
    Texas shoe shine (inhalant)
    Texas tea (cannabis)
    Thai sticks (cannabis)
    THC (nicotine; tobacco)
    The beast (heroin; opioid)
    The bomb (fentanyl; opioid)
    The C (amphetamine; methcathinone; stimulant)

drugs (street names)
    The devil (crack cocaine)
    The five way (re: smoking heroin/cocaine/meth/Rohypnol and drinking alcohol)
    The Ghost (LSD; hallucinogen)
    The Hawk (LSD; hallucinogen)
    The witch (heroin; opioid)
    therobolin (steroid compound)
    thing (re: cocaine; crack; heroin; or current drug of choice)
    thirst monsters (crack cocaine)
    thirteen (cannabis)
    thirty-eight (cannabis; crack cocaine)
    thrust (inhalant)
    thrusters (amphetamine; stimulant)
    thumb (cannabis)
    thunder (heroin; opioid)
    tic (methamphetamine; phencyclidine/PCP)
    tic tac (phencyclidine/PCP; hallucinogen)
    tick tick (methamphetamine; stimulant)
    ticket (LSD; hallucinogen)
    tigre (heroin; opioid)
    tigre blanco (heroin; opioid)
    tigre del norte (heroin; opioid)
    Timothy Leary (LSD; hallucinogen)
    tin (cannabis)
    Tina (stimulant
    tio (cannabis; cocaine)
    tish (phencyclidine/PCP; hallucinogen)
    tissue (crack cocaine)
    titch (phencyclidine/PCP; hallucinogen)
    tits (black tar heroin; opioid)

drugs (street names)
- TNT (designer drug; re: heroin plus fentanyl; opioid)
- Tohai (khat; stimulant)
- toilet water (inhalant)
- toke (cannabis; cocaine)
- toke up (cannabis)
- tolly (re: toluene used in many inhalants)
- Tom and Jerries (club drug; ecstasy/MDMA; stimulant)
- tongs (heroin; opioid)
- tooies (amobarbital; S-H-A)
- tooles (barbiturate; depressant; S-H-A)
- toonies (club drug; designer drug; Nexus; hallucinogen)
- toot (cocaine)
- tooties (barbiturate; depressant; S-H-A)
- Tootsie Roll (heroin; opioid)
- top drool (heroin; opioid)
- top gun (crack cocaine)
- topi (mescaline; hallucinogen)
- tops (mescaline/peyote; hallucinogen)
- torc (cannabis)
- torch (cannabis)
- torch up (cannabis)
- torpedo (cannabis; crack cocaine)
- toss up(s) (crack cocaine)
- totally spent (designer drug; re: hangover; adverse reaction to MDMA)
- touché (re: cocaine booster which is inhaled)
- toucher (crack cocaine)
- tout (opium; opioid)
- toxy (opium; opioid)
- toys (opium; opioid)
- TR-6s (amphetamine; stimulant)
- tragic magic (crack cocaine; phencyclidine/PCP)
- trails (re: LSD perceptions)
- train (heroin; opioid)

drugs (street names)
- trank (phencyclidine/PCP; hallucinogen)
- tranq (barbiturate; depressant) (S-H-A)
- trauma (cannabis)
- travel agent (re: drug supplier)
- tray (cannabis)
- trees (cannabis)
- trey (cocaine; crack cocaine)
- trip (designer drug; LSD; hallucinogen)
- triple A (cannabis)
- triple crowns (club drug; ecstasy/MDMA; stimulant)
- triple Rolexes (club drug; ecstasy/MDMA; stimulant)
- triple stacks (club drug; MDMA/ecstasy; stimulant)
- tripstacy (Nexus + ecstasy; S-H-A + stimulant)
- troll (club drug; re: use of MDMA and LSD)
- troop (crack cocaine)
- trophobolene (steroid compound)
- truck drivers (amphetamine; stimulant)
- trupence bag (cannabis)
- Ts and Rits (Talwin/Ritalin injection simulating heroin/cocaine effect)
- Ts and Rs (Talwin/Ritalin injection simulating heroin/cocaine effect)
- Tschat (khat; stimulant)
- TT1 (phencyclidine/PCP; hallucinogen)
- TT2 (phencyclidine/PCP; hallucinogen)
- TT3 (phencyclidine/PCP; hallucinogen)
- tuie (barbiturate; depressant; S-H-A)
- turbo (crack cocaine)
- turkey (amphetamine; cocaine; stimulant)

drugs (street names)
    turnabout (amphetamine;
        stimulant)
    tutti-frutti (cocaine)
    tutus (club drug;
        MDMA/ecstasy; stimulant)
    tweak mission (crack
        cocaine)
    tweaker (crack cocaine)
    tweaking (crack cocaine)
    tweaks (crack cocaine)
    tweeker (designer drug;
        methcathinone; stimulant)
    tweety birds
        (ecstasy/MDMA; stimulant)
    twenties (crack cocaine)
    twenty-five (LSD;
        hallucinogen)
    Twin Towers (heroin; opioid)
    Twinkie (cocaine)
    twist (cannabis)
    twisters (methamphetamine;
        stimulant)
    twists (re: twist-tied small
        bag of heroin)
    twistum (cannabis)
    two for nine (crack cocaine)
    U.P.S. (amphetamine;
        designer drug;
        ecstasy/MDMA; stimulant)
    ultimate (crack cocaine)
    ultimate xphoria (club drug;
        designer drug;
        ecstasy/MDMA; stimulant)
    Uncle Milty (barbiturate;
        depressant; S-H-A)
    unkie (morphine; opioid)
    unotque (cannabis)
    up against the stem
        (cannabis)
    uppers (amphetamine;
        stimulant)
    uppies (amphetamine;
        stimulant)
    ups and downs (barbiturate;
        depressant; S-H-A)
    uptown (cocaine)
    utopiates (hallucinogen)

drugs (street names)
    uzi (crack cocaine)
    V (depressant; S-H-A)
    valo (inhalant)
    vanilla sky (club drug;
        cocaine; designer drug; re:
        powdery substance with
        ecstasy effect)
    vega (cannabis)
    Venus (club drug; designer
        drug; Nexus; hallucinogen)
    vidrio (heroin; opioid)
    viper (cannabis)
    viper's weed (cannabis)
    Vita-G (club drug; GHB;
        depressant; S-H-A)
    vitamin K (designer drug;
        ketamine; dissociative
        hallucinogen)
    vitamin Q (depressant)
    vitamin R (Ritalin; stimulant)
    vodka acid (LSD;
        hallucinogen)
    wac (cannabis;
        phencyclidine/PCP;
        hallucinogen)
    wack (phencyclidine/PCP;
        hallucinogen)
    wacky weed (cannabis)
    wafers (club drug;
        ecstasy/MDMA; stimulant)
    waffle dust (club drug; re:
        combined MDMA and
        amphetamine; timulant)
    wagon wheels (depressant)
    wake and bake (cannabis)
    wake ups (amphetamine;
        stimulant)
    wash (methamphetamine;
        stimulant)
    water (club drug; re:
        cannabis/GHB/meth/PCP
        and other drug mixtures)
    water-water (cannabis;
        phencyclidine/PCP;
        hallucinogen)
    watercolors (LSD;
        hallucinogen)

drugs (street names)
waters (re: designer drug mixture)
wave (crack cocaine)
wedding bells (LSD; hallucinogen)
wedge (LSD; hallucinogen)
weed (cannabis; phencyclidine/PCP; hallucinogen)
weed tea (cannabis)
weightless (crack cocaine)
West Coast (Ritalin; stimulant)
West Coast turnarounds (designer drug; amphetamine; ecstasy/MDMA; stimulant)
wet (cannabis; methamphetamine; phencyclidine/PCP)
wet daddies (cannabis)
wet sticks (cannabis; phencyclidine/PCP; hallucinogen)
whack (re: cannabis with insecticides); (re: crack or heroin with PCP mixture)
whackatabacky (cannabis)
wheat (cannabis)
wheels (designer drug; ecstasy/MDMA; stimulant)
when-shee (opium; opioid)
whiffle dust (amphetamine; designer drug; ecstasy/MDMA; stimulant)
whippets (nitrous oxide; inhalant)
white (heroin; amphetamines)
white ball (crack cocaine)
white boy (heroin; powder cocaine)
white cloud (crack cocaine)
white cross (amphetamine; methamphetamine; stimulant)

drugs (street names)
white diamonds (ecstasy/MDMA; stimulant)
white dove (ecstasy/MDMA; stimulant)
white dragon (cocaine; heroin)
white dust (LSD; hallucinogen)
white ghost (crack cocaine)
white girl (cocaine; heroin)
white-haired lady (cannabis)
white horizon (phencyclidine/PCP; hallucinogen)
white horse (cocaine; heroin; opioid)
white junk (heroin; opioid)
white lady (cocaine; heroin)
white lightning (LSD; hallucinogen)
white mosquito (cocaine)
white nothing (ecstasy/MDMA; stimulant)
white nurse (heroin; opioid)
white Owsley's (LSD; hallucinogen)
white powder (cocaine; phencyclidine/PCP)
White Russian (cannabis)
white stick (crack cocaine)
white stuff (heroin; opioid)
white sugar (crack cocaine)
white tiger (synthetic cannabis)
white tornado (crack cocaine)
whiteout (inhalant)
whites (amphetamine; stimulant)
whiz bang (cocaine; heroin)
wicked (potent heroin; opioid)
wicky (cannabis; cocaine; phencyclidine/PCP)
wicky stick (cannabis) (phencyclidine/PCP; hallucinogen)

drugs (street names)
    wigits (ecstasy/MDMA; stimulant)
    wild cat (cocaine; designer drug; methcathinone; stimulant)
    window glass (LSD; hallucinogen)
    window pane (cocaine; crack cocaine; LSD)
    wings (cocaine; heroin)
    wired on (cocaine)
    witch (cocaine; heroin; opioid)
    witch hazel (heroin; opioid)
    wobble weed (phencyclidine/PCP; hallucinogen)
    wolf (phencyclidine/PCP; hallucinogen)
    wolfies (designer drug)
    wolla blunt (marijuana and heroin)
    wollas (nicotine; tobacco)
    wollie (cannabis; crack cocaine)
    wollies (marijuana and heroin; phencyclidine/PCP)
    wolly blunts (phencyclidine/PCP; hallucinogen)
    wonder star (designer drug; methcathinone; stimulant)
    wool blunts (cocaine)
    woolah (cannabis; crack cocaine)
    woolas (cannabis; cocaine; crack cocaine)
    woolie (cocaine; nicotine; tobacco)
    woolie blunt (cocaine; crack cocaine)
    woolies (cannabis; crack cocaine)
    wooly blunts (cannabis; crack cocaine)
    wooties (cocaine; crack cocaine)

drugs (street names)
    work (methamphetamine; stimulant)
    working (crack cocaine)
    working bags (cocaine; crack cocaine)
    working fifty (crack cocaine)
    working half (crack cocaine)
    working man's cocaine (methamphetamine; stimulant)
    worm (phencyclidine/PCP; hallucinogen)
    wrecking crew (crack cocaine)
    WTC (heroin; opioid)
    X (designer drug; amphetamine; cannabis; ecstasy/MDMA; methamphetamine; stimulant)
    X-ing (designer drug; ecstasy/MDMA; stimulant)
    X-plus (ecstasy/MDMA; stimulant)
    XTC (designer drug; ecstasy/MDMA; stimulant)
    Ya Ba (club drug; pure and powerful form of methamphetamine; stimulant)
    yaba (methamphetamine; stimulant)
    yahoo/yeaho (crack cocaine)
    Yale (crack cocaine)
    yam (crack cocaine)
    yao (cocaine)
    yarn (cocaine)
    yay (cocaine; crack cocaine)
    yayoo (crack cocaine)
    yeah-O (crack cocaine)
    yeh (cannabis)
    yellow (barbiturate; depressant; LSD; hallucinogen)
    yellow bam (methamphetamine; stimulant)

drugs (street names)
    yellow barn (stimulant)
    yellow bullets (depressant; S-H-A)
    yellow dimples (LSD; hallucinogen)
    yellow fever (phencyclidine/PCP; hallucinogen)
    yellow jackets (methamphetamine; stimulant)
    yellow powder (methamphetamine; stimulant)
    yellow submarine (cannabis)
    yellow sunshine (LSD; hallucinogen)
    yellows (depressant; S-H-A)
    yen pop (cannabis)
    Yen Shee Suey (opium wine; opioid)
    yen sleep (re: restless, drowsy state after LSD use)
    yeo (crack cocaine)
    yeola (crack cocaine)
    yerba (cannabis)
    yerba mala (cannabis; phencyclidine/PCP; hallucinogen)
    yerhia (cannabis)
    yesca (cannabis)
    yesco (cannabis)
    yeyo (cocaine)
    yimyom (crack cocaine)
    Ying Yang (LSD; hallucinogen)
    Zacatecas purple (cannabis)
    zambi (cannabis)
    zay (cannabis)
    Ze (opium; opioid)
    zen (LSD; hallucinogen)
    zero (opium)
    zig zag man (cannabis; LSD; hallucinogen)
    zip (cocaine)
    zol (cannabis)
    zombie (phencyclidine/PCP; hallucinogen)

drugs (street names)
    zombie weed (phencyclidine/PCP; hallucinogen)
    zooie (cannabis)
    zoom (cannabis; phencyclidine/PCP; hallucinogen)
    zoomer (crack cocaine)
    zoquete (heroin; opioid)
    zulu (crack cocaine)
drugs test
    blood level of anti-convulsant
    blood level of illicit
    blood screen for
    urine screen for
drum membrane
drumhead
"dry high" (street name, cannabis/marijuana)
dry hoarseness
DSC (Developing Skills Checklist)
DSM-5 (Diagnostic and Statistical Manual - 5; 2013)
DT/CEP (Differential Test of Conduct and Emotional Problems)
DTLA (Detroit Test of Learning Aptitude
DTLA-A (Detroit Test of Learning Aptitude—Adult)
DTLA-P (Detroit Test of Learning Aptitude—Primary
DTVP (Developmental Test of Visual Perception
dualism, mind/body
"duct" (street name, cocaine)
duct, cochlear
Dudsberry, Structured Photographic Articulation Test Featuring
"duji" (street name, heroin)
dull headache
dull pain
"dummy dust" (street name, phencyclidine)
duplication, syllable

"durabolin" (re: injectable steroid)
duration
    nocturnal sleep
    normal sleep
    recurrent
    reduced sleep
    short sleep
duration duty cycle
duration of drug action
duration of illness
duration of pain
duration of phonation, maximum
duration of sustained blowing, maximum
durations of intoxication, characteristic
"Durog" (street name, cannabis/marijuana)
"Duros" (street name, cannabis/marijuana)
Durrell Analysis of Reading Difficulty
"dust joint" (street name, phencyclidine)
"dust of angels" (street name, phencyclidine)
"dusted parsley" (street name, phencyclidine)
"dusting" (re: adding heroin or PCP to cannabis)
Dutch Association of Psychologists (NIP)
duties, neglect of household
duty cycle, duration
duty to warn
D-V (domestic violence)
Dx (diagnostic therapy)
Dyadic Parent-Child Interaction Coding System
"dymethzine" (re: injectable steroid)
dynamic ambulatory balance
dynamic aphasia
dynamic range
dynamic standing balance
"dynamite" (street name, heroin and cocaine)
dynamometer
dyne
"dyno" (street name, heroin)
"dyno-pure" (street name, heroin)
dysacusis
dysarthria
    apractic
    apraxic
    ataxic
    flaccid
    hyperkinetic
    hypokinetic
    laryngeal
    parkinsonian
    peripheral
    somesthetic
    spastic
Dysarthria Assessment, Frenchay
dysarthric
dysarthric behaviors
dysarthric speech assessment of intelligibility
dysaudia
dyscontrol
    affective
    behavioral
    emotional
    episodic
    impulsive
    temper
dysesthesic sensation
dysfluencies
    avoidance of speech
    emotional response to speech
    speech
dysfunction
    acquired sexual
    alcohol-induced sexual
    alcohol-induced sexual
    amphetamine-induced sexual
    arousal
    autonomic
    behavioral
    bilateral cerebral
    bilateral hemisphere
    bilateral hemispheric
    biological

dysfunction
    brain
    brain stem
    cocaine-induced sexual
    cognitive
    diffuse brain
    educational
    ejaculatory
    emotional
    erectile (ED)
    frontal lobe
    generalized sexual
    hemispheral
    hemispherical
    higher cerebral (HCD)
    higher cortical
    interpersonal
    language
    life-long sexual
    lingual airway
    male erectile
    manifestation of behavioral
    manifestation of biological
    manifestation of
      psychological
    mid brain
    neurological
    parietal lobe
    posttraumatic cortical
    psychological
    school
    self-care
    severe diffuse brain
    sexual
    situational sexual
    social
    substance-induced sexual
    swallowing
    sympathetic
    symptoms of behavioral
    symptoms of biological
    symptoms of psychological
    tongue
    work
dysfunction due to a substance, sexual
dysfunction due to combined factors, sexual
dysfunction due to GMC, sexual
dysfunction due to psychological factors, sexual
dysfunctional behavior, learned
dysfunctional relational functioning
dysfunctional relationship
Dysfunctions of Children, Neurological
dysglossia
dysgraphicus, status
dyskinesia
    disfluency
    neuroleptic-induced tardive
    tardive (G24,91)
    tardive orobuccal
dyskinetic cerebral palsy (CP)
dyskinetic movement
Dyslexia Determination Test
Dyslexia Screening Survey, The
dyslexic
dyslogia
dysmathia
dysmorphic defect, body
dysnomia, autonomic
dysostosis, mandibulofacial
dyspareunia
    acquired type
    female
    generalized type
    lifelong type
    male
    situational type
dyspareunia due to combined factors
dyspareunia due to psychological factors
dysphemia and biochemical theory of stuttering
dysphonia
    hyperkinetic
    spastic
    ventricular
dysphoria
    chronic irritable
    feeling of
    gender
    intense episodic

dysphoria disorder, premenstrual (N94.3)
dysphoria in children, gender
dysphoric affect
dysphoric disorder
    late luteal phase
    premenstrual
dysphrasia
dysplasia
dyspnea
dyspractic movement
dyspraxia
dyspraxic children, evaluation of movement and posture of
dysprosody
dysregulation, defensive
dysrhythmic movement
dysrhythmic speech
dyssocial personality disorder
dyssomnia
    delayed sleep phase type
    jet lag type
    shift work type
    unspecified type
dysthymia (persistent depressive disorder) in full remission (F34.1)
dysthymia (persistent depressive disorder) in partial remission (F34.1)
dysthymia (persistent depressive disorder) with early onset (F34.1)
dysthymia (persistent depressive disorder) with intermittent major depressive episode (F34.1)
dysthymia (persistent depressive disorder) with intermittent major depressive episode, without current episode (F34.1)
dysthymia (persistent depressive disorder) with late onset (F34.1)
dysthymia (persistent depressive disorder) with persistent major depressive episode (F34.1)
dysthymia (persistent depressive disorder) with pure dysthymic syndrome (F34.1)
dysthymic disorder, alternative criterion B for
dystonia
    body
    idiopathic
    medication-induced acute (G21.02)
    neuroleptic-induced acute
    nocturnal paroxysmal
    oropharyngeal
    substance-induced
    tardive (G24.09)
dystonic cerebral palsy (CP)
dystonic movement(s)
dystonic tremordystrophy, muscular

E

"E" (street name, ecstasy; MDMA)
"E-bombs" (street name, ecstasy; MDMA)
"E-puddle" (re: sleeping after MDMA use)
"E-tard" (re: under the influence of MDMA)
EA (educational age)
EAA (Educational Audiology Association)
EAAP (European Association for Aviation Psychology)
EADP (European Association for Developmental Psychology)
EAP (Employee Assistance Program)
EAPP (European Association of Personality Psychology)
EAWOP (European Association of Work and Organizational Psychology)
ear
    artificial
    Cargot
    external
    glue
    inner
    middle
    nose, throat (ENT)
    outer
ear canal
ear molds
ear muscle reflex, middle
ear training
eardrum
Early Academic and Language Skills
early-age trauma and PTSD
Early Child Development Inventory
early childhood disturbances in feeding and eating, infancy and
Early Communication Skills for Hearing-Impaired Children
Early Coping Inventory
early dementia
Early Development Scale for Preschool Children
early development tests *(see also* tests)
early full remission
Early Language Development Test
Early Language Milestone Scale
early-onset drinking
early onset of schizophrenia
early partial remission
early phase of dementia
Early Reading Ability Test (Deaf or Hard of Hearing)
early relationship
Early School Assessment (ESA)
Early Screening Inventory
Early Screening Profiles
early sign of schizophrenia
Early Socioemotional Development Test
Early Speech Perception Test (ESP)
early traumatic epilepsy
Early Years Easy Screen (EYES)
earmold
    nonoccluding
    open
    perimeter
    shell
    skeleton
    standard
    vented
earmuffs (hearing protection device)
earphone
earplugs (hearing protection device)
ears, low-set
"earth" (re: cannabis cigarette)

earwax
ease of fatigue
EASIC (Evaluating Acquired Skills in Communication)
easily disturbed sleep
"easing powder" (street name, opium)
eastern equine viral encephalitis
"Eastside player" (re: crack)
easy fatigability
"easy score" (re: easy drug acquisition)
"eating" (re: taking a drug orally)
eating disorders, gender differences in
Eating Disorder Inventory (EDI)
eating hairs
Eating Inventory
eating syndrome, nocturnal
EBL (estimated blood loss)
Ebonics (Black English)
ebolaphobia
EBPS (Emotional and Behavior Problem Scale)
Eby Elementary Identification Instrument
eccentric
eccentricities of behavior, pattern of
ecdemiomania (foreign sources/origins)
echo chamber
echoic operant
echokinesis
echolalia
    immediate
    mitigated
    unmitigated
echolocation
echo speech
e-cigarettes/e-cigs (electronic cigarettes)
eclamptic convulsion
eclecticism
ECochG (electrocochleography)
ECoG (electrocochleography)
ecology
ecomania (environment)

Economic Literacy Test
economic problem
economic self-sufficiency
Economic Understanding Test
economically depressed
economy reward, token
ECPA (European Community Psychology Association)
ECS (endocannabinoid system)
ecstasy (methylenedioxy-methamphetamine; MDMA) (street names)
    007s
    2C1
    2CE
    4 Dot
    69s
    Adam
    Batman
    B-bombs
    bean
    bens
    Benzedrine
    Bermuda triangles
    bibs
    biphetamine
    blue kisses
    blue lips
    blue Nile
    boat
    bump up
    bumping up
    Care Bears
    candy flipping on a string
    candy raver (re: club drug user)
    Cat in the Hats
    Charge+
    charity
    chocolate chip cookies
    clarity
    cloud nine
    Cristal
    crystal methadrine
    dead road
    debs
    decadence
    dex

ecstasy (street names)
- dexedrine
- diamonds
- disco biscuit(s)
- doctor
- dolls
- domex
- draf
- drivers
- E
- E-bombs
- E-puddle
- E-tard
- Egyptians
- elephant flipping
- elephants
- essence
- Eve
- exiticity
- fastin
- flipping
- flower flipping
- four leaf clover
- gaggler
- go
- green triangles
- greenies
- gum
- GWM
- H-bomb
- hammerheading
- happy drug
- happy pill
- hawkers
- herbal bliss
- hippieflip
- hug
- hug drug
- hugs and kisses
- hype
- iboga
- ice
- igloo
- ivory wave
- jellies
- Jerry Garcias
- kitty flipping

ecstasy (street names)
- Kleenex
- K-lots
- letter biscuits
- love drug
- love flipping
- love pill
- love trip
- lovers' special
- lovers' speed
- MAO
- MDM
- MDMA
- methedrine
- mini beans
- Mitsubishi
- Molly
- monoamine oxidase
- moonstone
- morning shot
- Nexus flipping
- nineteen
- NOX
- ocean burst
- on the ball
- orange bandits
- P and P
- parachute down
- party and play
- peace
- peepers
- piggybacking
- Pikachu
- Pink Panthers
- Playboy bunnies
- playboys
- pollutants
- pure ivory
- purple wave
- rave energy
- red devils
- rib
- ritual spirit
- roca
- rolling
- Rolls Royce
- running

ecstasy (street names)
  Scooby snacks
  sextasy (re: ecstasy used with Viagra)
  Shabu
  slammin'/slamming
  speed for lovers
  speedballing
  speedies (re: MDMA adulterated with amphetamine)
  spivias
  stacking (re: using 3 or more MDMA tablets at a time)
  stacks (re: adulterated MDMA with heroin or crack)
  stars
  strawberry shortcake
  super X (re: MDMA and methamphetamine combo)
  Superman
  swans
  sweeties
  tabs
  tachas
  tens
  Tom and Jerries
  totally spent (re: hangover, adverse reaction to MDMA)
  triple crowns
  triple Rolexes
  tweety birds
  U.P.S.
  ultimate xphoria
  vanilla sky (re: use of powdery substance with ecstasy effect)
  wafers
  waffle dust (re: combined MDMA and amphetamine)
  West Coast turnarounds
  wheels
  whiffledust
  white diamonds
  white dove
  white nothing
  wigits

ecstasy (street names)
  X
  X-ing
  X-plus
  XTC
ecstasy effect
EDA (electrodermal audiometry)
edema, cerebral
edeomania (genitalia)
EDI (Eating Disorder Inventory)
Edinburgh Functional Communication Profile
Edinburgh Picture Test
Edinburgh Reading Tests
Edinburgh Rehabilitation Status Scale
Edinburgh-2 Coma Scale
EDPA (Erhardt Developmental Prehension Assessment)
EDRA (electrodermal response audiometry) test
education
  age-appropriate
  speech
educational achievement tests *(see also* tests)
educational age (EA)
educational audiology
educational background, evaluation of
educational development tests *(see also* tests)
educational dysfunction
educational functioning
educational interest inventory *(see also* tests)
educational level, low
educational opportunity
educational prerequisite skills tests *(see also* tests)
educational problem(s)
educational progress
educational purposes
educational quotient (EQ)
educational screening tests *(see also* tests)
educational setting
educational situation(s)

educational skills test *(see also tests)*
educational tool
educational treatments
educational value
educationally mentally disabled
educationally mentally handicapped
EDVA (Erhardt Developmental Vision Assessment)
EEA (electroencephalic audiometry)
EEG
    beta pattern on
    beta rhythm on
    beta wave on
    phase lag on
    phase reversal on
    phase spike on
    sleep spindle on
    waking
EEG activity measurement
EEG activity, slow-frequency (delta)
EEG alpha activity
EEG delta activity
EEG potential
EFCP (Revised Edinburgh Functional Communication Profile)
effect
    abnormal perceptions due to drug
    acute toxic
    adaptation
    Bernoulli
    body baffle (hearing aid)
    central nervous system
    chronic toxic
    consistency
    desired
    diminished
    direct physiological
    Doppler
    dose-dependent
    drug
    extra pyramidal side
effect
    extrapyramidal medication side
    Fere
    fetal alcohol (FAE)
    halo
    head shadow
    "hit and run"
    laws of cause and
    long-term
    major
    maximal
    medication side
    occlusion
    off
    peripheral sympathomimetic
    possible
    potential adverse
    psychoactive
    sedative
    side
    spiral
    stimulant
    sympathomimetic
    unintended
    Wever-Bray
effective action
effective amplitude
effective communication, impaired
effective masking
Effective Reading Tests
Effective School Battery, The (ESB)
effectiveness, decreased
effector operation
effects of alcohol, toxic
effects of cocaine, toxic
effects of deception
effects of hallucinogens, toxic
effects of lithium, cellular
effects of medication, adverse
effects of narcotics, toxic
effects of other substances, toxic
effects of treatment, side
effects on soldiers in combat, trauma

efferent aphasia
efferent (kinetic) motor aphasia
efferent motor aphasia
efferent nerve
efficiency
    good sleep
    lack of
    masking
    sleep
    vocal
efficiency tests *(see also* tests)
effort
    new-work
    vocal
effort level
effusion ego egocentric
EFPA (European Federation of Psychologists' Associations)
"egg" (street name, crack)
ego boundaries
ego boundaries, loss of
ego-dystonia
ego-dystonic intrusions
ego-dystonic orientation
ego egocentric, effusion
Ego Function Assessment
ego integration
ego-syntonic traits
egocentric, effusion ego
egocentric language
egocentric speech
egocentric thought processes
egocentrism
egoïsme à deux
egomania (self-absorbed)
egomechanism of defense
EH (emotional handicap)
EHR (Electroacoustic Health Record)
eidetic imagery
"eight ball" (re:1/8 ounce of drugs)
Eight State Questionnaire
"eightball" (re: crack and heroin)
eighth nerve tumor
"eighth" (street name, heroin)
ejaculatory dysfunction
ejaculatory inevitability

elaborate dream sequence
elasticity
elation
elder abuse
elder maltreatment and PTSD
elderly, drug treatment for the
"el diablito" (street name, cannabis, cocaine, heroin and phencyclidine)
"el diablo" (street name, cannabis, cocaine and heroin)
elected mutism
elective mutism, relative
electric field
electric irritability
"Electric Kool Aid" (street name, lysergic acid diethylamide)
electric response audiometry (ERA)
electric shock sensation
electrical activity map, brain (BEAM)
electrical artificial larynx
electrical measurement of speech production
electrical potential
electrical shock
electricity
electricity, feeling of
Electroacoustic Health Record (EHR)
electroacoustical
electroacoustic
electrocochleography (ECochG; ECoG)
electrocochleography audiometry (ECoG; ECochG)
electroconvulsive therapy for mood disorders
electroconvulsive therapy use in affective disorders
electroconvulsive therapy-induced mood disorder
electrode
electrodermal audiometry (EDA)
electrodermal response audiometry (EDRA) test

electroencephalic audiometry (EEA)
electroencephalic response audiometer (ERA)^
electroencephalic response audiometry (ERA)^
electroencephalography
electroglottograph
electrolarynx
electrolyte
electrolyte abnormalities
electrolyte disturbance
electrolyte imbalance
electromagnetic wave
electromotive force (EMF)
electromyographic activity, peripheral
electromyography
electron
electronic artificial larynx
electronic cigarettes (e-cigarettes/e-cigs)
electronystagmography (ENG)
electrooculographic activity
electrophysiologic audiometry
electrophysiology
Elementary Identification Instrument
Elementary School Behavior Rating Scale, Hahnemann
elements of performance objective
elements, cultural
"elephant" (street name, phencyclidine/PCP)
"elephant flipping" (re: use of PCP and MDMA)
"elephant tranquilizer" (street name, phencyclidine/PCP)
eleuthromania (freedom)
elevated mood
elevated risk
elevation screen
elevator muscle of soft palate
elevator muscles of rib
elevators
ELI (Environmental Language Inventory)
Elicited Articulatory System Evaluation
elicited imitation
eligibility, benefit
Elihorn Maze Test
elimination disorder
    other specified, with fecal symptoms (R15.9)
    other specified, with urinary symptoms (N39.498)
    unspecified, with fecal symptoms (R15.9)
    unspecified, with urinary symptoms (R32)
elision
Elizur Test of Psycho-Organicity: Children & Adults
ellipsis (pl. ellipses)
elopement ideation
elurophobia
E/M (Evaluation Management services)
EMAS (Endler Multidimensional Anxiety Scales)
EMAS-P (Endler Multidimensional Anxiety Scales)
EMAS-S (Endler Multidimensional Anxiety Scales)
EMAS-T (Endler Multidimensional Anxiety Scales)
"embalming fluid" (street name, phencyclidine/PCP)
embarrassment, fear of
embedded clause
embedded command
embedded sentence
embedded sound
embezzlement
embolism
embryo
embryonic
EMDR (eye movement desensitization and reprocessing)

EMDR Europe
EMDR therapy
"emergency gun" (re: drug
  injection)
emergent language
Emergent Language Scale
Emergent Language Test
  (Receptive-Expressive)
EMF (electromotive force)
EMH (educationally mentally
  handicapped)
emission(s)
    nasal
    otoacoustic
emotion
    controlled
    diminished feeling of
    discomfort with
    disruptive
    disturbance of
    effect of trauma on
    exaggerated expression of
    expression of
    intense
    lack of
    negative
    positive
    powerful
    public display of
    prosocial
    rapid shifting of
    restricted range of
    shallow expression of
    strong
emotion as cause of seizure
emotion-laden situations
Emotional and Behavior Problem
  Scale (EBPS)
emotional anesthesia
"emotional anesthesia"
emotional
  attachment/commitment
emotional blocking
emotional climate
emotional coldness
emotional conflict
emotional deadness
emotional deficit(s)
emotional dependence
emotional detail, minimization of
emotional difficulties
emotional disinhibition
emotional distress
emotional disturbance
emotional dyscontrol
emotional dysfunction
emotional emptiness, feelings of
emotional explosivity
emotional expression
emotional expression, reduced
  range of
emotional handicap (EH)
emotional handicap, severe (SEH)
emotional incontinence
emotional issues, preexisting
  underlying
emotional lability
emotional maltreatment of
  children
emotional manipulation
emotional needs
emotional problems
emotional problems, differential
  test for *(see also* tests)
emotional reaction
emotional reciprocity
emotional regulation:
    interpersonal effectiveness
    mindfulness
    reality acceptance
emotional response to speech
  dysfluencies
emotional responses
emotional responsiveness
emotional shading
emotional state
emotional stimulus
emotional stress precipitating
  tremor
emotional symptoms
emotional tone
emotional turmoil
emotional undercontrol
emotionality
    excessive
    labile

emotionality
　　negative
　　positive
emotionally provoking stimulus
emotions/conduct, adjustment
　disorder with disturbance of
Emotions Profile Index
emotive energy
emotive energy, active
　displacement of
emotive language
emotive speech
empathic behavior
empathy
empathy, communicating
emphasis
empiric cognition
empirical data
empirical evidence
empirical process
empirical review
empirical support
empiricist theory
empiricist theory, language
empleomania (become involved)
Employability Inventory, The
employability skills *(see also*
　tests)
Employee Aptitude Survey Tests
Employee Assistance Program
　(EAP)
Employee Attitude Inventory
Employee Effectiveness Profile
Employee Reliability Inventory
　(ERI)
Employment Inventory
Employment Service, United
　States (USES)
employment skill competencies
　(see also tests)
empowered families
emptiness
　　chronic feelings of
　　feelings of deep
　　feelings of emotional
　　　sense of
emptiness of affect

EMR (educationally mentally
　retarded)
"emsel" (street name, morphine)
encephalitis (pl. encephalitides)
　　arthropod-borne viral
　　Australian X viral
　　biundulant viral
　　California viral
　　Central European viral
　　Czechoslovakian viral
　　diphasic
　　　meningoencephalitis viral
　　eastern equine viral
　　Far Eastern viral
　　Ilheus viral
　　Japanese B viral
　　Langat viral
　　louping ill viral
　　mosquito-borne viral
　　Murray Valley viral
　　Powassan viral
　　Russian spring-summer
　　　viral
　　slow-acting viral
　　St. Louis viral
　　tick-borne viral
　　western equine viral
encephalopathic
encephalopathy
　　AIDS
　　allergic
　　anoxic
　　childhood
　　delirium due to hepatic
　　demyelinating
　　diffuse
　　hepatic (HE)
　　hypertensive
　　hypoxic-ischemic (HIE)
　　idiopathic
　　painter's
　　postanoxic
　　posttraumatic
　　progressive subcortical
　　progressive traumatic
　　punch-drunk
　　static

encephalopathy
    thiamine deficiency (TDE)
    traumatic
    viral
    Wernicke-Korsakoff
encoder
encoding, impairment of new memory
encoding communication board
encopresis (F98.1)
encounter bats
encounter for mental health services:
    perpetrator of non-parental child abuse (Z69.021)
    perpetrator of non-parental child neglect (Z69.021)
    perpetrator of non-parental child psychological abuse (Z69.021)
    perpetrator of non-parental child sexual abuse (Z69.021)
    perpetrator of nonspousal adult abuse (Z69.82)
    perpetrator of parental child abuse (Z69.011)
    perpetrator of parental child neglect (Z69.011)
    perpetrator of parental child psychological abuse (Z69.011)
    perpetrator of parental child sexual abuse (Z69.011)
    perpetrator of spousal or partner neglect (Z69.12)
    perpetrator of spousal or partner physical violence (Z69.12)
    perpetrator of spousal or partner sexual violence (Z69.12)
    victim of child abuse by parent (Z69.010)
    victim of child neglect by parent (Z69.010)

encounter for mental health services:
    victim of child psychological abuse by parent (Z69.010)
    victim of child sexual abuse by parent (Z69.010)
    victim of non-parental child abuse (Z69.020)
    victim of non-parental child neglect (Z69.020)
    victim of non-parental child psychological abuse (Z69.020)
    victim of non-parental child sexual abuse (Z69.020)
    victim of nonspousal adult abuse (Z69.81)
    victim of spousal or partner neglect (Z69.11)
    victim of spousal or partner physical violence (Z69.11)
    victim of spousal or partner psychological abuse (Z69.12)
    victim of spousal or partner sexual violence (Z69.81)
encountered association, frequency of
encounters
    frequency of sexual
    indiscriminate sexual
    patient
    types of sexual
end point tremor
endangered, physically
endings, inflectional
Endler Multidimensional Anxiety Scales
"endo" (street name, cannabis)
endocannabinoid system (ECS)
endocentric construction
endocentric construction of phrases
endocrine assessment
endocrine conditions, dementia due to

endocrine system
endogenous
endogenous abnormalities in
   sleep-wake timing mechanisms
endogenous circadian pacemaker
endogenous circadian period
endogenous circadian rhythm
   phase
endogenous pain
endolymph
endolymphatic hydrops
end-organ of hearing
endoscope
endoscopy
end-stage renal disease
enduring pattern of inflexibility
"energizer" (street name,
   phencyclidine/PCP)
energy
      acoustic
      active displacement of
        emotive
      decreased
      emotive
      excess
      full of
      increased
      kinetic
      lack of
      low
      potential
      vital
energy expenditure, resting
energy level, high
ENG (electronystagmography)
engagement level
engineering, human
English
      manual
      pidgin Sign (PSE)
      signed
      Signing Exact (SEE)
      Test of Standard Written
      Test of Written
      TOEFL Test of Written
English as a Foreign Language
   Test

English Language Assessment
   Battery
English Language Institute
   Listening Comprehension Test
English phoneme
      anterior feature
      back feature
      consonantal feature
      continuant feature
      coronal feature
      high feature
      low feature
      nasal feature
      round feature
      strident feature
      tense feature
      vocalic feature
      voiced feature
English/Spanish Del Rio
   Language Screening Test
Enhanced ACT Assessment
Enjoying Sobriety, Youth (YES)
enjoyment, family
enjoyment of life
"enoltestovis" (re: injectable
   steroid)
enosimania (belief one's offenses
   are unpardonable)
ensuing
ENT (ear, nose, throat)
entering problem, school
entheomania (heightened
   enthusiasm)
entire period of illness
entities, controlling external
entitlement, sense of
entity-locative
entomomania (insects)
entopic vision
enunciate
enuresis
      diurnal only (F98.0)
      nocturnal and diurnal
        (F98.0)
      nocturnal only (F98.0)
enuretic events
envelope
envious behavior

environment(s)
    academically
      understimulating
    awareness of the
    complete unawareness of
    controlled
    dark
    decreased reactivity to
    distorted perception of
    domestic
    immediate
    in a controlled
    inadequate school
    inattention to the
    institutional
    multicultural
    natural
    perception of the
    physical
    problems related to the
    social
    scaffolded language-
      learning
    social
    vocational
environment questionnaire *(see also* tests)
environment scales *(see also* tests)
environment type, natural
environmental assessment
Environmental Assessment Procedure, Multiphasic (MEAP)
environmental deficiency
environmental deprivation
environmental deprivation, severe
Environmental Language Inventory (ELI)
Environmental Pre-Language Battery
environmental pressure
environmental problem
environmental problem, psychosocial and
Environmental Scale, Children's Version/Family
environmental stimulation
environmental stimuli, selective focusing on
environmental stimulus
environmental understatement
environmental understimulation
EOWPVT (Expressive One-Word Picture Vocabulary Test)
EP (evoked potential) brain test
ephaptic conduction
"ephedrone" (street name, methcathinone)
epidemic hysteria
epidemiological causation
epidemiological data
epidemiological study depression scale *(see also* tests)
epiglottis
epilepsia partialis continua seizure
epilepsy
    absence
    alcoholic
    alcohol-precipitated
    centrotemporal
    childhood
    chronic
    cortical
    depression in
    diurnal
    early traumatic
    extrinsic
    hippocampal
    impulsive petit mal
    Jackson
    Koshevnikoff
    laryngeal
    late traumatic
    nocturnal
    parasomnia type sleep disorder due to
    pattern-induced
    perceptive
    photic
    photosensitive
    postanoxic
    precipitation of
    reading
    sensorial
    situation-related
    sleep-related

epilepsy
    symptomatic
    television-induced
    thalamic
    visual
epilepsy in infancy, polymorphic (PMEI)
epilepsy in infancy, severe myoclonic (SMEI)
epileptic aphasia, acquired
epileptic automatism
epileptic convulsion
epileptic focus
epileptic fugue state
epileptic seizure
epileptics mania
epileptic syndrome
epilepticus
    convulsive status
    non-convulsive status
epileptogenic stimulation
epileptogenic stimulus
episode
    aphonic
    confusional
    current
    daytime sleep
    depressive
    first
    florid
    frequency of sleep terror
    gray-out
    hypomanic-like
    manic-like
    mixed manic-depressive-like
    mood
    most recent depressed mood
    most recent hypomanic mood
    most recent manic mood
    most recent mixed mood
    most recent unspecified mood
    non-substance-induced
    non-substance-related
    pattern of major depressive

episode
    prolonged nocturnal sleep
    prolonged sleep
    recent
    recurrent
    recurrent mood
    recurring psychotic
    schizoaffective
    second
    single
    single hypomanic
    single major depression
    single manic
    sleep onset
    unintentional daytime sleep
    untreated
episode of cataplexy
episode of depression
episode of illness
episode of intoxication
episode of mania, first
episode of schizophrenia, psychotic
episodic changes of consciousness
episodic confusion
episodic course
episodic dyscontrol
epithelium (pl. epithelia)
epochs, wakefulness
equal frequency
equal loudness contours
equal sex ratio
equilibratory ataxia
equilibrium
equine viral encephalitis
    eastern
    western
equipment
    "dirty" drug-injecting
    used drug-injecting
"equipoise" (re: veterinary steroid)
equivalence, complex
equivalent
    delusional
    grammatical
equivalent criteria
equivalent diagnosis

equivalent dosage
equivalent intoxication criteria
equivalent speech reception threshold
equivalent symptomatic presentation
equivalent symptoms
equivalent withdrawal criteria
ER (evoked response)
ER (evoked response) brain test
ERA (electric response audiometry)
ERA (electroencephalic response audiometer)
ERA (electroencephalic response audiometry)
ERA (evoked response audiometry)
Erb palsy
erectile arousal disorder, male
erectile disorder
    acquired type male
    generalized type male
    lifelong type male
    male
    situational type male
erectile disorder due to combined factors, male
erectile disorder due to psychological factors, male
erectile dysfunction (F52.21)
    acquired
    generalized
    lifetime
    mild
    moderate
    severe
    situational
erectile functioning, vasculogenic loss of
erectile problems, occasional
eremiomania (solitude/deserted places)
eremiophobia
ergasiomania (work)
ergomania (work)
ergometer
ergotism
Erhardt Developmental Prehension Assessment (EDPA)
Erhardt Developmental Vision Assessment (EDVA)
ERI (Employee Reliability Inventory)
erosion, dental
erotic arousal
erotic dream(s)
erotic feeling
erotic stimuli
eroticized behavior
eroticomania (sexual desire & behavior)
erotographomania (sexually explicit writing/erotica)
erotomania (sexual desire & behavior)
erotomanic-type delusions
erotomanic-type schizophrenia
erratic
erratic mood
erratic rhythm of speech
erratic speech rhythm
erroneous belief
erroneous impression
error
    anomic
    aphasic
    paralexic
    phonemic articulation
    phonetic articulation
error signal, therapeutic (TES)
errors of metabolism, inborn
errors of ordering of sounds
errors of selection of sounds
"erth" (street name, phencyclidine/PCP)
ERV (expiratory reserve volume)
erythromania (color red) (blushing)
ESA (Early School Assessment)
ESB (The Effective School Battery)
ESBRA (European Society for Biomedical Research on Alcoholism)

escalating pattern of substance use
escalative process
escape, nasal
escape learning
escape reaction
esketamine nasal spray (antidepressant)
ESL/Literacy Placement Test
esophageal speech
    breathing method of
    inhalation method of
    injection method of
    methods of
    sniff method of
    suction method of
    swallow method of
esophageal tears
esophageal voice
ESP (Early Speech Perception Test)
Español, MRT
"Esra" (street name, cannabis)
ESS (The ACT Evaluation/Survey Service)
"essence" (street name, methylenedioxy-methamphetamine; MDMA)
essential cerebellar tremor
essential cerebral tremor
essential convulsion
essential features
essential headache
essential tremor, benign
Essentials Test, Minimum (MET)
established delusion
esthesic(s)
estimated blood loss (EBL)
ESTSS (European Society for Traumatic Stress Studies)
"estuffa" (street name, heroin)
"ET" (street name, alpha-ethyltyptamine)
etat lacunaire (multiple small strokes)
etheromania (pure air)
ethical aspects of assaultive client care
ethical aspects of dementia
ethics, medical
ethmoid bone
ethmoid skull bone
ethnic background
ethnic reference group
ethnopsychology
etiological agent(s)
etiological association
etiological factor(s)
etiological neurological condition
etiological relationship
etiology
    generalized medical
    theories of
ETSA Tests
etymology
eugnathia
eunuchoid voice
euphemism
euphoria
euphoric, feeling
euphoric mood
eupnea
European Association for Aviation Psychology (EAAP)
European Association for Developmental Psychology (EADP)
European Association of Personality Psychology (EAPP)
European Association of Work and Organizational Psychology (EAWOP)
European Community Psychology Association (ECPA)
European Federation of Psychologists' Associations (EFPA)
European Federation of Sport Psychology (FEPSAC)
European Society for Biomedical Research on Alcoholism (ESBRA)
European Society for Traumatic Stress Studies (ESTSS)
eustachian tube
euthymia
euthymic mood

euthymic state
Evaluating Acquired Skills in
  Communication (EASIC)
Evaluating Communicative
  Competence
Evaluating Communicative
  Competence: A Functional
  Pragmatic Procedure
Evaluating Educational Programs
  for Intellectually Gifted
  Students
Evaluating Movement and
  Posture Disorganization in
  Dyspraxic Children
evaluation
    adolescents
    appropriate
    audiological
    clinical
    component of
    comprehensive
    condescending
    criterion
    cultural background
    cultural content of
    dementia
    educational background
    hearing aid (HAE)
    home
    indirect
    longitudinal
    mental capacity
    multiaxial
    need for continued
    negative
    neurological
    neuropsychologic
    process of clinical
    rehabilitation
    vocational (VE)
Evaluation and Screening Test of
  Aphasia
evaluation by others, anxiety due
  to potential
"Eve" (street name, MDEA)
evening headache
event
    antecedent

event
    force of
    interpretation of
    life
    life change
    negative life
    nuretic
    potential positive event,
      psychosocial
    reexperienced traumatic
    sense of reliving an
everyday activities, diminished
  pleasure in
everyday life
everyday memory questionnaire
evidence, empirical
evidence-based practices
evidence-based process
evidence of amnesia
evidence of dissociation disorder
evoked potential
    brain stem
    brain stem auditory
      (BAEP)
    visual (VEP)
evoked response (ER)
evoked response
    brain stem auditory
      (BAER)
    visual (VER)
evoked response audiometry
  (ERA)
    average (AERA)
    brain stem (BSER)
    cardiac (CERA)
evoked response test, visual
evoked somatosensory response
evolution of the disorder
evolution of the syndrome
evolutionary intervention
evolutionary phonetics
Evzio (naloxone HCl)
"Ewings" (street name,
  methaqualone)
exacerbated symptoms of a
  preexisting mental disorder
exacerbation of pain
exacerbation schizophrenia, acute

Exact English Signing
exaggerated achievements
exaggerated communication in
 schizophrenia
exaggerated defect
exaggerated expression of
 emotion(s)
exaggerated feeling of well being
exaggerated inferential thinking in
 schizophrenia
exaggerated language in
 schizophrenia
exaggerated negative qualities
exaggerated perception in
 schizophrenia
exaggerated startle response
exaggerated talent
exaggeration of deep tendon
 reflexes
exaggeration of inferential
 behavioral monitoring
exaggeration of inferential
 perception
exaggeration of inferential
 thinking
exaggeration of language and
 communication
exam *(see also* tests)
exam, visual field
examination
    associated physical
    longitudinal mental status
    microscopic
    neurobehavioral cognitive
     status
    neurological
    neuropsychological status
    oral peripheral
    psychiatric
    psychological
examining expressive morphology
Examining for Aphasia Test
exceptional child
excess energy
excessive admiration
excessive anger, feelings of
excessive anxiety
excessive concern for defect

excessive emotionality
excessive fatigue
excessive fear
excessive menstrual bleeding
excessive motor activity
excessive nasality
excessive need for advice
excessive need for approval
excessive need for care
excessive need for nurturance
excessive need for others to
 assume responsibility
excessive need for reassurance
excessive need for sexual
 expression
excessive need for support
excessive need to be cared for
excessive pride
excessive semen loss
excessive sleep, lack of
excessive sleepiness
excessive social anxiety
excessive use of abstract thinking
excessive worry
excessively impressionistic
 speech
excessively upset
excitation, wave of
excitatory state, central
excited delusion intoxication
excitement
    adequate sexual
    caffeine-induced
    disturbance in
    sexual
excitement phase of sexual
 response cycle
excitement-seeking tendency
excitotoxicity, glutamate
exclamatory sentence
excoriation (skin-picking)
 disorder (L98.1)
excrescence
executive aphasia
executive function
executive functioning, disturbance
 in
executive language

Executive Profile Survey
executive speech
exercise, journaling
exertional headache
exertional headache, benign
exhalation
exhalation muscles
exhaustion
exhibitionism, shock
exhibitionistic behavior
exhibitionistic disorder (F65.2)
existance of a problem
exocentric construction of phrases
exogenous
exogenous depression
exophoric
exophoric pronoun
exostosis (pl. exostoses)
expansion
expansive mood
expectable response
expectation, internal world of
expectation of death
expected speech sounds, developmentally
expenditure, resting energy
expense of treatment
experience
    clinical
    closed to
    common
    cultural
    culturally sanctioned
    depersonalization
    depressive
    disturbing
    dream
    fantasied sexual
    lack of
    life
    narcolepsy
    openness to
    physical
    repeated painful
    Schedule of Recent
    sexual
    social phobia
    stimulating

experience
    stressful life
    subjective
    terrifying
    traumatic
    troubling
    unconscious processing of affective
    unconscious processing of traumatic
experience and behavior, deviant pattern of inner
experienced feeling state, subjectively
experience from the past
experience of dissociative episode
experience of spiritual possession
experience of the external world
experience of the self
experience pleasure, inability to
experiences checklist *(see also* tests)
experience sleep paralysis
experiences questionnaire *(see also* tests)
experiences scale *(see also* tests)
experience the world as unreal
experimental audiology
experimental games
experimental phonetics
experimentally delayed auditory feedback
experimentation in childhood, developmental
expiration reserve volume (ERV)
expiratory volume, forced (FEV)
explanations for illness, cultural
explicit process
exploitation, interpersonal
exploratory behavior
"explorers club" (re: LSD users)
explosion
explosive behavior
explosivity, emotional
exposed, fear of being
exposure meter, noise
exposure to an object
expressed feelings, freely

expressed motivation
expression
    affective
    disorder of written
    emotional
    excessive need for sexual
    parenthetical
    passivity in anger
    reduced range of emotional
    signs of affective
    staring facial
expression of customs, acculturation problems with
expression of emotion
    exaggerated
    shallow
expression of habits, acculturation problems with
expression of political values, acculturation problems with
expression of religious values, acculturation problems with
expression of traumatic themes through repetitive play
expressive delusion(s)
expressive language
expressive language development
expressive language disorder
expressive language problem
Expressive One-Word Picture Vocabulary Test-Upper Extension
extended jargon paraphasia
Extended Merrill-Palmer Scale, The
extension semantics
extensor plantar response
exteriorized stuttering
external acoustic meatus
external auditory meatus
external awards, potential
external control
external ear
external entities, controlling
external force
external genitalia swelling
external incentive motivation
external intercostal muscles
external memory aids
external reality
external reality, abnormal perceptions of
external rewards, potential
external spirits, controlling
external stimulation
external stimulus
external stressor
external structure
external world
    experience of the
    perception of the
external world of reality
externalize blame, tendency to
externi, musculi intercostales
externus abdominis, musculus obliquus
exteroception, tactile
exteroceptor
extinction reinforcement schedule
extracerebral aneurysm
extracranial aneurysm
extradural hemorrhage
extramarital behavior
extramarital relations
extraneous movement
extraneous noise
extrapolation
extrapyramidal cerebral palsy (CP)
extrapyramidal medication side effect
extrapyramidal side effect
extrapyramidal symptoms, prevention of
extrapyramidal tract
extratensive coping style
extratensive personality style
extreme agitation
extreme anxiety
extreme hearing loss
extreme negativism
extreme stressor
extreme trauma
extremity, weakness of an
extremity pain
extrinsic epilepsy

extrinsic muscles
    infrahyoid
    suprahyoid
extrinsic muscles of the larynx
extrinsic muscles of the tongue
eye accessing cues
eye blinking
eye gouging
eye movement
    non-rapid (NREM)
    rapid (REM)
    reflex
    rhythmic slow
    saccadic
eye movement abnormality
eye movement desensitization and reprocessing (EMDR)
"eye opener" (street name, crack; amphetamine)
eye scanning
eye teeth
eyelid conditioning
EYES (Early Years Easy Screen)
eyes
    fluttering of the
    narrow-set
    wide-set
eyes staring
Eysenck Personality Questionnaire

F

15-Item Memorization Test
"45 minute psychosis" (re: dimethyltryptamine
4-MTA (4 methylthio-amphetamine) (street names)
    flatliners
    golden eagle
fabulized response(s)
face
    anthropomorphic
    staring
face pain, atypical
FACES (Family Adaptability and Cohesion Evaluation Scales)
Facial Action Coding System (FACS)
facial agnosia
facial asymmetry
facial expression, staring
facial expression automatism
facial nerve (cranial nerve VII)
facial pain
facial paralysis
facial paresis, center of
facial reflex
facial responsiveness
facial sensation
facial tic
facial tremor
facial twitch/twitching
facies (pl. facies)
    mask (of parkinsonism)
    masklike (mask-like)
    myasthenic
    myopathic
    myotonic
    parkinsonian
facilitated sexual assault, drug
facilitation, social
facilitation of resonance
facilities, health care
facioversion of teeth
FACS (Facial Action Coding System)
factitious disorder (F68.10)
factitious disorder by proxy
factitious disorder imposed on another (F68.10)
factitious disorder imposed on self (F68.10)
factitious disorder, "patient" role in
factitious interface disorder
factitive case (parts of speech)
factor
    causal
    disorganized
    etiological
    human growth (HGF)
    know organic
    negative
    nerve growth (NGF)
    physiological
    precipitating
    predisposing
    psychological
    psychosocial
    psychotic
    risk
    significant risk
    suicide-risk
factor in schizophrenia
    disorganized
    negative
    psychotic
factorial validity
factors
    biological
    cultural
    dyspareunia due to combined
    dyspareunia due to psychological
    etiological
    female orgasmic disorder due to combined
    female orgasmic disorder due to psychological

factors
    female sexual arousal
      disorder due to combined
    female sexual arousal
      disorder due to
      psychological
    hypoactive sexual desire
      disorder due to combined
    hypoactive sexual desire
      disorder due to
      psychological
    male erectile disorder due
      to combined
    male erectile disorder due
      to psychological
    male orgasmic disorder due
      to combined
    male orgasmic disorder due
      to psychological
    perpetuating
    psychological
    sexual aversion disorder
      due to combined
    sexual aversion disorder
      due to psychological
    unspecified psychological
    vaginismus due to
      combined
    vaginismus due to
      psychological
factors affecting medical
  conditions, psychiatric
factors for suicide, risk
factors that constitute health risks
factors that interfere with
  treatment
factors to increase tremor
"factory" (re: drug-making place)
faculty, mental
FAE (fetal alcohol effect)
fag, brain
failed suicide attempt
failing grades, pattern of
failure, chronic renal
failure theory, communication
failure to plan ahead
failure to resist a drive

failure to resist an impulse
failure to resist temptation
failure to speak, consistent
faith conversion problem
"fake STP" (street name,
  phencyclidine/PCP)
"fake-bad"
faking feelings
"fall" (re: to be arrested)
"Fallbrook red hair" (street name,
  cannabis/marijuana)
falling, gradual
falling curve
    gradual
    marked
falling curve, sharply
falling curve audiogram
  configurations
    gradual
    marked
    sharply
false accusations
false confessions
false fluency
false folds, hyperkinesia of the
false memories
false-negative response
false paracusis
false perceptions of movement
false-positive response
false role disorder
false threshold
false vocal folds
falsetto
falsetto voice
familial
familial dementia
familial migraine headache
familial pattern
familial seizure, benign neonatal
familial tendency
familial transmission of
  schizophrenia
familial tremor
families, empowered
Families with Chronically Ill or
  Handicapped Members

family
    blended
    functioning as a
Family Adaptability and Cohesion
    Evaluation Scales (FACES)
Family Apperception Test (FAT)
family caregiver
family connectedness
family counselor
family enjoyment
Family Environment Scale (FES)
family functioning, disruptive of
Family Inventory of Life Events
    and Changes (FILE)
family life
family medicine
family members
family neglect
family of health problems
family physician
family practice
family pursuits
family relations
Family Relations Test: Children's
    Version
Family Relationship Inventory
family routines
Family Satisfaction Scale
family separation
family situations
family stress
family/system research orientation
family treatments
family violence
"famous dimes" (street name,
    crack)
famous person, themes of special
    relationship to a deity or
Famous Sayings Test
"Fantasia" (re: bizarre fantasies)
"fantasia" (re: DMT
    (dimethyltryptamine),
    hallucinogen)
fantasies, intense sexual
fantasized sexual experience
fantasy
    autistic
    female object of sexual

fantasy
    grandiosity in
    internal world of
    masochistic sexual
    nonpathological sexual
    paraphiliac
    pathological sexual
    romantic
    sexual
    sexually arousing
    voyeuristic sexually
        arousing
fantasy figure, female
fantasy play
farad (electrical capacity unit)
Far Eastern viral encephalitis
fasciculations of tongue
fasciculus (pl. fasciculi)
fasciculus, arcuate (AF)
FASD (fetal alcohol spectrum
    disease)
FAST (Fein Articulation
    Screening Test
FAST (Flowers Auditory
    Screening Test)
FAST (Frenchay Aphasia
    Screening Test)
fast activity
"fastin" (street name,
    amphetamine)
FAT (Family Apperception Test)
fat, body
"fat bags" (street name, crack)
fatigability, easy
fatigue
    auditory
    chronic
    daytime
    ease of
    excessive
    marked
    perstimulatory
    sustained
    symptoms of
    vocal
    voice
fatigue as cause of seizure
fatigue strength

fatigue stress
fatigued, feeling
"fatty" (street name,
　cannabis/marijuana cigarette)
fauces, isthmus of
faulty judgment
fear(s)
　acute
　agoraphobic
　excessive
　focus of
　incapacitating
　intense
　marked
　maturity
　paranoid
　performance
　persistent
　reasonable
　sensations of
　subjective
　sudden
　unreasonable
fear of an object, irrational
fear of being exposed
fear of being shamed
fear of criticism
fear of death
fear of disapproval
fear of dying (panic attack
　indicator)
fear of embarrassment
fear of flaws revealed
fear of "going crazy" (panic
　attack indicator)
fear of helplessness
fear of humiliation
fear of imperfections revealed
fear of loneliness
fear of losing control (a panic
　attack indicator)
fear of loss of approval
fear of loss of support
fear of missing out
fear of rejection
fear of retribution
fear of ridicule
fear of scrutiny

fear of self-care
fear of separation
Fear Survey Schedule for
　Children
feared disease
feared object
feared single performance
　situation
feared situation
feared words
fearful, feeling suddenly
feature analysis, distal distinctive
feature contrasts processes
features
　age
　age-related
　age-specific
　agitative
　associated
　atypical
　catatonic
　characteristic
　clinical
　common shared
　cultural
　culture-related
　culture-specific
　delusional
　depressive
　descriptive
　diagnostic
　dominant
　essential
　gender-specific
　hysteroid
　junctural
　manic
　melancholic
　mixed
　mood disorders with
　　catatonic
　mood-congruent psychotic
　mood-incongruent
　　psychotic
　neurotic
　nondistinctive
　obsessive-compulsive
　paranoid

features
    personality
    phonetic
    psychotic
    schizoid
    semantic
    shared phenomenological
    similar shared
    specific age
    specific gender
features of insomnia
febrile convulsion
fecal continence
fecal incontinence
fecal symptoms with other specified elimination disorder (R15.9)
fecal symptoms with unspecified elimination disorder (R15.9)
Federation of the European Societies of Neuropsychology (FESN)
"feed bag" (re: cannabis container)
feedback
    acoustic
    afferent
    auditory
    biofeedback
    corrective
    delayed auditory (DAF)
    experimentally delayed auditory
    haptic
    inverse
    kinesthetic
    negative
    proprioceptive
    simultaneous auditory
    tactile
feedback audiometry, delayed (DFA)
feeding and eating, infancy and early childhood disturbances in
feeding behavior
feeding or eating disorder
    other specified (F50.8)
    unspecified (F50.9)

feeling
    absence of
    erotic
feeling "blah"
feeling "high"
feeling "keyed up"
feeling "on edge"
feeling anxious
feeling confident
feeling constantly threatened
feeling depressed
feeling detached
feeling detached from reality (a panic attack indicator)
feeling disgust
feeling dizzy
feeling euphoric
feeling faint (a panic attack indicator)
feeling fatigued
feeling guilty
feeling inadequate, pattern of
feeling irritable
feeling keyed up
feeling lethargic
feeling numb
feeling of dejection
feeling of detachment
feeling of dysphoria
feeling of electricity
feeling of emotion, diminished
feeling-of-knowing
feeling of tension
feeling of well being, exaggerated
feeling of well-being
feeling on edge
feeling out of control
feeling permanently damaged
feeling sad
feeling state
feeling state, subjectively experienced
feeling suddenly fearful
feeling suddenly sad
feeling superior to others
feeling tense
feeling threatened

feeling threshold
feelings
    associated
    chronic
    covert
    depressive
    disturbing
    faking
    freely expressed
    guilt
    intimate
    "keyed-up"
    loving
    maladaptive
    negative
    "on edge"
    rageful
    separation of ideas from
    subjective
    transference
    unacceptable
feelings of anxiety
feelings of choking (a panic attack indicator)
feelings of danger
feelings of deep emptiness
feelings of depersonalization (a panic attack indicator)
feelings of derealization
feelings of despair
feelings of dirtiness
feelings of dizziness
feelings of emotional emptiness
feelings of excessive anger
feelings of futility
feelings of guilt
feelings of incisiveness
feelings of ineffectiveness
feelings of inferiority to others
feelings of irritability
feelings of lack of self-confidence
feelings of loneliness
feelings of low self-worth
feelings of not fitting in
feelings of personal unappeal
feelings of pessimism
feelings of restlessness
feelings of sadness
feelings of self-disgust
feelings of shame
feelings of social ineptness
feelings of unreality (a panic attack indicator)
feigned symptoms
Fein Articulation Screening Test (FAST)
felinophobia
"Felix the Cat" (street name, LSD)
female dyspareunia
female fantasy figure
female object of sexual fantasy
female orgasmic disorder (F52.31)
    acquired type (F52.31)
    generalized type (F52.31)
    lifelong type (F52.31)
    never experienced orgasm (F52.31)
    situational type (F52.31)
female orgasmic disorder due to combined factors
female orgasmic disorder due to psychological factors
female sexual arousal disorder (F52.22)
    acquired type (F52.22)
    generalized type (F52.22)
    lifelong type (F52.22)
    situational type (F52.22)
female sexual arousal disorder due to combined factors
female sexual arousal disorder due to psychological factors
female sexual interest/arousal disorder (F52.22)
feminine clothing
feminine mannerisms
feminine speech patterns
femininity, construction of
femininity, traditional traits of:
    emotional sensitivity
    empathetic
    nurturing
fence, low
fenestra (pl. fenestrae)

fenestra cochlea
fenestra ovalis
fenestra rotunda
fenestra vestibuli
fenestration
fenethylline (brand names)
    Biocapton
    Captagon
    Fitton
fenetylline
fentanyl (street names)
    Apache
    China girl
    China town
    China white (heroin plus fentanyl)
    dance fever
    drop dean
    Fat Albert
    friend
    goodfellas
    great bear
    he-man
    incredible hulk
    jackpot
    keel (heroin laced with fentanyl)
    kill (heroin laced with fentanyl)
    king ivory
    lethal injection
    murder 8
    perc-a-pop (diverted from cancer patients)
    poison
    Tango and Cash
    The bomb
    TNT (heroin plus fentanyl)
FEPSAC (European Federation of Sport Psychology)
Fere effect
"ferry dust" (street name, heroin)
Fer-Will Object Kit
FES (Family Environment Scale)
FESN (Federation of the European Societies of Neuropsychology)
festinant quality in parkinsonian speech
festinating gait
fetal alcohol effect (FAE)
fetal alcohol spectrum disease (FASD)
fetal fetus
fetal movement
fetal movement, subjective sensation of
fetation
fetish object
fetishism, transvestic
fetishistic disorder (F65.0)
    body part(s) (F65.0)
    nonliving object(s) (F65.0)
    other (F65.0)
FEV (forced expiratory volume)
few activities, take pleasure in
fiber, nerve
fiberscope
fibrosis, cystic
fiddling with fingers, nonfunctional and repetitive
fidgeting behavior
"fi-do-nie" (street name, opium)
field
    electric
    free
    minimum audible (MAF)
    sound
    visual
field construction, visual
field cut, visual
field data
field defects, visual
field disturbance, visual
field dependence-independence
field exam, visual
field images, peripheral
field room, free
field test, visual
field-trial projects
field-trial results
field trials
Field Work Performance Report
"fields" (street name, lysergic acid diethylamide/LSD)

Psychiatric Words and Phrases 243

"fiend" (re: solo cannabis user)
"fifteen cents" (re: $15 worth of drugs)
"fifty-one" (street name, crack)
fights, recurrent physical
figural aftereffect
figural memory
figurative blind spot (scotoma)
Figurative Language Interpretation Test (FLIT)
figure, female fantasy
figure-ground
    auditory
    visual
figure-ground discrimination
    auditory
    visual
figure-ground distortion
figure of speech:
    allusion
    apostrophe
    hyperbole
    idiom
    irony
    litotes
    metaphor
    metonymy
    overstatement
    personification
    simile
    synecdoche
    understatement
Figure Preference Test, Welsh
figures
    attachment
    major attachment
FILE (Family Inventory of Life Events and Changes)
filled pauses in speech
filter
    active
    band-pass
    high-pass
    octave-band
    pass-band
    perceptual
    wave
filtered speech

FIM (Functional Independence Measure)
"finajet/finaject" (street name, veterinary steroid)
final consonant
    deletion of
    devoicing of
final consonant position
financial remuneration
findings, neurophysiological
fine motor
fine movements, rapid
fine postural tremor
"fine stuff" (street name, cannabis/marijuana)
fine tactile sensation
"finger" (street name, cannabis cigarette)
finger anomia
"finger lid" (street name, marijuana/cannabis)
Finger Localization Test (FLT)
fingerspelling
finger-tapping score(s)
finite grammar
"fir" (re: drug injection)
"fir" (street name, cannabis; crack/methamphetamine)
"fire it up" (re: cannabis/marijuana use)
"Fire line" (street name, morphine)
fire setting
    deliberate
    intentional
    juvenile
firing an anchor
first deciduous molar
first deciduous molar teeth
first-degree biological relatives
first episode of mania
first language
"first line" (street name, morphine)
first messengers, lithium's action on
first position
first premolar teeth

"first-rank symptoms",
    Schneider's list of
first sentences first words
first sign of schizophrenia
first-time drinkers
first words, first sentences
"fish scales" (street name, crack)
fissure
    longitudinal cerebral
    rectal
fissure of Rolando
fissure of Sylvius
fist clenching
fist rank symptoms of delusion(s)
fistula
    cleft palate
    rectovaginal
fit, psychomotor
fits (seizure), cerebellar
fitting in, feelings of not
Fitzgerald Key
five-axis system (DSM-IV
    system)
"five C note" (re: $500 bill)
"five cent bag" (re: $5 worth of
    drugs)
"five dollar bag" (re: $50 worth of
    drugs)
Five P's: Parent Professional
    Preschool Performance Profile,
    The
"fives" (street name,
    amphetamine)
"fix" (re: drug injection)
fix and focus attention
fixation in stuttering
fixed-ended session
fixed interval reinforcement
    schedule
fixed ratio reinforcement schedule
"fizzies" (street name,
    methadone)
F-JAS (Fleishman Job Analysis
    Survey)
flaccid cerebral palsy (CP)
flaccid dysarthria
flaccid paralysis
flaccid speech

flaccidity
"flag" (re: drug injection)
Flakka (designer drug; alpha-
    PVP)
flake" (street name, cocaine)
"flakes" (street name,
    phencyclidine/PCP)
flame, manometric
"flame cooking" (re: cocaine use)
"flamethrower" (street name,
    cocaine- and heroin-laced
    cigarette)
"flamingos" (street name,
    methaqualone)
flap, pharyngeal
flap consonant
flapping movement
flapping tremor
flare, axon
"flash" (street name, lysergic acid
    diethylamide/LSD)
flashbacks, acid
flashes of color
flat audiogram configurations
"flat blues" (street name, lysergic
    acid diethylamide/LSD)
"flat chunks" (re: crack cut with
    benzocaine)
flat consonant
flattening, affective
flattened affectivity
flaws revealed, fear of
"flea powder" (re: low quality
    heroin)
Fleishman Job Analysis Survey
    (F-JAS)
flesh-eating drug (re: "krocodil"
    opioid desomorphine
flexibility
    behavioral
    lack of
flexion reflex
flexor
flicker fusion
flight of ideas (FOI)
flirtatious behavior
flirting and coquetting

FLIT (Figurative Language Interpretation Test)
floating sensation, drug-induced
florid episode
Florida International Diagnostic-Prescriptive Vocational Competency Profile
Florida Kindergarten Screening Battery, The
"Florida snow" (street name, heroin; cocaine)
florimania (flowers/plants)
flow, cerebral blood (CBF)
"flower" (street name, cannabis/marijuana)
"flower flipping" (re: ecstasy with mushrooms)
"flower tops" (street name, cannabis/marijuana)
"flowers" (street name, methaqualone)
Flowers Auditory Screening Test (FAST)
Flowers-Costello Test of Central Auditory Abilities
FLT (Finger Localization Test)
fluctuating affect
fluctuating mood disturbance
fluctuations, weight
fluency
    basal
    disturbance in
    disturbance in rate of
    false
    reduced
    verbal
fluency disorder, adult-onset (F98.5)
fluency disorder, childhood-onset (stuttering) (F80.81)
fluency of speech
    decreased
    disturbance in the normal
fluency of thought
fluent aphasia, acquired
fluent aphasic speech
fluent paraphasic speech

Fluharty Speech and Language Screening Test
fluid disturbance
fluid overload
fluid retention
fluids, body
flunitrazepam (Rohypnol) (drug-facilitated sexual assault)
flutter
    alar
    auditory
flutter fusion, auditory
fluttering of the eyes
"flying" (re: under the influence of drugs)
flying, sensation of
Fly Mexican Airlines (re: to smoke marijuana)
FM (frequency modulation)
FNA (Functional Needs Assessment)
focal ability, impaired
focal contralateral routing of signals (FOCALCROS)
focal neurologic disturbance
focal neurologic signs
focal nonextrapyramidal neurologic signs
focal twitch/twitching
FOCALCROS (focal contralateral routing of signals)
focus
    characteristic paraphiliac
    epileptic
    mirror
    multiple
    principal
    somatic
    stationary
    tone
    unilateral
    vocal
focus groups
focus of activity
focus of anxiety
focus of attention
focus of avoidance
focus of clinical attention

focus of concern
focus of delusional system
focus of diagnosis
focus of fear
focus of the delusion
focus of treatment
focus of worry
focus on body parts
focusing on environmental stimuli, selective
FOI (flight of ideas)
folate-deficiency
fold, ventriculus
fold approximation, vocal
fold paralysis, vocal
folds
    aryepiglottic
    bowed vocal
    false vocal
    polypoid degenerative of the true
    true vocal
    vestibular
folic acid-deficiency
folie a deux (shared delusional belief)
folk illness
follicles, damaged hair
follicular phase
follicular phase of the menstrual cycle
following movement
"following that cloud" (re: searching for drugs)
Follow-up Drinker Profile
Folstein Mini-Mental Status Examination
"foo-foo dust" (street name, cocaine)
"foo foo stuff" (street name, heroin; cocaine)
food cravings, marked specific
food deprivation
food intake abnormality
food intake disorder, avoidant/restrictive (F50.8)
foods
    intolerance to different

foods
    low-calorie diet
"foolish powder" (street name, heroin; cocaine)
foot-pound
"footballs" (street name, amphetamine)
footplate
for sleep and dreaming, amnesia
foramen, incisive
fore-glide
force
    electromotive (EMF)
    external
    nerve
    outside
forced cross-gender
forced expiratory volume (FEV)
forced sex
forced sleep
forced vibration
forced whisper
force of events
foreign accent
forensic determination(s)
Forer Structured Sentence Completion Test
foreshortened future, sense of a
foreskin, reduced sensation of the
forgery
"forget me drug" (re: Rohypnol)
"forget pill" (re: Rohypnol)
forked tongue
form
    free
    language
form recognition, oral
form word
formal contract
formal method
formal operations period
Formal Reasoning, Arlin Test of
formal universals
formation
    affricate consonant
    brain stem reticular
    compromise
    continuant consonant

formation
    dark lateral consonant
    frictionless consonant
    glide consonant
    groove fricative consonant
    implosive consonant
    light lateral consonant
    liquid consonant
    nasal consonant
    new identity
    nonsonorant consonant
    obstruent consonant
    omen
    personality
    plosive consonant
    retroflex consonant
    scar tissue
    semi-vowel consonant
    sibilant consonant
    slit fricative consonant
    sonant consonant
    sonorant consonant
    spirant consonant
    stop consonant
    trill consonant
former identity
forms, informational *(see also tests)*
forms of pain, chronic
forms reliability coefficient, alternate
formulate a plan
formulation
    cultural
    language
formulations, psychodynamic
fornication
fortification scotoma
fortis consonant
forward coarticulation
forward digital span recall test
forward masking
"forwards" (street name, amphetamine)
fossa (pl. fossae)
foster care
Foster Mazes
Four Picture Test
four-point restraints
four-pointed, to be (restrained)
Fourier analysis
Fourier's law
fourteen-and-six Hertz positive spikes
foveal vision
FPR (Functional Performance Record)
fragile X syndrome
fragment
fragmentary delusions in schizophrenia
fragmentary dream image
fragmentary hallucinations in schizophrenia
fragmented nighttime sleep
"fraho/frajo" (street name, cannabis)
frame, analytic
Franceschetti's syndrome
Francomania (France/things French)
fraud
FRC (functional residual capacity)
free base cocaine
free field
free field room
free form
free mandibular movement
free morpheme
free radicals
free variation
free vibration
"freebase" (re: smoking crack cocaine)
freedom, loss of
freely expressed feelings
"freeze" (street name, cocaine)
freezing of movement
freezing phenomenon
Fregoli delusion
"French blue" (street name, amphetamine)
"French fries" (street name, crack)
French method

Frenchay Activities Index
Frenchay Aphasia Screening Test (FAST)
Frenchay Dysarthria Assessment
frenulum (pl. frenula)
frenum (pl. frena or frenums)
frenum, lingual
frequencies
    range of
    speech
frequency
    alpha
    band
    decreased
    dominant waking
    equal
    fundamental
    high (HF)
    high filter (HFF)
    increased
    infrasonic
    low (LF)
    low filter (LFF)
    mean peak
    modal
    natural
    resonant
    respiratory
    speech
    treatment
    ultrasonic
frequency-amplitude gradient
frequency audiometry, high
frequency CROS, high (HICROS)
frequency deafness, high
frequency encountered association
frequency hearing theory
frequency jitter
frequency modulation (FM)
frequency-modulation auditory trainer
frequency of anxiety
frequency of anxiety symptoms
frequency of depressive symptoms
frequency of drug use
    high
    low
frequency of episodes
frequency of headache
frequency of reinforcement
frequency of self-administration of drugs
frequency of sexual encounters
frequency of sleep terror episodes
frequency of violent acts
frequency range
frequency range, maximum
frequency response
frequency response curve
frequent derailment
frequent drug dosing, need for
"fresh" (street name, phencyclidine/PCP)
freudian theory
fricative(s)
    gliding of
    groove
    slit
    stopping of
fricative consonant formation
    groove
    split
fricative sounds
frictionless consonant formation
"friend" (street name, fentanyl)
friends, substance-using
"fries" (street name, crack)
fright, stage
frigophobia
"frios" (re: cannabis laced with phencyclidine)
"Frisco special" (street name, cocaine/heroin/LSD)
"Frisco speedball" (street name, cocaine/heroin/LSD)
"friskie powder" (street name, cocaine)
frog in the throat
from social affairs, withdrawal
front phoneme
front routing of signals (FROS)
"front-stabbing"
front vowel
frontal bone
frontal gyri

frontal headache
frontal lisp
frontal lobe
frontal lobe dementia
frontal lobe dysfunction
frontal plane
frontal release sign
frontal release signs, positive
frontal routing of signals,
  ipsilateral (IFROS)
frontal skull bone
frontal sulci
frontal sulcus
    inferior
    middle
    superior
fronting, palatal
frontocortical aphasia
frontolateral laryngectomy
frontolenticular aphasia
frontotemporal brain atrophy
frontotemporal hypometabolism
FROS (front routing of signals)
Frotteurism
Frotteuristic disorder (F65.81)
frustration, sense of
frustration-induced impaired
  social functioning
"fry" (street name, crack)
fry
    glottal
    vocal
"fry daddy" (street name, crack
  and cannabis; crack-laced
  cigarette)
FSI (Functional Status Index)
FSQ (Functional Status
  Questionnaire)
FTEQ (Functional Time
  Estimation Questionnaire)
"fu" (street name, cannabis)
"fuel" (street name, cannabis and
  insecticides; phencyclidine)
"fuete" (re: hypodermic needle)
fugue, dissociative
fugue state
    epileptic
    hysterical

Fuld Object-Memory Evaluation
full-blown delirium
full interepisode recovery
full of energy
full-on gain
  HF average
  high-frequency (HF)
    average
full panic attacks
Full-Range Picture Vocabulary
  Test
Full Range Picture Vocabulary
  Test, Ammons
full remission, sustained
Full Scale Scores
full symptom criteria
full wakefulness, state of
Fullerton Language Test for
  Adolescents
"fuma D'Angola" (street name,
  cannabis)
function
    acoustic measurement of
      auditory
    adequate sexual
    affective
    articulation-gain
    brain
    brain stem
    caloric stimulation test for
      vestibular
    central auditory
    cognitive
    deterioration of language
    differential
    discrepant intellectual
    executive
    hepatic
    higher level cognitive
    impaired immune
    impairment of cognitive
    inability to
    intact motor
    intact sensory
    integrity of brain
    intrapsychical
    language
    mapping of cortical

function
   neuroendocrine
   performance-intensity
   primary
   psychosocial
   referential
   renal
   reproductive
   role
   semi-autonomous systems concept of brain
   sensory
   speech-motor
   spiritual
   unable to
   ventricular
   verbally mediated
function word
Functional Ambulation Categories
functional aphonia
functional articulation disorder
functional assessment *(see also* tests)
Functional Assessment Inventory
functional brain imaging
functional capacity
Functional Communication Profile
functional deafness
functional disability
functional impairment
Functional Independence Measure (FIM)
Functional Limitation Profile
Functional Limitations Battery
functional loss
functional movement
Functional Needs Assessment (FNA)
functional neurological symptoms disorder
Functional Performance Record (FPR)
functional residual capacity (FRC)
Functional Status Index (FSI)
Functional Status Questionnaire (FSQ)

Functional Time Estimation Questionnaire (FTEQ)
functional variation, physiological
functionally impaired
functioning
   anxiety-induced impaired social
   body
   borderline intellectual (R41.83)
   competent relational
   defensive
   deterioration in
   discrepant intellectual
   disrupted relational
   disruptive of family
   disturbance in executive
   dysfunctional relational
   educational
   frustration-induced impaired social
   general intellectual
   hierarchical
   impaired cognitive
   impaired daytime
   impairment in adaptive
   impairment in cognitive
   impairment in occupational
   impairment in social
   independent
   interepisode
   interpersonal
   level of
   level of occupational
   level of social
   long-term
   low self-esteem as cause for impaired social
   major impairment of
   marked decline in academic
   marked decline in occupational
   normal neurological
   potential impairment of, immune
   premorbid level of
   psychosocial
   receptor

functioning
    serious impairment of
    slight impairment of
    stability of vocational
    subaverage academic
    vasculogenic loss of erectile
    voluntary motor
    voluntary sensory
functioning as a family
functioning in society
functioning scale *(see also* tests)
functor
fund of information
fund of information test
fundamental approach
fundamental frequency
fusion
    auditory flutter
    binaural
    flicker
futility
    feelings of
    medical
future
    foreshortened
    sense of a foreshortened
future pace
future perfect progressive tense
future perfect tense
future progressive tense, simple
future tense, simple
futuristic thinking

G

"G" (re: $1000 or 1 gram of drugs; an unfamiliar male)
"G.B." (street name, barbiturate)
GABA (gabapentin)
GAD (generalized anxiety disorder)
GAEL (Grammatical Analysis of Elicited Language)
GAFS score (Global Assessment of Functioning Scale)
"gaffel" (re: fake cocaine)
"gaffus" (re: hypodermic needle)
gag reflex
"gage/guage" (street name, cannabis)
"gagers" (street name, methcathinone)
"gaggers" (street name, methcathinone)
gain
    acoustic
    desire for personal
    high-frequency (HF) average full-on
    peak acoustic
    potential secondary
    prevention of weight
    secondary
gain control
    acoustic
    automatic
gain profit, manipulative behavior to
gait
    abnormal
    antalgic
    ataxic
    cerebral
    disturbances of
    festinating
    hysterical
    narrow-based
    Parkinsonian
    retropulsion of
    shuffling
    staggering
    stuttering
    swaying
    uncoordinated
    unsteady
    waddling
    wide-based
gait abnormalities
gait analysis
gait disorder
gait problem
galactosemia
Gallomania (things Gaelic)
"galloping horse" (street name, heroin)
galvanic skin resistance
galvanic skin response audiometry (GSRA)
galvanometer
Galveston Orientation and Awareness Test (GOAT)
gambling
    professional
    social
gambling behavior
gambling behavior, maladaptive
gambling disorder (mild, moderate/severe) (F63.0)
gambling strategy
game theory
games, experimental
gaming disorder
gamma-aminobutyric acid
gamma butyrolactone (GBL) (street names)
    Blue Nitrate Vitality (contains GBL)
    firewater (contains GBL)
    lactone (GBL)
    RenewTrient (contains GBL)

gamma butyrolactone (GBL)
  (street names)
    revivarant (GBL product)
    revivarant-G
gamma-glutamyltransferase
  (GGT)
gamma hydroxybutyrate (GHB)
  (street names)
    Candy raver
    caps
    cherry mein
    everclear
    fantasy
    G
    GBH
    GBL (GBL is used to make
      GHB)
    Georgia home boy
    GHB
    goop
    great hormones at bedtime
    grievous bodily harm
    G-riffic
    hawkers (re: sellers of
      GHB)
    Jib
    liquid E
    liquid ecstasy
    liquid G
    liquid X
    max (water-diluted
      GHB/amphetamine
      mixture)
    organic Quaalude
    Salty water
    scoop
    sleep
    sleep-500
    soap
    somatomax
    vita-G
    water (GHB and other drug
      mixtures)
gamomania (marriage)
"gamot" (street name, heroin)
"gange" (street name, synthetic
  cannabis)
ganglia, basal

ganglion (pl. ganglia or
  ganglions)
"gangster" (street name, cannabis)
"gangster pills" (street name,
  barbiturate)
"gank" (street name, fake crack)
GAP (Group for the Advancement
  of Psychiatry)
gap, air-borne
gaping
gaps, memory
gaps in memory, retrospective
"garbage" (re: poor quality drugs)
"garbage head" (re: crack user;
  multiple drug user)
"garbage rock" (street name,
  crack)
GARF (Global Assessment of
  Relational Functioning) Scale
Garliner tongue thrust
  classification
garrote
garrulous affect
"gash" (street name, cannabis)
"gasper" (street name, cannabis
  cigarette)
"gasper stick" (street name,
  cannabis cigarette)
gasping during sleep
gastric ruptures
gastrointestinal conditions and
  concurrent psychiatric problems
gastrointestinal pain
gastrointestinal symptom,
  somatization
gastrointestinal symptoms
Gate Theory of Pain
Gates-MacGinitie Reading Test
Gates-McKillop-Horowitz
  Reading Diagnostic Tests
"gato" (street name, heroin)
Gaucher's disease
"gauge butt" (street name,
  cannabis)
gaussian curve
gaussian distribution
gaussian noise
gaze deficit

gaze impairment
gaze palsy
GBH (amino acid concoction) dependence
GBL (gamma butyrolactone)
GCDAS (The Gesell Child Development Age Scale)
GCS (Glasgow Coma Scale)
GCT (General Clerical Test)
"gee" (street name, opium)
"geek" (street name, crack and cannabis)
"geeker" (re: crack user)
"geeze" (re: cocaine use)
"geezer" (re: drug injection)
"geezin a bit of dee gee" (re: drug injection)
GEI (The Grief Experience Inventory)
gender
    boundaries and
        multiple personality and
gender-based attitudes
gender confusion
gender differences in anxiety disorders
gender differences in eating disorders
gender differences in mood disorders
gender differences in schizophrenia
gender differences in sleep disorders
gender differences in somatoform disorders
gender differences in unipolar depression
gender dysphoria
gender dysphoria in adolescence and adults (F64.1)
gender dysphoria in adolescence/adults with a disorder of sex development (F64.1 + code for sex development)
gender dysphoria in children (F64.2)
gender dysphoria in children with a disorder of sex development (F64.2 + code for sex development)
gender dysphoria
    other specified (F64.8)
    unspecified (F64.9)
gender features, specific
gender identity
gender identity disorder (GID)
gender identity problem
gender identity psychosexual development
gender nonconformity
gender role
    persistent discomfort with social stereotypical
gender-sensitive psychopharmacology
gender-specific features
gene, autosomal dominant
General Ability Battery
General Clerical Test (GCT)
General Educational Development Tests
general hospital consultation/liaison services
general intellectual functioning
General Interest Survey
general linguistics
General Management In-Basket (GMIB)
general medical condition (GMC)
general medical condition, problems related to a
general oral inaccuracy articulation
general paresis
general phonetics
general population setting
general responsiveness
general rule
general semantics
generalization
    response
    stimulus
generalized anxiety disorder (GAD) (F41.1)

Generalized Anxiety Disorder Scale
generalized auditory agnosia
generalized convulsion
generalized headache
generalized hyperreflexia
generalized intellectual impairment
generalized medical etiology
generalized reinforcer
generalized sexual dysfunction
generalized tonic/clonic convulsion
generalized tonic-clonic seizure (GTC)
generalized type dyspareunia
generalized type female orgasmic disorder
generalized type female sexual arousal disorder
generalized type hypoactive sexual desire disorder
generalized type male erectile disorder
generalized type male orgasmic disorder
generalized type sexual aversion disorder
generalized type vaginismus
generational responsibility
generative intervention
generative semantics
generative transformational grammar
generator
    new behavior
    noise
genetic counselor
genetic vulnerability
genetics, behavioral
genioglossus, musculus
genioglossus muscle
geniohyoideus, musculus
geniohyoid muscle
genital pain
genital sexual contact
genital stimulation, tactile
genitalia, ambiguous
genitalia swelling, external
genitive case
genitor-pelvic pain/penetration disorder (F52.6)
genitourinary system
"genuines" (street name, methaqualone)
geometric designs test, copy
"George smack" (street name, heroin)
"Georgia home boy" (street name, GHB; gamma hydroxybutyrate)
gephyromania (bridges)
geranyl pyrophosphate (GPP)
gerascophobia
geriatric
geriatric audiology
Geriatric Depression Scale
geriatric neuropsychiatry
geriatrics
German measles
German method
German Psychological Society (DGPs)
Germanomania (Germany/things German)
gerontological
gerontology
Gerstmann syndrome
gerund (parts of speech)
GES (Gifted Evaluation Scale)
Gesell Child Development Age Scale, The (GCDAS)
Gesell Preschool Test
Gesell School Readiness Test
Gestalt tests *(see also* tests)
gestural automatism
gesture language
gestures
    body
    kinesic
    suicidal
gesture speech, social
"get a gage up" (re: cannabis use)
"get a gift" (re: drug acquisition)
"get down" (re: drug injection)
"get high" (re: cannabis use; drug influence)

"get lifted" (re: drug influence)
"get off" (re: drug injection; drug influence)
"get the wind" (re: cannabis use)
"get through" (re: drug acquisition)
geumophobia
GGT (state markers of heavy drinking)
GGT level
"Ghana" (street name, cannabis)
"GHB" (street name, gamma hydroxybutyrate)
"ghost" (street name, lysergic acid diethylamide/LSD)
"ghost busting" (re: crack acquisition; cocaine use)
gibberish
"gick monster" (re: crack user)
GID (gender identity disorder)
GID of adolescence
GID of adulthood
GID of childhood
Gifted and Talented Screening Form
gifted child
Gifted Evaluation Scale (GES)
Gifted Program Evaluation Survey, The
"gift-of-the-sun" (street name, cocaine)
"giggle smoke" (street name, cannabis)
giggling, nervous
Gillingham-Childs Phonics Proficiency Scales
Gilmore Oral Reading Test
"gimmick" (re: drug injection)
"gimmie" (street name, crack and cannabis)
"gin" (street name, cocaine)
"girlfriend" (street name, cocaine)
"give wings" (re: drug injection)
giving, transgenerational role of
"glad stuff" (street name, cocaine)
"glading" (re: inhalant use)
"glancines" (street name, heroin)
Glasgow Assessment Schedule

Glasgow Coma Scale (GCS)
Glasgow Outcome Scale
"glass" (re: hypodermic needle)
"glass" (street name, amphetamine)
"glass gun" (re: hypodermic needle)
glide consonant formation
glide, vocalic
gliding of fricatives
gliding of liquids
gliosis, astrocytic
"glo" (street name, crack)
global amnesia
global amnesic
Global Alliance for Behavioral Health and Social Justice
Global Assessment of Functioning Scale (GAFS) score
Global Assessment of Relational Functioning (GARF) Scale
global assessment of sensory disturbance
global cognitive deficit
global dementia
global developmental delay (F88)
global loss of language
global measures of disability
glossal catch
glossectomy
glossitis
glossograph
glossokinetic potential
glossopalatine arch
glossopalatine muscle
glossopharyngeal nerve (cranial nerve IX)
glossopharyngeal press
glossosteresis
glottal area
glottal area consonant placement
glottal attack, hard
glottal catch
glottal chink
glottal click
glottal cycle
glottal fry

glottal pulse
glottal replacement
glottal stop, ubiquitous
glottal stroke
glottal tone
glottal vibration
glottic
glottidospasm
glottis
glue ear
glue sniffer's rash
"gluey" (re: glue sniffer)
glutamate excitotoxicity
glutethimide and codeine cough syrup, "pancakes and syrup"
glutethimide group
glutethimide intoxication
Glycerol Test
GMC (general medical condition)
    anxiety disorder due to
    delirium due to
    insomnia type sleep disorder due to
    mental disorder affecting
    parasomnia type sleep disorder due to
    psychological disorder affecting
    sexual dysfunction due to
    sleep disorder due to
GMIB (General Management In-Basket)
gnathic
gnawing
"go into a sewer" (re: drug injection)
"go loco" (re: cannabis use)
goal-directed activity(ies)
goal-directed behavior
    diminution of
    initiation of
goal orientation, lack of
goal-oriented processes
goals, long-term
goals skills, negotiating
GOAT (Galveston Orientation and Awareness Test)

"God's drug" (street name, morphine)
"God's flesh" (street name, psilocybin/psilocin)
"God's medicine" (street name, opium)
God's voice, hearing
"go-fast" (re: methcathinone use)
going blank, mind
"gold" (street name, cannabis; crack)
"gold dust" (street name, cocaine)
"gold star" (street name, cannabis)
"golden dragon" (street name, lysergic acid diethylamide/LSD)
"golden girl" (street name, heroin)
"golden leaf" (street name, cannabis)
Goldman-Fristoe Test of Articulation
Goldman-Fristoe-Woodcock Auditory Skills Test Battery
Goldman-Fristoe-Woodcock Test of Auditory Discrimination
Goldstein-Scheerer Tests of Abstract and Concrete Thinking
"golf ball" (street name, crack)
"golf balls" (street name, barbiturate)
Golombok Rust Inventory of Marital State, The (GRIMS)
"golpe" (street name, heroin)
"goma" (street name, opium; black tar heroin)
"gondola" (street name, opium)
"gong" (street name, cannabis; opium)
"goob" (street name, methcathinone)
"good" (street name, phencyclidine/PCP)
"Good and Plenty" (street name, heroin)
"good butt" (street name, cannabis cigarette)

"good giggles" (street name, cannabis)
"good go" (re: drug dealing)
"good H" (street name, heroin)
"good lick" (re: high quality drugs)
good sleep efficiency
Goodenough "Draw-A-Man"
Goodenough-Harris Drawings Test
"goodfellas" (street name, fentanyl)
Goodman Lock Box
"goof butt" (street name, cannabis cigarette)
"goofy's" (street name, lysergic acid diethylamide/LSD)
"goon" (street name, phencyclidine/PCP)
"goon dust" (street name, phencyclidine/PCP)
"gopher" (re: drug dealing)
Gordon Personal Profile Inventory
"Goric" (street name, opium)
"gorilla biscuits" (street name, phencyclidine/PCP)
"gorilla pills" (street name, barbiturate)
"gorilla tab" (street name, phencyclidine/PCP)
GORT-3 (Gray Oral Reading Tests
"got it going on" (re: drug dealing)
gouging, eye
gown restrictions
GPP (geranyl pyrophosphate)
"G-rock" (re: 1 gram of rock cocaine)
"G-rock" (street name, cocaine)
Graded Naming Test
Graded Word Reading Test
Graded Word Spelling Test
grades, pattern of failing
gradient
    amplitude
    frequency-amplitude

gradual falling curve
gradual falling curve audiogram configurations
gradual rising curve
gradual rising curve audiogram configurations
gradual topic shift
"graduate" (re: ending drug usage)
Graduate and Managerial Assessment
"gram" (street name, hashish)
grammar
    finite
    generative
    generative transformational
    particular
    pedagogical
    phrase structure
    pivot
    prescriptive
    scientific
    traditional
    transformational generative
    universal
grammar case
grammatical analysis
Grammatical Analysis of Elicited Language (GAEL)
grammatical categories
grammatical component
grammatical equivalent
grammatical meaning
grammatical morpheme
grammatical structure
grammatic closure
grammatic method aural rehabilitation
grand mal (tonic-clonic) seizure
grand mal status
grandiose concepts
grandiose content
grandiose themes
grandiose type delusions
grandiose type schizophrenia
grandiosity, pattern of
grandiosity in fantasy
granulovascular degeneration

"grape parfait" (street name, LSD)
grapheme
graphic disorientation
graphic impairment
graphomania (writing)
Grashey aphasia
"grass brownies" (street name, cannabis)
Grassi Block Substitution Test
"grata" (street name, cannabis)
gratification, manipulative behavior for material
grave phoneme
"gravel" (street name, crack; alpha-PVP)
gravel voice
gravis, myasthenia
gravity (CG), center of
gravity perception
"gravy" (re: drug injection)
"gravy" (street name, heroin)
gray matter (of CNS)
gray matter
    center of
    cortical
    dorsal
Gray Oral Reading Tests (GORT)
gray-out episode
"grease" (re: currency)
"great bear" (street name, fentanyl)
"great tobacco" (street name, opium)
greater responsibility
Grecomania (Greece/things Greek)
"green" (street name, cannabis; phencyclidine/PVP; ketamine)
"green double domes" (street name, lysergic acid diethylamide/LSD)
"green frog" (street name, barbiturate)
"green goddess" (street name, cannabis)
"green gold" (street name, cocaine)
"green goods" (re: currency)
"green leaves" (street name, phencyclidine/PCP)
"green single domes" (street name, lysergic acid diethylamide/LSD)
"green stuff/greens" (re: currency)
"green tea" (street name, phencyclidine/PCP)
"green wedge" (street name, lysergic acid diethylamide/LSD)
"greeter" (street name, cannabis)
gregarious
Gregorc Style Delineator
"Greta" (street name, cannabis)
"grey shields" (street name, LSD)
"gridiron abdomen"
grief counselor
Grief Experience Inventory, The (GEI)
"griefo" (street name, cannabis)
"griff" (street name, cannabis)
"griffa" (street name, cannabis)
"griffo" (street name, cannabis)
grimace
grimacing
grimacing, prominent
GRIMS (The Golombok Rust Inventory of Marital State)
"grit" (street name, crack)
"groceries" (street name, crack)
grommet
grooming, deterioration in
groove fricative consonant formation
Grooved Pegboard Test
gross impairment in communication
gross impairment in reality testing
gross motor
Gross Motor Development Test
gross neurologic deficit
gross sound
grossly disorganized behavior
grossly pathogenic care
"ground control" (re: hallucinogenic drug use)

group
    age
    CNS disease
    diverse
    focus
    glutethimide
    heterogeneous
    high-risk
    primary support
    sensitivity training
    substance
    work
Group Achievement Identification Measure
group audiometer
group audiometry
group contract
Group Diagnostic Reading Aptitude and Achievement Tests
group diversity
Group for the Advancement of Psychiatry (GAP)
Group Inventory for Finding Creative Talent
group living
group "means"
group of disorders
group play
Group Reading Test (GRT)
group setting
group structure
Group Styles Inventory (GSI)
Group Test of High Grade Intelligence
Group Tests of High Level Intelligence
Group Tests of Musical Abilities
group therapies
    adolescent
    adult
    child
growing skills *(see also* tests)
growth, period of
growth chart, pediatric
growth factor
    human (HGF)
    nerve (NGF)

GRT (Group Reading Test
grudge bearing
grunting
"G-shot" (re: drug withdrawal)
"G-shot" (street name, cannabis)
GSI (Group Styles Inventory)
GSR (galvanic skin response)
GSR on EEG
GSRA (galvanic skin response audiometry)
GTC (generalized tonic-clonic seizure)
guarded manner
guardedness, adolescent
guidance
    child
    vocational
guides *(see also* tests)
Guilford-Zimmerman Interest Inventory, The (GZII)
guilt, patterns of pervasive proneness to
guilt feelings
guilty, feeling
Gulf War, Persian
"gum" (street name, opium)
"guma" (street name, opium)
"gun" (re: needle for drug injection)
"gungun" (street name, cannabis)
gunshot wound, self-inflicted
gustatory aura
gustatory sensory modality
"gutter" (re: drug injection)
"gutter junkie" (re: drug acquisition)
guttural voice
gutturotetany
Guyon canal
gymnomania (nakedness)
gynecomania (womanizing)
gyrus (pl. gyri)
    angular
    callosal
    frontal
    Heschl's
    postcentral
    precentral

gyrus (pl. gyri)
    supramarginal
    temporal
    transverse temporal
"gyve" (street name, cannabis cigarette)

H

"H & C" (street name, heroin and cocaine)
"H-bomb" (re: ecstasy mixed with heroin)
"H Caps" (street name, heroin)
habilitation, audiologic
habit
    acculturation problems with expression of
    alcohol
    benign
    temporary
    tongue
habit pattern, intensive
habitual pitch
habromania (clothing/dress)
"hache" (street name, heroin)
HAE (hearing aid evaluation)
Hahnemann Elementary School Behavior Rating Scale
Hahnemann High School Behavior Rating Scale
HAIC (Hearing Aid Industry Conference)
"hail" (street name, crack)
hair cells
hair denuding
hair follicles, damaged
hair loss
    non-normative
    noticeable
    self-induced
hair-pulling behavior
hairs, eating
"hairy" (street name, heroin)
"half" (re: 1/2 ounce quantity of drug)
"half-a-C" (re: currency)
"half a football field" (re: 50 rocks of crack)
"half G" (re: currency)
"half load" (re: bags [decks] of heroin)
"half moon" (street name, mescaline)
"half piece" (re: 1/2 ounce of heroin or cocaine)
half reliability coefficient, split
"half track" (street name, crack)
hallucination(s)
    alcohol-induced psychotic disorder with
    amphetamine-induced psychotic disorder with
    auditory
    cannabis-induced psychotic disorder with
    cocaine-induced psychotic disorder with
    dreamlike
    gustatory
    hypnagogic
    hypnopompic
    mood-congruent
    mood-incongruent
    nocturnal
    olfactory
    prominent
    simple
    sleep-related
    somatic
    structured
    tactile
    transient auditory
    transient tactile
    transient visual
    unpleasant
    visual
hallucinations in schizophrenia, fragmentary
hallucinatory experience, transient
hallucinatory mania
hallucinogen (see also "hallucinogens street names")
hallucinogen-induced anxiety disorder

hallucinogen intoxication
   with use disorder, mild
     (F16.129)
   with use disorder,
     moderate/severe (F16.229)
   with no use disorder
     (F16.929)
hallucinogen intoxication delirium
hallucinogen persistent perception
   disorder (F16.983)
hallucinogen-related disorder,
   unspecified (F16.99)
hallucinogen use disorder
   mild (F16.10)
     moderate/severe (F16.20)
     with hallucinogen-induced
       bipolar or related disease
     with hallucinogen-induced
       brief psychotic disorder
     with hallucinogen-induced
       delirium
     with hallucinogen-induced
       delusional disorder
     with hallucinogen-induced
       depressive disorder
     with hallucinogen-induced
       schizoaffective disorder
     with hallucinogen-induced
       schizophrenia
     with hallucinogen-induced
       schizophreniform disorder
     with hallucinogen-induced
       schizotypal (personality)
       disorder
hallucinogenic agents *(see also
   psychodysleptic agents)*
     Afghanistan black
       (hashish)
     bhang (cannabis sativa
       milk preparation)
     cannabis indica
     cannabis trichomes
     dogbane (Indian hemp)
     ecstasy (3-4-methylene-
       dioxy-
       methamphetamine/MDM
       A)

hallucinogenic agents
   fake pot (synthetic
     marijuana)
   ganja (cannabis indica)
   hashish (cannabis
     trichomes)
   Hawaiian wood rose seeds
   heavenly blue (morning
     glory seeds)
   hemp (cannabis indica)
   incense (synthetic
     cannabinoids)
   Indian hemp (cannabis
     indica)
   iporrea violacea (morning
     glory seeds)
   Lebanese red (hashish)
   lophophora williamsii
     seeds (peyote)
   LSD (lysergic acid
     diethylamide)
   lysergic acid diethylamide
     (LSD)
   lysergides
   magic mushrooms
     (mescaline)
   marijuana (cannabis)
   MDMA (methylenedioxy-
     methamphetamine)
   megahalluciogens
   mescal buttons (mescaline)
   mescaline
   methylenedioxymeth-
     amphetamine (MDMA)
   morning glory seeds
     (iporrea violacea)
   pearly gates (morning glory
     seeds)
   pot
   psilocin
   psilocybin
   Royal Afghani (high grade
     Afghan black)
   salvia divinorum
   STP (2,5-dimethyloxy-4-
     methylamphetamine)
   STP (pseudo-
     phencyclidine)

hallucinogenic agents
    tetrahydrocannabinol (THC)
    THC (tetrahydrocannabinol)
    2,5-dimethyloxy-4-methylamphetamine (STP)
    Turkish green (immature Morus plant sap)
    XTC (ecstasy; MDMA)
hallucinogens (street names)
    100s (LSD)
    25s (LSD)
    A (LSD)
    acid (LSD)
    acid cube (sugar cube with LSD)
    acid head (user of LSD)
    acido (LSD)
    aeon flux (LSD)
    animal (LSD)
    back breakers (LSD and strychnine)
    bad seed (marijuana with peyote)
    barrels (LSD)
    bath salts (synthetic cannabinoids)
    battery acid (LSD)
    beans (mescaline)
    beast (heroin plus LSD)
    Beavis & Butthead (LSD)
    Big D (LSD)
    birdhead (LSD)
    black acid (LSD and PCP)
    black star (LSD)
    black sunshine (LSD)
    black tabs (LSD)
    blotter (LSD)
    blotter acid (LSD)
    blotter cube (LSD)
    blow your mind (get high on hallucinogens)
    blue acid (LSD)
    blue barrels (LSD)
    blue caps (mescaline)
    blue chairs (LSD)
hallucinogens (street names)
    blue cheers (LSD)
    blue heaven (LSD)
    blue microdot (LSD)
    blue mist (LSD)
    blue moons (LSD)
    blue vials (LSD)
    book (100 dosage units of LSD)
    brown dots (LSD)
    buttons (mescaline)
    cactus (mescaline)
    cactus buttons (mescaline)
    cactus head (mescaline)
    California sunshine (LSD)
    cap (LSD)
    caps (psilocybin/psilocin)
    chief (LSD) (mescaline)
    chocolate chips (LSD)
    Cid (LSD)
    coffee (LSD)
    come home (end a "trip" from LSD)
    comic book (LSD)
    conductor (LSD)
    contact lens (LSD)
    crackers (LSD)
    crystal tea (LSD)
    cube (LSD – 1 ounce)
    cupcakes (LSD)
    D (LSD)
    deeds (LSD)
    diviner's sage (salvia divinorum)
    domes (LSD)
    dosure (LSD)
    dots (LSD)
    double dome (LSD)
    Electric Kool Aid (LSD)
    Elvis (LSD)
    Explorers Club (group of LSD users)
    Felix the Cat (LSD)
    fields (LSD)
    flash (LSD)
    flat blues (LSD)
    flower flipping (Ecstasy mixed with mushrooms)

hallucinogens (street names)
   grape parfait (LSD)
   green single dome (LSD)
   green wedge (LSD)
   grey shields (LSD)
   ground control (re: guide during a hallucinogenic "trip")
   half moon (peyote)
   hats (LSD)
   Hawaiian sunshine (LSD)
   hawk (LSD)
   head light (LSD)
   heavenly blue (LSD)
   Hikori (peyote)
   Hikuli (peyote)
   hippieflip (use of mushrooms and MDMA)
   hombrecitos (psilocybin/psilocin)
   Hyatan (peyote)
   instant zen (LSD)
   K2 (synthetic cannabis)
   L (LSD)
   las mujercitas (psilocybin/psilocin)
   lason sa daga (LSD)
   laze (LSD)
   LBJ (heroin) plus (LSD) plus (PCP)
   lens (LSD)
   lime acid (LSD)
   little smoke (LSD); (psilocybin/psilocin)
   logor (LSD)
   Loony Toons (LSD)
   love flipping (use of mescaline and MDMA)
   love trip (mescaline) and (MDMA)
   Lucy in the sky with diamonds (LSD)
   magic mink (salvia divinorum)
   magic mushroom (psilocybin/psilocin)
   Maria Pastora (salvia divinorum)

hallucinogens (street names)
   mellow yellow (LSD)
   mesc (mescaline)
   Mickey's (LSD)
   microdot (LSD)
   Mighty Quinn (LSD)
   mind detergent (LSD)
   moon (mescaline)
   mushrooms (psilocybin/psilocin)
   musk (psilocybin/psilocin)
   nubs (peyote)
   one way (LSD)
   optical illusions (LSD)
   orange barrels (LSD)
   orange cubes (LSD)
   orange haze (LSD)
   orange micro (LSD)
   orange wedges (LSD)
   Owsley (LSD)
   Owsley's acid (LSD)
   P (peyote)
   pane (LSD)
   paper acid (LSD)
   peace tablets (LSD)
   Pearly gates (LSD)
   pellets (LSD)
   peyote (mescaline)
   pink blotters (LSD)
   Pink Panther (LSD)
   pink robots (LSD)
   pink wedges (LSD)
   pink witches (LSD)
   potato (LSD)
   pure love (LSD)
   purple barrels (LSD)
   purple flats (LSD)
   purple gel tabs (LSD)
   purple haze (LSD)
   Purple Hearts (LSD)
   purple ozone (LSD)
   rainbow (LSD)
   royal blues (LSD)
   Russian sickles (LSD)
   sacrament (LSD)
   sacred mushroom (psilocybin/psilocin)

hallucinogens (street names)
    sage of the seers (salvia divinorum)
    Sally D (salvia divinorum)
    salvia (salvia divinorum)
    Sandos (LSD)
    seni (peyote)
    Sherm (psychedelic mushrooms)
    shrooms (psilocybin/psilocin)
    Silly Putty (psilocybin/psilocin)
    Simple Simon (psilocybin/psilocin)
    smears (LSD)
    snowmen (LSD)
    South Parks (LSD)
    spice (synthetic cannabinoids)
    squirrel (LSD)
    strawberry (LSD)
    strawberry fields (LSD)
    street rocking (crack) and (LSD)
    sugar (LSD)
    sugar cubes (LSD)
    sugar lumps (LSD)
    sunshine (LSD)
    Superman (LSD)
    tabs (LSD)
    tail lights (LSD)
    ten pack (1,000 dosage units of (LSD)
    The Ghost (LSD)
    The Hawk (LSD)
    topi (mescaline)
    tops (peyote)
    trip (LSD)
    twenty-five (LSD)
    utopiates (LSD)
    vodka acid (LSD)
    wedding bells (LSD)
    wedge (LSD)
    white dust (LSD)
    white lightning (LSD)
    white Owsley's (LSD)
    window glass (LSD)

hallucinogens (street names)
    window pane (LSD)
    yellow (LSD)
    yellow dimples (LSD)
    yellow sunshine (LSD)
    yen sleep (restless, drowsy state after LSD use)
    Ying Yang (LSD)
    zen (LSD)
    zig zag man (LSD)
hallucinogens toxic effects
hallucinosis, peduncular
halo around object
halo effect
halogenated inhalational anesthetics
"halos", object
Halstead Category Test
Halstead Russell Neuropsychological Evaluation System (HRNES)
Halstead-Reitan Battery
Halstead-Reitan Neurological Battery and Allied Procedures
Halstead-Reitan Neuropsychological Test Battery for Adults
Halstead-Wepman Aphasia Screening Test
halting speech
hamartomania (sin)
hamaxophobia
"hamburger helper" (street name, crack)
Hamilton Anxiety Rating Scale
Hamilton Anxiety Scale
Hamilton Depression Rating Scale
Hamilton Depression Scale
Hamilton Rating Scale for Depression
hammer
"hammerheading" (re: use of MDMA with Viagra)
hand tremor
hand tremor, increased
hand waving, nonfunctional and repetitive

handedness
handicap
    emotional (EH)
    severe emotional (SEH)
Handicap Scales - WHO
handicapped
    educationally mentally (EMH)
    perceptually
handle of malleus
handling of stressors
hands, cold clammy
"hand-to-hand" (re: drug dealing)
"hand-to-hand man" (re: drug dealing)
"hanhich" (street name, cannabis)
"hanyak" (street name, smokable amphetamine)
hapax legomenon
happiness
"happy cigarette" (street name, cannabis cigarette)
"happy powder" (street name, cocaine)
"happy trails" (street name, cocaine)
haptic feedback
haptic perception
haptic system
HAQ (Health Assessment Questionnaire)
"hard candy" (street name, heroin)
hard contacts
hard glottal attack
"hard line" (street name, crack)
hard-of-hearing
hard palate
"hard rock" (street name, crack)
hard-wire auditory trainer
"hardware" (street name, isobutyl nitrite)
harelip
Hare Psychopathy Checklist
"Harlequin" (street name, liquid cannabis)
harm, prevention of physical
harmonic distortion

harmonic motion, simple (SHM)
harmony processes
Harrington-O'Shea Career Decision-Making System
Harris-Lingoes Subscales - MMPI
"Harry" (street name, heroin)
harsh discipline
harshness
HAS (high-amplitude sucking technique)
hashish (street names)
    black hash
    black Russian
    chillum
    gram
    quarter moon
    soles
"hats" (street name, lysergic acid diethylamide/LSD)
haughty behavior
"have a dust" (street name, cocaine)
"Hawaiian sunshine" (street name, LSD)
"hawk" (street name, LSD)
"hawkers" (re: sellers of club drugs)
Haws Screening Test for Functional Articulation Disorders
Hay Aptitude Test Battery
"hay butt" (street name, cannabis)
"haze" (street name, LSD)
"Hazel" (street name, heroin)
HBI (Hutchins Behavior Inventory)
HCCA (Health Care Compliance Association)
HCD (higher cerebral dysfunction)
"HCP" (street name, phencyclidine/PCP)
HE (hepatic encephalopathy)
"he-man" (street name, fentanyl)
head and neck tremor
head banging, nonfunctional and repetitive
head-banging behavior

"head drugs" (street name, amphetamine)
head injury, closed (CHI)
head jerking
head pain
head shadow effect
head trauma
    closed
    occult
head turn technique
headache
    aching
    acute confusional migraine
    alarm-clock
    aphasic migraine
    band-like
    basilar migraine
    benign exertional
    bifrontal
    bilateral
    bilateral migraine
    bioccipital
    blind
    cataclysmic
    chronic
    circumstantial migraine
    classical migraine
    cluster
    cluster migraine
    cocaine-related
    combination
    common migraine
    complicated migraine
    confusional migraine
    disabling
    dull
    essential
    evening
    exertional
    familial migraine
    frequency of
    frontal
    generalized
    hemiparesthetic migraine
    hemiplegic migraine
    histamine
    ipsilateral
    late-life migraine
headache
    migraine
    morning
    muscle contraction
    nitrite
    nonpulsating
    ocular migraine
    paroxysmal migraine
    postconcussion
    posttraumatic
    psychogenic
    pulsating
    recurrent
    recurrent migraine
    seasonal
    seasonal migraine
    severe
    severity of
    sex
    suboccipital
    sudden-onset
    temporal
    tension migraine
    tension-type
    tension-vascular
    throbbing
    traumatic
    unilateral
    unilateral migraine
    vascular
    vascular-type
    vasomotor
    vestibular migraine
    weekend
headache pain
headache syndrome
"headlights" (street name, LSD)
healing, ritual
healing rituals
health
    attitude to
    neglect of basic
    physical
    public
Health and Human Services, U.S. Department of (DHHS)
Health Assessment Questionnaire (HAQ)

health behavior
health behavior, maladaptive
health care, patient acceptance of
health care accountability
health care facilities, unavailability/inaccessibility of (Z75.3)
Health Care Financing Administration
health care provider(s)
Health Care Questionnaire
health care services, problems with access to
health concern
health personnel, attitude of
health problems, family of
Health Problems Checklist
health profile *(see also* tests)
health-related area
health-related consequence
health resource, mental
health risks, factors that constitute
health service encounters for counseling and medical advice
health surveys *(see also* tests)
Healy Pictorial Completion Test
hearing
    central
    cross
    end-organ of
    loss of
    visual
hearing aid
    air-conduction
    binaural
    body
    bone-conduction
    canal
    contralateral routing of signals (CROS)
    digital
    in-the-ear
    monaural
    pseudobinaural
    vibrotactile
    Y-cord
hearing aid assessment
hearing aid evaluation (HAE)
Hearing Aid Industry Conference (HAIC)
hearing aid selection
hearing aid systems
hearing center
hearing conduction test *(see also* tests)
hearing conservation
hearing deficiency
hearing disorder
hearing God's voice
hearing-impaired children, scales for C
hearing impairment
hearing impairment
    mild
    moderate
    moderately severe
    profound
    severe
hearing level (LH)
    threshold
    zero
hearing loss
    extreme
    mild
    moderate
    moderately severe
    perceptive
    profound
    severe
Hearing Loss Association of America (HLAA)
hearing protection device (HPD)
    canal caps
    circumaural
    earmuffs
    earplugs
    insert
    semiaural
hearing science, speech and
hearing sensation
hearing tests, behavioral
hearing theories
hearing theory
    frequency
    place
    telephone

hearing theory
    traveling wave
    volley
hearing threshold level (HTL)
heart disease
    atherosclerotic
    chronic pulmonary
    hypertensive
"heart-on" (street name, inhalant)
heat sensations (a panic attack indicator)
"heaven and hell" (street name, phencyclidine and LSD)
"heaven dust" (street name, heroin; cocaine)
heavy drinking, state markers of (GGT)
heavy metal screen
heavy use, long-term
hebephrenic schizophrenia
hedonic capacity
hedonic drive
hedonic volition
hedonistic activity
hedonomania (pleasure)
"heeled" (re: having lots of money)
height, tongue
heightened attention, state of
heightened awareness, state of
"Helen" (street name, heroin)
heliomania (sun)
helix
"hell dust" (street name, heroin)
help-rejecting complaining
help-seeking behavior
helping agencies, unavailability/inaccessibility of other (Z75.3)
helping behavior
helping verb
helplessness, learned
hemianopsia, bitemporal
hemangioma of the brain
hemiballismic movements
hemifacial spasm
hemifield of vision
hemilaryngectomy

hemiparesthetic migraine headache
hemiplegia, hysterical
hemiplegic migraine headache
hemisensory loss
hemispheral dysfunction
hemisphere dominance
    left
    left/right
    right
hemisphere dysfunction, bilateral
Hemispheric Abilities and Brain Improvement Training
hemispheric dysfunction, bilateral
hemispherical dysfunction
hemochromatosis
hemorrhage
    extradural
    intracerebral
    subarachnoid
    subdural
"hemp" (street name, cannabis)
hemp, industrial
hemp oil
Henderson-Moriarty ESL/Literacy Placement Test
Henmon-Nelson Ability Test
Henmon-Nelson Tests of Mental Ability
"henpicking" (re: crack acquisition)
"Henry" (street name, heroin)
"Henry VIII" (street name, cocaine)
hepatic conditions, dementia due to
hepatic encephalopathy (HE)
hepatic encephalopathy, delirium due to
hepatic encephalophy tremor
hepatic function
hepatitis, toxic
hepatorenal syndrome
"her" (street name, cocaine)
"Herb" (street name, cannabis)
"Herb and Al" (street name, cannabis and alcohol)
"herba" (street name, cannabis)

hereditary
heredofamilial tremor
"herms" (street name, phencyclidine/PCP)
"hero" (street name, heroin)
"hero of the underworld" (street name, heroin)
heroin (street names)
    A-bomb (marijuana cigarette with heroin or cocaine)
    AIP (heroin from Afghanistan, Iran, or Pakistan)
    Al Capone
    antifreeze
    Aries
    atom bomb (marijuana mixed with heroin)
    Aunt Hazel
    back to back (smoking crack after injecting heroin or
    bad bundle (inferior quality of heroin)
    bad seed
    bag (a package of drugs, usually marijuana or heroin)
    ball (Mexican Black Tar heroin)
    balloon (heroin supplier; a penny balloon containing heroin)
    ballot
    bars (heroin mixed with alprazolam/Xanax)
    Bart Simpson
    Batman
    beast (heroin + LSD)
    Belushi (combination of cocaine and heroin)
    big bag
    big doodig
    big H
    big Harry
    bin Laden (heroin after 9/11)
    bindle
    bipping (re: snorting heroin/cocaine alone or together)
    birdie power
heroin (street names)
    black eagle
    black pearl
    black stuff
    black tar
    blanco (heroin + cocaine)
    blue star
    bomb
    bombido
    bombita (heroin + amphetamine)
    bombs away
    bone (re: high purity heroin)
    Bonita
    boy
    boy-girl (heroin mixed with cocaine)
    Bozo
    brain damage
    Brea
    brick gum
    broja
    brown
    brown crystal
    brown rhine
    brown sugar
    brown tape
    bull dog
    bundle
    Butu
    caballo
    caca
    calbo
    canade (heroin and marijuana combination)
    Capital H
    caps
    carga
    carne
    channel swimmer (re: one who injects heroin)
    chapopote
    Charley
    chasing the dragon (crack mixed with heroin)
    chasing the tiger (re: smoking heroin)
    chiba

heroin (street names)
   chicle
   chieva
   China cat (re: high potency heroin)
   China white (heroin + Fentanyl; synthetic heroin)
   Chinese red
   chip
   chipper (re: occasional heroin user)
   chiva
   choco-fan
   chocolate chip cookies (heroin + MDMA)
   chocolate rock (crack/heroin smoked together)
   chucks (re: hunger following withdrawal from heroin)
   cigarette paper (re: packet of heroin)
   climax
   cocofan (Brown Tar heroin)
   cook (re: heating heroin before injecting it)
   cook down (re: liquefying heroin before inhaling it)
   cotics
   cotton brothers (cocaine/heroin/morphine)
   courage pills
   crank
   crap (re: low quality heroin)
   crisscrossing (re: process of snort cocaine and heroin)
   crown crap
   cura
   cut-deck (re: heroin mixed with dry milk)
   dead on arrival
   dead president
   deck (re: 1 to 15 grams of heroin)
   deuce
   dinosaurs (re: users in their 40s, 50s and older)
   dirt
   DOA

heroin (street names)
   dog food
   dogie
   dogs
   doogie/doojee/dugie
   dooley
   doosey
   dope
   double breasted dealing (re: dealing cocaine with heroin)
   Dr. Feelgood
   dragon rock (mixture of heroin & crack)
   dreck
   duji
   dujra
   dujre
   dust
   dusting (re: adding heroin or another drug to marijuana)
   dynamite (cocaine mixed with heroin)
   dyno
   dyno-pure
   eightball (crack mixed with heroin)
   eighth
   el diablito
   el diablo
   estuffa
   ferry dust
   five-way (re: snorting heroin/cocaine/meth/Rohypnol and drinking alcohol)
   flamethrowers (re: heroin/cocaine/tobacco combo)
   flee powder (re: low purity heroin)
   Florida snow
   foil
   foo foo stuff
   foolish powder
   Frisco special (cocaine, heroin, LSD)
   Frisco speedball (cocaine, heroin, and a dash of LSD)
   galloping horse
   gallup

Psychiatric Words and Phrases

heroin (street names)
  gamot
  garbage (re: low quality heroin)
  gato
  George
  George smack
  get off houses (re: places drug users buy/use for a fee)
  getting snotty
  girl
  give wings (re: to inject or teach someone to inject heroin)
  glacines
  glass
  goat
  gold
  golden girl
  golpe
  goma (black tar heroin plus opium)
  good
  Good and Plenty
  good H
  good horse
  goofball (cocaine mixed with heroin)
  gravy
  H
  H & C (heroin and cocaine)
  H caps
  hache
  hairy
  half load (re: 15 bags/decks of heroin)
  half piece (re: 1/2 ounce of heroin or cocaine)
  hard candy
  hard stuff
  Harry
  Hayron
  Hazel
  H-bomb (ecstasy mixed with heroin)
  heaven dust
  Helen
  hell dust

heroin (street names)
  Henry
  hera
  hero
  hero of the underworld
  heroina
  herone
  hessle
  him
  hitters (re: people who inject others, in exchange for drugs)
  holly terror
  hombre
  homicide
  hong-yen
  horning
  horse
  horsebite
  hospital heroin (Dilaudid)
  hot dope
  hot heroin (re: given as poison to a police informant)
  HRN
  hype
  Isda
  jee gee
  Jerry Springer
  jive
  jive doo jee
  joharito
  jojee
  jojee
  Jones
  joy
  joy flakes
  joy powder
  kabayo
  Karachi
  keel (narcotic, possibly heroin, laced with fentanyl)
  kill (narcotic, possibly heroin, laced with fentanyl)
  la Buena
  la chiva
  lady
  LBJ (heroin + LSD + PCP)

heroin (street names)
    lemonade (blunts mixed with marijuana & heroin)
    little bomb
    little boy
    load (re: 25 bags of heroin)
    love boat
    mac
    manteca
    Matsakow
    mayo
    meth speedball (methamphetamine and heroin)
    Mexican brown
    Mexican horse
    Mexican mud
    Mojo
    mone
    money talks
    monkey
    moonrock (crack mixed with heroin)
    moonstone (re: MDMA shaved into a bag of heroin by dealer)
    Morotgara
    mortal combat (re: high potency heroin)
    mud (heroin plus opium)
    murder one
    murotugora
    muzzle
    nanoo
    New Jack Swing (heroin and morphine)
    nice and easy
    nickel bag
    nickel deck
    noise
    nose
    nose drops
    number 3
    number 4
    number 8
    nurse
    ogoy
    oil

heroin (street names)
    old garbage
    old navy
    Old Steve
    on the ball (MDMA shaved into bag of heroin by a dealer)
    one on one house (re: place to purchase cocaine and heroin)
    one plus one sales (re: selling cocaine and heroin together)
    one way
    orange line
    pack
    Pangonadalot
    paper (re: a dosage unit of heroin)
    paperboy (re: heroin peddler)
    parachute
    parachute down (re: use of MDMA after heroin)
    P-dope (re: 20-30% pure heroin)
    Peg
    Perfect High
    perias (re: street dealer)
    P-funk
    Pluto
    poison
    polo (re: mixture of heroin and motion sickness drugs)
    polvo
    poppy
    poro (heroin plus PCP)
    powder
    pulborn
    pure
    quill
    Racehorse Charlie
    ragweed
    Rambo
    rane
    raw (re" high purity heroin)
    raw fusion
    raw hide
    ready rock
    red chicken

heroin (street names)
- red devil
- red eagle
- red rock
- red rock opium (heroin, barbital, strychnine, & caffeine)
- red rum (heroin, barbital, strychnine, & caffeine)
- red stuff (heroin, barbital, strychnine, & caffeine)
- reindeer dust
- Rhine
- rider (re: 5 kilos heroin given with purchase of 100 kilo of cocaine)
- rush hour
- sack
- salt
- sandwich (2 cocaine layers with a middle layer of heroin)
- scag
- scat
- scate
- Scott
- scramble (re: low quality heroin plus crack cocaine)
- second to none
- serial speedballing (re: sequencing cocaine/cough syrup/heroin over a 1-2 day period)
- shit
- shmeck/schmeek
- skag
- skid
- skunk
- sleeper
- sleeper & red devil (heroin and a depressant)
- slime
- smack
- smoke (heroin and crack)
- smoking gun (heroin & cocaine)
- sniffer bag (re: $5 bag of heroin – for inspection)

heroin (street names)
- snotty
- snow
- snowball (cocaine & heroin)
- speedball (crack/heroin smoked together)
- speedballing (to smoke a mixture of cocaine & heroin)
- spider
- spider blue
- spike (re: heroin cut with strychnine or scopolamine)
- spoon (1/16 oz of heroin)
- stacks (re: MDMA adulterated with heroin or crack)
- stuff
- sugar
- sweet dreams
- Sweet Jesus
- sweet stuff
- T.N.T. (heroin + fentanyl)
- tar
- taste
- tecate
- the beast
- the five way (heroin/cocaine/meth/ Rohypnol snorting plus drinking alcohol)
- the witch
- thing
- thunder
- tigre
- tigre blanco
- tigre del norte
- tits (black tar heroin)
- tongs
- Tootsie Roll
- top drool
- train
- Twin Towers
- twists (re: small bag of heroin secured with a twist tie)
- vidrio
- whack
- white

heroin (street names)
    white boy
    white dragon
    white girl
    white horse
    white junk
    white lady
    white nurse
    white stuff
    whiz bang
    wicked
    wings
    witch
    witch hazel
    wolla blunt (marijuana and heroin)
    wollies (marijuana and heroin)
    WTC
heroin and cocaine (street names)
    dynamite
    H & C
    number one
    smoking gun
    speedball
heroin and crack, "smoke"
heroin and morphine, "New Jack Swing"
heroin and phencyclidine, "oil"
herpes simplex virus meningitis
herpes zoster meningitis
hertz (Hz)
Hertz positive spikes, fourteen-and-six
Hertz positive spikes, six
Hertz positive spike-waves, six
Heschl's gyri
hesitation phenomena
"hessle" (street name, heroin)
heterocyclic antidepressant
heterogeneous
heterogeneous group
heterogeneous word
heterophemy
heterosexual marriage
heterosexual orientation
heterotopy
hexing, illness ascribed to

HF (high frequency)
HF audiometry
HF average full-on gain
HF average SSPL 90
HF average SSPL output
HF deafness
HFF (high filter frequency)
HHF (Hearing Health Foundation)
HIA (Hearing Industries Association)
HICROS (high frequency CROS)
hiding behavior, cunning and
HIE (hypoxic-ischemic encephalopathy)
hierarchical functioning
hierarchical scale of ADL's
hierarchical structure
hierarchy
    response
    social
hieromania (religious items)
high adaptive level
high affectivity ratio
high energy level
high expressed emotion level within family (Z63.8)
high feature English phoneme
high filter frequency (HFF)
high frequency (HF)
high frequency audiometry
high frequency CROS (HICROS)
high frequency deafness
high frequency of drug use
high level intelligence test *(see also* tests)
high level perceptual disturbance
High Level SISI
high potential for painful consequences
high risk activity(ies)
high risk behavior
high risk for suicide
High School Career-Course Planner (HSCCP)
high score
high standards of performance, self-imposed

high tolerance potential
high value
high vowel
"high", feeling
high-amplitude sucking technique (HAS)
"highbeams" (re: crack use)
high-dose drug
high-dose use of substance
higher cerebral dysfunction (HCD)
higher cognitive processes *(see also* tests)
higher cortical dysfunction
higher integrative language processing
higher level cognitive function
high-frequency (HF) average full-on gain
high-frequency average full-on gain
high-frequency average saturation sound pressure level 90
high-frequency average SSPL 90
high-pass filter
high-risk group
high-stimulus speech
"hikori" (street name, mescaline)
"hikuli" (street name, mescaline)
Hilson Adolescent Profile
Hilson Personnel Profile/Success Quotient (HPP/SQ)
"him" (street name, heroin)
"Hinkley" (street name, phencyclidine/PCP)
HIP (Hypnotic Induction Profile)
"hippie crack" (street name, inhalant)
"hippieflip" (re: use of MDMA with mushrooms)
hippocampal amnesia
hippocampal amnesic
hippocampal epilepsy
hippomania (horses)
"Hiropon" (street name, smokable methamphetamine)
Hirshprung disease

HIS (International Hearing Society)
histamine headache
histogram
historical linguistics
historical phonetics
history
    detailed
    drinking
    family
    known
    life
    lifetime
    neuro-ophthalmologic
    premorbid
    previous
    prior
    psychosexual
history of depression
history of medication use
history of pain
history of seizure(s)
history of suicide attempts
histrionic character
histrionic personality disorder (F60.4)
"hit" (re: cannabis cigarette use)
"hit" (street name, crack)
HIT (health information technology)
"hit and run" effect
"hit of acid" (re: LSD use)
"hit the hay" (re: cannabis use)
"hit the main line" (re: drug injection)
"hit the needle" (re: drug injection)
hitting one's own body, nonfunctional and repetitive
HIV (human immuno-deficient virus)
HIV-based dementia
HIV disease (infection) (B20)
HIV infection and concurrent psychiatric problems
HKNC (Helen Keller National Center for Deaf-Blind Youths and Adults)

HL (hearing level)
HLAA (Hearing Loss Association of America)
HMT (Hodkinson Mental Test)
hoarding disorder (F42)
hoarding disorder with excessive acquisitions (F42)
hoarseness
    dry
    rough
    wet
"hocus" (street name, opium; cannabis)
Hodkinson Mental Test (HMT)
hodomania (traveling)
hole, bore
holophrastic utterances
"hombre" (street name, heroin)
"hombrecitos" (street name, psilocybin)
home, run away from
home assessment
Home Environment Questionnaire
home evaluation
home language
Home Observation for Measurement of the Environment
Home Screening Questionnaire
home setting
homelessness (Z59.0)
homemaking responsibilities
homeostatic balance
homicidal behavior
homicidomania (murder)
homocysinuria
homogeneous scintillating scotoma
homogeneous word
homograph
homonym
homonymy, analysis of
homophene
homophone
homorganic
homosexual marriage
homosexual orientation
homovanillic acid, plasma (HVA)

"honey" (re: currency)
"honey blunts" (re: cannabis cigars sealed with honey)
"honey oil" (street name, ketamine; inhalant)
"honeymoon" (re: drug use)
"hong-yen" (re: heroin in pill form)
"hooch" (street name, cannabis)
Hood masking technique
Hood technique
"hooked" (re: addicted to drugs)
Hooper Visual Organization Test
"hooter" (street name, cocaine; cannabis)
"hop/hops" (street name, opium)
"hopped up" (re: drug influence)
horizontal canal
horizontal nystagmus
horizontal plane
hormonal level
hormonal self-treatment
hormonal sex-reassignment
hormone ingestion
"horn" (street name, cocaine)
"horning" (re: cocaine use)
"horning" (street name, heroin)
horrific impulses
"horse heads" (street name, amphetamine)
"horse tracks" (street name, phencyclidine/PCP)
"horse tranquilizer" (street name, phencyclidine/PCP)
Hospital Anxiety and Depression Scale
hospital-based psychiatry
hospital-based study
hospital consultation/liaison service
hospital-patient relations
hospital-physician relations
hospital regulations, noncompliance of
hospital routine
hospital unit, locked
hospitalization, need for
host culture

hostage status
hostile behavior
hostile identity
hostile response
hostility, voice
"hot dope" (street name, heroin)
"hot heroin" (re: poisoned heroin given to a police informant)
"hot ice" (street name, smokable methamphetamine)
"hot load/hot shot" (re: drug injection)
"hot stick" (street name, cannabis cigarette)
"hotcakes" (street name, crack)
House – Person – Tree Test
"house fee" (re: crack use)
"house piece" (re: crack use)
house test, draw a
household duties, neglect of
household responsibilities
housing, inadequate (Z59.1)
housing or economic problem, unspecified (F59.9)
Houston Test for Language Development
"How do you like me now?" (street name, crack)
Howell Prekindergarten Screening Test
"hows" (street name, morphine)
HPD (hearing protection device)
HPNT (The Hundred Pictures Naming Test)
HPP/SQ (Hilson Personnel Profile/Success Quotient)
"HRN" (street name, heroin)
HRNES (Halstead Russell Neuropsychological Evaluation System)
HSCCP (High School Career-Course Planner)
HTL (hearing threshold level)
"hubba pigeon" (re: crack user)
"Hubba, I am back" (street name, crack)
"hubbas" (street name, crack)
"huff" (street name, inhalant)

"huffer" (re: inhalant user)
huffing
"hug drug" (street name, MDMA/ecstasy)
"hugs and kisses" (re: MDMA and methamphetamine hydro)
"hulling" (re: stealing drugs)
hum, sixty-cycle
hum noise, sixty-cycle
human design
human development
human engineering
human evolution
human growth factor (HGF)
Human Information Processing Survey
human movement responses
human-pet bonding
humiliation, fear of
humor, sense of
hunches, tendency to play
hundred (100) test, count backwards from
Hundred Pictures Naming Test (HPNT)
hunger drive
"hunter" (street name, cocaine)
Huntington's disease, dementia due to
Hunt's syndrome
huskiness
"hustle" (re: drug dealing)
Hutchins Behavior Inventory (HBI)
HVA (homovanillic acid)
HVA (plasma homovanillic acid)
HVA levels in schizophrenia, plasma
hyalophobia
"hyatari" (street name, mescaline)
hydrargyromania (Mercury poisoning)
hydrocephalus
    communicating
    congenital
    dementia due to normal-pressure
    obstructive

hydrodipsomania (uncontrollable thirst)
hydromania (water)
hydrops
    endolymphatic
    labyrinthine
    vestibular
hygiene
    deterioration in
    impaired personal
    inadequate sleep
    lack of minimal
    lapses in
    mental
    minimal personal
    sleep
hylomania (substances)
hyoglossal (hyoglossus) muscle
hyoglossus, musculus
hyoglossus muscle
hyoid bone
hypacusic
"hype" (re: an addict; a heroin user)
"hype stick" (re: hypodermic needle)
hypemania (extravagant promotion)
hyperactive behavior
hyperactive-impulsive attention-deficit/hyperactivity disorder
hyperactive-impulsive combined behavior
hyperactive sexual desire
hyperactivity, autonomic
hyperactivity disorder
hyperactivity-impulsivity
hyperactivity indices
hyperactivity signs, autonomic
hyperadrenocorticism
hyperarousal, autonomic
hyperbole (figure of speech)
hypercalcemia
hypercarbia
hypercorrect language
hyperdefensive attitude
hyperdopaminergic state
hyperemotional

hyperesthesia, laryngeal
hypergraphia
hyperkalemia
hyperkeratosis
hyperkinesia of the false folds
hyperkinesis
hyperkinesis index *(see also* tests)
hyperkinetic dysarthria
hyperkinetic dysphonia
hyperkinetic speech
hypermania (heightened state of mania)
hypernasality voice disorder
hypernatremia
hyperplasia
hyperplasia, congenital adrenal
hyperplastic laryngitis
hyperpyrexia
hyperrecruitment
hyperreflexia
    autonomic
    generalized
hyperresponsible worries
hyperrhinolalia voice disorder
hyperrhinophonia voice disorder
hypersensitivity to negative evaluation, pattern of
hypersomnia, primary
hypersomnia related to another mental disorder
hypersomnolence disorder
    acute, persistent, subacute (G47.10)
    with another sleep disorder (G47.10)
    with medical condition (G47.10)
    with mental disorder (G47.10)
hypersomnolent
hypertensive encephalopathy
hypertensive heart disease
hypertensive renal disease
hyperthermia, malignant
hypertonia
hypertonic tongue
hypertrophic pyloric stenosis, congenital

hypervalvular phonation
hyperventilation
   autonomic
   central neurogenic
hypervigilance
hypnomania (sleep)
hypnosis
   diagnostic use of
   suggestion
   symptom relief through
hypnotic abuse
hypnotic agents (psychotropics)
   Ativan
   Dalmane
   flunitrazepam
   flurazepam
   Halcion
   lorazepam
   oxazepam
   Restoril
   Serax
   Sereen
   temazepam
   T-Quil
   triazolam
   Valium
   Valium Injection
hypnotic and sedative agents (non-psychotropics)
   Alurate
   aprobarbital (barbiturate)
   butabarbital (barbiturate)
   divalproex sodium
   Duralith
   Epitol
   Epival
   Imovane
   Lotusate
   Nembutal
   pentobarbital (barbiturate)
   secobarbital (barbiturate)
   Seconal
   talbutal (barbiturate)
   zopiclone
hypnotic drug
hypnotic-induced anxiety disorder
Hypnotic Induction Profile (HIP)
hypnotic interview
hypnotic intoxication delirium
hypnotic intoxication with use disorder
   mild (F13.129)
   moderate/severe (F13.229)
hypnotic intoxication with no use disorder (F13.929)
hypnotic-related disorder
hypnotic relaxation technique training
hypnotic-type withdrawal
hypnotic use disorder
   mild (F13.10)
   moderate/severe (F13.20)
hypnotic use disorder with hypnotic-induced anxiety disorder
hypnotic use disorder with hypnotic-induced bipolar or related disease
hypnotic use disorder with hypnotic-induced brief psychotic disorder
hypnotic use disorder with hypnotic-induced delirium
hypnotic use disorder with hypnotic-induced delusional disorder
hypnotic use disorder with hypnotic-induced depressive disorder
hypnotic use disorder with hypnotic-induced major and mild neurocognitive disorder
hypnotic use disorder with hypnotic-induced schizoaffective disorder
hypnotic use disorder with hypnotic-induced schizophrenia
hypnotic use disorder with hypnotic-induced schizophreniform disorder
hypnotic use disorder with hypnotic-induced schizotypal (personality) disorder
hypnotic use disorder with hypnotic-induced sexual dysfunction

hypnotic use disorder with hypnotic-induced sleep disorder
hypnotic withdrawal delirium
hypnotic withdrawal symptom, sedative
hypnotic withdrawal with perceptual disturbance
hypnotic withdrawal with no perceptual disturbance
hypnotizability
hypoactive sexual desire disorder
    acquired type
    generalized type
    lifelong type
    situational type
hypoactive sexual desire disorder due to combined factors
hypoactive sexual desire disorder due to psychological factors
hypocalcemia
hypocretin deficiency
hypofunction
hypoglossal (cranial nerve XII)
hypoglossal nerve
hypoglottis
hypoglycemic delirium
hypogonadism
hypokalemia
hypokinesis
hypokinetic dysarthria
hypokinetic speech
hypologia
hypomania (mild degree of mania)
hypomanic episode, single
hypomanic-like episode
hypometabolism
    frontotemporal
    striatal
hyponatremia
hypopharynx
hypophonia
hypophonic aphasia
hypophrasia
hypoplasia
    lingual
    mandibular

hypopnea, obstructive sleep apnea (G47.33)
hypoprosody
hypothermia
hypothesis, Whorf's
hypotonic cerebral palsy (CP)
hypoventilation
    comorbid sleep-related (G47.36)
    congenital central alveolar (G47.35)
    idiopathic (G47.34)
    sleep-related, comorbid (G47.36)
hypoventilation syndrome, central alveolar
hypoxia, toxic
hypoxic-ischemic encephalopathy (HIE)
hypoxyphilia
hypoxyphilia-caused deaths
hypsiphobia
hysteria, epidemic
hysteric coma-like state
hysterical aphonia
hysterical aura
hysterical blindness
hysterical fugue state
hysterical gait
hysterical hemiplegia
hysterical mania
hysterical mutism
hysterical overbreathing, voluntary
hysterical pregnancy
hysterical seizure
hysterical stuttering
hysterical trance
hysterical tremor
hysterical visual loss
hysterical voluntary overbreathing
hysteroid defenses
hysteroid features
hysteromania (psychogenic symptoms)
Hz (Hertz or cycles per second)

I

I marker (intentional marker)
I tracing (interrupted tracing)
"I" statements
I.P.I. Aptitude-Intelligence Test Series
IAAT (Iowa Algebra Aptitude Test)
IABP (Indian Association of Biological Psychiatry)
IACP (Indian Association of Clinical Psychologists)
iambic stress
IAPP (Indian Association of Private Psychiatry)
IAS (Integrated Assessment System)
IASP (International Association for the Study of Pain)
iatrogenic induction
iatrogenic seizure
iatrophobia
IC (inspiratory capacity)
ICA (Infancy, Childhood and Adolescence)
ICD-9-CM system
ICD-10-CM system
"ice" (street name, cocaine; smokable amphetamine; MDMA and PCP)
"ice cream habit" (re: occasional drug use)
"ice cube" (street name, crack)
ICF (International Classification of Functioning, Disability and Health)
ichthyomania (fish)
"icing" (street name, cocaine)
iconomania (image worship)
icons
ICRT (Individualized Criterion Referenced Testing)
ICRTM (Individualized Criterion Referenced Testing - Mathematics)
ICRTR (Individualized Criterion Referenced Testing - Reading)
ICSD (International Classification of Sleep Disorders)
ictal amnesia
ictal amnesic
ictal automatism
ictal confusional seizure
ictal depression phase of seizure, past
ictal period
idea(s)
    flight of (FOI)
    intrusive distressing
    overvalued
    persistent inappropriate
    persistent intrusive
    separation of feelings from
    strongly held
    unreasonable
    unwarranted
idea of persecution
IDEA Oral Language Proficiency Test
IDEA System
idealized value
IDEAS (Interest Determination, Exploration and Assessment)
ideas of reference, transient
ideation
    AWOL
    elopement
    recurrent suicidal
    stress-related paranoid
    suicidal
    suspicious
    transient
ideatory apraxia
identifiable being
identifiable pattern of sleep and wakefulness
identifiable stressor

identification
    cross-gender
    deep trance
    projective
    social
identification audiometry
Identification Instrument, Eby Elementary
Identification of Language Learning Strengths and Weaknesses
Identifying Children with Specific Language Disability
identities, multiple distinct
identity
    adolescent sexual
    alternate
    controlling
    cultural
    former
    gender
    hostile
    new
    particular
    personal
    primary
    "protector"
    sense of personal
    traditional feminine
    traditional masculine
identity, traditional feminine (normal oxytocin levels)
    emotional sensitivity
    empathetic
    nurturing
identity, traditional masculine (extreme/high testosterone level)
    aggression
    dominance
    female abuse
    female oppression
    violent temper
identity, traditional masculine (normal/neutral testosterone level)
    aggressiveness
    assertiveness

identity, traditional masculine (normal/neutral testosterone level)
    competitiveness
    protective vigilance
    stoicism
identity disorder
    dissociative
    gender (GID)
    sexual
    sexual and gender
identity disturbance
identity problem
    adolescent
    gender
identity states
ideographs
ideokinetic apraxia
ideomotor apraxia
idiom (figure of speech)
idiopathic central sleep apnea (G47.31)
idiopathic dystonias
idiopathic encephalopathy
idiopathic hypoventilation (G47.34)
idiopathic insomnia
idiopathic language retardation
idiopathic sleep-related hypoventilation (G47.34)
idiosyncratic intoxication, alcohol
idiosyncratic meaning
idiosyncratic processes
idiosyncratic reaction
"idiot pills" (street name, barbiturate)
idolomania (idol worship)
(I/E)initial encounter
IFROS (ipsilateral frontal routing of signals)
ILA (Inventory of Language Abilities)
ILEAD (Instructional Leadership Evaluation and Development Program)
Ilheus viral encephalitis
iliocostal muscle, lumbar
iliocostal muscle of thorax

iliocostalis dorsi, musculus
iliocostalis lumborum, musculus
iliocostalis thoracis, musculus
ill, commitment of mentally
illegal drug purchases
illegal drugs *(see also* drugs, street names)
illeism
illeist
illicit drugs test, blood level of
illicit stimulants *(see also* drugs, street names)
illicit psychoactive substance
Illinois Children's Language Assessment Test
illness
    consequence of
    continuous period of
    course of
    duration of
    entire period of
    episodes of
    folk
    individual episode of
    length of
    life-threatening
    onset of
    period of
    progressive dementing
    psychotic
    residual period of
    same period of
    serious
    total period of
    uninterrupted period of
illness anxiety disorder, care avoidance or seeking type (F45.21)
illness ascribed to hexing
Illness Behavior Questionnaire
illness behavior(s)
illness during pregnancy, psychiatric
illness phase
illusion, bodily
illusionary misconceptions
illusions
    optic

illusions
    transient auditory
    transient tactile
    transient visual
ILSA (Interpersonal Language Skills and Assessment)
image
    distorted body
    persistence of visual
    splitting of
    transient
IMAGE-CA (Imagery and Disease)
image control
IMAGE-DB (Imagery and Disease)
image distortion, body
image-distorting level
image intensification
image intensifier
image of others
image of others, splitting of
IMAGE-SP (Imagery and Disease)
imagery
    eidetic
    paraphiliac
Imagery and Disease (IMAGE-CA; IMAGE-DB; IMAGE-SP)
Imagery of Cancer
images
    peripheral field
    persistent inappropriate
    persistent intrusive
    trailing
imaginary playmate
imaginative play
imagined abandonment
imagined defect
imaging
    functional brain
    structural brain
imaging studies, brain
imbalance
    central language
    developmental
    electrolyte
    orofacial muscle

IMI (Impact Message Inventory)
imitation, spontaneous
imitative and auditory
  discrimination tests *(see also*
  tests)
imitative behavior
imitative movement, repetitive
imitative word repetition,
  senseless
immaturity, perceptual
immediate anxiety
immediate echolalia
immediate environment
immediate memory test *(see also*
  tests)
immediate sentence constituents
immigrant status
immittance measurement test,
  acoustic
immobility
    motor
    motoric
immune disorders, dementia due
  to
immune function, impaired
immune functioning, potential
  impairment of
immune mechanism
impact, potential
Impact Message Inventory (IMI)
Impact of Event Scale-Revised
impact of illness profile test *(see*
  also tests)
impact of stress scale *(see also*
  tests)
impacted cerumen
impaired
    communicatively
    functionally
impaired affect
impaired affect modulation
impaired arousal, sexual
  dysfunction with
impaired attention ability
impaired attention skills
impaired balance
impaired cognitive functioning
impaired communication ability

impaired communication skills
impaired condition
impaired consciousness
impaired control
impaired coordination
impaired daytime functioning
impaired desire
impaired desire, sexual
  dysfunction with
impaired development
impaired effective communication
impaired focal ability
impaired immune function
impaired intellectual ability
impaired language
impaired learning ability
impaired linguistic skills
impaired mathematical skills
impaired memory ability
impaired motor performance
impaired occupational functioning
impaired orgasm, sexual
  dysfunction with
impaired perceptual skills
impaired performance
impaired personal hygiene
impaired rapid repetitive
  movements
impaired relationships
impaired sensation
impaired social functioning
    anxiety-induced
    frustration-induced
    low self-esteem as cause
      for
impaired social interaction
impaired speech
impaired thinking ability
impaired ventilation
impaired ventilation during sleep
impaired vision
impairment
    adaptive functioning
    aphasic
    cognitive functioning
    communication
    developmental
    disproportionate

impairment
    functional
    gaze
    generalized intellectual
    graphic
    hearing
    immune functioning
    intellectual
    judgment
    language
    level of cognitive
    marked
    measurable
    memory
    mild hearing
    moderate hearing
    moderately severe hearing
    motor
    new memory encoding
    objective symptoms of
    occupational functioning
    organic
    perceptual-motor
    perceptual-motor abilities
    permanent residual
    profound hearing
    reading comprehension
    reality testing, gross
    reciprocal social interaction
    residual
    reversible memory
    school functioning
    sensory
    severe hearing
    severe memory
    significant
    social functioning
    speech
    subjective symptoms of
    visual
impairment-based measurement
impairment criterion
impairment of consciousness
impairment of dementia
impedance
    acoustic
    static acoustic
impedance matching

impedance measures
impediment, speech
impediment of speech
impending death
imperative mood
imperative sentence
imperception, auditory
imperfections revealed, fear of
implant, cochlear
implication
    semantic
    management
implicit language
implicit stuttering
implosive consonant formation
important responsibilities
important role
imposition of legal sanctions
imposition of social sanctions
impostors
impoverished speech
impoverished thoughts
impoverishment, personality
impoverishment in thinking
impression, erroneous
impressionable/impressionability
impressionistic phonetics
impressionistic speech
impressionistic speech,
    excessively
imprisonment or other
    incarceration (Z65.1)
improper diet
Improvement Cards (Speech)
Improving Writing, Thinking, and
    Reading Skills (ACO)
impulse, failure to resist an
impulse-control disorder
impulse-control, disruptive, and
    conduct disorders
impulse-control interface disorder
impulse-control problems
impulse regulation, lack of
impulses
    aggressive
    horrific
    persistent inappropriate
    persistent intrusive

impulsive activity
impulsive behavior
impulsive/compulsive
   psychopathology
impulsive dyscontrol
impulsive petit mal epilepsy
impulsive tendencies
impulsiveness
impulsivity
      lack of
      self-damaging
      tendency toward
IMQ (Inquiry Mode
   Questionnaire: A Measure of
   How You Think and Make
   Decisions)
"in" (re: drug suppliers)
in a controlled environment
in a "dream world," living
In-Basket, General Management
   (GMIB)
in-the-ear hearing aid
in the opposite sex role, living
inability to experience pleasure
inability to function
inability to sleep
inaccuracy
      general oral
      oral
inaccuracy articulation, general
   oral
inadequate discipline
inadequate housing (Z59.1)
inadequate information
inadequate school environment
inadequate sleep hygiene
inanimate
inappropriate compensatory
   behavior
inappropriate dependent care
inappropriate ideas, persistent
inappropriate images, persistent
inappropriate impulses, persistent
inappropriate passage of feces,
   repeated
inappropriate posture
inappropriate quality of
   obsessions

inappropriate sexual behavior
inappropriate social relatedness,
   developmentally
inappropriate thoughts, persistent
inappropriate urges, persistent
inappropriate voiding of urine,
   repeated
inappropriate words
inappropriateness, social
inarticulate
inattention
inattention to the environment
inattentive behavior
inattentive type attention-
   deficit/hyperactivity disorder
"inbetweens" (street name,
   barbiturate; LSD; amphetamine)
inborn errors of metabolism
"Inca message" (street name,
   cocaine)
incapacitating fear
incarceration
incentive motivation, external
incestual
incestual relationship
incestuous
incident wave
incipient stuttering
incisive foramen
incisiveness, feelings of
incisor teeth
      central
      lateral
inclusion bodies, intraneuronal
   argentophilic Pick
incoherent patient
incoherent speech
incompatible behavior
incompetence, velopharyngeal
incomplete cleft palate
incomplete phrases
incomplete recruitment
Incomplete Sentences Task
incomprehensible speech
incongruent
inconsistent contact with reality
inconsistent laboratory test results
inconsistent manner

inconsistent parental discipline
incontinence
    affective
    emotional
    fecal
    urinary
incoordination
increase tremor, factors to
increased arousal
increased arousal from sleep
increased autonomic signs
increased energy
increased frequency
increased hand tremor
increased interpersonal conflicts
increased muscle tension
increased responsibility
increased risk for schizophrenia
increased sensitivity to rejection
increased sleep
increased sleep disruption
increasing sense of tension
Increment Sensitivity Index, Short (SISI)
incus
indecisiveness
indefinite vowel
independence, physical
Independent Behavior Scales
independent clause
independent functioning
independent living
independent living, capacity for
Independent Living Behavior Checklist
indeterminate sex
indeterminate sleep
index (pl. indices) *(see also* tests)
    ADL
    alpha
    alphabetical
    ambulation
    articulation
    beta
    body mass (BMI)
    delta
    hyperactivity
    Insomnia Severity

index (pl. indices)
    maturation
    multi-item
    shift referential
    switch referential
    tabular
    theta
index of physiological sleepiness
index/position, self
Indian Association of Biological Psychiatry (IABP)
Indian Association of Clinical Psychologists (IACP)
Indian Association of Private Psychiatry (IAPP)
"Indian boy" (street name, cannabis)
"Indian hay" (street name, cannabis)
Indian School Psychology Association (InSPA)
"Indica" (street name, cannabis)
indicative mood
indicator(s)
    activity pattern
    rehabilitation *(see also* tests)
    skill *(see also* tests)
    thyration
indicator of occupational stress *(see also* tests)
indictment
indifference, sexual
indirect laryngoscopy
indirect motor system
indirect object
indiscriminate sexual encounters
individual(s)
    age-matched
    androgynous
    insightless
    self-stimulatory behaviors in
individual care
individual counselor
individual episode of illness
Individual Phonics Criterion Test
individual psychotherapy

individual responsibility
individual screen for basic
    achievement skills individual
    skills
individuality
Individualized Criterion
    Referenced Testing - Reading
    (ICRTR)
Individualized Criterion
    Referenced Testing (ICRT)
Individualized Criterion
    Referenced Testing -
    Mathematics (ICRTM)
individual's age
individual's culture
individuation problem
"Indo" (street name, cannabis)
indoctrination while captive
"Indonesian bud" (street name,
    cannabis; opium)
inductance
induction auditory trainer, loop
induction coil
induction loop
Induction Profile, Hypnotic (HIP)
induction, iatrogenic
inductive reactance
inductor
industrial audiometry
industrial deafness
industrial hemp
industrialized culture
ineffective anger
ineffective decision making
ineffectiveness
ineffectiveness, feelings of
ineffectual parent
inertial bone conduction
inevitability
    ejaculatory
    sensation of ejaculatory
Infancy, Childhood and
    Adolescence (ICA)
infancy and early childhood
    disturbance(s)
infancy and early childhood
    disturbances in feeding and
    eating
infant behavior *(see also* tests)
infant development inventory *(see
    also* tests)
infant development scales *(see
    also* tests)
Infant Reading Tests, The
Infant/Toddler Environment
    Rating Scale (ITERS)
infantile affect
infantile aphasia
infantile behavior
infantile convulsion
infantile perseveration
infantile speech
infantile swallowing
infarct, lacunar
infection
    HIV (B20)
    skin
    upper respiratory (URI)
infectious disorders, dementia due
    to
Inference Ability in Reading
    Comprehension Test
inferential behavioral monitoring
    distortion of
    exaggeration of
inferential perception
    distortion of
    exaggeration of
inferential thinking
inferential thinking in
    schizophrenia
    distorted
    exaggerated
inferential thinking
    distortion of
    exaggeration of
inferior
    musculus constrictor
        pharyngis
    musculus serratus posterior
inferior constrictor muscle of
    pharynx
inferior frontal sulcus
inferior laryngotomy
inferior linguae, musculus
    longitudinalis

inferior longitudinal muscle of
  tongue
inferior maxillary bone
inferior meatus, nasi
inferior nasal concha
inferior pharyngeal constrictor
inferior sibling lifestyle
inferior temporal sulcus
inferiority to others, feelings of
Inferred Self-Concept Scale
infestation, sensation of insect
infibulation (pinning and
  piercing)
infinitive
infinitive (parts of speech)
inflammatory croup
inflated identity
inflated knowledge
inflated power
inflated worth
inflection
inflectional endings
inflexibility
inflexibility, enduring pattern of
inflexible attitude
inflexible pattern
informal contract
informal method
Informal Reading Comprehension
  Placement Test
informal reading inventory *(see
  also* tests)
information
  additional
  analyzing
  assimilating
  auditory
  autobiographical
  clinical
  contradictory
  cultural
  diagnostic
  disturbance in learning new
  disturbance in rapidity of
    analyzing
  disturbance in rapidity of
    assimilating

information
  disturbance in recalling
    new
  domain of
  fund of
  inadequate
  insufficient
  learning
  personal
  recall of
  recalled
  source of
  statistical
  unbiased
Information Form
  Policy and Program
  Resident and Staff
information-memory-
  concentration test *(see also*
  tests)
information processing,
  disturbance in speed of
information test
  fund of
  recall of
information theory
information with motor activity
  disturbance in integrating
    tactile
  disturbance in integrating
    visual
  disturbance in integrating
    auditory
informational support
infraglottic
infrahyoid extrinsic muscles
infrahyoid muscles
infrasonic
infrasonic frequency
infraversion
infraversion of teeth
ingestion, hormone
inhalant (street names)
  aimies
  air blast
  ames
  amyl nitrate
  amys

inhalant (street names)
  aroma of men
  bagging (using inhalants)
  bang
  bolt
  boppers
  bullet
  bullet bolt
  butyl nitrate
  buzz bomb
  climax
  discorama
  dusting (re: using inhalants)
  glading (re: using inhalants)
  gluey (glue sniffer or inhaler)
  hardware
  heart-on
  hiagra in a bottle
  highball
  hippie crack
  honey oil
  huff
  huffer (inhalant abuser)
  huffing (to sniff an inhalant)
  isobutyl nitrite
  kick
  laughing gas (nitrous oxide)
  locker room
  Medusa
  moon gas
  nitrate
  Oz
  pearls
  poor man's pot
  poppers
  satan's secret
  snappers
  sniff (to inhale drugs)
  snort (to use inhalants)
  snorting (using inhalants)
  snotballs (re: inhaling fumes from burned rubber cement)

inhalant (street names)
  spray
  Texas shoe shine
  thrust
  toilet water
  tolly (toluene used in many inhalants)
  touché (octane booster which is inhaled)
  valo
  whippets (nitrous oxide)
  whiteout
inhalant abuse
inhalant dependence
inhalant-induced anxiety disorder
inhalant-induced disorder
inhalant intoxication delirium
inhalant intoxication with use disorder
    mild (F18.129)
    moderate/severe (F18.229)
inhalant intoxication with no use disorder (F18.929)
inhalant-related disorder, unspecified (F18.99)
inhalant substance use disorder with inhalant substance-induced brief psychotic disorder
inhalant substance use disorder with inhalant substance-induced delusional disorder
inhalant use disorder
    mild (F18.10)
    moderate/severe (F18.20)
inhalant use disorder with inhalant substance-induced anxiety disorder
inhalant use disorder with inhalant substance-induced delirium
inhalant use disorder with inhalant substance-induced depressive disorder
inhalant use disorder with inhalant substance-induced major or mild neurocognitive disorder
inhalant use disorder with inhalant substance-induced psychotic disorder

inhalant use disorder with inhalant substance-induced schizoaffective disorder
inhalant use disorder with inhalant substance-induced schizophreniform disorder
inhalant use disorder with inhalant substance-induced schizophrenia
inhalant use disorder with inhalant substance-induced schizotypal (personality) disorder
inhalants, pulmonary absorption of
inhalation (forced) muscles
inhalation (quiet) muscles
inhalation method
inhalation method of esophageal speech
inhalation of drug
inhalational anesthetics, halogenated
inhaling intoxicating vapors, method of
inherent vulnerability to psychosis
inherited abnormality
inherited disease
inherited progressive degenerative disease
inhibited mania
inhibited type
inhibited type reactive attachment disorder
inhibition
inhibition, reactive
inhibitions level, mental
inhibitory tone
initial consonant, deletion of
initial consonant position
initial encounter (I/E)
initial insomnia
initial lag
initial masking
initial phase of insomnia
initial string
initial teaching alphabet
initiating and maintaining sleep, disorder of (DIMS)
initiating insomnia
initiation of goal-directed behavior
injectable and oral steroid, primobolan
injectable steroid
    anatrofin
    bolasterone
    deca-duabolin
    delatestryl
    dep-testosterone
    dihydrolone
    durabolin
    dymethzine
    enoltestovis
    methatriol
    quinolone
    therobolin
    trophobolene
injection drug users
injection method
injection method, cross-consonant
injection method of esophageal speech
injury
    brain
    dementia due to traumatic brain
    Mini Inventory of Right Brain (MIRBI)
    potential for
    self-induced
    self-inflicted bodily
    toxic
    traumatic
    traumatic brain (TBI)
inkblot series, somatic
inkblot test *(see also* tests)
innateness theory
    language
    speech
inner barrenness
inner battery clusters
inner child issues
inner ear
inner language
inner life
inner speech

inner tension
innervation
innervation, patterns of motor
innervation apraxia
inpatient, psychiatric
inpatient patient populations
inpatient psychiatric setting
in phase
input
inquiry forensic psychiatry *(see also* tests)
Inquiry Mode Questionnaire: A Measure of How You Think and Make Decisions (IMQ)
insanity, dread of
insect infestation, sensation of
insecticide, organophosphate
insecurity, social
insensitivity syndrome, androgen
insert hearing protection device
insertion loss
insidious onset
insight
    myopic
    poor
insightless individuals
insightless tendency
insincerity
insomnia
    chronic
    cocaine-produced
    complaints of
    features of
    idiopathic
    initial
    initial phase of
    initiating
    maintenance
    middle
    mild
    prevalence of
    primary
    psychophysiological
    significant
    sleep disorder
    sleep-onset
    symptoms of

insomnia
    terminal
    withdrawal
insomnia disorder
    episodic, persistent, recurrent (G47.00)
    with non-sleep disorder mental comorbidity (G47.00)
    with other medical comorbidity (G47.00)
    with other sleep disorder (G47.00)
insomnia related to another mental disorder
Insomnia Severity Index
insomnia type caffeine-induced sleep disorder
insomnia type sleep disorder due to GMC
insomnia type substance-induced sleep disorder
InSPA (Indian School Psychology Association)
inspiration
inspiratory capacity (IC)
inspiratory reserve volume (IRV)
inspiratory voice
instability in interpersonal relationships
"instant zen" (street name, LSD)
instantaneous power
institutes (see *Associations, Professional)*
institution, religious
institution of marriage
institution of treatment
institutional environments
institutional setting
Instructional Environment Scale, The (TIES)
Instructional Leadership Evaluation and Development Program (I*LEAD*)
Instructional Leadership Inventory
instructional measurement systems *(see also* tests)

instructional objective inventories
  (see also tests)
instructional tests *(see also* tests)
instructions, voice
instrument for educational
  screening *(see also* tests)
Instrument for the Identification
  of Potential Learning Risks
Instrument Timbre Preference
  Test
instrumental ADL measurement
instrumental affair
instrumental avoidance act theory
  of stuttering
instrumental case (parts of
  speech)
instrumental conditioning
instrumental support
instrumental tasks
insufficiency
  basilar
  cerebrovascular
  corticoadrenal
  mitral valve
  palatal
  role
  velar
  velopharyngeal
  vertebrobasilar
insufficient data
insufficient information
insufficient nocturnal sleep
insufficient stimulation
insults, nutritional
intact, naming
intact motor function
intact reflexes
intact sensory function
intangible benefits of the
  "sick"role
Integrated Assessment System
  (IAS)
Integrated Literature and
  Language Arts Portfolio
  Program
integrating auditory information
  with motor activity, disturbance
  in

integrating responses/anchors
integrating tactile information
  with motor activity, disturbance
  in
integrating visual information
  with motor activity, disturbance
  in
integration
  binaural
  competing messages
  ego
  social
integration and praxis tests *(see
  also* tests)
integrative language processing,
  higher *(see also* tests)
integrative learning *(see also*
  tests)
integrity of brain function
integumentary system
intellect learning abilities tests
  (see also tests)
intellectual ability, impaired
intellectual capacity
intellectual deterioration
intellectual developmental
  disorders
intellectual disability
  mild (F70)
  moderate (F71)
  profound (F73)
  severe (F72)
  unspecified (F79)
intellectual function, discrepant
intellectual functioning
  borderline (R41.83)
  discrepant
  general
  subaverage
intellectual impairment
  accompanying
  generalized
intelligence
  above-average
  low
intelligence period, sensorimotor
intelligence quotient (IQ)
intelligence scales *(see also* tests)

intelligence tests *(see also* tests)
intelligibility, speech
intelligibility tests *(see also* tests)
intelligibility threshold
intelligible threshold
intense affect
intense anger
intense anxiety
intense autonomic arousal
intense desire
intense emotion
intense episodic dysphoria
intense fear
intense intoxication
intense pain
intense painful affect
intense psychological distress
intense relationship
intense sexual behavior
intense sexual fantasies
intense sexual urges
intense wish
intensification, image
intensified action
intensifier, image
intensity, sound
intensive habit pattern
intention semantics
intention tremor
intentional fire setting
intentional marker (I marker)
intentional stereotyped
  movements
intentional tremor
intentionally produced symptoms
interaction
        communicative
        impaired social
        impairment in reciprocal
          social
        interpersonal
        occupational
        sexual
        social
interaction with the legal system,
  problems related to
interactive phenomenon
interaural attenuation

intercalation
interceptor
interconsonantal vowel
intercostal muscle(s)
    internal
    external
intercostales externi, musculi
intercostalis internus, musculus
intercourse
    anal
    sexual
intercurrent anxiety
interdental lisp
interdepartmental relations
interepisode functioning
interepisode recovery, full
interepisode residual symptoms of
  schizophrenia
interest
        cross-gender
        decreased
        low sexual
        stereotyped
Interest Check List
interest in usual activities,
  decreased
interest indices *(see also* tests)
interest inventories *(see also* tests)
interest measurements *(see also*
  tests)
interest profiles *(see also* tests)
interest scales *(see also* tests)
interest surveys *(see also* tests)
interface, acoustic
interface disorder
    adjustment
    dissociative
    factitious
    impulse-control
    psychiatric system
    somatoform
interference, semantic
interference level
    noise (NIL)
    speech (SIL)
interference modification
Interference Procedure for the
  Bender Gestalt Test

intergenerational relations
interhemispheric asymmetry
interictal behavior
interictal period
interinstitutional relations
interior turbinated bone
interiorized stuttering
interjection (parts of speech)
interjections
Intermediate Booklet Category Test
intermediate string
intermediate structure
intermetamorphosis, syndrome of
intermittent aphonia
intermittent explosive disorder (F63.81)
intermittent pain
intermittent reinforcement schedule
intermittent wakefulness
intermodulary distortion
internal acoustic meatus
internal auditory canal
internal auditory meatus
internal-external control
internal intercostal muscle
internal juncture
internal speech
internal stressor
internal world of belief
internal world of expectation
internal world of fantasy
internal world of perception
internalizing style of conflict resolution
International Association for the Study of Pain (IASP)
International Classification of Functioning, Disability and Health (ICF)
International Classification of Sleep Disorders (ICSD)
International Diagnostic-Prescriptive Vocational Competency
International Organization for Standardization (ISO)
International Phonetic Alphabet (IPA)
International Society for Biomedical Research on Alcoholism (ISBRA)
International Standard Manual Alphabet
International Stress and Behavior Society (ISBS)
International Stress Management Association (ISMA)
International Test for Aphasia
International Version of the Mental Status Questionnaire
internet addiction
internet games and game makers
internus, musculus intercostalis
internus abdominis, musculus obliquus
interoceptive awareness, lack of
interpersonal behavior
interpersonal control
interpersonal difficulty
interpersonal distrust
interpersonal dysfunction
interpersonal exploitation
interpersonal functioning
interpersonal interaction
Interpersonal Language Skills Assessment (ILSA)
interpersonal personality traits
interpersonal rapport, poor
interpersonal rejection
    pathological sensitivity to perceived
    perceived
interpersonal relations
interpersonal research orientation
interpersonal responsibilities
interpersonal roles
interpersonal strain
Interpersonal Style Inventory
interpersonal style, dramatic
"interplanetary mission" (re: crack acquisition)
interpretation
    differences in psychoanalytic

interpretation of a perceptual
  disturbance, delusional
interpretation of events
interpretation of test results
interpretation test, proverb
interprofessional relations
interpsychic relationship
interrogative sentence
interrupted tracing (I tracing)
interrupter device
intersensory transfer
intersex condition
  congenital
  physical
interstitial word
interval reinforcement schedule
  fixed
  variable
intervention
  associated
  barriers to
  cognitive-behavioral
  evolutionary
  generative
  outpatient
  paradoxical
  pharmacotherapeutic
  psychosocial
  remedial
interventions for mental disorders
interview
  barbiturate-facilitated
  hypnotic
  psychological
intervocalic consonant position
intimate feelings
intimidating behavior
intimidating others
intolerance, drug
intonation contour
intoxicating vapors, method of
  inhaling
intoxication *(see also* intoxication
  delirium)
  acute
    alcohol, with mild
      comorbid alcohol use
      disorder (F10.129)

intoxication
  alcohol, with moderate-to-
    severe comorbid alcohol
    use disorder (F10.229)
  alcohol, with no
    comorbidity (F10.929)
  alcohol idiosyncratic
  amphetamine, with mild
    comorbid amphetamine
    use disorder with
    perceptual disturbance
    (F15.122)
  amphetamine, with mild
    comorbid amphetamine
    use disorder with no
    perceptual disturbance
    (F15.129)
  amphetamine, with
    moderate-to-severe
    comorbid amphetamine
    use disorder with
    perceptual disturbance
    (F15.222)
  amphetamine, with
    moderate-to-severe
    comorbid amphetamine
    use disorder with no
    perceptual disturbance
    (F15.229)
  amphetamine, with no
    comorbidity, with
    perceptual disturbance
    (F15.922)
  amphetamine, with no
    comorbidity, with no
    perceptual disturbance
    (F15.929)
  anticonvulsant
  anxiolytic, with mild
    comorbid anxiolytic use
    disorder (F13.129)
  anxiolytic, with moderate-
    to-severe comorbid
    anxiolytic use disorder
    (F13.229)
  anxiolytic, with no
    comorbidity (F13.929)

intoxication
- caffeine, with no comorbidity (F15.929)
- cannabis, with mild comorbid cannabis use disorder with perceptual disturbance (F12.122)
- cannabis, with mild comorbid cannabis use disorder with no perceptual disturbance (F12.129)
- cannabis, with moderate-to-severe comorbid cannabis use disorder with perceptual disturbance (F12.222)
- cannabis, with moderate-to-severe comorbid cannabis use disorder with no perceptual disturbance (F12.229)
- cannabis, with no comorbidity, with perceptual disturbance (F12.922)
- cannabis, with no comorbidity, with no perceptual disturbance (F12.929)
- carbon dioxide
- carbon monoxide
- characteristic durations of
- cocaine, with mild comorbid cocaine use disorder with perceptual disturbance (F14.122)
- cocaine, with mild comorbid cocaine use disorder with no perceptual disturbance (F14.129)
- cocaine, with moderate-to-severe comorbid cocaine use disorder with perceptual disturbance (F14.222)

intoxication
- cocaine, with moderate-to-severe comorbid cocaine use disorder with no perceptual disturbance (F14.229)
- cocaine, with no comorbidity, with perceptual disturbance (F14.922)
- cocaine, with no comorbidity, with no perceptual disturbance (F14.929)
- episodes of
- glutethimide
- hallucinogen, with mild comorbid hallucinogen use disorder (F16.129)
- hallucinogen, with moderate-to-severe comorbid hallucinogen use disorder (F16.229)
- hallucinogen, with no comorbidity (F16.929)
- hypnotic, with mild comorbid hypnotic use disorder (F13.129)
- hypnotic, with moderate-to-severe comorbid hypnotic use disorder (F13.229)
- hypnotic, with no comorbidity (F13.929)
- inhalant, with mild comorbid inhalant use disorder (F18.129)
- inhalant, with moderate-to-severe comorbid inhalant use disorder (F18.229)
- inhalant, with no comorbidity (F18.929)
- intense level of manganese
- opioid, with mild comorbid opioid use disorder with perceptual disturbance (F11.122)

intoxication
    opioid, with mild comorbid opioid use disorder with no perceptual disturbance (F11.129)
    opioid, with moderate-to-severe comorbid opioid use disorder with perceptual disturbance (F11.222)
    opioid, with moderate-to-severe comorbid opioid use disorder wit no perceptual disturbance (F11.229)
    opioid, with no comorbidity, with perceptual disturbance (F11.922)
    opioid, with no comorbidity, with no perceptual disturbance (F11.929)
    other/unknown substance, with mild comorbid other/unknown substance use disorder (F19.129)
    other/unknown substance, with moderate-to-severe comorbid other/unknown substance use disorder (F19.229)
    other/unknown substance, with no comorbidity (F19.929)
    phencyclidine/PCP, with mild comorbid phencyclidine/PCP use disorder (F16.129)
    phencyclidine/PCP, with moderate-to-severe comorbid phencyclidine/PCP use disorder (F16.229)
    phencyclidine/PCP, with no comorbidity (F16.929)
    physiological

intoxication
    sedative, with mild comorbid sedative use disorder (F13.129)
    sedative, with moderate-to-severe comorbid sedative use disorder (F13.229)
    sedative, with no comorbidity (F13.929)
    signs of alcohol
    stimulant, with mild comorbid stimulant use disorder with perceptual disturbance (F15.122)
    stimulant, with mild comorbid stimulant use disorder with no perceptual disturbance (F15.129)
    stimulant, with moderate-to-severe comorbid stimulant use disorder with perceptual disturbance (F15.222)
    stimulant, with moderate-to-severe comorbid stimulant use disorder with no perceptual disturbance (F15.229)
    stimulant, with no comorbidity, with perceptual disturbance (F15.922)
    stimulant, with no comorbidity, with no perceptual disturbance (F15.929)
    water
intoxication criteria, equivalent
intoxication delirium
    alcohol (mild use disorder) (F10.121)
    alcohol (moderate/severe use disorder) (F10.221)
    alcohol (no use disorder) (F10.921)
    amphetaminc (mild use disorder) (F15.121)

intoxication delirium
   amphetamine
      (moderate/severe use
      disorder) (F15.221)
   amphetamine (no use
      disorder) (F15.921)
   anxiolytic (mild use
      disorder) (F13.121)
   anxiolytic (moderate/severe
      use disorder) (F13.221)
   anxiolytic (no use disorder)
      (F13.921)
   cannabis (mild use
      disorder) (F12.121)
   cannabis (moderate/severe
      use disorder) (F12.221)
   cannabis (no use disorder)
      (F12.921)
   cocaine (mild use disorder)
      (F14.121)
   cocaine (moderate/severe
      use disorder) (F14.221)
   cocaine (no use disorder)
      (F14.921)
   hallucinogen (mild use
      disorder) (F16.121)
   hallucinogen
      (moderate/severe use
      disorder) (F16.221)
   hallucinogen (no use
      disorder) (F16.921)
   hypnotic (mild use
      disorder) (F13.121)
   hypnotic (moderate/severe
      use disorder) (F13.221)
   hypnotic (no use disorder)
      (F13.921)
   inhalant (mild use disorder)
      (F18.121)
   inhalant (moderate/severe
      use disorder) (F18.221)
   inhalant (no use disorder)
      (F18.921)
   opioid (mild use disorder)
      (F11.121)
   opioid (moderate/severe
      use disorder) (F11.221)

intoxication delirium
   opioid (no use disorder)
      (F11.921)
   other/unknown substance
      (mild use disorder)
      (F19.121)
   other/unknown substance
      (moderate/severe use
      disorder) (F19.221)
   other/unknown substance
      (no use disorder)
      (F19.921)
   phencyclidine (mild use
      disorder) (F16.121)
   phencyclidine
      (moderate/severe use
      disorder) (F16.221)
   phencyclidine (no use
      disorder) (F16.921)
   sedative (mild use disorder)
      (F13.121)
   sedative (moderate/severe
      use disorder) (F13.221)
   sedative (no use disorder)
      (F13.921)
   stimulant (mild use
      disorder) (F15.121)
   stimulant (moderate/severe
      use disorder) (F15.221)
   stimulant (no use disorder)
      (F15.921)
intoxication syndrome
intra-aural reflex
intracerebral hemorrhage
intracorporeal pharmacological
   testing
intracranial abscess
intracranial aneurysm
intractable pain
intrafamilial relationships
intramedullary canal
intranasal drug
intraneuronal argentophilic Pick
   inclusion bodies
intraoral pressure
intrapleural pressure
intrapsychic personality traits

intrapsychical function
intrapulmonic pressure
intratest scatter
intrathoracic pressure
intravenous drug
Intrex Questionnaires
intriguing manner
intrinsic muscles of the larynx
intrinsic muscles of the tongue
intropunitive view
introspective and ruminative
introversive tendencies
intrusion
    linguistics
    ego-dystonic
intrusive distressing idea
intrusive ideas, persistent
intrusive images, persistent
intrusive impulses, persistent
intrusive quality of obsessions
intrusive thoughts, persistent
intrusive urges, persistent
intubation
invasive operation
inventory (pl. inventories) *(see also* tests)
    adaptive behavior
    adolescent personality
    adult career
    adult personality
    agency planning
    analytical reading
    assessment
    association adjustment
    athletic motivation
    basic concept
    basic personality
    biographical
    bipolar psychological
    brief symptom
    career assessment
    career development
    child abuse potential
    child care
    children's depression
    client
    communication sensitivity
    cooperation

inventory (pl. inventories)
    coping
    counseling
    culture shock
    decision making
    development
    driver risk
    early child development
    early coping
    early screening
    eating
    employee attitude
    employee reliability
    environmental language
    family relationship
    functional assessment
    impact message
    individual
    instructional leadership
    interpersonal style
    language abilities
    leadership practices (LPI)
    leadership skills
    learning styles
    life styles (LSI)
    management styles
    marital satisfaction
    marriage adjustment
    military environment
    motivational patterns
    organizational
    parent opinion
    partner relationship
    perceptual skills
    personal relationship
    personality assessment
    personnel selection
    problem solving
    psychological distress
    school climate
    school interest
    self-report personalities
    self-report psychological
    social behavior
    speech
    stress evaluation
    student adjustment
    substance abuse

inventory (pl. inventories)
   suicide intervention
   supervisory
   teacher opinion
   Teacher Stress
   teaching style
   temperament and values
   time perception
   time problems
inverse feedback
inverse-square law
investigation
   Luria's Neuropsychological
   principal
"invisible, better infamous than"
   (serial killer attitude)
in vivo magnetic resonance
   spectroscopy in psychiatric
   brain disorders
involuntary movement
involuntary state of trance
involuntary twitch/twitching
involuntary whispering
involvement, cranial nerve
Inwald Personality Inventory
ion
     negative
     positive
Iowa Algebra Aptitude Test
Iowa Tests of Basic Skills
Iowa Tests of Educational
   Development
Iowa's Severity Rating Scales for
   Speech and Language
   Impairments
IPA (International Phonetic
   Alphabet)
IPA (International Phonetic
   Association)
IPAT Anxiety Scale
IPAT Depression Scale
IPI (Inwald Personality Inventory
IPS (Inventory of Perceptual
   Skills)
ipsilateral cerebellar ataxia
ipsilateral frontal routing of
   signals (IFROS)
ipsilateral headache

ipsilateral loss
ipsilateral palsy
ipsilateral reflex, acoustic
ipsilateral routing of signals
   (IROS)
IQ (intelligent quotient)
IRI (Burns/Roe Informal Reading
   Inventory: Preprimer to Twelfth
   Grade)
iron deficiency anemia
irony (figure of speech)
IROS (ipsilateral routing of
   signals)
irradiation-induced mental
   deterioration
irrational fear of an object
irrationality
irregular menses
irregular movement
irregular sleep patterns
irregular sleep-wake pattern
irrelevant speech
irrelevant stimuli, screen out
irresponsibility, consistent
irresponsible work behavior
irritability
     electric
     feelings of
     marked
     myotatic
irritable, feeling
irritable dysphoria, chronic
irritable mood, prominent
IRV (inspiratory reserve volume)
Is This Autism? A Checklist of
   Behaviors and Skills for
   Children
ISBRA (International Society for
   Biomedical Research on
   Alcoholism)
ISBS (International Stress and
   Behavior Society)
ischemic attack, transient (TIA)
"Isda" (street name, heroin)
Islam phobia
Islamophile
Islamophilia
Islamophobe

Islamophobia
Islamophobic
island of control
ISMA (International Stress
  Management Association)
ISMHO (International Society for
  Mental Health Online)
ISO (International Organization
  for Standardization)
isobutyl nitrite (inhalant) (street
  names)
    aroma of men
    bolt
    bullet
    climax
    hardware
    locker room
    poppers
    quicksilver
    rush
    rush snappers
    snappers
    thrust
    whiteout
isochronal
isogloss
isolation
isolation aphasia
isolation of affect
isolation syndrome
isopterophobia
ISSTD (International Society for
  the Study of Trauma and
  Dissociation)
"issues" (street name, crack)
issues
    inner child
    preexisting underlying
      emotional
    to process
isthmus of fauces
ISTSS (International Society for
  Traumatic Stress Studies)
Italomania (Italy/things Italian)
"itch-like" sensation of the scalp
ITERS (Infant/Toddler
  Environment Rating Scale)
IWB (Index of Well-Being)

J

J (symbol for joule)
"J" (street name, cannabis cigarette)
"jab/job" (re: drug injection)
jabbing pain
"jack" (re: to steal drugs)
"jack-up" (re: drug injection)
"jackpot" (street name, fentanyl)
Jackson epilepsy
Jackson Evaluation System
Jackson syndrome
jacksonian seizure
"jag" (re: drug influence)
"jam" (street name, amphetamine; cocaine)
"jam cecil" (street name, amphetamine)
jamais vu aura
James Language Dominance Test
"Jane" (street name, cannabis)
Japanese B viral encephalitis
jargon paraphasia, extended
"jay" (street name, cannabis cigarette)
"jay smoke" (street name, cannabis)
JDI (Job Descriptive Index and Retirement Descriptive Index)
jealousy
    delusional
    obsessive (F42)
jealous type delusions
jealous type schizophrenia
"jee gee" (street name, heroin)
"Jefferson Airplane" (re: cannabis equipment)
"jellies" (re: MDMA and depressants in gel form)
"jellies" (street name, barbiturate; temazepam)
"jelly" (street name, cocaine)
"jelly baby" (street name, amphetamine)
"jelly beans" (street name, crack)
Jena method
Jenkins Non-Verbal Test
jerking, head
jerking movement
"jet" (street name, ketamine)
"jet fuel" (street name, phencyclidine/PCP)
jet lag type dyssomnia
Jette Functional Status Index
Jewett wave
Jikoshu-kyofu (olfactory reference syndrome) (F42)
"Jim Jones" (street name, cannabis, cocaine and phencyclidine)
JIRI (Johnston Informal Reading Inventory)
jitter, frequency
"jive" (street name, heroin; cannabis; illicit drugs)
"jive doo jee"(re: need for drugs)
"jive doo jee" (street name, heroin)
"jive stick" (street name, cannabis)
JLO (Judgment of Line Orientation)
JND (just noticeable difference)
job, loss of
job analysis survey *(see also* tests)
Job Descriptive Index and Retirement Descriptive Index (JDI; RDI)
JOB-O (Judgment of Occupational Behavior-Orientation)
job performance *(see also* tests)
job responsibilities
job satisfaction *(see also* tests)
Job Seeking Skills Assessment
"Johnson" (street name, crack)

Johnston Informal Reading Inventory (JIRI)
"joint" (street name, cannabis cigarette)
joint
    cricoarytenoid
    temporomandibular (TMJ)
joint pain
joint syndrome, temporomandibular
"joints" (re: cannabis use)
"jojee" (street name, heroin)
Joliet 3-Minute Speech and Language Screen
"jolly bean" (street name, amphetamine)
"jolly green" (street name, cannabis)
"jolly pop" (re: heroin user)
"jolt" (re: drug injection; drug reaction)
Jonah words
"Jones" (street name, heroin)
"Jonesing" (re: needing drugs)
Jordan Left-Right Reversal Test
Joseph Pre-School and Primary Self-Concept Screening Test
joule (J)
journaling exercise
"joy flakes" (street name, heroin)
"joy juice" (street name, barbiturate)
"joy plant" (street name, opium)
"joy pop" (re: drug injection)
"joy popping" (re: drug use)
"joy powder" (street name, heroin; cocaine)
"joy smoke" (street name, cannabis)
"joy stick" (street name, cannabis cigarette)
"Juan Valdez" (street name, cannabis)
"Juanita" (street name, cannabis)
Judaeophobia
judgment
    clinical
    diagnostic

judgment
    faulty
    lack of
    poor
    value
judgment and insight
Judgment Form 62 *(see also* tests)
Judgment of Line Orientation (JLO)
Judgment of Occupational Behavior-Orientation (JOB-O)
judgments, negative
Judophobia
"juggle" (re: drug dealing)
"juggler" (re: drug dealer)
"jugs" (street name, amphetamine)
"juice" (street name, steroids, phencyclidine/PCP)
"juice joint" (street name, cannabis and crack cigarette)
"ju-ju" (street name, cannabis cigarette)
"jum" (re: crack container)
jumbling of teeth
"jumbos" (re: crack containers)
junction, pharyngoesophageal (PE)
junctural feature
juncture
    closed
    internal
    open
    phonetics of
    plus
    terminal
Jungian theory
"junkie" (re: a drug addict)
just noticeable difference (JND)
justifiable reaction
Juul (brand name, e-cigarette)
Juul pod
juvenile fire setting
juvenile papillomatosis

K

"K" (street name, phencyclidine/PCP)
"K-lots" (re: bags of 1000 MDMA pills)
"K2" (street name, synthetic cannabis)
K & 1 screening *(see also* tests)
"kabayo" (street name, heroin)
KABC (Kaufman Assessment Battery for Children)
"Kabuki" (re: crack equipment)
kainomania (newness/freshness)
KAIT (Kaufman Adolescent and Adult Intelligence Test)
"Kaksonjae" (street name, smokable methamphetamine)
"Kali" (street name, cannabis)
"kangaroo" (street name, crack)
kappa opiate receptors
kappa receptors
"kaps" (street name, phencyclidine/PCP)
"Karachi" (street name, heroin)
Kasanin-Hanfmann Concept Formation Test
kathisomania (sitting down)
Katz ADL Index
Kaufman Adolescent and Adult Intelligence Test (KAIT)
Kaufman Assessment Battery for Children (KABC)
Kaufman Brief Intelligence Test (K-BIT)
Kaufman Development Scale (KDS)
Kaufman Infant and Preschool Scale
Kaufman Survey of Early Academic and Language Skills (K-SEALS)
Kaufman Test of Education Achievement
"kaya" (street name, cannabis)
K-BIT (Kaufman Brief Intelligence Test)
"K-blast" (street name, phencyclidine/PCP)
kc (kilocycle)
KCI (Kolbe Cognitive Index)
K-complex
KDS (Kaufman Development Scale)
Keegan Type Indicator
Kendrick Cognitive Tests for the Elderly
Kenny ADL Index
Kenny Self-Care Evaluation
Kenny Self-Care Questionnaire
Kent Infant Development Scale
"Kentucky blue" (street name, cannabis)
keratosis
keratotic lesions
Kerby Learning Modality Test
kernel sentence
ketamine (street names)
    black hole (re: depressant high due to ketamine use)
    bump (re: hit of ketamine - $20)
    candy raver (re: rave attendees wearing candy jewelry)
    cat killer
    cat Valium
    green (re: inferior quality of ketamine)
    honey oil
    jet
    ket
    K-hole (depressant high associated with ketamine)
    kit kat
    kitty flipping (re: use of ketamine and MDMA)
    purple
    Special K

ketamine (street names)
    special la coke
    speedballing (re: ecstasy mixed with ketamine)
    super acid
    Super C
    vitamin K
Ketanest (esketamine)
ketoacidosis, diabetic
Key, Fitzgerald
KeyMath Revised: A Diagnostic Inventory of Essential Mathematics
key word method
"keyed up," feeling
"KGB" (killer green bud) (street name, cannabis)
khat (street names)
    Abyssinian tea
    African salad
    bushman's tea
    Mirra
    Somali tea
    Tohai
    Tschat
Khatena-Torrance Creative Perception Inventory
"K-hole" (re: ketamine-induced confusion)
"Kibbles & Bits" (street name, small crumbs of crack)
"kick" (re: drug withdrawal)
"kick" (street name, inhalant)
"kick stick" (street name, cannabis cigarette)
"kiddie dope" (street name, prescription drugs)
kidnapping
kidney disease and concurrent psychiatric problems
"killer" (street name, cannabis; phencyclidine/PCP)
killer cults
"killer weed" (street name, cannabis)
killers
    serial
    serial sexual

kilo (2.2 pounds)
kilocycle (kc)
"kilter" (street name, cannabis)
"kind" (street name, cannabis)
kindergarten interest tests *(see also* tests)
kindergarten inventory of skills *(see also* tests)
kindergarten readiness scales *(see also* tests)
Kindergarten Readiness Test (KRT)
kindergarten screening batteries *(see also* tests)
kindergarten word lists *(see also* tests)
kinesic gestures
kinesigenic ataxia
kinesiology
kinesis
kinesomania (movement)
kinesthesia
kinesthesis
kinesthetic analysis
kinesthetic cue
kinesthetic feedback
kinesthetic method
kinesthetic perception, tactile
kinesthetic technique
kinetic analysis
kinetic energy
kinetic tremor
"king ivory" (street name, fentanyl)
"King Kong pills" (street name, barbiturate)
"king's habit" (street name, cocaine)
kinky hair disease
KIPS (Kaufman Infant and Preschool Scale)
"kit" (re: drug injection paraphernalia)
"kitty flipping" (re: use of ketamine and MDMA)
"KJ" (street name, phencyclidine/PCP)

"Kleenex" (street name, analog of amphetamine/methamphetamine; MDMA)
Klein's death wish
kleptomania (stealing) (F63.2)
"Klingons" (street name, crack addicts)
Klismaphilia
knowledge, inflated
knowledge of results
known environmental factors
known history
known medical or general conditions
known organic factor
Knox's Cube Test
Kohs Block Design
"Kokomo" (street name, crack)
Kolbe Cognitive Index (KCI)
"koller joints" (street name, phencyclidine/PCP)
"kools" (street name, phencyclidine/PCP)
Korean Psychological Association (KPA)
Koro (Dhat syndrome) (F42)
Korsakoff amnesia
Korsakoff amnesic
Korzybski, Alfred (1879-1950) (psychoanalyst)
Koshevnikoff epilepsy
KPA (Korean Psychological Association)
Krabbe's disease
"krocodil" (street name, desomorphine derivative; a flesh-eating opioid)
KRT (Kindergarten Readiness Test)
"Kryptonite" (street name, crack)
"krystal" (street name, phencyclidine/PCP)
"krystal joint" (street name, phencyclidine/PCP)
K-SEALS (Kaufman Survey of Early Academic and Language Skills)
Kuder General Interest Survey

Kufs' disease
"Kumba" (street name, cannabis)
Kuru
Kussmaul aphasia
"KW" (street name, phencyclidine/PCP)
Kwell bath
kymogram
kymograph
kynophobia

L

"L" (street name, lysergic acid diethylamide/LSD)
"L.A." (re: long-acting amphetamine)
"L.A. glass" (street name, smokable methamphetamine)
"L.A. ice" (street name, smokable methamphetamine)
LA (long-acting)
labeling
labial
labial assimilation
labial cleft
labile emotionality
labile range of affect
labile type personality disorder
lability
    affective
    emotional
lability of mood
labiodental area consonant placement
labioglossolaryngeal paralysis
labioglossopharyngeal paralysis
labioversion of teeth
laboratory abnormality
laboratory data
laboratory test results, inconsistent
labored speech
labyrinth
    bony
    membranous
    osseous
labyrinthine aplasia
labyrinthine deafness
labyrinthine disorder
labyrinthine hydrops
labyrinthine vertigo

"lace" (street name, cocaine and cannabis)
lack of abandonment concerns
lack of adequate food (Z59.4)
lack of boundaries
lack of control
lack of desire
lack of drive
lack of efficiency
lack of emotion
lack of empathy
lack of energy
lack of excessive sleep
lack of experience
lack of flexibility
lack of goal orientation
lack of impulse regulation
lack of impulsivity
lack of interoceptive awareness
lack of judgment
lack of meaningful relationships
lack of minimal hygiene
lack of motivation
lack of nurturance
lack of openness
lack of pleasure
lack of remorse
lack of responsibility
lack of safe drinking water (Z59.4)
lack of self-confidence, feelings of
lack of self-esteem
lack of self-respect
lack of self-responsibility
lack of spontaneity
lack of stimulation
lack of structure
lack of support
lacrimal bone
lacrimal skull bone
lacunae
lacunaire, etat (multiple small strokes)
lacunar dementia
lacunar infarct
lacunar state
lacunar stroke

lacunar syndrome
ladder, abstraction
laddergram
"lady caine" (street name, cocaine)
"lady snow" (street name, cocaine)
lag
    initial
    jet
    maturational
    terminal
"lakbay diva" (street name, cannabis)
lalomania (talkativeness)
lambdacism
Lambeth Disability Screening Questionnaire
"Lamborghini" (re: crack equipment)
laminograph
Landau-Kleffner syndrome (acquired epileptic aphasia)
Langat viral encephalitis
language
    automatic
    clarity of
    common
    computer
    configuration confused
    confused
    delayed
    deviant
    difficulties in speech or
    disturbance in
    dominant
    egocentric
    emergent
    emotive
    executive
    expressive
    first
    gesture
    global loss of
    home
    hypercorrect
    impaired
    impairment in

language
    implicit
    inner
    integrative
    native
    negotiating
    nonspecific
    nonstandard
    oral
    organ
    peculiar thoughts and
    peculiarities of
    prelinguistic
    primary
    rationalist theory of
    receptive
    reduced body
    school
    sign
    standard
    subcultural
    substandard
    transmission of ideas by
    true
    twin
    written
language abilities
Language Abilities and Inventory of Language Abilities
language and communication
    distortion of
    exaggeration of
language and speech characteristics of cleft palate
language aptitude tests *(see also* tests)
language areas of brain, mapping of
language arts
language assessment batteries *(see also* tests)
language Assessment Scales - Reading and Writing (LAS-R/W)
Language Assessment Scales - Oral (LAS-O)
language assessment tests *(see also* tests)

language barriers
language boundary
language centers
language characteristics of cleft palate, speech and
language clinician
language clinician, speech and
language competence tests *(see also* tests)
language comprehension tests *(see also* tests)
language concepts test *(see also* tests)
language content
language deficit, central
language development
    expressive
    receptive
    slow rate of
language development tests *(see also* tests)
language difference
language difficulties
language disability screening tests *(see also* tests)
language disorder (F80.9)
    central (CLD)
    expressive
    mixed receptive-expressive
    receptive
    schizophrenic speech and
    speech and
language disorder in dementia
language disorders in psychiatry, speech and
language disturbance tests *(see also* tests)
language dominance test *(see also* tests)
language dysfunction
language empiricist theory
language evaluation *(see also* tests)
language form
language formulation
language function, deterioration of
language function tests *(see also* tests)
language grammar tests *(see also* tests)
language imbalance, central
language impairment, accompanying
language impairment tests *(see also* tests)
language in schizophrenia
    distorted
    exaggerated
language innateness theory
language instructional test *(see also* tests)
language inventories *(see also* tests)
language learning theory
language mixture theory
Language Modalities Test for Aphasia
language nativist theory
language of lying
language pathologist, speech and
language pathology, speech and
language problem
    expressive
    receptive
language processing, higher integrative
language processing disorder
    expressive
    receptive
Language Processing Test
language proficiency tests *(see also* tests)
language rationalist theory
language retardation, idiopathic
language sample
language scales *(see also* tests)
language screening tests *(see also* tests)
Language Sentence Imitation Diagnostic Inventory - Oral (OLSIDI)
language skills assessment tests *(see also* tests)
language structure

language theories
language theory, biolinguistic
language therapist
language use
lapse of awareness
lapses in hygiene
laryngeal anesthesia
laryngeal anomaly
laryngeal atresia
laryngeal dysarthria
laryngeal epilepsy
laryngeal hyperesthesia
laryngeal motor paralysis
laryngeal oscillation
laryngeal paralysis
laryngeal paralysis, bilateral
laryngeal paresthesia
laryngeal-pharyngeal spasm
laryngeal prominence
laryngeal reflex
laryngeal respiration
laryngeal sensory paralysis
laryngeal stuttering
laryngeal web
laryngectomee
laryngectomy
    anterior partial
    frontolateral
    subtotal
    total
larynges (pl. of larynx)
laryngis, ventriculus
laryngismus
laryngitic
laryngitis
    acute
    chronic
    chronic subglottic
    croupous
    hemorrhagic
    hyperplastic
    hypertrophic
    membranous
    spasmodic
    stridulous
    traumatic
laryngocele
laryngofissure
laryngograph
laryngology
laryngomalacia
laryngoparalysis
laryngopathy
laryngophantom
laryngopharyngeal
laryngopharyngectomy
laryngopharyngitis
laryngopharynx
laryngophony
laryngophthisis
laryngoplasty
laryngoplegia
laryngoptosis
laryngorhinology
laryngoscope
laryngoscopist
laryngoscopy
    direct
    indirect
    suspension
laryngospasm
laryngostenosis
laryngostomy
laryngostroboscope
laryngotome
laryngotomy
    inferior
    median
    superior
laryngotracheal
laryngotracheitis
laryngotracheobronchitis
laryngotracheotomy
laryngoxerosis
larynx (pl. larynges)
    electrical artificial
    electronic artificial
    extrinsic muscles of the
    intrinsic muscles of the
    pneumatic artificial
    reed artificial
larynx muscles
"las mujercitas" (street name, psilocybin)
LAS-O (Language Assessment Scales - Oral)

"lason sa daga" (street name, LSD)
LASSI (Learning and Study Strategies Inventory)
last relationship
late adolescence
late-age trauma and PTSD
late-life migraine headache
late luteal phase dysphoric disorder
late luteal phase of menstrual cycle
late onset of schizophrenia
late speech development
late traumatic epilepsy
latency
    acoustic reflex
    mean sleep
    prolonged sleep
    reduced rapid eye movement
    short sleep
    sleep
latency period psychosexual development
latency responses
    long
    middle
latent response
lateral, dark
lateral adenoidectomy
Lateral Awareness and Directionality Test
lateral canal
lateral consonant formation
    dark
    light
lateral cricoarytenoid muscle
lateral dominance
lateral gaze palsy
lateral incisor teeth
lateral lisp
lateral occipital sulcus
lateral sclerosis, amyotrophic (ALS; Lou Gehrig's disease)
lateral sulcus
lateral trim of the adenoid
lateralis, musculus cricoarytenoideus
laterality
    crossed
    mixed
Laterality Preference Schedule
laterality theory of stuttering
lateralization, cortical
latissimus dorsi muscle
"laugh and scratch" (re: drug injection)
"laughing grass" (street name, cannabis)
"laughing weed" (street name, cannabis)
law
    Bernoulli's
    conflict with the
    difficulties with the
    Fourier's
    inverse-square
    Ohm's
    Semon-Rosenbach
    Semon's
lawful behavior
LAW R/W (Language Assessment Scales, Reading and Writing)
laws of cause and effect
lax consonant
lax phoneme
lax toilet training
lax vowel
"lay back" (street name, barbiturate)
"lay-out" (re: drug equipment)
LBA-II (Leader Behavior Analysis II)
"LBJ" (street name, LSD; phencyclidine; heroin)
LCT (Listening Comprehension Test)
LD (learning disabled)
LDES (Learning Disability Evaluation Scale)
L-dopa, on-off effect of
"lead-pipe" rigidity

lead poisoning
lead system
leaden paralysis
Leader Behavior Analysis II (LBA-II)
Leadership Ability Evaluation
Leadership and Management Styles
leadership behavior
leadership index *(see also* tests)
leadership inventories *(see also* tests)
leadership management *(see also* tests)
Leadership Practices Inventory (LPI)
leadership questionnaire *(see also* tests)
Leadership Skills Inventory
leadership survey *(see also* tests)
"leaf" (street name, cannabis; cocaine)
"leaky bolla" (street name, phencyclidine/PCP)
"leaky leak" (street name, phencyclidine/PCP)
"leapers" (street name, amphetamine)
"leaping" (re: drug influence)
learned dysfunctional behavior *(see also* tests)
learned helplessness
learning
    association
    avoidance
    critical period of
    discrimination
    escape
    integrative
    maze
    operant
    paired-associate
    probability
    problem-based
    reversal
    serial
    serial list
    verbal

learning abilities tests *(see also* tests)
learning ability, impaired
learning and behavioral disabilities test *(see also* tests)
Learning and Study Strategies Inventory (LASSI)
learning aptitude tests *(see also* tests)
learning cues
learning difficulties
learning disability assessment *(see also* tests)
Learning Disability Evaluation Scale (LDES)
Learning Disability Rating Procedure
learning disabled (LD)
learning disorder
    specific, with impairment in mathematics (F81.2)
    specific, with impairment in reading (F81.0)
    specific, with impairment in written expression (F81.81)
Learning Efficiency Test-II (LET-II)
learning information
Learning Inventory of Kindergarten Experiences (LIKE)
learning modality tests *(see also* tests)
learning new information, disturbance in
learning skills tests *(see also* tests)
Learning Style Profile (LSP)
Learning Styles Inventory
learning tests *(see also* tests)
learning theory
    language
    social
    stuttering
leather restraints
Leatherman Leadership Questionnaire (LLQ)
leaving parental control problem

LEC (Life Experiences Checklist)
Leeds Scales for the Self-
 Assessment of Anxiety and
 Depression
left bundle branch block
left hemisphere dominance
left-out sibling profile
left-right hemisphere dominance
Left-Right Reversal Test
legal action
legal aspects of assaultive client
 care
legal aspects of dementia
legal contract
legal counselor
legal responsibilities
legal sanctions, imposition of
"legal speed" (re: over the counter
 asthma drug)
legal system, problems related to
 interaction with the
legalized recreational cannabis
legomenon, hapax
Leisure Diagnostic Battery
Leiter Adult Intelligence Scale
Leiter International Performance
 Scale
Leiter Recidivism Scale
"lemon 714" (street name,
 phencyclidine/PCP)
"lemonade" (re: poor quality
 drugs)
"lemonade" (street name, heroin)
"lemons" (street name,
 methaqualone)
length, mean sentence (MSL)
length of hospital stay
length of illness
length of response, mean (MLR)
length of utterance, mean (MLU)
Lengthened-Off-Time (LOT)
lengths of action
lenis consonant
lenis phoneme
"Lennons" (street name,
 methaqualone)
Lennox-Gastaut (petit mal variant
 seizure) syndrome

"lens" (street name, lysergic acid
 diethylamide/LSD)
lenticular aphasia
lepraphobia
Lesch-Nyham syndrome
lesion
 brain
 brain stem
 callosal
 keratotic
LET (Learning Efficiency Test)
lethal catatonia
"lethal weapon" (street name,
 phencyclidine/PCP)
lethargic, feeling
lethargic patient
letheomania (forgetfulness)
"Let's Talk" Inventory for
 Adolescents
letter cancellation test
letter reversal
letter symbols
"lettuce" (re: currency)
leukodystrophy, metachromatic
leukoencephalopathy, progressive
 multifocal
levator veli palatini, musculus
levatores costarum, musculi
level
 action
 activity
 alcohol
 alertness
 anticonvulsant drugs test,
  blood
 automatic phrase
 blood alcohol
 cognitive impairment
 consciousness, change in
 current defense
 defense
 defensive dysregulation
 demarcation in sensory
  testing
 denervation
 desire
 difficulty
 disability

level
    disavowal
    discomfort, tolerance
    effort
    engagement
    functioning
    functioning, premorbid
    GGT
    hearing (LH)
    hearing threshold (HTL)
    high adaptive
    high energy
    hormonal
    image-distorting
    illicit drugs test, blood
    intoxication
    loudness
    low educational
    mental inhibition
    noise interference (NIL)
    occupational functioning
    operant
    overall sound
    peak and trough
    perceived noise (PNdB)
    predominant defense
    psychopathology
    reference zero
    saturation sound pressure
      (SSPL)
    sensation (SL)
    sensory loss
    serum calcium
    social functioning
    society
    speech interference (SIL)
    tolerance
    toxic
    uncomfortable loudness
      (UCL)
    zero hearing
level difference, masking
level masking technique,
  sensorineural acuity
level meter, sound
level 90, high-frequency average
  saturation sound pressure
level perceptual disturbance, high

Levine-Pilowsky Depression
  Questionnaire
Lewy body disease (G31.83)
Lewy body disease, diffuse
lexical agraphia
lexical categories
lexical measuring
lexical morpheme
lexical word
lexicography
lexicon
LF (low frequency)
LFF (low filter frequency)
LH (hearing level)
"lib" (street name, Librium;
  barbiturate)
libido, diminished
library/media skills test *(see also
  tests)*
licensing board, state
"lid" (re: 1 ounce of cannabis)
"lid poppers" (street name,
  amphetamine)
lidocaine
lidocaine, "Blow up" (crack cut
  with lidocaine to increase size,
  weight or value)
lie, living a
lie detection
Liepmann apraxia
life
    adult
    enjoyment of
    everyday
    family
    inner
    late
    later in
    loss of
    ordinary demands of
    satisfaction with
life activity, major
life change events
life circumstances, difficult
life-cycle adjustment
life-cycle change(s)
life-cycle transition
life-cycling transition

life difficulties, multiple
life event, negative
Life Event Scale: Adolescents
Life Event Scale: Children
life events and changes inventory
    (see also tests)
life experiences, stressful
Life Experiences Checklist (LEC)
life goals evaluation *(see also*
    tests)
life history inventory *(see also*
    tests)
life problem, phase of
life quality questionnaire *(see also*
    tests)
Life Satisfaction Index (LSI)
life skills *(see also* tests)
life span
life stress, severe
life's stressors, state of
    vulnerability to
Life Styles Inventory (LSI)
life-threatening disease
life-threatening illness
life-threatening medical condition
lifelong sexual dysfunction
lifelong type dyspareunia
lifelong type female orgasmic
    disorder
lifelong type female sexual
    arousal disorder
lifelong type hypoactive sexual
    desire disorder
lifelong type male erectile
    disorder
lifelong type male orgasmic
    disorder
lifelong type sexual aversion
    disorder
lifelong type vaginismus
lifestyle
    inferior sibling
    problem related to (Z72.9)
    sedentary
lifetime history
lift, palatal
light, cone of
light lateral consonant formation
"light stuff" (street name,
    cannabis)
light therapy-induced mood
    disorder
light touch sensation
light voice
light vowel
lightheadedness (a panic attack
    indicator)
"ligthning" (street name,
    amphetamine)
LIKE (Learning Inventory of
    Kindergarten Experiences)
"Lima" (street name, cannabis)
limbic system disorders
limbs, abnormal positioning of
    distal
"lime acid" (street name, lysergic
    acid diethylamide/LSD)
limen, difference (DL)
limit-setting for adolescents
limitations battery *(see also* tests)
limited activity
limited diet
limited range audiometry
limited range speech audiometry
limited speech
limited support
limited-symptom attacks
limited to pain
limiter, noise
limits, to press
Lincoln-Oseretsky Motor
    Development Scale
"line" (street name, cocaine)
lingua-alveolar area
lingua-alveolar area consonant
    placement
linguadental area consonant
    placement
linguae
    musculus longitudinalis
        inferior
    musculus longitudinalis
        superior
    musculus transversus
    musculus verticalis
lingual airway dysfunction

lingual frenum
lingual hypoplasia
lingual lisp
lingual paralysis
lingual raphe
lingual sulcus
    medial
    median
linguist
linguistic aspects
Linguistic Awareness in Reading Readiness
linguistic borrowing
linguistic competence
linguistic component
    morphological
    phonological
    pragmatic
    semantic
    syntactic
linguistic deficit
linguistic determinism
linguistic disorganization
linguistic disorganization in schizophrenia
linguistic intrusion
linguistic mechanisms
linguistic performance
linguistic phonetics
linguistic relativity
linguistic retention
linguistic set of disturbances
linguistic skills, impaired
linguistic stimulation
linguistic universals theory
linguistic variation
linguistics
    anthropological
    applied
    comparative
    contrastive
    descriptive
    diachronic
    general
    historical
    structural
    synchronic
    theoretical

linguodental area
linguoversion of teeth
Link Between Phonology and Articulation: Assessment
link, causal
linking verb
lip
    bilateral cleft
    median cleft
    unilateral cleft
lip rounding
lip tremor
lipidosis, cerebral
lipoid metabolism
lipreading
lipreading aural rehabilitation
"Lipton tea" (re: poor quality drugs)
liquid consonant formation
liquids, gliding of
lisp
    dental
    frontal
    interdental
    lateral
    lingual
    nasal
    occluded
    protrusion
    strident
    substitutional
list learning, serial
list of "first-rank symptoms"
listening
    auditory selective
    dichotic
    diotic
    selective
    visual
Listening Accuracy in Children Test
Listening Comprehension Test (LCT)
listening tasks, dichotic
lists, preoccupation with
"lit up" (re: drug influence)
literacy tests *(see also* tests)
literal paraphasia

literature review
lithium
    cellular effects of
    clinical action of
    therapeutic action of
    toxic action of
lithium for mood disorders
lithium-induced postural tremor
lithium's action on first messengers
lithium's action on membranes
lithium's action on second messengers
lithium toxicity
lithium tremor
    nontoxic
    toxic
lithium use in affective disorders
litotes (figure of speech)
"little bomb" (street name, amphetamine; heroin; barbiturate)
"little ones" (street name, phencyclidine)
little sense of other people's boundaries
"little smoke" (street name, cannabis; psilocybin/psilocin)
"live ones" (street name, phencyclidine/PCP)
live voice audiometry
live voice audiometry, monitored
liver function tests
living
    daily
    group
    independent
    normal activities of daily
    standard of
living a lie
living alone, problem related to (Z60.2)
living circumstances
living conditions
living in a "dream world"
living in a crime-ridden neighborhood
living in the opposite sex role
living skills checklist *(see also* tests)
"L.L." (street name, cannabis)
"llesca" (street name, cannabis)
LLQ (Leatherman Leadership Questionnaire)
LOA (loosening of associations)
"load" (re: 25 bags of heroin)
"loaded" (re: drug influence)
"loaf" (street name, cannabis)
lobe
    frontal
    occipital
    parietal
    temporal
lobe dysfunction
    frontal
    parietal
"lobo" (street name, cannabis)
LOC (loss of consciousness)
local convulsion
localis paracusis
localization
    auditory
    cerebral
    sound
localized weakness
locative case (parts of speech)
locked hospital unit
locked in state
locked seclusion
locomotion
locomotor ataxia
"locoweed" (street name, cannabis)
locutions
Loevinger's Washington University Sentence Completion Test
loft register
"log" (street name, phencyclidine/PCP; cannabis cigarette)
logical memory test
logical operations
logomania (speaking/words)
"Logor" (street name, lysergic acid diethylamide/LSD)

logospasm
Lombard Test
loneliness
    fear of
    feelings of
long-acting drug (LA)
long-distance counseling
long-half-life anxiolytic
  substances
long latency responses
long sleepers
long spinal white matter
long-term cannabis abuse
long-term chase (gambling)
long-term cocaine dependence
long-term counseling
long-term course of abuse
long-term data
long-term dependence
long-term dependency
long-term effect
long-term functioning
long-term goals
long-term heavy use
long-term memory
long-term mortality rate
long-term neuroleptic treatment
long-term occupational exposure
long-term outcome
long-term pattern
long-term patterns of functioning
long-term relationships
long-term remissions
long-term sobriety
longitudinal cerebral fissure
longitudinal evaluation
longitudinal mental status
  examination
longitudinal muscle of tongue
    inferior
    superior
longitudinal observation
longitudinal raphe, median
longitudinal wave
longitudinalis inferior linguae,
  musculus
longitudinalis superior linguae,
  musculus

Look and Say Articulation Test
loop
    calibrated
    induction
loop-induction auditory trainer
loquacity
Lorge-Thorndike Intelligence
  Test/Cognitive Abilities Test,
  The
losing control
"losing one's mind"
loss
    axon
    appetite
    bilateral muscle
    central sensory
    complete visual
    cortical sensory
    dense sensory
    dissociated sensory
    estimated blood (EBL)
    excessive semen
    extreme hearing
    functional
    global language
    hemisensory
    hysterical visual
    insertion
    ipsilateral
    job
    level of sensory
    mechanical functional
    memory
    mild hearing
    mild sleep
    moderate hearing
    moderately severe hearing
    monocular visual
    motor
    nerve
    neuronal
    partial visual
    perceptive hearing
    peripheral sensory
    profound hearing
    sensory
    severe hearing
    speech

loss
    stocking-glove sensory
    visual
loss aids, weight-
loss of approval, fear of
loss of belief
loss of biographical memory
loss of bladder control
loss of body control
loss of bowel control
loss of consciousness (LOC)
loss of control
loss of control of the mind
loss of desire
loss of ego boundaries
loss of erectile functioning, vasculogenic
loss of faith problem
loss of freedom
loss of hearing
loss of life
loss of memory
    amnesia
    anterograde
    retrograde
loss of pain sensation
loss of pleasure
loss of sensory modalities
loss of sexual desire
loss of significant supporting persons
loss of spontaneity
loss of stable social situations
loss of support, fear of
loss of touch
losses, "chasing" one's
lost performative
LOT (Lengthened-Off-Time)
LOTE Reading and Listening Tests
Lou Gehrig's disease (ALS/ amyotrophic lateral sclerosis)
loud snoring
loud speech
loudness
    Bekesy comfortable (BCL)
    most comfortable (MCL)

loudness balance tests *(see also* tests)
loudness contours, equal
loudness level, uncomfortable (UCL)
loudness perception
loudness range, most comfortable (MCLR)
loudness unit
loudspeaker
Louisville Behavior Checklist
louping ill viral encephalitis
"loused" (re: drug injection)
"love" (street name, crack)
"love affair" (street name, cocaine)
"love boat" (street name, cannabis; phencyclidine/PCP)
"love drug" (street name, analog of amphetamine/methamphetamine; barbiturate; MDMA)
"love flipping" (re: use of mescaline and MDMA)
"love pearls" (street name, alpha-ethyltyptamine)
"love pills" (street name, alpha-ethyltyptamine)
"love trip" (street name, methylenedioxy-methamphetamine and mescaline)
"love weed" (street name, cannabis)
"lovelies" (street name, cannabis laced with phencyclidine/PCP)
"lovely" (street name, phencyclidine/PCP; hallucinogen)
"lovers" (street name, depressant)
"lovers' special" (street name, club drug; ecstasy/MDMA; stimulant)
"lovers' speed" (street name, ecstasy (MDMA; stimulant)
loving feelings
low-activity situation
low back pain, radicular
low-calorie diet foods
low-complexity movements
"low" desire

low educational level
low energy
low feature English phoneme
low fence
low filter frequency (LFF)
low frequency (LF)
low frequency of drug use
low income, problems relating to
low self-confidence
low self-esteem
low self-esteem as cause for impaired social functioning
low self-worth, feelings of
low-set ears
low sexual desire
low sexual interest
low-stimulation situation
low tolerance potential
low tone deafness
low-tyramine diet
low vowel
LPI (Leadership Practices Inventory)
LPT (Language Proficiency Test)
LSA (Linguistic Society of America)
LSD (lysergic acid diethylamide)
LSD-type perceptions
LSES (Salamon-Conte Life Satisfaction in the Elderly Scale)
LSI (Life Satisfaction Index)
LSI (Life Styles Inventory)
LSP (Learning Style Profile)
LSV (Vocational Learning Styles)
L-theanine (A2X ingredient)
"lubage" (street name, cannabis)
lubrication, vaginal
"Lucy in the sky with diamonds" (street name, LSD)
"ludes" (street name, methaqualone)
"luding out" (street name, barbiturate)
"luds" (street name, barbiturate)
lumbar iliocostal muscle
lumborum, musculus iliocostalis
"lump in the throat"
lung capacity, total
lung volume
Luria-Nebraska Neuropsychological Battery
Luria's Neuropsychological Investigation
luteal phase dysphoric disorder, late
lycomania (wolves)
lying, repetitive
lysergic acid diethylamide (street names)
    100s
    25s
    A
    acid
    acid cube
    acid freak
    acid head
    acido
    aeon flux
    amp head
    animal
    backbreakers (LSD and strychnine)
    banana split (Nexus and LSD)
    barrels
    battery acid
    beast
    Beavis and Butthead
    big D
    birdhead
    black acid
    black star
    black sunshine
    black tabs
    blotter
    blotter acid
    blotter cube
    blue acid
    blue barrels
    blue caps
    blue chairs
    blue cheers
    blue heaven
    blue microdot
    blue mist

lysergic acid diethylamide (street names)
- blue moons
- blue vials
- brown bombers
- brown dots
- California sunshine
- candy flipping (LSD and Ecstasy)
- candy flipping on a string
- candy raver (rave clubbers wearing candy jewelry)
- cap
- chief
- chocolate chips
- Cid
- coffee
- come home
- comic book
- conductor
- contact lens
- crackers
- crystal tea
- cube
- cupcakes
- D
- deeda
- domes
- doses
- dosure
- dots
- double dome
- Electric Kool Aid
- Elvis
- explorers club
- Felix the cat
- fields
- flash
- flat blues
- frisco special
- frisco speedball
- ghost
- golden dragon
- goofy's
- grape parfait
- green double domes
- green single domes
- green wedge

lysergic acid diethylamide (street names)
- grey shields
- hats
- Hawaiian sunshine
- hawk
- haze
- head light
- heavenly blue
- inbetweens
- instant zen
- L
- lason sa daga
- LBJ (heroin + LSD + PCP)
- lens
- lime acid
- little smoke
- Logor
- Looney Toons
- LSD
- Lucy in the sky with diamonds
- mellow yellow
- Mickey's
- microdot
- Mighty Quinn
- mind detergent
- one way
- optical illusions
- orange barrels
- orange cubes
- orange haze
- orange micro
- orange wedges
- outerlimits (crack and LSD)
- Owsley
- Owsley's acid
- pane
- paper acid
- peace tablets
- peace (LSD and phencyclidine)
- pearly gates
- pellets
- pink blotters
- Pink Panther
- pink robots

lysergic acid diethylamide (street names)
- pink wedges
- pink witches
- potato
- pure love
- purple barrels
- purple flats
- purple gel tabs
- purple haze
- purple hearts
- purple ozoline
- rainbow
- recycle
- red lips
- royal blues
- Russian sickles
- sacrament
- sandoz
- sheet rocking
- smears
- snowmen
- south parks
- squirrel
- strawberry
- strawberry fields
- sugar
- sugar cubes
- sugar lumps
- sunshine
- Superman
- tabs
- tail lights
- The Hawk
- ticket
- Timothy Leary
- trails (LSD perception of moving objects with trails behind them)
- travel agent (LSD supplier)
- trip
- troll
- twenty-five
- utopiates
- vodka acid
- watercolors
- wedding bells
- wedge

lysergic acid diethylamide (street names)
- white dust
- white lightning
- white Owsley's
- window glass
- window pane
- yellow
- yellow dimples
- yellow sunshine
- yen sleep
- ying yang
- zen
- zig zag man

"M" (street name, cannabis)
"M&M" (street name, barbiturate)
MAC (Minimum Auditory Capabilities) Test
machiavellianism
"machinery" (street name, cannabis)
"macho" manner
MACI (Millon Adolescent Clinical Inventory)
MacKenzie syndrome
Macmillan Graded Word Reading Test
"Macon" (street name, cannabis)
macrocheilia
macroglossia
macrognathia
macromania (overvaluation of self)
macrostomia
"mad dog" (street name, phencyclidine/PCP)
"madman" (street name, phencyclidine/PCP)
MAF (minimum audible field)
"magic" (street name, phencyclidine/PCP)
"magic dust" (street name, phencyclidine/PCP)
"magic mushroom" (street name, psilocybin/psilocin)
"magic smoke" (street name, cannabis)
magical thinking and paganism
magnet resonance imaging
magnetic apraxia
magnetic resonance spectroscopy in psychiatric brain disorders, in vivo
magnitude, response
MAI (Marriage Adjustment Inventory)
main clause
"main line" (re: drug injection)
"mainliner" (re: drug injection)
mainstreaming
mainstreaming scale *(see also tests)*
maintaining sleep difficulty
    disorder of initiating and (DIMS)
maintenance insomnia
maintenance of pain
major, musculus pectoralis
major attachment figures
major depression, postpartum
major depression episode, single
major depressive disorder
    recurrent episode, with anxiety distress (F33.3)
    recurrent episode, with peripartum onset (F33.3)
    recurrent episode, in full remission (F33.42)
    recurrent episode, in partial remission (F33.41)
    recurrent episode, mild (F33.0)
    recurrent episode, moderate (F33.1)
    recurrent episode, severe (F33.2)
    recurrent episode, unspecified (F33.9)
    recurrent episode, with atypical features (F33.3)
    recurrent episode, with catatonia (F33.3) and (F06.1)
    recurrent episode, with melancholic features (F33.3)
    recurrent episode, with mixed psychotic features (F33.3)

major depressive disorder
    recurrent episode, with mood-congruent psychotic features (F33.3)
    recurrent episode, with mood-incongruent psychotic features (F33.3)
    recurrent episode, with psychotic features (F33.3)
    recurrent episode, with rapid cycling features (F33.3)
    recurrent episode, with seasonal pattern (F33.3)
    single episode, in full remission (F32.5)
    single episode, in partial remission (F32.4)
    single episode, mild (F32.0)
    single episode, moderate (F32.1)
    single episode, severe (F32.2)
    single episode, unspecified (F32.9)
    single episode, with anxiety distress, mild/moderate/severe (F32.3)
    single episode, with atypical features (F32.3)
    single episode, with catatonia (F32.3) and (F06.1)
    single episode, with melancholic features (F32.3)
    single episode, with mixed psychotic features (F32.3)
    single episode, with mood-congruent psychotic features (F32.3)
    single episode, with mood-incongruent psychotic features (F32.3)
    single episode, with peripartum onset (F32.3)

major depressive disorder
    single episode, with psychotic features (F32.3)
    single episode, with rapid cycling features (F32.3)
    single episode, with seasonal pattern (F32.3)
major depressive episode, pattern of
major effect
major image-distorting level
major impairment of functioning
major life activity
major mental disorders, biology of
major motor aphasia
major motor seizure
major neurocognitive disorder
    mild, due to Alzheimer's disease (G31.84)
    possibly due to Alzheimer's disease (G31.9)
    with behavioral disturbance, due to Alzheimer's disease (G30.9) and (F02.81)
    without behavioral disturbance, due to Alzheimer's disease (G30.9) and (F02.80)
major point of activity
major role obligations
majority society
make amends symbolically
make-believe play
"make up" (re: drugs acquisition)
makeup application, ritualization
malabsorption, disaccharide
maladaptive behavior, absence of
maladaptive behavioral changes
maladaptive feelings
maladaptive gambling behavior
maladaptive health behavior
maladaptive pattern
maladaptive pattern of substance use

maladaptive personality traits,
  pervasive and persistent
maladaptive psychological
  changes
maladaptive reaction to a stressor
maladaptive response
malar bones
malar skull bones
male delayed ejaculation (F52.32)
male dyspareunia
male (early) ejaculation (F52.4)
male erectile arousal disorder
male erectile disorder, acquired,
  generalized, lifelong, situational
  type (F52.21)
male erectile dysfunction (F52.8)
male hypoactive sexual desire
  disorder, lifetime, acquired,
  generalized, situational (F52.0)
male orgasmic disorder
male unspecified sexual
  dysfunction (F52.9)
malignant brain neoplasm
malignant hyperthermia
malignant syndrome, neuroleptic
malinger
malingering (Z76.5)
malingering disorder
mallet, anger
malleus, handle of
malnutrition, potential risks for
malocclusion, teeth
malpositions, teeth
maltreatment and PTSD, elder
maltreatment of children,
  emotional
maltreatment problems
    adolescent
    adult
    child
"mama coca" (street name,
  cocaine)
management
    case
    clinical
    contingency
    crisis
    time

management appraisal
management by medication
management cleft palate,
  prosthetic
Management Development Profile
management development skills
  (see also tests)
management implications
Management Inventory on
  Leadership
management inventory styles
management of aggressive
  behavior, multidisciplinary
management of cleft palate,
  prosthetic
management of dementia
    behavioral
    pharmacological
    psychological
management of dementia-related
  behavior
management of pregnancy
management of recurrent suicidal
  behavior, crisis
management of violence,
  multidisciplinary
management plan
Management Position Analysis
  Test
Management Readiness Profile
Management Styles Inventory
Manager Profile Record
Manager Style Appraisal
managerial position questionnaire
managing stress, understanding
  and
mandible, alveolar border of
mandible skull bone
mandibular hypoplasia
mandibular movement, free
mandibular restriction
mandibulofacial dysostosis
"Mandies" (street name,
  methaqualone)
manganese intoxication
"Manhattan silver" (street name,
  cannabis)

mania
  ablutomania (cleanliness/washing/bathing)
  abulomania (indecision/lack of willpower)
  acromania (heights)
  acute
  agoramania (open spaces)
  agyiomania (being in the street)
  aidoiomania (genitalia)
  ailuromania (cats)
  akinetic
  alcoholomania (alcohol)
  amaxomania (vehicles)
  amenomania (lack of/diminished menses)
  Americamania (America/things American)
  andromania (men/males)
  Anglomania (England/things English)
  anthomania (flowers)
  aphrodisiomania (excessive erotic interest)
  apimania (bees)
  arithmomania (mathematics/figures)
  automania (self/solitude)
  autophonomania (one's own voice)
  ballistomania (missiles)
  Bell
  bibliokleptomania (theft of books)
  bibliomania (books)
  bruxomania (grinding of teeth)
  cacodemonomania (possession by evil spirits)
  callomania (beauty)
  cheromania (heavenly desire)
  Chinamania (China/things Chinese)

mania
  chionomania (snow)
  choreomania (dance)
  chronic
  clinomania (bending)
  compulsive
  coprolalomania (foul language)
  cremnomania (precipices)
  cresomania (dramatic buildup/climax)
  cryomania (cold)
  cynomania (dogs)
  dancing
  Dantomania (writings of Dante)
  delirious
  demomania (people)
  demonomania (demons)
  dinomania (terror/fright)
  dipsomania (alcohol consumption)
  doramania (animal skin/fur)
  doubting
  drapetomania (running away from home)
  dromomania (wander or travel)
  ecdemiomania (foreign sources/origins)
  ecomania (environment)
  edeomania (genitalia)
  egomania (self-absorbed)
  eleuthromania (freedom)
  empleomania (become involved)
  enosimania (belief one's offenses are unpardonable)
  entheomania (heightened enthusiasm)
  entomomania (insects)
  epileptics
  eremiomania (solitude/deserted places)
  ergasiomania (work)
  ergomania (work)

mania
- eroticomania (sexual desire and behavior)
- erotographomania (sexually explicit writing/erotica)
- erotomania (sexual desire & behavior)
- erythromania (color red) (blushing)
- etheromania (pure air)
- florimania (flowers/plants)
- Francomania (France/things French)
- Gallomania (things Gaelic)
- gamomania (marriage)
- gephyromania (bridges)
- Germanomania (Germany/things German)
- graphomania (writing)
- Grecomania (Greece/things Greek)
- gymnomania (nakedness)
- gynecomania (womanizing)
- habromania (clothing/dress)
- hallucinatory
- hamartomania (sin)
- hedonomania (pleasure)
- heliomania (sun)
- hieromania (religious items)
- hippomania (horses)
- hodomania (traveling)
- homicidomania (murder)
- hydrargyromania (Mercury poisoning)
- hydrodipsomania (uncontrollable thirst)
- hydromania (water)
- hylomania (substances)
- hypemania (extravagant promotion)
- hypermania (heightened state of mania)
- hypnomania (sleep)

mania
- hypomania (mild degree of mania)
- hysterical
- hysteromania (psychogenic symptoms)
- ichthyomania (fish)
- iconomania (image worship)
- idolomania (idol worship)
- inhibited
- Italomania (Italy/things Italian)
- kainomania (newness/freshness)
- kathisomania (sitting down)
- kinesomania (movement)
- kleptomania (stealing)
- lalomania (talkativeness)
- letheomania (forgetfulness)
- logomania (speaking/words)
- lycomania (wolves)
- macromania (overvaluation of self)
- megalomania (overvaluation of self)
- melomania (music/song)
- mentulomania (counseling/mentoring)
- mesmeromania (hypnosis)
- methomania (alcoholic beverages)
- metromania (incessant verse writing)
- micromania (self-depreciation)
- monomania (solitude)
- morphinomania (addiction to morphine)
- morphiomania (aphrodisiacs)
- musicomania (music)
- musomania (meditation/dreamy abstraction)

mania
- mythomania (myths/untruths)
- narcomania (craving a drug to deaden pain)
- narcosomania (narcotic addiction)
- necromania (corpses/death)
- noctimania (night/darkness)
- nosomania (disease)
- nostomania (home)
- nudomania (nakedness)
- nymphomania (excessive female sex drive)
- ochlomania (crowds)
- oestromania (female state of sexual excitability)
- oikomania (household/family)
- oligomania (mild form of mania)
- oniomania (compulsive shopping)
- onomatomania (names)
- onychotillomania (picking one's nails)
- ophidiomania (snakes)
- opiomania (addiction to opium)
- opsomania (longing for specific/high seasoned foods)
- orchidomania (men/males)
- orinthomania (birds)
- paramania (related to mania)
- parousiamania (birth)
- pathomania (disease)
- peotillomania (pseudo masturbation)
- peracute
- periodical
- phagomania (eating)
- phaneromania (preoccupation with visible body parts)

mania
- pharmacomania (drugs/medicine)
- philopatridomania (patriotism)
- phonomania (voices/sounds)
- photomania (light)
- phronemomania (thoughts/the mind)
- phthiriomania (lice)
- plutomania (delusions of great wealth)
- politicomania (politics)
- poriomania (wander or journey from home)
- pornographomania (pornography)
- potomania (drinking)
- pseudomania (factitious mental disorder)
- pyromania (fire)
- Ray
- reasoning
- recurrent episode
- religious
- Russiomania (Russia/things Russian)
- satyromania (excessive male sex drive)
- scribblemania (incessant scribbling)
- scribomania (writing)
- senile
- siderodromomania (astrology)
- single episode
- sitomania (eating/food)
- sophomania (belief in personal great wisdom)
- squandermania (squandering)
- stupor
- submania (mild form of mania)
- symmetromania (balanced beauty)

mania
- Teutonomania (things Teutonic)
- thalassomania (sea)
- thanatomania (death)
- theomania (God)
- theotromania (speculation)
- timbromania (recognizing speech variances)
- tomomania (sections/parts)
- toxicomania (poisons)
- transitory
- trichomania (hair)
- trichorrhexomania (splitting hairs)
- trichotillomania (pulling out one's hair)
- tristimania (sad/mournful)
- tromomania (delirium tremors)
- Turkomania (Turkey/things Turkish)
- typomania (impressions/designs)
- unproductive
- uteromania (things maternal)
- verbomania (excessive talkativeness)
- xenomania (strangers)
- zoomania (animals)

Mania "9" Scale
manic-depressive-like episodes, mixed
manic episode, single
manic features
manicky
manic-like episodes
manic phase
manic reaction
manic speech
manic symptoms
manifest anxiety scale for children (*see also* tests)
manifestation of behavioral dysfunction
manifestation of biological dysfunction
manifestation of pain, physical
manifestation of psychological dysfunction
manifestations of pathology
manifested disability
manipulation
- digital
- emotional

manipulative aptitude test
manipulative behavior for material gratification
manipulative behavior to attain power
manipulative behavior to gain profit
manipulatory tasks
man-machine systems
man-made disasters
manner
- devious
- guarded
- inconsistent
- intriguing
- "macho"
- patronizing
- secretive
- superior
- sustained
- unkempt
- unusual

mannerisms
- feminine
- speech

"mannitol, comeback" (street name, benzocaine/mannitol adulteration of cocaine)
manometer, oral
manometric flame
Manual Alphabet
- American
- International Standard (ISMA)

manual communication
manual dexterity test
manual English
manual method aural rehabilitation
manual stimulation

manual volume control
manubrium (pl. manubria)
manufacturing amphetamines
MAOI-meperidine
MAOI-serotonergic agents
MAOI-tricyclides
MAP (minimum audible pressure)
map
    brain
    brain electrical activity (BEAM)
map of reality
mapping
    behavioral
    cognitive
    cortical
mapping of apraxia, cerebral
mapping of cortical function
mapping of language areas of brain
"marathons" (street name, amphetamine)
Marfan syndrome
marginal member of society
"Mari" (street name, marijuana cigarette)
marijuana (see *cannabis for street drug names*)
marijuana smoking
Marital Communication Scale
marital counselor
marital disruption
marital dissatisfaction
Marital Satisfaction Inventory
marked affective lability
marked and excessive specific phobia
marked and persistent specific phobia
marked and unreasonable specific phobia
marked anger
marked anxiety
marked change in appetite
marked decline in academic functioning
marked decline in occupational functioning
marked depression
marked distress in occupational functioning
marked distress in social functioning
marked disturbances in social relatedness
marked drowsiness
marked falling curve audiogram configurations
marked fatigue
marked fear
marked impairment
marked impulsivity, pattern of
marked interference with school/work activities
marked interference with social activities
marked irritability
marked lack of energy
marked overeating
marked shift in mood
marked specific food cravings
marked tension
markedly depressed mood
marker
    I (intentional marker)
    sign
markers of heavy drinking, state (GGT)
marking, analog
marks, bite
marriage
    heterosexual
    homosexual
    institution of
    related by
    same-sex
Marriage Adjustment Inventory (MAI)
Marriage and Family Attitude Survey
marriage counselor
marriage problem
marriage readiness (*see also* tests)
"marshmallow reds" (street name, barbiturate)

Martinez Assessment of the Basic
  Skills
"Mary" (street name, cannabis)
"Mary and Johnny" (street name,
  cannabis)
"Mary Ann" (street name,
  cannabis)
"Mary Jonas" (street name,
  cannabis)
"Mary Warner" (street name,
  cannabis)
"Mary Weaver" (street name,
  cannabis)
Maryland Parent Attitude Survey
MAS (Memory Assessment
  Scales)
masculine constructs in:
    contextual setting
    cultural setting
    social setting
masculine hostility
masculinity, toxic
masculinity, traditional traits of:
    aggressiveness
    competition
    dominance
    stoicism
Masculinity-Femininity "5" Scale
"Maserati" (re: crack equipment)
mask (of parkinsonism) facies
masking
    backward
    central
    effective
    forward
    initial
    maximum
    perceptual
    peripheral
    upward
masking efficiency
masking level difference
masking technique
    Hood
    plateau
    sensorineural acuity level
    shadowing
    threshold shift

masklike facies
Maslach Burnout Inventory
  (MBI)
masochism
    sadism and (S&M)
    sexual (F65.51)
masochistic sexual activity
masochistic sexual behavior
masochistic sexual fantasy
masochistic sexual urges
mass, cerebellar
mass behavior
mastery tests *(see also* tests)
mastication
mastoid, artificial
mastoid process
mastoidectomy
    modified
    radical
masturbation
masturbatory activity
MAT (Metropolitan Achievement
  Tests
MAT (Music Achievement Tests
  1, 2, 3, and 4)
match, perceptual-motor
"matchbox" (re: 1/4 ounce of
  cannabis; 6 cannabis cigarettes)
matching, impedance
mate, age
material aspects of the body
material gratification,
  manipulative behavior for
maternal addiction clinics
maternal behavior
mathematical ability
mathematical problem solving
  (see also tests)
mathematical skills, impaired
mathematical symbols
mathematics *(see also* tests)
mathematics disorder
Mathematics Systems
  Instructional Objectives
  Inventory, DMI
matrices *(see also* tests)
matrix (pl. matrices or matrixes)
Matrix Analogies Test

matrix sentence
"Matsakow" (street name, heroin)
matter
    central gray
    cortical gray
    dorsal gray
    gray (of CNS)
    long spinal white
    midbrain
    periventricular white
    subcortical white
    white (of CNS)
maturation, rate of
maturation index
maturational lag
maturity, sexual
maturity fears
Maudsley Personality Inventory
"Maui wauie" (street name, cannabis)
"Max" (street name, gamma hydroxy butyrate (GHB) and amphetamines)
Maxfield-Buchholz Social Maturity Scale for Blind Preschool
maxibolin (oral steroid)
maxilla, alveolar process of
maxilla skull bone
maxillary bone
    inferior
    superior
maxillary skull bone
    inferior
    superior
maximal contrasts
maximal effect
maximum acoustic output
maximum amplitude
maximum duration of phonation
maximum duration of sustained blowing
maximum frequency range
maximum masking
maximum power output (MPO)
max score, PB
"mayo" (street name, cocaine; heroin)

maze learning
Mazes, Foster
maze test *(see also* tests)
MBD (minimal brain dysfunction) syndrome
MBHI (Millon Behavioral Health Inventory)
MBI (Maslach Burnout Inventory)
MBSP (Monitoring Basic Skills Progress)
McCarthy Screening Test
McGill Pain Questionnaire
MCLR (most comfortable loudness range)
McMaster Health Index Questionnaire
MCMI (Milan Multiaxial Clinical Inventory)
McNaughton Rules
MCRE (The Mother-Child Relationship Evaluation)
MDM (methylenedioxy-methamphetamine)
MDMA (methylenedioxymeth-amphetamine) (street names)
    007s
    69s
    Adam
    Batman
    B-bombs
    bean
    bens
    Benzedrine
    Bermuda triangles
    bibs
    biphetamine
    blue kisses
    blue lips
    blue Nile
    bump up (re: bolstering MDMA with cocaine)
    bumping up (re: combining MDMA with cocaine)
    Cat in the Hat
    candy flipping on a string (re: mixing LSD/MDMA/cocaine)

MDMA (street names)
- candy ravers (re: rave attendees wearing candy necklaces)
- Care Bears
- charge + (re: powdery substance with effects like ecstasy)
- cloud nine
- Cristal
- dead road
- debs
- decadence
- dex
- Dexedrine
- diamonds
- disco biscuit(s)
- doctor
- dolls
- domex
- drivers
- E (ecstasy)
- E-bombs
- ecstasy
- E-puddle (re: sleeping after MDMA use)
- essence
- E-tard (re: under the influence of MDMA)
- Eve
- exiticity
- fastin
- flipping
- flower flipping (re: ecstasy with mushrooms)
- four leaf clover
- gaggler
- go
- green triangles
- greenies
- gum
- GWM
- hammerheading (re: MDMA mixed with Viagra)
- happy drug

MDMA (street names)
- hawkers (re: seller of club drugs (MDMA/GHB/LSD)
- H-bomb (re: ecstasy/MDMA mixed with heroin)
- herbal bliss
- hippieflip (re: use of MDMA with mushrooms)
- hug drug
- hugs and kisses
- hydro
- hype (re: MDMA addict)
- iboga
- ice
- igloo
- ivory wave
- jellies (re: MDMA and depressants in gel form)
- Jerry Garcias
- kitty flipping (re: ketamine and MDMA)
- Kleenex
- K-lots (re: bags of 1000 MDMA pills)
- letter biscuits
- love drug
- love flipping (re: use of mescaline and MDMA)
- love pill
- love trip
- lovers' special
- lovers' speed
- MAO
- MDM
- methedrine
- mini beans
- Mitsubishi
- Molly
- monoamine oxidase
- moonstone (re: dealer shaves MDMA into a bag of heroin)
- morning shot
- Nexus flipping (re: use of Nexus (2-CB) and MDMA)

MDMA (street names)
  nineteen
  NOX (re: use of nitrous oxide and MDMA)
  ocean burst (re: powdery substance mimics effect of ecstasy)
  on the ball (re: a dealer shaves MDMA into a bag of heroin)
  orange bandits
  P and P (re: MDMA combined with Viagra)
  parachute down (re: use of MDMA after heroin)
  party and play (re: MDMA combination with Viagra)
  party pack (Combine Nexus with MDMA - ecstasy)
  peace (re: PCP; LSD; MDMA)
  peepers
  piggybacking (simultaneously injecting two drugs)
  Playboy bunnies
  pollutants
  pure ivory (re: substance with effects similar to ecstasy)
  purple wave (re: substance with effects similar to ecstasy)
  rave energy
  red devils
  rib
  ritual spirit
  roca
  rolling
  Rolls Royce
  running
  Scooby snacks
  Sextasy (re: Ecstasy used with Viagra)
  Shabu
  slammin'/slamming
  Smurfs

MDMA (street names)
  snackies (re: MDMA adulterated with mescaline)
  speed for lovers
  speedballing
  spivias
  stacking (re: 3 or more MDMA tablets in combination)
  stacks (re: adulterated MDMA with heroin or crack)
  stars
  strawberry shortcake
  super X (re: MDMA and methamphetamine combined)
  Supermans
  swans
  sweeties
  tabs
  tachas
  tens
  Tom and Jerries
  totally spent (re: hangover, adverse reaction to MDMA)
  triple crowns
  triple Rolexes
  triple stacks
  troll (re: use of MDMA and LSD)
  tutus
  tweety birds
  vanilla sky (re: powdery substance with ecstasy effect)
  wafers
  waffle dust (re: combined MDMA and amphetamine)
  West Coast turnarounds
  wheels
  whiffledust
  white diamonds
  white dove
  wigits

MDMA (street names)
    X
    X-ing
    X-plus
    XTC
MDQ (Menstrual Distress Questionnaire)
"mean green" (street name, phencyclidine/PCP)
mean length of response (MLR)
mean length of utterance, "1" (MLU)
mean peak frequency
mean relational utterance (MRU)
mean sentence length (MSL)
mean sleep latency
meaning
    grammatical
    idiosyncratic
    transferred
meaning reframing
meaningful, psychologically
meaningful language assessment *(see also* tests)
meaningful relationship
meaningful relationships, lack of
"means," group
MEAP (Multiphasic Environmental Assessment Procedure)
measles, German
measurable impairment
Measure of How You Think and Make Decisions Questionnaire
measured capacity
measurement(s)
    EEG activity
    global (of disability)
    instrumental ADL
    physiological
    probe microphone
    reproductive hormonal
    core body temperature
measurement of auditory function, acoustic
Measurement of Language Development
measurement of speech production, electrical
measurement systems
measurement test, acoustic immittance
measurement tests *(see also* tests)
measures
    assessment and monitoring
    impedance
    psychotherapeutic
measures of disability, global
Measures of Music Audiation - Advanced
Measures of Music Audiation - Primary
Measures of Musical Abilities
Measures of Musical Talents
Measures of Psychosocial Development (MPD)
measuring, lexical
meatus (pl. meatus)
    acoustic
    acusticus externus
    acusticus internus
    external acoustic
    external auditory
    internal acoustic
    internal auditory
    nasi inferior
    nasi medius
    nasi superior
    nasopharyngeus
mechanical functional loss
Mechanical Technology (NOCTI Teacher Occupational Competency Test)
mechanics, body
mechanism
    balance
    direct causative pathophysiological
    endogenous abnormalities in sleep-wake timing
    immune
    linguistic
    pathophysiological
    physiologic
    shared

mechanism
　　specific pathophysiological
　　speech
　　triggering
media
　　adhesive otitis
　　chronic suppurative otitis
　　mental disorder due to
　　mucoid otitis
　　nonsuppurative otitis
　　psychiatric factors affecting
　　psychological factors
　　　affecting
　　scala
　　serous otitis (SOM)
　　suppurative otitis
media push back, purulent otitis
medial consonant position
medial nasal concha
medial turbinate bone
median age
median cleft lip
median laryngotomy
median lingual sulcus
median longitudinal raphe
median sagittal plane
mediated function, verbally
mediated response,
　psychologically
mediation, verbal
medical care
medical condition, life-
　threatening
medical ethics
medical etiology, generalized
medical futility
medically related position
medical management of violence
medical marijuana (legal cannabis
　use)
medical marriages
medical/neurological disorder
Medical Outcomes Study Short
　Form-36
medical/psychiatric sleep disorder
medical psychology
medical services
medical sociology

medical stress
medical treatment
medical treatment, nonadherence
　to (Z91.19)
Medicare system
medication (descriptive terms)
　　adverse effects of
　　agonist
　　antagonist
　　beta-adrenergic
　　cessation of a
　　cheeking
　　management by
　　NSAID
　　overuse of
　　psychoactive
　　tricyclic antidepressants
medication-induced acute
　akathisia (G25.71)
medication-induced acute
　dystonia (G21.02)
medication-induced delirium
medication-induced movement
　disorder, other (G25.79)
medication-induced movements
medication-induced
　Parkinsonism, other (G21.19)
medication-induced postural
　tremor (G25.1)
medication-induced postural
　tremor (anticonvulsant)
medication-induced postural
　tremor (antidepressant)
medication-induced postural
　tremor (beta-adrenergic)
medication-induced postural
　tremor (dopaminergic)
medication-induced postural
　tremor
　(neuroleptic/antipsychotic0
medication madmen
medications (drugs) (*see also*
　illicit drugs *under* drugs, street)
　　Abilify (neuroleptic/
　　　antipsychotic)
　　Alilitat (neuroleptic/
　　　antipsychotic)

medications (drugs)
    acarbose (anti-diabetic agents)
    acecarbromal (anxiolytic)
    acepromazine (tranquilizer)
    acetaminophen (with butalbital and caffeine) (barbiturate)
    acetaminophen (with caffeine) (psychostimulant)
    acetazolamide (carbonic acid inhibitor)
    acetophenazine maleate (tranquilizer)
    acetylcarbromal (sedative)
    acetylsalicylic acid (salicylate)
    Aches-N-Pain (anti-rheumatic)
    Acutrim (autonomic nervous system drug)
    Adapin (antidepressant)
    Adderall (psychostimulant)
    Adderall XR (psychostimulant)
    ADH (antidiuretic hormone)
    Advil (anti-rheumatic)
    Akineton (biperiden) (anti-parkinsonism drug)
    Aldactone (diuretic)
    Aleve (anti-rheumatic)
    Allegron (antidepressant)
    alprazolam (benzodiazepine tranquilizer)
    Alurate (barbiturate)
    Amaphen (barbiturate)
    amantadine HCl (anti-parkinsonism agent)
    Ambien (sedative)
    Americet (barbiturate)
    amfebutamone HCl (antidepressant)
    aminophenylpyridone (tranquilizer)
    amitriptyline (antidepressant)

medications (drugs)
    amobarbital sodium (barbiturate)
    amoxapine (antidepressant)
    amphenidone (tranquilizer)
    amphetamine (psychostimulant)
    amylobarbitone (barbiturate)
    Amytal Sodium (barbiturate)
    Amytl nitrite vapors (inhalant)
    Anacin (with caffeine) (psychostimulant)
    Anacin-3 (with caffeine) (psychostimulant)
    Anafranil (tricyclic) (antidepressant)
    Anaprox (NSAID)
    Anoquan (barbiturate)
    Antabuse (alcohol deterrent)
    antidiuretic hormone (ADH)
    Antispasmodic (barbiturate)
    Antivert (meclizine) (anti-vertigo drug)
    Antrocol (barbiturate)
    Anx (tranquilizer)
    Anxanil (tranquilizer)
    Anzenet (tranquilizer)
    APF (arthritis pain formula)
    aprobarbital (barbiturate)
    Aquachloral (sedative)
    Aricept (cholinergic)
    Arco-Lase Plus (barbiturate)
    aripiprazole (neuroleptic/antipsychotic)
    Artane (trihexyphenidyl) (antispasmodic)
    arthritis pain formula (APF)
    Arthropan (NSAID)
    Ascriptin A/D (NSAID)

medications (drugs)
  Asendin (tricyclic)
    (antidepressant)
  aspirin (with butalbital and
    caffeine) (barbiturate)
  ataractics (tranquilizer)
  Atarax (tranquilizer)
  Atarax 100 (tranquilizer)
  Atenolol (analgesic for
    migraine)
medications (drugs)
  Ativan (benzodiazepine
    tranquilizer)
  atomoxetine (diagnostic
    agent)
  atomoxetine (Strattera)
    (contrast/diagnostic agent)
  Atretol (antimanic0
  atropine sulfate (anesthetic)
  Aventyl HCl (tricyclic)
    (antidepressant)
  Axocet (barbiturate)
  Axotal (with butalbital)
    (barbiturate)
  azacyclonol (tranquilizer)
  baclofen (muscle relaxant)
  Bancap HCl (analgesic)
  Banthine (antispasmodic)
  Barbidonna (barbiturate)
  Barbidonna-N (barbiturate)
  barbital (barbiturate)
  barbitone (barbiturate)
  Bayer aspirin (analgesic)
  Bellacane (barbiturate)
  Bellacane SR (barbiturate)
  belladonna and Opium
    (antispasmodic)
  Bellatal (barbiturate)
  Bellergal S (with P-B) (bar-
    biturate)
  Bel-Phen-Ergot SR (bar-
    biturate)
  benactyzine HCl (anti-
    depressant)
  Benadryl (anti-allergy
    drug)
  Bentyl (dicyclomine HCl)
    (antispasmodic)

medications (drugs)
  benzedrine (amphetamine/
    psychostimulant)
  benzodiapin (tranquilizer)
  benzodiazepine (tran-
    quilizer)
  benzperidol (tranquilizer)
  benzphetamine HCl
    (appetite depressant)
  benztropine mesylate (anti-
    parkinsonism agent)
  bethanechol chloride
    (cholinergic)
  Biocapton (psycho-
    stimulant)
  biperiden HCl (antiparkin-
    sonism agent)
  biphetamine (psychostim-
    ulant)
  Bontril (appetite depress-
    sant)
  bromide (sedative)
  bromine (sedative)
  brompheniramine (anti-
    emetic)
  Bucet/butalbital (barbitur-
    ate)
  buclizine (tranquilizer)
  Bufferin (analgesic)
  bufotenine (hallucinogen)
  Bunavail (opioid
    antagonist)
  Bupap (barbiturate)
  bupivacaine (anesthetic)
  Buprenex (antipyretic)
  buprenorphine HCl (antipy-
    retic)
  buprenorphine/naloxone
    (opioid antagonist)
  bupropion (antidepressant)
  bupropion/naloxone
    (opioid antagonist)
  BuSpar (anxiolytic)
  buspirone HCl (anxiolytic)
  buspirone (transdermal
    patch) (anxiolytic)
  butabarbital (barbiturate)

medications (drugs)
- butabarbital sodium (barbiturate)
- butabarbitone (barbiturate)
- butalbital (barbiturate)
- butalbital (with acetaminophen and caffeine) (barbiturate)
- butalbital (with aspirin and caffeine) (barbiturate)
- butalbital (with caffeine) (psychostimulant)
- Butalbital Compound (barbiturate)
- butaperazine (tranquilizer)
- Butex Forte (barbiturate)
- Butibel (barbiturate)
- Butisol sodium (barbiturate)
- butorphanol tartrate (analgesic)
- butriptyline (antidepressant)
- butyrophenone (tranquilizer)
- Cafatine with caffeine (psychostimulant)
- Cafatine PB (barbiturate)
- Cafergot with caffeine (psychostimulant)
- Cafergot PB (barbiturate)
- Cafetrate with caffeine (psychostimulant)
- caffeine (psychostimulant)
- calcium carbimide (antacid)
- Cama (salicylate)
- cannabis (hallucinogen)
- Captagon (psychostimulant)
- carbamazepine (anticonvulsant/antimanic)
- Carbatrol (anticonvulsant/antimanic)
- carbidopa (anticonvulsant)
- Carbolith (antimanic)
- carbromal (barbiturate)

medications (drugs)
- carisoprodol (muscle-tone depressant)
- carphenazine maleate (tranquilizer)
- Cassipa (opioid antagonist)
- Catatrol (antidepressant)
- cefadroxil (cephalosporin/antibiotic)
- Celexa (SSRI) (antidepressant)
- Celontin (anticonvulsant)
- Centrax (tranquilizer)
- Cephulac (psychotherapeutic agent)
- Chardonna-2 (barbiturate)
- chloral hydrate (sedative/hypnotic)
- chlordiazepoxide HCl (tranquilizer)
- chlordiazepoxide/ amitriptyline (antidepressant)
- chlorpromazine (tranquilizer)
- Cibalith-S (psychostimulant)
- citalopram hydrobromide (antidepressant)
- clobazam (sedative/hypnotic)
- clomipramine HCl (antidepressant)
- clonazepam (tranquilizer)
- clorazepate (tranquilizer)
- chlordiazepoxide (anxiolytic)
- chlordiazepoxide HCl (anxiolytic)
- chlormezanone (anxiolytic)
- Cholac (psychotherapeutic agent)
- Clindex (anxiolytic)
- clobazam (anxiolytic)
- clorazepate dipotassium (anxiolytic)
- clozapine (neuroleptic/antipsychotic)

medications (drugs)
    Clozaril (neuroleptic/ antipsychotic)
    Concerta (psychostimulant)
    Contrave (opioid antagonist)
    Cymbalta (SSRI) (antidepressant)
    Cyprolidol (antidepressant)
    Dalmane (tranquilizer/ sedative)
    Daytrana (patch) (psychostimulant)
    Depade (opioid antagonist)
    Depakote (anticonvulsant/ antimanic)
    Depakote ER (anticonvulsant/antimanic)
    Depitol (antimanic)
    desipramine HCl (antidepressant)
    Desoxyn (psychostimulant)
    Desyrel (antidepressant)
    Dexedrine (psychostimulant)
    dexmedetomidine HCl (sedative/hypnotic)
    dexmethylphenidate HCl (psychostimulant)
    dextroamphetamine (psychostimulant)
    DextroStat (psychostimulant)
    diazepam (tranquilizer/ anxiolytic)
    dichloralphenazone (sedative/hypnotic)
    Diprivan (sedative/ hypnotic)
    disulfiram (alcohol deterrent)
    divalproex sodium (barbiturate)
    Dizac (anxiolytic/sedative)
    Dolgic (barbiturate)
    Donna-Sed (barbiturate)
    Donnatal (barbiturate)

medications (drugs)
    Doral (tranquilizer/ sedative)
    dothiepin HCl (antidepressant)
    doxepin HCl (antidepressant)
    duloxetine (antidepressant)
    Duralith (barbiturate)
    Edronax (antidepressant)
    Effexor (SSRI) (antidepressant)
    Effexor XR (antidepressant)
    Elavil (tricyclic) (antidepressant)
    Emsam (antidepressant)
    Encyprate (antidepressant)
    Endep (antidepressant)
    Endolor (barbiturate)
    Enulose (psychotherapeutic agent)
    Epitol (barbiturate)
    Epival (barbiturate)
    Equagesic (anxiolytic/ sedative)
    Equanil (anxiolytic)
    escitalopram oxalate (antidepressant)
    Esgic (barbiturate)
    Eskalith (psychotropic/ antimanic)
    esketamine nasal spray (antidepressant)
    estazolam (sedative/ hypnotic)
    ethchlorvynol (sedative/ hypnotic)
    Etrafon/amitriptyline (antidepressant)
    Etrafon Forte (antidepressant)
    Etrafon/perphenazine (tranquilizer)
    etryptamine (antidepressant)
    E-Vista (tranquilizer)
    Evzio (opioid antagonist)

medications (drugs)
- Exparel (analgesic)
- Fanapt (antipsychotic)
- Femcet (barbiturate)
- Fentazine (tranquilizer)
- Fioricet (barbiturate)
- Fiorinal (barbiturate)
- Fiorpap (barbiturate)
- Fiortal (barbiturate)
- Fitton (psychostimulant)
- Fluanxol Depot injection (neuroleptic)
- flunitrazepam (tranquilizer)
- fluoxetine HCl (antidepressant)
- flupenthixol (neuroleptic/antipsychotic)
- fluphenazine decanoate (tranquilizer)
- fluphenazine enanthat (antipsychotic)
- fluphenazine HCl (antipsychotic)
- flurazepam HCl (tranquilizer/sedative)
- fluvoxamine maleate (antidepressant)
- Focalin (psychostimulant)
- Folergot-DF (barbiturate)
- fosphenytoin sodium (anticonvulsant)
- Frisium (anxiolytic/sedative)
- gabapentin (anticonvulsant)
- Gamma OH (antidepressant/sedative)
- Gen-Xene (tranquilizer/anxiolytic)
- Geodon (neuroleptic/antipsychotic)
- glutethimide (sedative/hypnotic)
- Gustase (barbiturate)
- halazepam (tranquilizer/anxiolytic)
- Halcion (tranquilizer)
- Haldol Injection (tranquilizer)

medications (drugs)
- Haldol decanoate (tranquilizer)
- haloperidol (tranquilizer)
- haloperidol decanoate (tranquilizer)
- haloperidol lactate (tranquilizer)
- heptachlor (chlorinated hydrocarbon)
- hydroxyzine HCl (tranquilizer/anxiolytic)
- hydroxyzine pamoate (tranquilizer/anxiolytic)
- Hyosophen (barbiturate)
- Hyzine-50 (tranquilizer)
- iloperidone (neuroleptic/antipsychotic)
- imipramine HCl (antidepressant)
- imipramine pamoate (antidepressant)
- Imovane (sedative/hypnotic)
- iproniazid (antidepressant)
- isocarboxazid (antidepressant)
- Isocet (barbiturate)
- Isocom (sedative/hypnotic)
- Isopap (sedative/hypnotic)
- Janimine Oral (antidepressant)
- Kadian (opioid)
- Kalcinate (electrolytic agent)
- Kemadrin (antiparkinsonism agent)
- ketamine (anesthetic)
- Ketanest (antidepressant)
- Ketoprofen (anti-rheumatic agent)
- Klonopin (tranquilizer)
- lactulose (psychotherapeutic agent)
- lamotrigine (succinimide)
- Lanorinal (barbiturate)
- Largactil (tranquilizer)
- Largon (sedative/hypnotic)

medications (drugs)
    Laroxyl (antidepressant)
    levacecarnine (neuroleptic)
    Levoprome (sedative/
      hypnotic)
    Levsin PB (barbiturate)
    Lexapro (SSRI) (antide-
      pressant)
    Librax (psychotropic/
      anxiolytic)
    Libritabs (tranquilizer/
      anxiolytic)
    Librium (tranquilizer/
      anxiolytic)
    Limbitrol-amitriptyline
      (antidepressant)
    Limbitrol-chlordiazepoxide
      (tranquilizer)
    Limbitrol DS 10-25 (anti-
      depressant/anxiolytic)
    lisdexamfetamine
      dimesylate (psychostimu-
      lant)
    Lithane (psychotropic/
      antimanic)
    lithium carbonate (psycho-
      tropic/antimanic)
    lithium citrate (psychotro-
      pic/antimanic)
    Lithizine (psychotropic/
      antidepressant)
    Lithobid (psychotropic/
      antimanic)
    Lithonate (psychotropic/
      antimanic)
    Lithotabs (psychotropic/
      antimanic)
    lorazepam (tranquilizer/
      anxiolytic)
    Lotusate (barbiturate)
    Loxapac (neuroleptic/anti-
      psychotic)
    loxapine HCl (neuroleptic/
      antipsychotic)
    loxapine succinate (neuro-
      leptic/antipsychotic)
    Loxitane C (neuroleptic/
      antipsychotic)

medications (drugs)
    Loxitane IM (neuroleptic/
      antipsychotic)
    Ludiomil (tricyclic) (anti-
      depressant)
    Lufyllin-EPG (barbiturate)
    Luminal Sodium (barbitur-
      ate)
    Luvox (SSRI) (antide-
      pressant)
    Manerix (antidepressant)
    Mangesic (barbiturate)
    MAO inhibitor (antidepres-
      sant)
    maprotiline HCl (antide-
      pressant)
    Marplan (MAOI) (antide-
      pressant)
    Marsilid (antidepressant)
    Marten-Tab (barbiturate)
    Mebanazine (antidepres-
      sant)
    Mebaral (barbiturate)
    medazepam (tranquilizer)
    Medigesic (barbiturate)
    Mellaril (tranquilizer)
    Mellaril S (tranquilizer)
    meloxicam (anti-
      inflammatory)
    mephobarbital (barbiturate)
    meprobamate
      (tranquilizer/sedative)
    mesoridazine (tranquilizer)
    Metadate CD (psychostim-
      ulant)
    Metadate ER (psychostim-
      ulant)
    methamphetamine (psycho-
      stimulant)
    methotrimeprazine (seda-
      tive)
    Methylin (psychostimulant)
    methylmorphine (opioid)
    methylphenidate (psycho-
      stimulant)
    metronidazole (anti-
      infective)

medications (drugs)
- Micrainin (anxiolytic/sedative)
- midazolam HCl (sedative)
- Midchlor (sedative)
- Midrin (sedative)
- Migratine (sedative)
- Miltown (anxiolytic)
- Miltown 600 (anxiolytic)
- mirtazepine (antidepressant)
- Mitran Oral (antianxiolytic)
- Moban (neuroleptic/antipsychotic)
- moclobemide (antidepressant)
- modafinil (psychostimulant)
- Modecate (neuroleptic/antipsychotic)
- Mogadon (sedative)
- molindone HCl (neuroleptic/antipsychotic)
- moperone (tranquilizer)
- Mudrane (barbiturate)
- Mysoline (anticonvulsant)
- nalmefene HCl (analeptic stimulant)
- naloxone HCl (opioid antagonist)
- naltrexone (opioid antagonist)
- Narcan (opioid antagonist)
- Nardil (MAOI) (antidepressant)
- Navane (neuroleptic/antipsychotic)
- nefazodone HCl (antidepressant)
- Nembutal (barbiturate)
- Nembutal Sodium (barbiturate)
- Neuramate (anxiolytic)
- Nialamide (antidepressant)
- nicotine nasal spray (tobacco)
- Nicotrol NS (tobacco)

medications (drugs)
- nitrazepam (tranquilizer/sedative)
- Norpramine (tricyclic) (antidepressant)
- nortriptyline (antidepressant)
- Nozinan (neuroleptic/antipsychotic)
- olanzepine (neuroleptic/antimanic)
- Orap (neuroleptic/antipsychotic)
- Ormazine (neuroleptic/antipsychotic)
- oxazepam (tranquilizer/sedative)
- oxycodone/naltrexone (opioid antagonist)
- oxypertine (antidepressant)
- Pamelor (tricyclic) (antidepressant)
- Paral (sedative)
- paraldehyde (sedative)
- Parnate (MAOI) (antidepressant)
- paroxetine HCl (antidepressant)
- paroxetine mesylate (antidepressant)
- Paxarel (sedative)
- Paxil (SSRI) (antidepressant)
- Paxil CR (antidepressant)
- Paxipam (tranquilizer)
- pentobarbital (barbiturate)
- pentobarbital sodium (barbiturate)
- pentobarbitone (barbiturate)
- pericyazine (tranquilizer)
- Permitil Oral (tranquilizer)
- perphenazine (tranquilizer)
- Pertofrane (antidepressant)
- Pexeva (SSRI) (antidepressant)
- phenaglycodol (tranquilizer)

medications (drugs)
  phencyclidine (I.V. anesthetic)
  phenelzine sulfate (antidepressant)
  pheniprazine (antidepressant)
  phenobarbitone (barbiturate)
  Phenobel-S (barbiturate)
  phenobarbital (barbiturate)
  phenobarbital sodium (barbiturate)
  phenothiazine (tranquilizer)
  Phrenilin (barbiturate)
  Phrenilin Forte (barbiturate)
  pimozide (neuroleptic/antipsychotic)
  Placidyl (sedative)
  Plegicil (tranquilizer)
  prazepam (tranquilizer/sedative)
  Precedex (sedative)
  Prexa (SSRI) (antidepressant)
  primidone (anticonvulsant)
  procalmidol (tranquilizer)
  prochlorperazine (antidepressant)
  Prolixin Oral (tranquilizer)
  Promacet (barbiturate)
  promazine (tranquilizer)
  propiomazine HCl (sedative)
  propofol (sedative)
  ProSom (sedative)
  Prothiaden (antidepressant)
  Prothipendyl (tranquilizer)
  protriptyline HCl (antidepressant)
  Prozac (SSRI) (antidepressant)
  Pyridium Plus (barbiturate)
  Quaalude (sedative/hypnotic)
  Quadrinal (barbiturate)

medications (drugs)
  quazepam (tranquilizer/sedative)
  quetiapine fumarate (neuroleptic/antimanic)
  Quiess (tranquilizer/anxiolytic)
  quinalbarbitone (barbiturate)
  Raudixin (antihypertensive)
  rauwolfia serpentina (neuroleptic/antipsychotic)
  reboxetine mesylate (antidepressant)
  Redux (weight loss agent)
  Remeron (antidepressant)
  Reminyl (cholinergic)
  remoxipride (neuroleptic/antipsychotic)
  Repan (barbiturate)
  Repan CF (barbiturate)
  Reposans-10 Oral (anxiolytic)
  Reserpine (neuroleptic/antipsychotic)
  Restoril (tranquilizer/sedative)
  Revex (opioid)
  ReVia (opioid antagonist)
  Risperdal Oral (neuroleptic/antipsychotic)
  risperidone (neuroleptic/antipsychotic)
  Ritalin LA (psychostimulant)
  Ritalin SK (psychostimulant)
  Ritalin SR (psychostimulant)
  ritanserin (psychotherapeutic agent)
  Sabril (antiepileptic)
  Saphris (antipsychotic/antimanic)
  Saroten (antidepressant)
  secobarbital sodium (barbiturate)

medications (drugs)
- Seconal Sodium (barbiturate)
- Sedapap (barbiturate)
- selegiline (antiparkinsonism drug)
- Serafem (psychotherapeutic agent)
- Serax (anxiolytic/sedative)
- Sereen (tranquilizer)
- Serentil (neuroleptic/antipsychotic)
- Seroquel (neuroleptic/antipsychotic)
- serotonin-specific reuptake inhibitor (SSRI)
- sertraline HCl (antidepressant)
- Serzone (antidepressant)
- sildenafil (vasodilator)
- Sinequan Oral (antidepressant)
- sodium oxybate (sedative/hypnotic)
- Solfoton (barbiturate)
- Sonata (sedative/hypnotic)
- Sparine (neuroleptic/antipsychotic)
- Spasmolin (barbiturate)
- spiperone (tranquilizer)
- Spravata (antidepressant)
- SSRI (selective serotonin reuptake inhibitor)
- Stelazine Oral (antipsychotic/anxiolytic)
- Strattera (diagnostic agents)
- Suboxone (opioid antagonist)
- sulpiride (antipsychotic)
- Surmontil (antidepressant)
- Susano (barbiturate)
- Symbyax (Prozac & Zyprexa) (antidepressant)
- synthetic delta-9-THC (cannabin/antiemetic)
- talbutal (barbiturate)
- Talwin Nx (analgesic)

medications (drugs)
- tanezumab (analgesic)
- Tegretol (anticonvulsant/antimanic)
- Tegretol XR (anticonvulsant/antimanic)
- temazepam (sedative/hypnotic)
- Tencon (barbiturate)
- thiazesim (antidepressant)
- thioridizine (neuroleptic/antipsychotic)
- thiothixene HCl (neuroleptic/antipsychotic)
- thiothixene (neuroleptic/antipsychotic)
- Thixol
- Thorazine (neuroleptic/antipsychotic)
- tizanidine HCl (CNS depressant)
- Tofranil Oral (tricyclic) (antidepressant)
- Tofranil-PM (tricyclic) (antidepressant)
- Topamax (anticonvulsant)
- topiramate (anticonvulsant)
- tramadol (analgesic)
- Trancopal (anxiolytic)
- Tranxene (anticonvulsant/anxiolytic)
- Tranxene SD (anticonvulsant/anxiolytic)
- tranylcypromine (MAOI) (antidepressant)
- trazodone HCl (antidepressant)
- Triad (barbiturate)
- Triavil (antidepressant)
- Triavil 4-50 (antidepressant)
- triazolam (sedative/hypnotic)
- tricyclic antidepressants
- trifluoperazine HCl (neuroleptic/antipsychotic)
- triflupcridol (tranquilizer)

medications (drugs)
    triflupromazine HCl (neuroleptic/antipsychotic)
    Trilafon (neuroleptic/antipsychotic)
    trimethadione (anticonvulsant)
    trimipramine (antidepressant)
    trimipramine maleate (antidepressant)
    Triptan (anti-migraine agent)
    Troxyca ER (opioid antagonist)
    Truvada (antiviral drug - AIDS prevention)
    tryptizol (antidepressant)
    Tuinal (barbiturate)
    Ultram (analgesic)
    Uendex (antiviral drug – AIDS prevention)
    Unisom (sedative/hypnotic)
    Valium (anxiolytic)
    Valium injection (anxiolytic)
    valproate sodium (salicylate)
    Vesprin (neuroleptic/antipsychotic)
    venlafaxine (antidepressant)
    Versed (sedative/hypnotic)
    Vestra (antidepressant)
    Vicodin (narcotic analgesic)
    vigabatrin (antiepileptic)
    viloxazine (antidepressant)
    Vistacon-50 (anxiolytic)
    Vistaject-25 (tranquilizer)
    Vistaject-50 (tranquilizer)
    Vistaril (tranquilizer)
    Vistazine-50 (anxiolytic)
    Vivactil (tricyclic) (antidepressant)
    Vivitrol (opioid antagonist)
    Vyvanse (ADHD agent)
    Wellbutrin (antidepressant)

medications (drugs)
    Wellbutrin SR (antidepressant)
    Wolfina
    Wygesic (narcotic analgesic)
    Xanax (anxiolytic/antipanic)
    Xyrem (sedative/hypnotic)
    zaleplon (sedative/hypnotic)
    Zanaflex (CNS depressant)
    Zetran Injection (tranquilizer)
    zidovudine (antiviral drug – AIDS prevention)
    Zilretta (injectable analgesic)
    ziprasidone HCl (neuroleptic/antipsychotic)
    ziprasidone mesylate (neuroleptic/antipsychotic)
    zolmaril (neuroleptic/antipsychotic)
    Zoloft (antidepressant/antipanic)
    zolpidem tartrate (sedative/hypnotic)
    Zonalon topical cream (anti-pruritic)
    zonisamide (anticonvulsant)
    zopiclone (sedative/hypnotic)
    Zubsolv (opioid antagonist)
    Zyprexa (antipsychotic/antimanic)
medication side effect, extrapyramidal
medication-specific treatment (see *psychotropic agents*)
medication trial, placebo
medicine
    behavioral
    concepts in
    family
    history of

medius
    musculus scalenus
    musculus constrictor
      pharyngis
medius meatus, nasi
medulla oblongata
medullary canal
"Meg" (street name, cannabis)
Mega Test, The
megalomania (overvaluation of
  self)
"Megg" (street name, cannabis
  cigarette)
"Meggie" (street name, cannabis)
mel (tone pitch unit)
melancholic features
"mellow yellow" (street name,
  lysergic acid
  diethylamide/LSD)
melomania (music/song)
member of society, marginal
members, family
membrane
    basilar
    drum
    mucous
    Reissner's
    vestibular
membrane ion channel
membranes, lithium's action on
membranous labyrinth
membranous laryngitis
memories, false
memories of childhood trauma
Memorization Test (15-Items)
memory
    amnesia loss of
    anterograde loss of
    auditory
    body
    disturbance in
    effect of trauma on
    figural
    gaps in
    loss of biographical
    poor
    recognition
    recurrence of a

memory
    retrograde loss of
    retrospective gaps in
    rote
    semantic
    sequence
    sequence of sounds and
    sequential
    verbal
    visual-spatial
memory ability, impaired
Memory Assessment Scales
  (MAS)
memory difficulties
memory encoding, impairment of
  new
memory for digits test
memory gaps
memory impairment
    reversible
    severe
memory loss
memory problems
memory questionnaire, everyday
memory recall
memory retention
memory scale
memory sequencing tests
memory span, auditory
memory span tests
memory test
    draw a picture from
    immediate
    logical
    recent
    remote
memory tests *(see also* tests)
men, gay
Meniere's disease
meningitis
    bacterial
    cryptococcal
    herpes simplex virus
    herpes zoster
    syphilitic
    viral
meningoencephalitis viral
  encephalitis, diphasic

meniscus (pl. menisci)
menses, irregular
menstrual bleeding, excessive
menstrual cycle
    follicular phase of the
    late luteal phase of
Menstrual Distress Questionnaire (MDQ)
menstruation, pain during
mental abilities test *(see also* tests)
mental activity, stream of
mental alertness test *(see also* tests)
mental capacity, evaluation of
mental changes
mental competency
mental condition, problems related to a
mental control, pattern of
"mental defect"
mental deficit
mental deterioration
    irradiation-induced
    radiation-induced
mental development screen *(see also* tests)
mental disability
mental disorder(s)
    anxiety-related
    biology of major
    co-occurring
    delirium-related
    dementia-related
    depression-related
    exacerbated symptoms of a preexisting
    hypersomnia related to another
    insomnia related to another
    interventions for
    non-substance-induced
    other specified, due to another medical condition (F06.8)
    primary
    substance-induced

mental disorder(s)
    unspecified, due to another medical condition (F09)
    wandering associated with a (Z91.83)
mental disorder affecting GMC
Mental Disorders Manual *(see* Diagnostic and Statistical Manual of Mental Disorders-5 DSM-5)
mental disturbance in children
mental faculty
mental function in the elderly *(see also* tests)
mental health resources
mental health services, community
mental hygiene
mental inhibition(s) level of
mental obtundation
mental processes
mental scotoma
mental state, transient
mental status
    altered
    disordered
mental status changes
mental status examination, longitudinal
Mental Status Questionnaire
mental status test
    mini
    similarities
mental syndrome, organic
mental tests *(see also* tests)
mentalize
mentally, obtunded
mentally disordered offenders
mentally handicapped, educationally (EMH)
mentally ill, commitment of
mentally retarded
    education of
    educationally (EMR)
mentation
    change in
    normal

mentation rate
mentulomania (counseling/mentoring)
MEP (multimodality evoked potential) brain test
"merchandise" (re: drugs)
mercurial behavior
merinthophobia
"merk" (street name, cocaine)
Merrill-Palmer Scale
"mescal" (street name, mescaline)
mescaline (street names)
    bad seed
    beans
    blue caps
    britton
    buttons
    cactus
    cactus buttons
    cactus head
    chief
    half moon
    hikori
    hikuli
    hyatari
    love flipping (mescaline & MDMA)
    love trip (mescaline & MDMA)
    mesc
    mescal
    mese
    mezc
    moon
    nubs
    peyote
    seni
    snackies (MDMA adulterated with mescaline)
    topi
    tops
"mese" (street name, mescaline)
mesioclusion of teeth
mesioversion of teeth
mesmeromania (hypnosis)
message inventory
messages
    dichotic
    diotic
messages integration, competing
messengers
    chemical
    lithium's action on first
    lithium's action on second
"messorole" (street name, cannabis)
MET (Minimum Essentials Test)
meta-model
meta-outcome
meta-person
metabolic abnormalities
metabolic acidosis
metabolic alkalosis
metabolic amyloidosis
metabolic conditions, dementia due to
metabolic derangements
metabolic disturbance
metabolic rate
metabolic tremor
metabolic volume depletion
metabolics, neurotransmitter
metabolism
    dopamine
    inborn errors of
    lipoid
    mineral
    myelin
    neuronal
    plasma protein
    porphyrin
    purine
    pyrimidine
metachromatic leukodystrophy
metal screen, heavy
metalanguage
metalinguistics
metallurgic syndrome
metaphor (figure of speech)
metaphorical speech
metathesis
meteorophobia

Psychiatric Words and Phrases

meter
- vibration
- volume unit (VU meter)

"meth head" (re: methamphetamine user)

"meth monster" (re: methamphetamine user)

methadone (street names)
- amidone
- chocolate chip cookies (MDMA with heroin or methadone)
- fizzies

methamphetamine (street names)
- 5-way (heroin/cocaine/meth/Rohypnol/alcohol)
- batak
- Bathtub crank
- batu
- beanies
- biker coffee (methamphetamine mixed with coffee)
- black
- Black Beauty
- blade (crystal methamphetamine)
- bling bling
- blue devils
- blue meth
- boo
- box labs (small labs that make meth)
- brown
- cha
- chicken feed
- Christmas tree
- Christmas tree meth (using Draino for color)
- chrome (crystal methamphetamine)
- cinnamon
- clear
- cook/cooker (meth manufacturer)
- CR
- crank

methamphetamine (street names)
- crankster (user or maker of meth)
- crink
- cris
- Cristina
- croak
- crush and rush (re: manufacturing process)
- crypto
- crystal
- crystal glass (crystal shards of meth)
- crystal meth
- crystals
- desocsins
- desogtion
- domes
- dropping (wrapping meth in bread & eating it)
- elbows (1 lb of methamphetamine)
- fast
- fire (crack and methamphetamine)
- gangster (user/maker of methamphetamine)
- geep
- geeter
- get-go
- getting glassed (snorting methamphetamine)
- glass
- go-fast
- granulated orange
- half elbows (1/2 lb of methamphetamine)
- hanyak (smokable methamphetamine)
- hironpon (smokable methamphetamine)
- hiropon (smokable methamphetamine)
- holiday meth (green colored meth using Draino)
- hot ice (smokable methamphetamine)

methamphetamine (street names)
- hot railing (heat, then inhale meth)
- hot rolling (liquefying meth to inhale it)
- hugs and kisses (methamphetamine and MDMA)
- ice (methamphetamine; smokable methamphetamine)
- jet fuel (methamphetamine combined with PCP)
- Kaksonjae
- L.A. glass (smokable methamphetamine)
- L.A. ice (smokable methamphetamine
- lemon drop (meth with a dull yellow tint)
- lithium (better grade of methamphetamine)
- lithium (skin lesions due to meth abuse)
- load of laundry
- Maui-wowie
- meth
- meth head (regular methamphetamine user)
- meth monster (violent reaction to meth)
- meth speedball (methamphetamine and heroin)
- methlies Quik
- methnecks (methamphetamine addicts)
- Mexican crack
- Mexican speedballs (crack and methamphetamine)
- Nazimeth
- OZs
- P and P (methamphetamine, MDMA, and Viagra)
- Paper (1/10 dosage unit of methamphetamine)

methamphetamine (street names)
- Peanut butter
- Pink
- Pink elephants
- Pink hearts
- Quartz (smokable methamphetamine)
- quill
- Red
- Redneck cocaine
- Rock
- Schmiz
- Scootie
- Shabu (powder cocaine and methamphetamine)
- Sketch
- soap
- soap dope (methamphetamine with a pinkish tint)
- spackle
- Sparkle (methamphetamine with a shiny appearance)
- Speckled birds
- Speed
- Speed freak (habitual user of meth)
- spoosh
- Stove top (crystal methamphetamine)
- Strawberry Quik (strawberry-flavored meth)
- super ice (smokable methamphetamine)
- Super X (MDMA and methamphetamine)
- Superlab (hidden labs making meth in 24 hrs.)
- tic
- tick tick
- twisters
- wash
- water
- wet
- white cross
- work
- working man's cocaine

methamphetamine (street names)
    X
    ya ba (pure, powerful form
      of methamphetamine)
    yaba
    yellow bam
    yellow jackets
    yellow powder
methamphetamine abuse
methaqualone (street names)
    714s
    bandits
    Beiruts
    Blou Bulle
    disco biscuits
    Ewings
    flamingos
    flowers
    genuines
    Karachi (heroin/phenobar-
      bital/methaqualone)
    Lemmon 714
    lemons
    Lennons
    lovers
    ludes
    Mandies
    Qua
    Quaaludes
    quack
    quad
    Randy Mandies
    soaper
    sopes
    sporos
    Vitamin Q
    wagon wheels
methaqualone compound
methatriol (injectable steroid)
methcathinone (street names)
    bathtub speed
    Cadillac express
    cat
    crank
    ephedrone
    gagers
    gaggers
    go-fast

methcathinone (street names)
    goob
    Qaat
    slick superspeed
    sniff (inhaling
      methcathinone)
    Somali tea
    star
    stat
    The C
    tweeker
    wild cat
    wonder star
method
    acoupedic
    acoustic
    analytic
    artificial
    assessment
    auditory
    bisensory
    breathing
    chewing
    combined
    consonant-injection
    cross-consonant injection
    formal
    French
    German
    informal
    inhalation
    injection
    key word
    kinesthetic
    manual
    nonpurging
    numerical cipher
    optimal
    oral-aural
    plateau
    plosive-injection
    poor
    preferred
    purging
    review
    shadowing
    sniff
    synthetic

method
    systematic
    verbotonal
    visual
method of administration
method of ascertainment
method of assessment
method of aural rehabilitation
    bimodal
    natural
method of defining criteria
method of esophageal speech
    breathing
    inhalation
    injection
    sniff
    suction
    swallow
method of inhaling intoxicating vapors
method of monitoring
method of purging
method of rehabilitation, acoupedic
method of retrieval
method of weight loss
method sine wave, simultaneous
method threshold shift
methods of esophageal speech
methomania (alcoholic beverages)
methylene chloride
methylenedioxymethamphetamine *(see also* MDMA, street names*)*
methylmorphine (street name, codeine)
methylphenidate (Ritalin) (street names)
    crackers (re: Ritalin/Talwin combined injections simulate heroin/cocaine effect)
    one and ones (re: Ritalin/Talwin combined injections simulate heroin/cocaine effect)
    pharming (re: consuming a mixture of prescription substances)

methylphenidate (street names)
    poor man's heroin (re: Ritalin/Talwin combined injections simulate heroin/cocaine effect)
    set (re: Ritalin/Talwin combined injections simulate heroin/cocaine effect)
    speedball (re: Ritalin mixed with heroin)
    Ts and Rits (re: Talwin/Ritalin combined injections simulate heroin/cocaine effect)
    Ts and Rs (re: Talwin/Ritalin combined injections simulate heroin/cocaine effect)
    vitamin R (Ritalin)
    West Coast (Ritalin)
methyltestosterone (oral steroid)
methylxanthime-induced postural tremor
meticulously detailed plan
metonymy (figure of speech)
metromania (incessant verse writing)
Metropolitan Achievement Tests (MAT)
Metropolitan Language Instructional Test
Metropolitan Readiness Tests (MRT)
"Mexican brown" (street name, cannabis; heroin)
"Mexican horse" (street name, heroin)
"Mexican mud" (street name, heroin)
"Mexican mushroom" (street name, psilocybin/psilocin)
"Mexican red" (street name, cannabis)
"Mexican reds" (street name, barbiturate)
Meyer-Kendall Assessment Survey (MKAS)

"mezc" (street name, mescaline)
MHACA (Mental Health Association of Central Australia)
MHAQ (Modified Health Assessment Questionnaire)
MI (mentally impaired)
Michigan English Language Assessment Battery
Michigan Picture Inventory
Michigan Picture Test Revised
Michigan Screening Profile of Parenting
"Mickey Finn" (street name, barbiturate)
"Mickey's" (street name, barbiturate)
microcephalus
microcephaly
microcheilia
microglossia
micrognathia
micromania self-depreciation)
microphone
    directional
    nondirectional
    omnidirectional
    probe tube
microphone measurements, probe
microphonia, cochlear
microphonics
microscopic examination
microstomia
microtia
MICS (Mother/Infant Communication Screening)
mid vowel
midbrain deafness
midbrain dysfunction
midbrain matter
middle childhood, examination of educational readiness
middle constrictor muscle of pharynx
middle ear
middle ear muscle reflex
middle frontal sulcus
middle insomnia

middle latency responses
middle pharyngeal constrictor
"midnight oil" (street name, opium)
"Mighty Joe Young" (street name, barbiturate)
"mighty mezz" (street name, cannabis cigarette)
"Mighty Quinn" (street name, lysergic acid diethylamide/LSD)
migraine
    classical
    common
migraine aura
migraine headache
    acute confusional
    aphasic
    basilar
    bilateral
    circumstantial
    classical
    cluster
    common
    complicated
    confusional
    familial
    hemiparesthetic
    hemiplegic
    late-life
    ocular
    paroxysmal
    recurrent
    seasonal
    tension
    unilateral
    vestibular
migrainous syndrome
migration, cultural adjustment following
Milan Multiaxial Clinical Inventory (MCMI)
mild ataxia
mild bipolar I disorder
mild disability
mild hearing impairment
mild hearing loss
mild insomnia

mild neurocognitive disorder
mild sleep loss
milestone scales *(see also* tests)
military combat
military deployment, personal history of (Z91.82)
Military Environment Inventory
military psychiatry
military psychology
Mill Hill Vocabulary Scale
Miller Assessment for Preschoolers
Miller-Yoder Language Comprehension Test
milligram catch, CBD oil
Millon Adolescent Clinical Inventory (MACI)
Millon Adolescent Personality Inventory
Millon Behavioral Health Inventory (MBHI)
Millon Clinical Multiaxial Inventory
MILMD (Management Inventory on Leadership: Motivation and Decision-Making)
Milton-model
mimetic addiction, sympathic
mimic speech
mimics of schizophrenia
mind
    loss of control of the
    psychoanalysis and the
mind/body dualism
mind control
"mind detergent" (street name, lysergic acid diethylamide/LSD)
mind going blank
mind reading
mindedness, psychological
mineral metabolism
Mini Inventory of Right Brain Injury (MIRBI)
mini mental status test
"minibennie" (street name, amphetamine)
MINICROS (contralateral routing of signals)
minimal articulation competence *(see also* tests)
minimal contrasts
minimal pair
minimal personal hygiene
minimal prosody of speech
minimal residual symptoms
minimal role
minimization of emotional detail
minimum acceptable skill
minimum audible field (MAF)
minimum audible pressure (MAP)
Minimum Auditory Capabilities (MAC) Test
Minimum Essentials Test (MET)
minimum self-support
Minnesota Clerical Assessment Battery
Minnesota Clerical Test
Minnesota Importance Questionnaire
Minnesota Infant Development Inventory
Minnesota Manual Dexterity Test
Minnesota Multiphasic Personality Inventory (MMPI)
Minnesota Multiphasic Personality Inventory-- Adolescent (MMPI-A)
Minnesota Preschool Scales
Minnesota Rate of Manipulation Tests
Minnesota Test for Differential Diagnosis of Aphasia
Minnesota Test of Aphasia
minor, musculus pectoralis
minor depressive disorder
minor image-distorting level
minor stimuli, angry reaction to
"mint leaf" (street name, phencyclidine/PCP)
"mint weed" (street name, phencyclidine/PCP)
"mira" (street name, opium)
MIRBI (Mini Inventory of Right Brain Injury)

mirror focus
mirroring, cross-over
misattribute
misattribution
misconceptions, illusionary
misdirected urinary stream
Miskimins Self-Goal-Other Discrepancy Scale
misophobia
misperception, sleep state
misplaced objects test
mispronunciation
"missile basing" (street name, crack liquid and phencyclidine/PCP)
"mission" (re: crack acquisition)
Missouri Kindergarten Inventory of Developmental Skills
Missouri Occupational Card Sort
"mist" (street name, crack smoke; phencyclidine/PCP)
"mister blue" (street name, morphine)
MIT (Motor Impersistence Test)
mitigated echolalia
mitral valve insufficiency
mixed anxiety/depressed mood, adjustment disorder with
mixed anxiety-depressive disorder
mixed aphasia, transcortical
mixed cerebral dominance
mixed deafness
mixed episode
mixed features
mixed laterality
mixed manic-depressive-like episodes
mixed-mood state
mixed nasality voice disorder
mixed presentation
mixed receptive-expressive language disorder
mixed sedative
mixed sleep apnea
mixed symptom picture with perceptual disturbances
mixed type delusions
mixed type of symptom

mixed type schizophrenia
mixture approach
mixture theory, language
"MJ" (street name, cannabis)
MKAS (Meyer-Kendall Assessment Survey)
MLB (Monaural Loudness Balance) Test
MLQ (Multifactor Leadership Questionnaire)
MLR (mean length of response)
MLU (mean length of utterance)
MMPI (Minnesota Multiphasic Personality Inventory)
MMPI-A (Minnesota Multiphasic Personality Inventory--Adolescent)
MMTIC (Murphy-Meisgeier Type Indicator for Children)
"MO" (street name, cannabis)
moaning
mobility disability
Mobility Index *(see also* tests)
mobilization, stapes
Mobius syndrome
modal auxiliary verb
modal frequency
modal operators
modal tone
modal verb
modality
    auditory
    auditory sensory
    gustatory sensory
    language
    olfactory sensory
    sensory
    tactile sensory
    therapeutic
    visual sensory
modality test
"modams" (street name, cannabis)
mode, vocal
model
    biopsychosocial
    categorical
    dimensional

model of schizophrenia, 3-factor dimensional
modeled (not mottled) behavior
modeling
models, psychological
moderate ataxia
moderate bipolar I disorder
moderate depression
moderate drinking pattern
moderate hearing impairment
moderate hearing loss
moderate one's drinking pattern, to
moderate substance use disorder
moderate to severe (m/s)
moderately severe hearing impairment
moderately severe hearing loss
Modern Language Aptitude Test
Modern Occupational Skills Test (MOST)
modes of action
modification
    active
    behavior
    carbonyl
    interference
Modified Health Assessment Questionnaire (MHAQ)
modified mastoidectomy
modified self-report measure of social adjustment
Modified Vygotsky Concept Formation Test
modifier
    nonrestrictive
    restrictive
modulated affect
modulation
    amplitude (AM)
    impaired affect
modules of auditory discrimination (see also tests)
"Mohasky" (street name, cannabis)
"Mojo" (street name, cocaine; heroin)
mokita

molar
    first deciduous
    second deciduous
molar teeth
molds, ear
molecular neurobiology
"Molly" (re: purest form of MDMA)
moment, product
monaural hearing aid
Monaural Loudness Balance (MLB) Test
monauralis diplacusis
Mondini deafness
monetary value
mongolism
monitored live voice audiometry
monitoring
    behavioral
    method of
monitoring audiometry
Monitoring Basic Skills Progress
"monkey" (re: drug dependency)
"monkey" (street name, cocaine-laced cigarette)
"monkey dust" (street name, phencyclidine/PCP)
"monkey tranquilizer" (street name, phencyclidine/PCP)
monoamine oxidase inhibitor agent(s) (MOI agents)
monoamine oxidase inhibitor-serotonergic agent(s)
monoamine oxidase inhibitor-tricyclic agent(s)
monoamine oxidase inhibitors (MOI) for mood disorders
monocular visual loss
monocyclic antidepressant
monogamous relationship
monologue, collective
monomania (solitude)
monoplegia
"monos" (street name, cocaine-laced cigarette)
monosyllabic processes
monosyllabic speech

monosyllabic whole word
    repetition
monosyllabic word
monothematic delusion
monotone
"monte" (street name, cannabis)
month of year test
month test, day of
"mooca/moocah" (street name,
    cannabis)
mood
    abnormal
    adjustment disorder with
        depressed
    changes in
    cranky
    dejected
    depressed
    deterioration of
    elevated
    erratic
    euphoric
    euthymic
    expansive
    imperative
    indicative
    lability of
    marked shift in
    markedly depressed
    nondepressed
    prominent irritable
    sad
    subjunctive
mood-altering substance
mood assessment scale *(see also
    tests)*
mood changes, unpredictable
mood-congruent hallucination
mood-congruent psychotic
    features
mood disorder(s)
    alpha-methyldopa-induced
    amitriptyline-induced
    amphetamine-induced
    carbamazepine for
    clozapine for
    cocaine-induced
    electroconvulsive therapy for

mood disorder(s)
    electroconvulsive therapy-
        induced
    gender differences in
    light therapy-induced
    lithium for
    neuroleptics for
    substance-induced
    unknown substance-induced
mood disorder with catatonic
    features
mood disorder with psychotic
    features, primary
mood disorder with rapid cycling
mood disorder with seasonal
    pattern
mood disturbance
    fluctuating
    predominant
mood episode
    most recent depressed
    most recent hypomanic
    most recent manic
    most recent mixed
    most recent unspecified
    recurrent
mood-incongruent hallucination
mood-incongruent psychotic
    features
mood stabilizer agents:
    anticonvulsants
        carbamazepine
        Depakote
        Divalproex sodium
        gabapentin
        Lamictal
        lamotrigine
        Neurontin
        oxcarbazepine
        Tegretol
        Topamax
        Topiramate
        Trileptal
        valproic acid
mood stabilizer agents:
    psychotropics, benactyzine
        Eskalith
        lithium carbonate

mood stabilizer agents:
   psychotropics, benactyzine
      lithium citrate
      Lithobid
mood swings
mood symptomatology
mood symptoms, prominent
mood symptoms in schizophrenia
"moon" (street name, mescaline)
"moonrock" (street name, crack and heroin)
"moonstone" (re: dealer shaves MDMA into a bag of heroin)
"mooster" (street name, cannabis)
"moota/mutah" (street name, cannabis)
"mooters" (street name, cannabis cigarette)
"mootie" (street name, cannabis)
"mootos" (street name, cannabis)
"mor a grifa" (street name, cannabis)
moral injury
morale
morals
morbid responses
morbid rumination
"more" (street name, phencyclidine/PCP)
"morf" (street name, morphine)
moribund state
morning headache
"morning shot" (street name, ecstasy/MDMA)
"morning wake-up" (re: crack use)
Moro reflex
"Morotgara" (street name, heroin)
morpheme
      bound
      free
      grammatical
      lexical
      structural rule
      zero (0)
morphinan

morphine (street names)
   C and M
   cotton brothers
   double yoke
   dreamer
   emsel
   first line
   God's drug
   hows
   M
   Miss Emma
   Mister Blue
   morf
   morpho
   M.S.
   New Jack Swing
   unkie
morphine derivative (desomorphine)
morphine derivative, krocodil (street name)
morphine-like action
morphinomania (addiction to morphine)
morphiomania (aphrodisiacs)
morphological
morphometric analysis
morphophonemic component
"mortal combat" (street name, heroin)
mortality rate, long-term
mosquito-borne viral encephalitis
"mosquitos" (street name, cocaine)
MOST (Modern Occupational Skills Test)
most comfortable loudness (MCL)
most comfortable loudness range (MCLR)
most recent depressed mood episode
most recent hypomanic mood episode
most recent manic mood episode
most recent mixed mood episode
most recent unspecified mood episode

Mot (motility-related)
Mot-dysphagia patient
"mota/moto" (street name, cannabis)
"moth-eaten" teeth
"mother" (street name, cannabis)
Mother Card
Mother-Child Relationship Evaluation, The (MCRE)
Mother/Infant Communication Screening (MICS)
"mother's little helper" (street name, barbiturate)
motility-related (Mot)
motion
    brownian
    simple harmonic (SHM)
motion perception
motion rate, alternate (AMR)
motion studies, time and
motivating operation
motivation
    decreased
    deterioration of
    expressed
    external incentive
    lack of
    presence of
    psychological
    suicide
motivation and decision-making inventory
motivation for cross-dressing
motivation for self-injury
Motivational Patterns Inventory
motives, conflicting
motokinesthetics
motor abilities, disturbance in perceptual
motor ability, perceptual
motor activity
    disturbance in integrating auditory information with
    disturbance in integrating tactile information with
    disturbance in integrating visual information with
    excessive

motor activity
    pharyngeal
    purposeless
motor aphasia
    afferent (kinetic)
    efferent (kinetic)
    subcortical
    transcortical
motor apraxia
motor area
motor assessment *(see also* tests)
motor behavior
    catatonic
    driven
    nonfunctional
    nonfunctional and repetitive
motor center
motor coordination, subaverage
motor cortex
motor deficit
motor development
motor development scale *(see also* tests)
motor disorders
motor evoked potential (MEP)
motor function, intact
motor functioning, voluntary
motor immobility
motor impairment
Motor Impersistence Test (MIT)
motor innervation, patterns of
motor loss
motor movement
    nonrhythmic stereotyped
    stereotypic
    synkinetic
motor nerve conduction
motor neuron
motor or vocal tic disorder, persistent (chronic) (F95.1)
    with motor tics only (F95.1)
    with vocal tics only (F95.1)
motor paralysis, laryngeal
motor pathways disease, central
motor performance, impaired
motor problems inventory

motor proficiency test
motor restlessness
motor scales, developmental *(see also* tests)
motor skill disturbances
motor skills
    fine
    gross
motor skills disorder
Motor Steadiness Battery
motor symptom(s)
motor system
    direct
    indirect
motor tic(s)
    complex
    simple
motor type of symptom
motor-vocal tic disorder, chronic
motor vocalization, nonrhythmic stereotyped
motoria
motoric immobility
motoric phenomenon
motorically
motorphobia
mouth breathing, daytime
"mouth worker" (re: drug user)
mouthing movement
movement
    abdominal wall
    abnormal
    adventitious
    anomalous
    arcuate
    athetoid
    ballistic
    brownian
    cardinal ocular
    choreiform
    clonic
    compensatory
    complex whole body
    disjugate
    dyskinetic
    dyspractic
    dysrhythmic
    dystonic

movement
    extraneous
    false perceptions of
    fetal
    flapping
    following
    free mandibular
    freezing of
    functional
    hemiballismic
    impaired rapid repetitive
    intentional stereotyped
    involuntary
    irregular
    jerking
    low-complexity
    mandibular
    medication-induced
    mouthing
    muscle
    myoclonic
    non-rapid eye (NREM)
    nonrhythmic stereotyped motor
    oscillatory
    paucity of
    perseverative
    poverty of
    purposeless
    pursuit
    quasipurposive
    random
    rapid
    rapid eye (REM)
    rapid fine
    rapid-alternating (RAM)
    reflex eye
    reflexive
    repetitive imitative
    rhythmic
    rhythmic slow eye
    roving eye
    roving ocular
    saccadic eye
    stereotyped
    stereotyped body
    stereotyped motor
    stereotypical

movement
    subjective sensation of fetal
    synkinetic motor
    tonic-clonic
    tremulous
    vermicular
    vestibular
    visual pursuit
    volitional
    volitional oral
    voluntary
    voluntary muscle
    withdrawal
movement abnormality, eye
movement and posture disorganization *(see also* tests)
movement disorder
    medication-induced
    neuroleptic-induced acute
    neuropsychiatric
    stereotypic
movement of tongue, vermiform
movement peculiarities, voluntary
movement symptoms
movement toward the community
"movie star drug" (street name, cocaine)
moving object
"mow the grass" (re: cannabis use)
MPD (Measures of Psychosocial Development)
MPD (multiple personality disorder)
MPO (maximum power output)
MRT (Metropolitan Readiness Tests)
MRT Español
MRU (mean relational utterance)
"MS" (street name, morphine)
m/s (moderate to severe)
MSCS (Multidimensional Self-Concept Scale)
MSL (mean sentence length)
MSLT (Multiple Sleep Latency Test)
"MU" (street name, cannabis)
mu opiate receptors

mu receptors
mucoid otitis media
mucosa
mucous membrane
"muggie" (street name, cannabis)
mugging
"mujer" (street name, cocaine)
"mule" (re: drug dealing)
Mullen Scales of Early Learning
multiaxial evaluation
multiaxial system
MULTICROS (contralateral routing of signals)
multicultural environment
Multidimensional Anxiety Scales
Multidimensional Aptitude Battery
Multidimensional Functional Assessment Questionnaire
Multidimensional Self-Concept Scale (MSCS)
multidisciplinary group psychiatry
multidisciplinary management of aggressive behavior
multidisciplinary management of violence
Multifactor Leadership Questionnaire (MLQ)
multifocal leukoencephalopathy, progressive
multi-item index
multi-item test
Multilevel Informal Language Inventory
multiparity
Multiphasic Environmental Assessment Procedure (MEAP)
Multiphasic Personality Inventory - Adolescent
Multiple Affect Adjective Check List
multiple cognitive deficits
multiple distinct identities
multiple focus
multiple life difficulties
multiple personality and gender
multiple personality crime

multiple personality disorder (MPD)
multiple psychotherapy
multiple sclerosis
Multiple Sleep Latency Test (MSLT)
multisensory
MULTISOCRE
multistep task, complex
mumbling automatism
"murder 8" (street name, fentanyl)
"murder one" (street name, heroin and cocaine)
murmuring, voice
Murphy-Meisgeier Type Indicator for Children (MMTIC)
Murray Valley viral encephalitis
muscle *(see also* muscles)
    anterior digastric
    anterior omohyoid
    anterior scalene
    aryepiglottic
    arytenoid
    cricoarytenoid
    cricothyroid
    genioglossal
    genioglossus
    geniohyoid
    glossopalatine
    greater pectoral
    hyoglossal (hyoglossus)
    hyoglossus
    internal intercostal
    lateral cricoarytenoid
    latissimus dorsi
    lumbar iliocostal
    middle scalene
    mylohyoid
    oblique arytenoid
    palatoglossus
    pharyngopalatine
    posterior cricoarytenoid
    posterior digastric
    posterior omohyoid
    posterior scalene
    salpingopharyngeal
    serratus anterior
    serratus posterior inferior
muscle
    serratus posterior superior
    smaller pectoral
    sternoclavicular
    sternocleidomastoid
    sternohyoid
    sternothyroid
    styloglossus
    stylohyoid
    stylopharyngeal
    subclavian
    thyroarytenoid
    thyroepiglottic
    thyrohyoid
    transverse arytenoid
    uvular
    vocal
muscle contraction headache
muscle imbalance, orofacial
muscle movement, voluntary
muscle of abdomen
    external oblique
    internal oblique
muscle of pharynx
    inferior constrictor
    middle constrictor
    superior constrictor
muscle of soft palate
    elevator
    tensor
muscle of the uvula
muscle of thorax, iliocostal
muscle of tongue
    inferior longitudinal
    superior longitudinal
muscle reflex, middle ear
muscle relaxants, depolarizing
muscle rigidity
muscle strength, antagonistic
muscle tone, normal
muscle twitch/twitching
muscles *(see also* muscle)
    exhalation
    external intercostal
    infrahyoid
    infrahyoid extrinsic
    inhalation (forced)
    inhalation (quiet)

muscles *(see also* muscle)
    intrinsic
    larynx
    palate
    pharynx
    suprahyoid extrinsic
muscles of respiration
muscles of rib, elevator
muscles of the larynx
    extrinsic
    intrinsic
muscles of the palate
muscles of the pharynx
muscles of the tongue
    extrinsic
    intrinsic
muscular dystrophy
muscular relaxation, sense of
muscular rigidity, parkinsonian
muscular tension
musculi intercostales externi and interni
musculi levatores costarum
musculus (musculi) *(see also* lists in the Appendix)
musculus aryepiglotticus
musculus arytenoideus transversus
musculus constrictor pharyngis inferior
musculus constrictor pharyngis medius
musculus constrictor pharyngis superior
musculus cricoarytenoideus lateralis
musculus cricoarytenoideus posterior
musculus cricothyroideus
musculus digastricus anterior
musculus digastricus posterior
musculus genioglossus
musculus geniohyoideus
musculus hyoglossus
musculus iliocostalis dorsi
musculus iliocostalis lumborum
musculus iliocostalis thoracis
musculus intercostalis internus
musculus latissimus dorsi
musculus levator veli palatini
musculus longitudinalis inferior linguae
musculus longitudinalis superior linguae
musculus mylohyoideus
musculus obliquus externus abdominis
musculus obliquus internus abdominis
musculus omohyoideus anterior
musculus omohyoideus posterior
musculus palatoglossus
musculus palatopharyngeus
musculus pectoralis major
musculus pectoralis minor
musculus salpingopharyngeus
musculus scalenus anterior
musculus scalenus medius
musculus scalenus posterior
musculus serratus anterior
musculus serratus posterior inferior
musculus serratus posterior superior
musculus sternoclavicularis
musculus sternocleidomastoideus
musculus sternohyoideus
musculus sternothyroideus
musculus styloglossus
musculus stylohyoideus
musculus stylopharyngeus
musculus subclavius
musculus tensor palati
musculus tensor veli palatini
musculus thyroarytenoideus
musculus thyroepiglotticus
musculus thyrohyoideus
musculus transversus linguae
musculus uvulae
musculus verticalis linguae
musculus vocalis
Music Achievement Tests 1, 2, 3, and 4 (MAT)
music audiation *(see also* tests)
musical abilities *(see also* tests)
musical abilities, measures of

musical stimulus
musical talents, measures of
musicomania (music)
"musk" (street name, psilocybin/psilocin)
musomania (meditation/dreamy abstraction)
mutation voice
mute, deaf
"mutha" (street name, cannabis)
mutilation, sadistic
mutism
    catatonic
    elected
    hysterical
    relative elective
    selective
muttering
mutual affective responsiveness
"muzzle" (street name, heroin)
My Vocational Situation
myasthenia gravis
myasthenic facies
myelin metabolism
myelination
myelinization
myelogram
Myers – Briggs Type Indicator
Myerson reflex
mylohyoid muscle
mylohyoideus, musculus
myoclonic convulsion
myoclonic movements
myoclonic seizure, bilateral
myoelastic-aerodynamic theory of phonation
myofunctional therapy
myopathic facies
myopathic paralysis
myopic insight
myotatic irritability
myotatic reflex
myotonic facies
myringitis
myringoplasty
myringotomy
myrinx
mythomania (myths/untruths)

N

N (newton)
NAADAC (National Association for Alcoholism & Drug Addiction Counselors)
NAAPA (National Association of Academic Psychiatry Administrators)
NABH (National Association for Behavioral Healthcare)
NAD (National Association for the Deaf)
nadir
NAFC (National Association of Forensic Counselors)
"nail" (street name, cannabis cigarette)
"nailed" (re: being arrested)
naloxone HCl
naloxone hydrochloride injection
naloxone-pentazocine
Naltrexone
name, categorical
name the date test
NAMI (National Alliance for the Mentally Ill)
naming common objects test
naming intact
naming test
    confrontation
    graded
    hundred pictures (HPNT)
"nanoo" (street name, heroin)
NAOP (National Academy of Psychology)
napping phenomenon, normal voluntary
Narcan (naloxone HCl)
Narcan Nasal Spray
narcissistic personality disorder (F60.81)
narcissistic vulnerability
narcolepsy, autosomal dominant, obesity, and type 2 diabetes (G47.419)
narcolepsy cataplexy syndrome
narcolepsy experience
narcolepsy secondary to another medical condition (G47.429)
narcolepsy with cataplexy but without hypocretin deficiency (G47.411)
narcolepsy without cataplexy but with hypocretin deficiency (G47.419)
narcomania (craving a drug to deaden pain)
narcosomania (narcotic addiction)
narcotic agonist drug
narcotic drugs (street names)
    40 (OxyContin)
    40-bar (OxyContin)
    80 (OxyContin)
    AC/DC (cocaine)
    Ah-pen-yen (heroin)
    AIP (heroin)
    Al Capone (heroin)
    antifreeze (heroin)
    Aries (heroin)
    atom bomb (heroin)
    Aunt Emma (opium)
    Aunt Hazel (heroin)
    Aunti (opium)
    bad bundle (inferior heroin)
    bad seed (marijuana combo)
    bag man (drug pusher)
    balloon (heroin supplier)
    ballot (heroin)
    barr (codeine cough syrup)
    Bart Simpson (heroin)
    beast (heroin and LSD)
    Belushi (cocaine/heroin)
    big bag (heroin)
    Big H (heroin)
    Big Henry (heroin)
    Big O (opium)
    bindle (heroin; small packet)

narcotic drugs (street names)
   birdie powder (cocaine; heroin)
   black (marijuana; opium, methamphetamine)
   black hash (opium and hashish)
   black pearl (heroin)
   black pill (opium)
   black Russian (opium and hashish)
   black stuff (heroin; opium)
   black tar (heroin)
   bombita (heroin and amphetamine; depressants)
   bombs away (heroin)
   Bonita (heroin)
   boy (cocaine; heroin)
   Bozo (heroin)
   brain damage (heroin)
   brea (heroine)
   brick gum (heroin)
   broja (heroin)
   brown (marijuana, heroin, meth)
   brown crystal (heroin)
   brown rhine (heroin)
   brown sugar (heroin)
   bundle (heroin)
   Butu (heroin)
   caballo (heroin)
   caca (heroin)
   calbo (heroin)
   Capital H (heroin)
   carga (heroin)
   carne (heroin)
   chandoo/chandu (opium)
   channel swimmer (a heroin injector)
   chapopote (heroin)
   Charley (heroin)
   chasing the dragon (crack and heroin mix)
   chasing the tiger (smoking heroin)
   chatarra (heroin)
   chicle (heroin)
   chieva (heroin)

narcotic drugs (street names)
   China cat (heroin)
   China white (synthetic heroin)
   Chinese molasses (opium)
   Chinese red (heroin)
   Chinese tobacco (opium)
   chip (heroin)
   chipper (occasional heroin user)
   chucks (hunger after heroin withdrawal)
   cigarette paper (packet of heroin)
   climax (crack heroin, isobutyl, inhalants)
   cocofan (brown tar heroin)
   cook (heroin prep for injection)
   cotica (heroin)
   coties (cocaine)
   cotton brothers (cocaine, heroin, morphine)
   courage pills (heroin, depressants
   crackers (LSD, Talwin, Ritalin mix)
   crank (crack cocaine, heroin, others)
   crap (low quality heroin)
   crown crap (heroin)
   Cruz (opium from Vera Cruz, Mexico)
   cura (heroin)
   cut-deck (heroin mixed with powdered milk)
   dead on arrival (heroin)
   deuce (heroin; $2 of drugs)
   dinosaurs (older population of heroin users)
   dirt (heroin)
   DOA (crack, heroin, PCP)
   doctor shopping (using doctors to obtain meds)
   dog food (heroin)
   doggie (heroin)
   doogie/doojee/dugic (heroin)

narcotic drugs (street names)
- dooley (heroin)
- dope (marijuana, heroin, other drugs)
- dopium (opium)
- dors and 4s (Doriden and Tylenol #4 combo)
- Dover's deck (opium)
- Dover's powder (opium)
- dream stick (opium)
- dreams (opium)
- dreck (heroin)
- duji (heroin)
- dust (marijuana; cocaine; heroin; PCP)
- dynamite (cocaine mixed with heroin)
- dyno (heroin)
- dyno-pure (heroin)
- easing powder (opium)
- eightball (crack with heroin)
- eighth (heroin)
- el diablito (cocaine; marijuana, heroin, PCP)
- el diablo (cocaine, marijuana, heroin)
- estuffa (heroin)
- ferry dust (heroin)
- Fi-do-nie (opium)
- flamthrowers (heroin, cocaine, tobacco)
- flea powder (low purity heroin)
- foolish powder (cocaine; heroin)
- furra (heroin)
- gallop (heroin)
- galloping horse (heroin)
- gamut (heroin)
- garbage (low quality marijuana, heroin)
- gato (heroin)
- gee (opium)
- George (heroin)
- George smack (heroin)
- girl (cocaine, crack cocaine, heroin)

narcotic drugs (street names)
- give wings (to inject heroin)
- glacines (heroin)
- glass (heroin; amphetamine; meth; hypodermic needle)
- God's medicine (opium)
- gold (marijuana, crack cocaine, heroin)
- golden girl (heroin)
- good (PCP; heroin)
- Good and Plenty (heroin)
- good H (heroin)
- good horse (heroin)
- goofball (cocaine with heroin; depressants)
- goric (opium)
- gravy (heroin; to inject a drug)
- great tobacco opium;
- gum (opium)
- guma (opium)
- H (heroin)
- H caps (heroin)
- H&C (heroin and cocaine)
- hache (heroin)
- hairy (heroin)
- hard candy (heroin)
- hard stuff (heroin; opium)
- Hazel (heroin)
- heaven (cocaine; heroin)
- heaven dust (cocaine; heroin)
- Helen (heroin)
- hell dust (heroin)
- Henry (heroin)
- Hera (heroin)
- hero (heroin)
- hero of the underworld (heroin)
- Heroina (heroin)
- Herone (heroin)
- hessle (heroin)
- him (heroin)
- hocus (marijuana; opium)
- hombre (heroin)

narcotic drugs (street names)
- homicide (heroin cut with scopolamine/strychnine)
- hong-yen (heroin in pill form)
- hop/hops (opium)
- hot heroin (poisoned heroin for informant)
- HRN (heroin)
- hype (re" an addict)
- Indonesian bud (marijuana; opium)
- Isda (heroin)
- jee gee (heroin)
- jive (marijuana; heroin; drugs)
- jive doo gee (heroin)
- Joharito he (heroin)
- Jojee (heroin)
- jolly pop (casual heroin user)
- Jones (heroin)
- joy (heroin)
- joy flakes (heroin)
- joy plant (opium)
- joy powder (cocaine; heroin)
- junk (cocaine; heroin)
- kabayo (heroin)
- Karachi (heroin; phenobarbital, and methaqualone)
- Karo (cocaine cough syrup)
- keel (possibly heroin with fentanyl)
- kicker (OxyContin)
- kill (possibly heroin with fentanyl)
- La Buena (heroin)
- LBJ (heroin plus LSD and PCP)
- lean (cocaine cough syrup)
- lemonade (heroin; poor quality drugs)
- little bomb (heroin; amphetamine; depressants)
- mansakow (heroin)
- manteca (heroin)

narcotic drugs (street names)
- mayo (cocaine; heroin)
- Mexican brown (marijuana; heroin)
- Mexican horse (heroin)
- Mexican mud (heroin)
- Morotgara (heroin)
- mortal combat (high potency heroin)
- mud (heroin and opium)
- murder one (heroin and cocaine)
- Murotugora (heroin)
- muzzle (heroin)
- nanoo (heroin)
- New Jack Swing (heroin and morphine)
- nice and easy (heroin)
- nickel bag ($5 worth of heroin)
- nickel deck (heroin)
- nod (effect of heroin)
- nods (codeine cough syrup)
- noise (heroin)
- nose (cocaine; heroin)
- nose drops (liquid heroin)
- number 3 (cocaine; heroin)
- number 4 (heroin)
- number 6 (heroin)
- O (opium)
- OCs (OxyContin)
- ogoy (heroin)
- oil (heroin; PCP)
- Old Steve (heroin)
- on the nod (under influence of narcotics)
- on the nod (under the influence of depressants)
- OP (opium)
- ope (opium)
- pack (marijuana; heroin)
- pangonadalot (heroin)
- paper (1/10 of gram of a drug; methamphetamine)
- paper (a dosage unit of heroin)
- paper boy (heroin peddler)

narcotic drugs (street names)
  parachute (crack/PCP
    smoked heroin)
  P-dope (20-30% pure
    heroin
  P-funk (crack with PCP;
    heroin)
  pin gon (opium)
  pin yen (opium)
  poison (heroin; fentanyl)
  polvo (heroin; PCP)
  poor man's heroin
    (Talwin/Ritalin injection)
  poppy (heroin)
  powder (cocaine; heroin;
    amphetamine)
  pox (opium)
  predator (heroin)
  primo-1 (mixture of crack,
    marijuana & cocaine)
  primo-2 (mixture of crack
    and heroin)
  primo-3 (mixture of heroin,
    cocaine, tobacco)
  pulborn (heroin)
  pure (heroin)
  purple drank (mixture:
    promethazine/cocaine
    syrup
  quill (cocaine; heroin;
    methamphetamine)
  Racehorse Charlie
    (cocaine; heroin)
  ragweed (inferior
    marijuana; heroin)
  Rambo (heroin)
  rane (cocaine; heroin)
  raw fusion (heroin)
  raw hide (heroin)
  red chicken (heroin)
  red eagle (heroin)
  red rock (heroin)
  reindeer dust (heroin)
  Rhine (heroin)
  sack (heroin)
  salt (heroin)
  sandwich (cocaine/heroin/
    cocaine layers)

narcotic drugs (street names)
  scag (heroin)
  scat (heroin)
  scate (heroin)
  Scott (heroin)
  second to none (heroin)
  set (place where drugs are
    sold)
  shoot (heroin)
  skag (heroin)
  skee (opium)
  skid (heroin)
  skunk (marijuana; heroin)
  sleeper (heroin; depress-
    sants)
  slime (heroin)
  smack (heroin)
  smoke (marijuana; heroin/
    crack; crack cocaine)
  smoking gun (heroin and
    cocaine)
  snow (cocaine; heroin;
    amphetamine)
  snowball (cocaine and
    heroin)
  speedball (cocaine/heroin
    mix)
  speedball (crack/heroin
    smoked together)
  speedball (Ritalin/heroin
    mix); amphetamine
  spider blue (heroin)
  spoon (1/16 oz. of heroin)
  spoon (heroin injection
    paraphernalia)
  stuff (heroin)
  sugar (cocaine; crack
    cocaine; heroin; LSD)
  sweet dreams (heroin)
  Sweet Jesus (heroin)
  sweet stuff (cocaine;
    heroin)
  T.N.T. (heroin; fentanyl)
  tar (crack/heroin smoked
    together; heroin; opium)
  taste (heroin; small sample
    of drugs)
  tecata (heroin)

narcotic drugs (street names)
    tecatos (Hispanic heroin addict)
    The beast (heroin)
    The witch (heroin)
    thing (cocaine; crack; heroin; or any current drug of choice)
    thunder (heroin)
    tigre (heroin)
    tigre blanco (heroin)
    tigre del norte (heroin)
    tongs (heroin)
    tootsie roll (heroin)
    Ts and Rits (Talwin and Ritalin injection)
    Ts and Rs (Talwin and Ritalin injection)
    vidrio (heroin)
    whack-1 (crack; or crack and PCP mixture)
    whack-2 (heroin and PCP mixture)
    whack-3 (marijuana with insecticides)
    when-shee (opium)
    white (heroin; amphetamines)
    white boy (heroin; powder cocaine)
    white girl (cocaine; heroin)
    white junk (heroin)
    white lady (cocaine; heroin)
    white nurse (heroin)
    white stuff (heroin)
    whiz bang (cocaine; heroin/cocaine)
    wicked (potent heroin)
    wings (cocaine; heroin)
    witch hazel (heroin)
    Yen Shee Suey (opium wine)
    Ze (opium)
    zero (opium)
    zoquete (heroin)
narcotics, toxic effects of
Narcotics Anonymous
nares constriction
naris (pl. nares)
narrative speech
narrow-band noise
narrow-based gait
narrow phonetic transcription
narrow range audiometer
narrow-set eyes
narrow transcription
narrow vowel
NART (National Adult Reading Test)
nasal alae
nasal assimilation
nasal bone
nasal cavity
    inferior
    medial
    nasal bone
    superior
    supreme
nasal concha skull bone
    inferior
    medial
    superior
    supreme
    sphenoidal
nasal conchae, sphenoidal
nasal consonant formation
nasal coupling
nasal emission
nasal escape
nasal feature English phoneme
nasal lisp
nasal Narcan
nasal port
nasal resonance
nasal respiration
nasal rustle
nasal septum
nasal skull bones
nasal snort
nasal tract
nasal turbulence
nasal twang
nasal uncoupling
nasality
    assimilated

nasality
   excessive
   mixed
   voice disorder of
     assimilated
nasality voice disorder, mixed
nasalization of vowels
NASEN (National Association for Special Education Needs)
NASET (National Association of Special Education Teachers)
nasi inferior meatus
nasi medius meatus
nasi superior meatus
naso-ocular
naso-oral
nasopalatine
nasopharyngeal pathology
nasopharyngeus meatus
nasopharyngoscope
nasopharynx
NASP (National Association of School Psychologists)
NASW (National Association of Social Workers)
NAT (Non-Verbal Ability Tests)
natal
National Academy of Psychology (India)
National Adult Reading Test (NART)
National Alliance for the Mentally Ill (NAMI)
National Association for the Deaf
National Association for the Visually Handicapped
National Association of School Psychologists (NASP)
National Association of Social Workers (NASW)
National Association of Veterans Affairs Chiefs of Psychiatry
National Business Competency Tests
National Center for Health Statistics (NCHS)
National Commission for Certifying Agencies) (NCCA)
National Committee on Vital and Health Statistics (NCVHS)
National Council of Community Mental Health Centers (NCCMHC)
National Council on Alcoholism & Drug Dependence
National Depressive and Manic Depressive Association (NDMDA)
National Down Syndrome Society (NDSS)
National Drug Intelligence Center (NDIC)
National Educational Development Tests
National Institute of Mental Health (NIMH)
National Institute of Neurological Disorders and Stroke (NINDS)
National Institute on Aging (NIA)
National Institute on Alcohol Abuse and Alcoholism (NIAAA)
National Institute on Deafness and Other Communication Disorders (NIDCD)
National Institute on Drug Abuse (NIDA)
National Institutes of Health (NIH)
National Medical Association (NMA)
National Medical Services (*now* NMS Labs)
National Mental Health Association (NMHA)
National Multiple Sclerosis Society (NMSS)
National Organization of Forensic Social Work (NOFSW)
National Police Officer Selection Test (POST)
National Student Speech Language Hearing Association (NSSLHA)
National Youth Tobacco Survey (NYTS)

native language
nativist theory, language
natural disasters as major childhood stressors
natural environment type
natural frequency
natural language inventory *(see also* tests)
natural method of aural rehabilitation
natural phonological processes
natural pitch
Natural Process Analysis
nausea (a panic attack indicator)
nausea/vomiting
NAVACP (National Association of Veterans Affairs Chiefs of Psychiatry)
NBAS (The Neonatal Behavioral Assessment Scale)
NBAS-K (Neonatal Behavioral Assessment Scale with Kansas Supplement
NCCA (National Commission for Certifying Agencies)
NCCMHC (National Council of Community Mental Health Centers)
NCHS (National Center for Health Statistics)
NCI (National Captioning Institute)
NCVHS (National Committee on Vital and Health Statistics)
NDIC (National Drug Intelligence Center)
NDMDA (National Depressive and Manic Depressive Association)
NDSS (National Down Syndrome Society)
NDT (noise detection threshold)
NEAT (Norris Educational Achievement Test)
necessary task
neck, bent-over
necromania (corpses/death)
necrosis negation

Nederlands Instituut van Psychologen (NIP)
need
   effective
   emotional
   excessive
   instrumental
   personal inventory of psychological
   repressed (theory in stuttering)
   unmet dependency
need a sentence test
need for admiration, pattern of
need for approval
need for care
need for care, excessive
Need for Cognition Scale
need for constant attention
need for continued evaluation
need for frequent drug dosing
need for hospitalization
need for prophylactic treatment
need for reassurance
need for sexual expression, excessive
need for sleep, decreased
need for supervision
need for support
need for treatment
need to be self-sufficient
need to control others
needs assessments *(see also* tests)
negation, necrosis
negative behavior
negative command
negative conditioning for sleep
negative correlation
negative effect of drug
negative emotion
negative emotionality
negative evaluation
negative factor
negative factor in schizophrenia
negative feedback
negative feelings
negative ion
negative judgments

negative life event
negative practice
negative qualities, exaggerated
negative reinforcer
negative relationship, perfect
negative response
negative scotoma
negative self-image
negative spike wave
negative spikes
negative symptoms of schizophrenia, prominent
negative symptoms scale *(see also* tests)
negativism
    catatonic
    extreme
negativistic behavior
negativistic personality disorder
neglect
    auditory
    child *(see also* child neglect)
    family
    perceived
    problems related to
    spatial
    spousal or partner (Confirmed/Initial) encounter (T74.01XA)
    spousal or partner (Confirmed/Subsequent) encounter (T74.01XD)
    spousal or partner (Suspected/Initial) encounter (T76.01XA)
    spousal or partner (Suspected /Subsequent) encounter (T76.01XD)
    unilateral
    unilateral organic
    unilateral spatial
    unilateral visual
    victim of child
    visual
neglect of basic health
neglect of elder adult
neglect of household duties
neglect of pleasurable activities
neglect of responsibilities
neglect of school work
neglect problems
    adult
    child
neglect syndrome, contralateral
negotiating goals skills
negotiating language
negotiating routines skills
negotiating rules skills
negotiation, problem-solving
Nelson-Denny Reading Test
Nelson Reading Skills Test, The
"nemmies" (street name, barbiturate)
NEO Personality Inventory (NEO-PI)
neonatal abstinence syndrome
neonatal auditory response cradle audiometry
Neonatal Behavioral Assessment Scale with Kansas Supplements
Neonatal Behavioral Assessment Scale, The (NBAS)
neonatal familial seizure, benign
neonate
NEO-PI (NEO Personality Inventory)
neoplasm
    benign brain
    malignant brain
nerve
    acoustic
    afferent
    alveolar
    cochlear
    efferent
    facial
    glossopharyngeal
    hypoglossal
    motor
    olfactory
    sensory
    vagus
    vestibulocochlear
nerve cell death
nerve cell destruction

nerve cell survival
nerve deafness
nerve fiber
nerve force
nerve growth factor (NGF)
nerve impulse, simultaneous
nerve loss
nerve tumor, eighth
nervous giggling
nervous system
    peripheral (PNS)
    visceral
network, delusional
neural deficit
neuralgia, trigeminal
neuralgic pain
neurilemoma, acoustic
neurinoma
neuroanatomy of aging
Neurobehavioral Cognitive Status Exam (Cognistat)
Neurobehavioral Rating Scale
neurobehavioral syndrome
neurobiology
    behavioral
    molecular
neurobiology in aging
neurocognitive disorder
    major, due to another medical condition with behavioral disturbance (code condition) and (F02.81)
    major, due to another medical condition without behavioral disturbance (code condition) and (F02.80)
    major, due to HIV infection with behavioral disturbance (B20) and (F02.81)
    major, due to HIV infection without behavioral disturbance (B20) and (F02.80)

neurocognitive disorder
    major, due to Huntington's disease with behavioral disturbance (G10) and (F02.81)
    major, due to Huntington's disease without behavioral disturbance (G10) and (F02.80)
    major, due to multiple etiologies (except vascular) with behavioral disturbance (code conditions) and (F02.81)
    major, due to multiple etiologies (except vascular) without behavioral disturbance (code conditions) and (F02.80)
    major, due to prior disease with behavioral disturbance (A81.9) and (F02.81)
    major, due to prior disease without behavioral disturbance (A81.9) and (F02.80)
    major, possibly due to Alzheimer's disease (G31.9)
    major, possibly due to Parkinson's disease (G31.9)
    major, probable, due to Parkinson's disease with behavioral disturbance (G20) and (F02.81)
    major, probable, due to Parkinson's disease without behavioral disturbance (G20) and (F02.80)
    major, with behavioral disturbance, due to Alzheimer's disease (G30.9) and (F02.81)

neurocognitive disorder
- major, without behavioral disturbance, due to Alzheimer's disease (G30.9) and (F02.80)
- mild, due to Alzheimer's disease (G31.84)
- mild, due to another medical condition (G31.84)
- mild, due to frontotemporal lobe degeneration (G31.84)
- mild, due to HIV infection (G31.84)
- mild, due to Huntington's disease (G31.84)
- mild, due to multiple etiologies (G31.84)
- mild, due to Parkinson's disease (G31.84)
- mild, due to prior disease (G31.84)
- mild, due to traumatic brain injury (G31.84)
- mild, vascular (G31.84)
- mild, with Lewy body disease (G31.84)
- possible major, due to Alzheimer's disease (G31.9)
- possible major, due to another medical condition (G31.9)
- possible major, due to frontotemporal lobe degeneration (G31.9)
- possible major, due to vascular disease (G31.9)
- possible major, with Lewy body disease (G31.9)
- probable major, due to Alzheimer's disease, with behavioral disturbance (G30.9) and (F02.81)

neurocognitive disorder
- probable major, due to Alzheimer's disease, without behavioral disturbance (G30.9) and (F02.80)
- probable major, due to frontotemporal lobe degeneration, with behavioral disturbance (G31.09) and (F02.81)
- probable major, due to frontotemporal lobe degeneration, without behavioral disturbance (G31.09) and (F02.80)
- probable major, vascular, with behavioral disturbance (F01.51)
- probable major, vascular, without behavioral disturbance (F01.50)
- probable major, with Lewy body disease, with behavioral disturbance, (G31.83) and (F02.81)
- probable major, with Lewy body disease, without behavioral disturbance, (G31.83) and (F02.80)
- probable major, without Lewy body disease, without behavioral disturbance, (G31.83) and (F02.80)
- substance/medication-induced, with use disorder (other or unknown)
- unspecified (R41.9)
- vascular, mild (G31.84)
- vascular, possible major (G31.9)

neurodegenerative disease
neurodevelopmental disorder, unspecified (F89)
neuroendocrine challenge

neuroendocrine function
neurofeedback
neurofibrillary tangles
neurogenic claudication
neurogenic hyperventilation,
  central
neurogenic shock
neuroimaging
neuroleptic agents (names of
  medications)
   butyrophenone
   chlorpromazine
   clozapine
   Clozaril
   Etrafon
   Fluanxol
   flupenthixol
   fluphenazine decanoate
   Haldol
   haloperidol
   Largactil
   Loxapac
   loxapine
   Loxitane
   Mellaril
   mesoridazine
   methtrimeprazine
   Modecate
   Navane
   nozinan
   olanzepine
   Orap
   Permitil
   perphenazine
   phenothiazine
   pimozide
   Piportil
   pipotiazine palmitate
   Prolixin
   quetiapine
   Risperdal
   risperidone
   Serentil
   Stelazine
   sulpiride
   thioridizine
   thiothixene
   Thixol

neuroleptic agents (names of
  medications)
   Thorazine
   trifluoperazine
   Trilafon
neuroleptic dose-dependent
  akathisia
neuroleptic-induced acute
  akathisia
neuroleptic-induced acute
  dystonia
neuroleptic-induced acute
  movement disorder
neuroleptic-induced akinesia
neuroleptic-induced Parkinson
  tremor
neuroleptic-induced parkinsonism
  (G21.11)
neuroleptic-induced postural
  tremor
neuroleptic-induced tardive
  dyskinesia
neuroleptic malignant syndrome
  (G21.0)
neuroleptic medication-induced
  postural tremor
neuroleptic treatment, long-term
neuroleptic treatment of
  childhood autism
neuroleptic treatment of
  childhood conduct disorders
neuroleptic treatment of
  childhood schizophrenia
neuroleptic treatment of
  childhood Tourette's syndrome
neuroleptics
   butyrophenone-based
   phenothiazine-based
neuroleptics for mood disorders
neurolinguistic programming
neurolinguistics
neurologic deficit, gross
neurologic deterioration
neurologic disability
neurologic disturbance, focal
neurologic signs
   focal
   focal nonextrapyramidal

neurological batteries *(see also* tests)
neurological condition
    dementia due to a
    etiological
neurological control
neurological dysfunction
Neurological Dysfunctions of Children
neurological evaluation
neurological examination
neurological functioning, normal
neurological scales/screening *(see also* tests)
neurological signs, soft
neurological soft signs
neurology, behavioral
neuroma, acoustic
neurometric analysis
neuromotor
neuromuscular
neuron(s)
    cholinergic
    motor
neuronal circuit
neuronal loss
neuronal metabolism
neuro-ophthalmologic history
neuro-otology
neuropathology of aging
neuropathy
    autonomic
    peripheral autonomic
neurophonia
neurophysiological assessment
neurophysiological findings
neurophysiological testing
neuropsychiatric disorder
neuropsychiatric movement disorder
neuropsychiatry, geriatric
neuropsychological assessment
Neuropsychological Battery: Luria-Nebraska
neuropsychological evaluation of dementia
neuropsychological evaluation systems *(see also* tests)
neuropsychological investigation
Neuropsychological Questionnaire – Adult (ANQ)
Neuropsychological Questionnaire – Child (CNQ)
Neuropsychological Screening Exam
Neuropsychological Status Examination
neuropsychological test batteries *(see also* tests)
neuropsychological testing
neuropsychologic evaluation
neuropsychologist
neuropsychometric test
neuropsychopharmacology of stroke
neuroses, psychoanalysis and
neurosis (pl. neuroses)
neurotic (theory in stuttering)
neurotic direction profile
neurotic features
neuroticism
neurotransmitter metabolics
neurotransmitter systems
neurotransmitters
neutralization, vowel
neutralize an obsession
neutralized anxiety
neutral stimulus
neutral vowel
neutroclusion of teeth
"new acid" (street name, phencyclidine/PCP)
new behavior generator
new career problem
new identity
new identity formation
new information
    disturbance in learning
    disturbance in recalling
"New Jack Swing" (street name, heroin and morphine)
New Jersey Test of Reasoning Skills
"new magic" (street name, phencyclidine/PCP)

new memory encoding,
  impairment of
new-onset seizure
new responsibilities
New Sucher-Allred Reading
  Placement Inventory, The
new-work effort
newborn opioid withdrawal
  syndrome
NewGAP
news of death
newton (N)
Nexus (hallucinogen) (street
  names)
    2CB
    2-CT-7
    7-up
    banana split (Nexus with
      LSD or other illicit
      substances)
    BDMPEA
    bromo
    CB
    MFT
    Nexus flipping (re: use of
      2CB and MDMA)
    party pack (re: Nexus with
      MDMA or other illicit
      drugs)
    spectrum
    T-7
    toonies
    tripstacy (Nexus and
      ecstasy)
    Venus
"Nexus flipping" (re: use of 2CB
  and MDMA)
NGF (nerve growth factor)
NIA (National Institute on Aging)
NIAAA (National Institute on
  Alcohol Abuse and Alcoholism)
niacin-deficiency
"nice and easy" (street name,
  heroin)
"nickel bag" (re: heroin use; $5
  worth of drugs)
"nickel deck" (re: heroin use)
"nickel note" (re: currency)

NicoDerm CQ (nicotine patch)
nicotine (street names)
  B-40
  banano
  basuco
  bazooka
  beedies
  chips
  cocktail
  cooler
  coolie
  crimmie
  dank
  flamethrowers
  geek-joints
  monos
  primo
  primos
  Smurf
  THC
  woolas
  woolie
nicotine addiction (tobacco abuse)
nicotine-delivery e-cigarettes
nicotine gum
nicotine intoxication
nicotine lozenges
Nicotine patch
nicotine-related disorder
Nicotine replacement therapy
  (NRT)
nicotine use disorder
nicotine withdrawal
NIDA (National Institute on Drug
  Abuse)
NIDCD (National Institute on
  Deafness and Other
  Communication Disorders)
"niebla" (street name,
  phencyclidine/PCP)
night, staying out at
night eating disorder (50.8)
nightmare disorder
    acute, persistent, subacute
      (F51.5)
    during sleep onset, acute,
      persistent, subacute
      (F51.5)

nightmare disorder
    with associated non-medical condition, acute, persistent, subacute (F51.5)
    with associated non-sleep disorder, acute, persistent, subacute (F51.5)
    with associated other sleep disorders, acute, persistent, subacute (F51.5)
nightmares, recurrent
nighttime activity
nighttime agitation
nighttime sleep
    alcohol-induced
    fragmented
nigrostriatal system
NIH (National Institutes of Health)
NIH Stroke Scale
NIL (noise interference level)
"nimbies" (street name, barbiturate)
NIMH (National Institute of Mental Health)
NIMH data
NINDS (National Institute of Neurological Disorders and Stroke)
nine-digit SDL task (SD9)
Ninjitsu
NIP (Nederlands Instituut van Psychologen, Dutch Association of Psychologists)
nitric oxide
nitrite headache
nitrite inhalant (amyl)
nitrite inhalant (butyl)
nitrite inhalant (isobutyl)
nitrous oxide (street names)
    buzz bomb
    laughing gas
    NOX (nitrous oxide and MDMA)
    shoot the breeze
    whippets
"nix" (re: stranger in the group)
NMA (National Medical Association)
NMDA receptor alterations
NMHA (National Mental Health Association)
NMS Labs (formerly National Medical Services)
NMSS (National Multiple Sclerosis Society)
nociceptive control
noctimania (night/darkness)
NOCTI Teacher Occupational Competency Test: Child Care and Guidance
NOCTI Teacher Occupational Competency Test: Mechanical Technology
nocturnal confusion
nocturnal drinking syndrome
nocturnal eating syndrome
nocturnal enuresis
nocturnal epilepsy
nocturnal hallucination
nocturnal panic attacks
nocturnal paroxysmal dystonia
nocturnal penile tumescence study
nocturnal sleep
    insufficient
    undisturbed
nocturnal sleep duration
nocturnal sleep episodes, prolonged
"nod" (re: heroin reaction)
node of Ranvier
nodes
    singer's
    speaker's
nodosa, chorditis
nodularity
nodule
    polyploid vocal
    sessile vocal
    vocal
no-echo chamber
NOFSW (National Organization of Forensic Social Work)
"noise" (street name, heroin)

noise
    acoustic
    ambient
    background
    complex
    extraneous
    feedback
    gaussian
    narrow-band
    pink
    random
    raw-tooth
    sixty-cycle hum
    speech
    speech discrimination in
    speech reception in
    thermal
    white
    wide-band
noise analyzer
noise detection threshold (NDT)
noise exposure meter
noise generator
noise hum, sixth cycle
noise-induced deafness
noise interference level (NIL)
noise level, perceived (PNdB)
noise limiter
noise pollution
noise ratio, signal to (S/N)
nomatophobia
nomenclature, psychiatric
nominal aphasia, partial
nominal compound
nominalization
nominative, predicate
nominative case
non-acidic cannabinoid
nonadherence to medical treatment (Z91.19)
non-bizarre delusion
noncognitive subscale, ADAS
noncoital stimulation
noncompliance of hospital regulations
noncompliance with treatment
nonconformity
noncontrastive distribution

nonconvulsive status epilepticus
nondepressed mood
nondirectional microphone
nondirective therapy
nondistinctive features
nonelaborative speech
nonextrapyramidal neurologic signs, focal
nonfluency
nonfluent aphasic speech
nonfunctional and repetitive fiddling with fingers
nonfunctional and repetitive hand waving
nonfunctional and repetitive head banging
nonfunctional and repetitive hitting one's own body
nonfunctional and repetitive motor behavior
nonfunctional and repetitive picking at bodily orifices
nonfunctional and repetitive picking at skin
nonfunctional and repetitive playing with hands
nonfunctional and repetitive rocking
nonfunctional and repetitive self-biting
nonfunctional and repetitive twirling of objects
nonfunctional motor behavior
noninvasive operation
Non-Language Learning Test
Non-Language Multi-Mental Test
nonlinear distortion
NONM (nonobstructive non-motility-related)
NONM-dysphagia patient
non-motility-related, nonobstructive (NONM)
non-nasal sound
non-neuroleptic-induced tremor
non-normative hair loss
no-no tremor
nonobstructive non-motility-related (NONM)

nonobtrusive text
nonoccluding earmold
nonorganic deafness
non-parental child abuse
nonparkinsonian tremor
nonpathological amnesia
nonpathological anxiety
nonpathological reaction
nonpathological reactions to stress
nonpathological sexual fantasy
nonpathological substance use
nonperiodic wave
nonpharmacologically induced tremor
non-problematic drinking
nonproductive activity
nonpropositional speech
nonpulsating headache
nonpurging methods
non-rapid eye movement (NREM)
non-rapid eye movement sleep arousal disorders
    sleep terror type (F51.4)
    sleepwalking type (F51.3)
    sleepwalking type with sleep-related eating (F51.3)
    sleepwalking type with sleep-related sexual behavior (sexomnia) (F51.3)
non-rapid-cycling pattern
Non-Reading Intelligence Tests (NRIT)
non-reduplicated babbling
non-REM (deep sleep), stage III of
non-REM (drowsiness), stage I of
non-REM (light sleep), stage II of
non-REM (very deep sleep), stage IV of
non-REM period
non-REM sleep
non-REM to REM, descent through
nonresponsive state
nonrestorative sleep
nonrestrictive modifier

nonrhythmic stereotyped motor movement
nonrhythmic stereotyped motor vocalization
nonsense syllable
nonsense word
nonsensical speech
nonsensical words
nonsexual boundary violations
nonspecific language
nonspeaking autism
nonspeech sounds
nonspousal abuse
nonstandard language
non-substance-induced disorder
non-substance-induced mental disorder
non-substance-related disorder
non-substance-related episodes
non-suppression, dexamethasone
nonsuppurative otitis media
nonsyllabic speech sounds
"nontoucher" (re: affectionless crack user)
nontoxic lithium tremor
nontrivial value
non-24 hour sleep-wake pattern
non-24-hour sleep-wake syndrome
Non-Verbal Ability Tests (NAT)
Nonverbal Form, SRA
nonverbal intellectual capacity
Nonverbal Intelligence Test
Nonverbal Performance Scale
Non-Verbal Reasoning Test
nonverbal tests *(see also* tests)
nonverbal testing
nonvocal communication
norm(s)
    adaptive scale
    cultural
    deviation from physiological
    physiological
    subculture
    violation of age-appropriate societal
norm-assertive stance

norm-referenced tests
normal activities of daily living
normal affect
normal curve
normal development
normal distribution
normal fluency of speech,
  disturbance in the
normal mentation
normal muscle tone
normal neurological functioning
normal-pressure hydrocephalus,
  dementia due to
normal probability curve
normal sleep duration
normal swallowing habit
normal transition
normal voluntary napping
  phenomenon
Normative Adaptive Behavior
  Checklist
normative aging process
normative behavior
normative data
normative phonetics
Norris Educational Achievement
  Test (NEAT)
North American Depression
  Inventories for Children and
  Adults
Northwestern University
  Children's Perception of Speech
  Test
Northwick Park Index of
  Independence in ADL
"nose" (street name, heroin)
nose cleft
"nose drops" (street name,
  liquified heroin)
"nose powder" (street name,
  cocaine)
"nose stuff" (street name,
  cocaine)
nosomania (disease)
nostomania (home)
nostophobia
nostril
not fitting in, feelings of

not in control
not otherwise specified disorder
notched wave
noticeable difference, just (JND)
noticeable hair loss
Nottingham Extended ADL Index
Nottingham Health Profile
Nottingham Ten-Point ADL Scale
noun (parts of speech)
noun, predicate
novel coronavirus pneumonia
novel setting
novel stimulus
novelty drugs
novelty seeking
"NOX" (re: use of nitrous oxide
  and MDMA)
noxious responsibilities
noxious stimulus
NREM (non-rapid eye movement)
NREM sleep, stage 1-4
NRIT (Non-Reading Intelligence
  Tests
NSSLHA (National Student
  Speech Language Hearing
  Association)
NU Auditory Test Lists
"nubs" (street name, mescaline)
nucleus (pl. nuclei)
nucleus
    dorsal cochlear
    ventral cochlear
nudomania (nakedness)
"nugget" (street name,
  amphetamine)
"nuggets" (street name, crack)
null
numb, feeling
"number" (street name, cannabis
  cigarette)
number 3 traced on patient's palm
  test
"number 3" (street name, cocaine,
  heroin)
"number 4" (street name, heroin)
"number 8" (street name, heroin)
numbing
    psychic

numbing
    sense of
numbing sensation
numerical cipher method
numerical reasoning skills
numerical symbols
Nurse Aide Practice Test
nurse-patient relations
nursing, psychiatric
nurturance
    excessive need for
    lack of
nutritional deficiency(ies)
nutritional insults
nutritional psychiatry
nymphomania (excessive female sex drive)
nystagmus
    horizontal
    toxic
    vertical
nystagmus tests
NYTS (National Youth Tobacco Survey)

O

"O" (street name, opium)
OARS Multidimensional Functional Assessment Questionnaire (OMFAQ)
OASIS-AS (Occupational Aptitude Survey and Interest Schedule)
OASIS-IS (Occupational Aptitude Survey and Interest Schedule)
OAT (Optometry Admission Testing Program)
obesity
    autosomal dominant narcolepsy, and type 2 diabetes (G47.419)
    overweight or (E66.9)
object(s)
    analytic
    avoidance of an
    cued by an
    direct
    exposure to an
    feared
    fetish
    halo around
    indirect
    irrational fear of an
    moving
    paraphiliac
    perception of
    substitute
object agnosia
object attachment
object blindness
object concept
object "halos"
object-memory evaluation *(see also* tests)
object of a delusion
object of sexual fantasy, female
object permanence
object reality testing inventory *(see also* tests)
object relations, psychoanalysis and
Object Relations Technique
object shadow
objective
    behavioral
    elements of performance
    instructional
    operational
    performance
    predicate
    principal
Objective-Analytic Batteries
objective case (parts of speech)
objective complement
objective quantity
objective signs of pregnancy
objective symptoms of impairment
objectives inventories *(see also* tests)
objects test
    misplaced
    naming common
obligations, major role
obligatory occurrence
oblique arytenoid muscle
oblique muscle of abdomen
    external
    internal
obliquus, arytenoideus
obliquus externus abdominis, musculus
obliquus internus abdominis, musculus
oblongata, medulla
O'Brien Vocabulary Placement Test, The
obscure vowel
observable disability
observation
    continuous
    direct
    longitudinal
    serial

Psychiatric Words and Phrases

observation audiometry, behavioral (BOA)
observation guides *(see also* tests)
observation scale *(see also* tests)
observer position
obsession
    alien
    inappropriate quality of
    intrusive quality of
    neutralize an
    trigger an
obsessional thoughts
obsessive-compulsive and related disorder
    other specified (F42)
    substance/medication-induced, with use disorder
    unspecified (F42)
obsessive-compulsive and related disorder due to another medical condition (F06.8)
obsessive-compulsive and related disorder due to another medical condition with obsessive-compulsive disorder-like symptoms (F06.8)
obsessive-compulsive and related disorder due to another medical condition with appearance preoccupations (F06.8)
obsessive-compulsive and related disorder due to another medical condition with hoarding symptoms (F06.8)
obsessive-compulsive and related disorder due to another medical condition with hair-pulling symptoms (F06.8)
obsessive-compulsive and related disorder due to another medical condition with skin-picking symptoms (F06.8)
obsessive-compulsive disorder (F42)
obsessive-compulsive disorder, tic related (F42)
obsessive-compulsive features
obsessive-compulsive personality disorder (F60.5)
obsessive-compulsive reaction
obsessive-compulsive scale *(see also* tests)
obsessive jealousy (F42)
Obst (obstruction)
Obst-dysphagia patient
obstruction, visual
obstruction (Obst)
obstruction sleep apnea syndrome
obstructive apnea
obstructive hydrocephalus
obstructive sleep apnea
obstructive sleep apnea hypopnea (G47.33)
obstructive sleep apnea syndrome
obstruent consonant formation
obstruent omission
obstruent singleton omissions, postvocalic
obtrusive text *(see also* tests)
obtundation, mental
obtunded mentally
obturator
occasional erectile problems
occasional orgasmic problems
occasional sexual aversion
occipital lobe
occipital skull bone
occipital sulcus, lateral
occluded lisp
occlusion effect
occult cleft palate
occult head trauma
occupational activity
Occupational Aptitude Survey and Interest Schedule--Aptitude Survey (OASIS-AS)
Occupational Aptitude Survey and Interest Schedule--Interest Survey (OASIS-IS)
occupational basic skills tests *(see also* tests)
occupational behavior-orientation test *(see also* tests)
occupational card sort *(see also* tests)

Occupational Check List
occupational competency tests
  (see also tests)
occupational deafness
occupational environment scales
  (see also tests)
occupational exposure, long-term
occupational functioning
  impairment in
  level of
  marked decline in
  marked distress in
occupational functioning
  assessment scale (see also tests)
occupational impairment
occupational interaction
Occupational Interests Explorer,
  The (OIE)
Occupational Interests Surveyor,
  The (OIS)
occupational literacy test (see also
  tests)
Occupational Roles Questionnaire
  (ORQ)
Occupational Safety and Health
  Act (OSHA)
occupational skill training
occupational skills test (see also
  tests)
Occupational Stress Indicator
  (OSI)
occupational therapist (OT)
occurrence, obligatory
occurrence of pain, pattern of
occurrence of seizure, sleep-
  waking cycle and
OCD (obsessive compulsive
  disorder)
OCD behavioral avoidance tests
  (BATs)
"ocean burst" (re: powdery
  substance mimics ecstasy
  effect)
ochlomania (crowds)
OCI (Organizational Culture
  Inventory)
"octane" (street name, phencyclidine laced with gasoline)

octave band analyzer
octave-band filter
octave filter, third
octave twist
ocular apraxia
ocular migraine headache
ocular movement
  cardinal
  roving
oculogyric crisis
oculomotor (cranial nerve III)
oculomotor apraxia
oculomotor disturbance
odd beliefs
odd-eccentric cluster
odd-even method reliability
  coefficient
odd thinking
odor, distorted perception of
oenopnobia
oestromania (female state of
  sexual excitability)
off-balance
off effect
off-glide
offending agent(s)
Offer Parent-Adolescent
  Questionnaire, The
Offer Self-Image Questionnaire
  for Adolescents
Offer Self-Image Questionnaire
  (OSIQ)
Office of Indian Alcohol and
  Substance Abuse (OIASA)
office seclusion
Office Skills Test
officer, probation (p.o.)
"ogoy" (street name, heroin)
Ohio Tests of Articulation and
  Perception of Sounds (OTAPS)
Ohio Vocational Interest Survey
ohm
Ohm's law
OIASA (Office of Indian Alcohol
  and Substance Abuse)
OIE (The Occupational Interests
  Explorer)
oikomania (household/family)

Psychiatric Words and Phrases 391

"oil" (street name, heroin; phencyclidine/PCP)
oinophobia
OIS (The Occupational Interests Surveyor)
"O.J." (street name, cannabis)
OLA (olivetolic acid)
old age psychiatry
"Old Steve" (street name, heroin)
olfactory (cranial nerve I)
olfactory area
olfactory aura
olfactory nerve
olfactory psychomotor seizure
olfactory sensory modality
oligodontia
oligomania (mild form of mania)
olivetolic acid (OLA)
olivopontocerebellar degeneration
OLSIDI (Oral Language Sentence Imitation Diagnostic Inventory)
OMC (short orientation-memory-concentration test)
Omega sign (+ or - for suicide)
omen formation
OMFAQ (OARS Multidimensional Functional Assessment Questionnaire)
omission, obstruent
omission articulation
omissions, postvocalic obstruent singleton
omnidirectional microphone
omnipotence
omohyoid muscle
    anterior
    posterior
omohyoideus anterior, musculus
omohyoideus posterior, musculus
"on a mission" (re: crack acquisition)
"on a trip" (re: drug influence)
on edge, feeling
on-glide
"on ice" (re: being in jail)
on-off effect of L-dopa
on-off phenomenon

"on the ball" (re: dealer shaving MDMA into heroin bag)
"on the bricks" (re: walking the streets)
"on the go"
"on the nod" (re: drug influence)
"on top of the world"
"one and one" (re: cocaine use)
"one box tissue" (re: one ounce of crack)
"one-fifty-one" (street name, crack)
one's drinking pattern, to moderate
one's own control
one-to-one situation
"one way" (street name, lysergic acid diethylamide/LSD)
One-Word Picture Vocabulary Test - Expressive (EOWPVT)
One-Word Picture Vocabulary Test - Receptive (ROWPVT)
One-Word Picture Vocabulary Test - Upper Extension, Expressive
oneirophobia
oniomania (compulsive shopping)
only child
onomatomania (names)
onomatopoeia
onset
    abrupt
    adolescent
    age at
    insidious
    pattern of
onset during withdrawal, with
onset episode, sleep
onset of agitation
onset of dementia
onset of illness
onset of pain
onset of schizophrenia
    early
    late
    pathophysiological significance of age at
onset of sleep

onset REM period, sleep (SOREMP)
onset time, voice (VOT)
ontogenesis
ontogeny
onychotillomania (picking one's nails)
OOB (out of bed)
OOBE (out of body experience)
OOC (out of control)
"O.P." (street name, opium)
OP or O/P (outpatient)
"ope" (street name, opium)
open (parts of speech)
open bite malposition of teeth
open earmold
open-ended session
open juncture
open quotient
open seclusion restrictions
open syllable
open vowel
open word
openness, lack of
openness to experience
operant
    autoclitic
    echoic
    tact
    textual
    verbal
operant behavior (theory in stuttering)
operant conditioning audiometry, tangible reinforcement (TROCA)
operant learning
operant level
operant procedures
operant therapy
operation
    effector
    invasive
    motivating
    noninvasive
    sensor
operational objectives
operational signs

operations, logical
operations period
    concrete
    formal
operators, modal
ophidiomania (snakes)
opiate receptors
    delta
    kappa
opiate receptors, mu
opinion, public
opinion inventory
opinion surveys
opioid, synthetic
opioid antagonist
    Bunavail
    buprenorphine/naloxone
    bupropion/naloxone
    Cassipa
    Contrave
    Depade
    Evzio
    naloxone HCl
    naltrexone
    Narcan
    ReVia
    Suboxone
    Troxyca ER
    Vivitrol
    Zubsolv
opioid crisis
opioid descriptors
    desomorphine
    diacetylmorphine (heroin)
    meperidine
    methadone
    methylmorphine (codeine)
    morphine
    opium
opioid epidemic
opioid-induced anxiety disorder
opioid-induced constipation
opioid intoxication
opioid intoxication delirium
opioid intoxication with perceptual disturbance
    with use disorder, mild (F11.122)

opioid intoxication with
  perceptual disturbance
    with use disorder, moder-
      ate/severe (F11.222)
    without use disorder
      (F11.922)
opioid intoxication without
  perceptual disturbance
    with use disorder, mild
      (F11.129)
    with use disorder, moder-
      ate/severe (F11.229)
    without use disorder
      (F11.929)
opioid overdose
opioid overdose crisis
opioid overdose deaths
opioid problem
opioid-related disorder,
  unspecified (F11.99)
opioid use disorder in a controlled
  environment
    mild (F11.10)
    moderate/severe (F11.20)
opioid use disorder with central
  sleep apnea comorbid with
  opioid use
    mild (F11.10) and (G47.37)
    moderate/severe (F11.20)
      and (G47.37)
opioid withdrawal with use
  disorder, moderate/severe
  (F11.23)
opiomania (addiction to opium)
opisthotonos
opium (street names)
    A-bomb
    ah-pen-yen
    Aunt Emma
    aunti
    big O
    black
    black hash
    black jack (injecting
      opium)
    black pill
    Black Russian
    black stuff

opium (street names)
    Budda
    chandoo/chandu
    chillum
    Chinese molasses
    Chinese tobacco
    chocolate
    Cruz
    dopium
    Dover's neck
    Dover's powder
    dream gun
    dream stick
    dreams
    easing powder
    fi-do-nie
    gee
    God's medicine
    goma
    gondola
    gong
    Goric
    great tobacco
    gum
    guma
    hocus
    hop/hops
    Indonesian bud
    joy plant
    midnight oil
    mira
    mud
    O
    O.P.
    ope
    pen yan
    pin gon
    pin yen
    pox
    skee
    tar
    tout
    toxy
    toys
    when-shee
    Yen Shee Suey
    ze
    zero

"O.P.P." (street name, phencyclidine/PCP)
opportunities for intervention
opportunity
    educational
    sexual
opposite affect state
opposite phase
opposites, polar
opposition breathing
opposition respiration
oppositional attitude, primary
oppositional-defiant disorder (F91.3)
opsomania (longing for specific/high seasoned foods)
optic (cranial nerve II)
"optical illusions" (street name, lysergic acid diethylamide/LSD)
optic illusions
opticochiasmatic depression
optimal development
optimal method
optimal relational functioning
optimal therapeutic intervention
optimistic atmosphere, situationally
optogenetics
oral apraxia
oral atresia
oral-aural method aural rehabilitation
oral cavity
oral character
oral form recognition
oral inaccuracy, general
oral inaccuracy articulation, general
Oral Language Evaluation
Oral Language Proficiency Test
Oral Language Sentence Imitation Diagnostic Inventory (OLSIDI)
oral language tests (see also tests)
oral manometer
Oral-Motor/Feeding Rating Scale
oral movement, volitional
oral-nasal acoustic ratio, the (TONAR)
oral peripheral examination
oral reading tests (see also tests)
oral respiration
oral sensory discrimination
oral stage psychosexual development
oral stereognosis
oral steroid
    Anadrol
    Anavar
    maxibolin
    methyltestosterone
    proviron
    winstrol
oral stimulation
Oral Structures and Functions Test (TOSF)
oralism
orality
"orange bandits" (street name, ecstasy/MDMA)
"orange barrels" (street name, lysergic acid diethylamide/LSD)
"orange crystal" (street name, phencyclidine/PCP)
"orange cubes" (street name, lysergic acid diethylamide/LSD)
"orange haze" (street name, lysergic acid diethylamide/LSD)
"orange micro" (street name, lysergic acid diethylamide/LSD)
"orange wedges" (street name, lysergic acid diethylamide/LSD)
"oranges" (street name, amphetamine)
orchidomania (men/males)
order
    birth
    preoccupation with
    rank
ordering of sounds, errors of

Ordinal Scales of Psychological
 Development
ordinary demands of life
organ language
organ of Corti
organic articulation disorder
organic brain syndrome, acute
organic brain syndrome with
 psychosis
organic deafness
organic delusional syndrome
organic impairment
Organic Integrity Test
organic neglect, unilateral
organization
  care
  disrupt sleep
  preoccupation with
  temporal
Organization Health Survey
organization of perception test
organization tests *(see also* tests)
Organizational Climate Index,
 The
Organizational Culture Inventory
 (OCI)
organizational plan
organizational skills
organizational structure
organizational surveys
Organizational Test for
 Professional Accounting
organized activity
organized-care psychiatry
organizer, decision-making
organizing principle
organophosphate insecticide
organs, vocal
orgasm
  coital
  sensation of
orgasmic capacity
orgasmic disorder
  acquired type female
  acquired type male
  female
  generalized type female
  generalized type male

orgasmic disorder
  lifelong type female
  lifelong type male
  male
  situational type female
  situational type male
orgasmic disorder due to
 combined factors
  female
  male
orgasmic disorder due to
 psychological factors
  female
  male
orgasmic phase of sexual response
 cycle
orgasmic problems, occasional
orientation
  biological
  bisexual
  coronal
  dextral
  disturbed
  ego-dystonic
  heterosexual
  homosexual
  lack of goal
  psychodynamic
  right-left
  sagittal
  sexual
  spatial
  temporal
  transgender
  transverse
Orientation and Awareness Test
orientation-memory-concentration
 test *(see also* tests)
orientation reflex audiometry,
 conditioned (COR)
Orientation Test for Professional
 Accounting, AICPA
orientation tests *(see also* tests)
oriented times three, alert and
 (A+Ox3)
orienting reflex (OR)
orifices, body
origin, culture of

original trauma
Orleans-Hanna Algebra Prognosis Test
orinthomania (birds)
ornithophobia
orobuccal dyskinesia, tardive
orofacial muscle imbalance
orolingual
oronasal
oro-ocular
oropharyngeal dystonia
oropharynx
ORQ (Occupational Roles Questionnaire)
orthodontics
orthographic
orthography
orthomolecular therapy
oscillating tremor
oscillation, laryngeal
oscillator, bone-conduction
oscillatory movement
oscilloscope
OSHA (Occupational Safety and Health Act)
OSI (Occupational Stress Indicator)
OSIQ (Offer Self-Image Questionnaire)
OSOT Perceptual Evaluation
osseous labyrinth
ossicle
ossicular chain
osteoma (pl. osteomas, osteomata)
osteoporosis, senile
Osterrieth Complex Figure Test
ostracism, peer
OTAPS (Ohio Tests of Articulation and Perception of Sounds)
OTC drugs *(see also* medications)
other people's boundaries, little sense of
other position
other or unknown substances, toxic effects of
other type personality disorder, nonspecific

others
    anxiety due to potential evaluation by
    feeling superior to
    image of
    need to control
Otis-Lennon School Ability Test
otitis media
    adhesive
    chronic suppurative
    mucoid
    nonsuppurative
    serous (SOM)
    suppurative
otitis media push back, purulent
otological screening
otology
otorhinolaryngology
otosclerosis
otoscope
otoscopy
ototoxic
out-of-body sensation
out of character
out of control
    feeling
    sense of being
out-of-control drinking behavior
out of control subjectivity
out-of-mind sensation
out of phase
outcome
    long-term
    well-formed
outcome scale
outer ear
"outerlimits" (street name, crack and lysergic acid diethylamide/LSD)
outflow tremor, cerebral
outlook, future
outpatient-based psychiatry
outpatient occupational therapy
outpatient patient populations
outpatient physical therapy
outpatient setting
outpatient speech therapy

Psychiatric Words and Phrases

output
    HF average SSPL
    maximum acoustic
    maximum power (MPO)
    saturation
outside control
outside force
outside stimulus
oval window
ovalis, fenestra
over-dependent attitude
over-elaborate speech
over-the-counter drug-related disorder
overabstract speech
overall severity of psychiatric disturbance
overall sound level
overbite malposition of teeth
overbreathing, voluntary hysterical
overconcern with sleep
overconcrete speech
overconscientious
overdependenvcy
overdose (OD)
overdose, opioid
overeating, marked
overflow incontinence
overinclusiveness
overindependence
overinvolvement
overjut, horizontal
overjut of teeth
overlapping
overlay
    emotional
    psychogenic
    supratentorial
overlearning
overload
    fluid
    role
overmasking
overprotectiveness
overreact, tendency to
overreaction, emotional
overresponse
oversleeping
overstatement (figure of speech)
overstimulation
overtalkative
overt compliance masking covert resistance
overt response
overtone
overuse of medication
overvalued idea
overweight or obesity
overwhelmed, sense of being
overwhelmed subjectivity
"Owsley" (street name, lysergic acid diethylamide/LSD)
"Owsley's acid" (street name, lysergic acid diethylamide/LSD)
oxidants
oxide
    nitric
    nitrous
oxycodone (street names)
    blue (OxyContin)
    cotton (OxyContin)
    doctor shopping (re: shopping for prescription meds)
    hillbilly heroin (OxyContin)
    OCs (OxyContin)
    Os (OxyContin)
    Ox (OxyContin)
    Oxicotton (semi-synthetic opiate)
    Oxy 80s (semi-synthetic opiate)
    Oxycet (semi-synthetic opiate)
    pills (OxyContin)
OxyContin (street names)
    40
    40-bar
    80
    blue
    cotton
    doctor shopping
    hillbilly heroin

OxyContin (street names)
    kicker
    OCs
    Os
    Ox
    Oxycotton
    Pharming
    Pill ladies
    pills
oxygen-carrying capacity
oxygen-deprived sexual arousal
oxygen-depriving activities
oxyhemoglobin saturation
"Oz" (street name, inhalant)
"ozone" (street name, phencyclidine/PCP)

P

"P" (street name, mescaline; phencyclidine/PCP)
"P and P" (re: MDMA combined with Viagra)
PAAT (Parent as a Teacher Inventory)
pace, future
pacemaker, endogenous circadian
PACG (The Prevocational Assessment and Curriculum Guide)
PACG Inventory
pacing behavior
"pack" (street name, cannabis; heroin)
"pack of rocks" (street name, cannabis cigarette)
PACL (Personality Adjective Check List)
P-ACT
paddling
paganism, magical thinking and
PAI (Personality Assessment Inventory)
pain
    abdominal
    aching
    acute
    anatomical site of
    atypical
    atypical face
    back
    burning
    causalgic
    chest
    chronic forms of
    complaints of
    continuous
    cramping
    diffuse

pain
    diminished response to
    dull
    duration of
    endogenous
    exacerbation of
    extremity
    facial
    gastrointestinal
    Gate Theory of
    genital
    head
    headache
    history of
    intense
    intermittent
    International Association for the Study of
    intractable
    jabbing
    joint
    limited to
    low back
    maintenance of
    minimal
    neuralgic
    onset of
    pattern of occurrence of
    pelvic
    persistent
    phantom
    physical manifestation of
    posttraumatic
    pounding
    pulsating
    radicular
    radicular low back
    reaction to
    recalcitrant
    rectal
    referred
    residual
    searing
    severity of
    sexual
    sharp
    shooting
    stabbing

pain
    steady
    stinging
    superficial
    temporal characteristics of
    temporomandibular joint
      (TMJ)
    throbbing
    unexplained
    vice-like
pain avoidance
pain behavior
pain complaints
pain disorder, sexual
pain during menstruation
pain during sexual intercourse
pain during urination
pain presentation
Pain Questionnaire (see also tests)
pain relievers (see also
  medications)
pain sensation
    loss of
    somatization
pain symptoms
pain syndromes
pain threshold
painful affect, intense
painful consequences, high
  potential for
painful stimulus
painful symptom
painkiller addiction
painter's encephalopathy
paired associate learning
paired syllable(s)
"Pakalolo" (street name,
  cannabis)
"Pakistani black" (street name,
  cannabis)
palatal area consonant placement
palatal fronting
palatal insufficiency
palatal lift
palatal paralysis
palate
    bilateral cleft
    classifications of the cleft

palate
    cleft
    complete cleft
    elevator muscle of soft
    hard
    incomplete cleft
    occult cleft
    partial cleft
    primary
    prosthetic management of
      cleft
    secondary
    soft
    speech and language
      characteristics of cleft
    submucous cleft
    subtotal cleft
    total cleft
    unilateral cleft
palate cleft, soft
palate muscles
palati, musculus tensor
palatine
    musculus levator veli
    musculus tensor veli
palatine bones
palatine raphe
palatine skull bones
palatine tonsil
palatoglossus, musculus
palatoglossus muscle
palatogram
palatography
palatopharyngeal muscle
palatopharyngeus, musculus
paliacusis
palipraxia
palpitations (a panic attack
  indicator)
palsy
    ataxic cerebral
    Bell
    bilateral gaze
    cerebral
    cranial nerve
    diplegic
    dyskinetic cerebral
    Erb

palsy
- gaze
- hemiplegic
- infantile cerebral
- ipsilateral
- lateral gaze
- Lennox-Gastaut (petit mal variant seizure)
- monoplegic
- progressive
- progressive supranuclear
- pseudobulbar
- quadriplegic
- shaking
- spastic cerebral
- supra nuclear gaze
- tetraplegic
- vertical-gaze

"Panama cut" (street name, cannabis)
"Panama gold" (street name, cannabis)
"panatella" (street name, cannabis cigarette)
"pancakes and syrup" (street name, glutethimide and codeine cough syrup)
"pane" (street name, lysergic acid diethylamide/LSD)
panencephalitis, subacute sclerosing
panendoscope
panendoscopy
"Pangonadalot" (street name, heroin)
"panic" (re: unavailability of drugs)
panic attack(s)
- full
- nocturnal
- recurrent, unexpected, multiple (4) (panic disorder) (F41.0)
- situationally bound (cued)
- situationally predisposed
- unexpected (uncued)

panic attack indicator
- abdominal distress

panic attack indicator
- chest discomfort
- chest pain
- chills
- derealization
- dizziness
- fear of "going crazy"
- fear of dying
- fear of losing control
- feeling detached from reality
- feeling faint
- feelings of choking
- feelings of depersonalization
- feelings of unreality
- heat sensations
- lightheadedness
- nausea
- palpitations
- paresthesias
- pounding or racing heart
- sensation of numbness
- sensation of shortness of breath (SOB)
- sensation of smothering
- sensation of tingling
- shaking
- sweating
- trembling
- unsteady

panic disorder
- agoraphobia without history of
- recurrent, unexpected multiple (4) panic attacks (F41.0)

panic disorder with agoraphobia
panic disorder without agoraphobia
panicky
PANSS (Positive and Negative Syndrome Scale)
Pantomime Recognition Test (PRT)
"paper acid" (street name, lysergic acid diethylamide/LSD)
"paper bag" (re: drug container)

"paper blunts" (street name, cannabis cigarettes)
"paper boy" (re: heroin dealer)
papilla, acoustic
papilloma (pl. papillomas, papillomata)
papillomatosis, juvenile
PAR (Proficiency Assessment Report)
PAR Admissions Testing program
parabolin (veterinary steroid)
paracentesis
paracentral scotoma
"parachute" (street name, crack and phencyclidine smoked; heroin)
"parachute down" (re: use of MDMA after heroin)
paracusis
    false
    localis
    Willis
paradigm
paradigmatic response
paradigmatic shift
paradigmatic word
"paradise" (street name, cocaine)
"paradise white" (street name, cocaine)
paradoxical intervention
paradoxical sleep
paragraph recall test *(see also* tests)
paralambdacism
paralanguage
paraldehyde
paralexic errors
paralinguistics
paralipophobia
parallel distribution
parallel spelling tests *(see also* tests)
parallel talk
paralysis
    abductor
    adductor
    Bell
    bilateral abductor

paralysis
    bilateral adductor
    bilateral laryngeal
    bulbar
    cricothyroid
    facial
    flaccid
    labioglossolaryngeal
    labioglossopharyngeal
    laryngeal
    laryngeal motor
    laryngeal sensory
    leaden
    lingual
    myopathic
    palatal
    postdormital sleep
    predormital sleep
    pseudobulbar
    pseudolaryngeal
    sensory
    sleep
    spastic
    unilateral
    unilateral abductor
    unilateral adductor
    vocal fold
paramania (related to mania)
paranoia, querulous
Paranoia "6" Scale
paranoia scale
paranoid behavior *(see also* tests)
paranoid belief system
paranoid disorder
paranoid fears
paranoid features
paranoid ideation, stress-related
paranoid personality disorder (F60.0)
paranoid states, psychoanalysis and
paranoid type schizophrenia
    extended jargon
    literal
    phonemic
    thematic
    verbal
paraphasic speech, fluent

paraphernalia
    paraphiliac
        shared drug
paraphilia
paraphiliac behavior
paraphilic disorder
        other specific (F65.89)
        unspecified (F65.9)
paraphiliac fantasy
paraphiliac focus, characteristic
paraphiliac imagery
paraphiliac objects
paraphiliac paraphernalia
paraphiliac pornography
paraphiliac preferences
paraphiliac stimulus
paraplegia, cerebral
parasigmatism (lisp)
parasomnia type sleep disorder due to epilepsy
parasomnia type sleep disorder due to GMC
parasomnia type substance-induced sleep disorder
parasomniac conscious state
parathyroid disease
parent
        ineffectual
        rejecting
        single
        ungiving
        weak
Parent-Adolescent Communication Scale *(see also tests)*
Parent-Adolescent Questionnaire
Parent as a Teacher Inventory (PAAT)
Parent Attachment Structured Interview
Parent Attitude Survey *(see also tests)*
Parent Awareness Skills Survey (PASS)
Parent-Child Interaction Coding System
parent-child relational problem (Z62.820)
Parent Diabetes Opinion Survey
parent evaluation of custody scale
Parent Opinion Inventory
Parent Perception of Child Profile (PPCP)
Parent Professional Preschool Performance Profile (The Five P's)
Parent Rating of Student Behavior
parent rating scale *(see also tests)*
Parental Acceptance-Rejection Questionnaire
parental control problem, leaving
parenthetical expression
parenthetical remarks
Parenting Stress Index
parents
        adoptive
        biological
paresis, general
paresthesia, laryngeal
paresthesias (a panic attack indicator)
parietal association area
parietal lobe dysfunction
parietal skull bones
parietotemporal area
Parkinson disease
        dementia due to
        primary
Parkinson tremor, neuroleptic-induced
parkinsonian crisis
parkinsonian dysarthria
parkinsonian facies
parkinsonian gait
parkinsonian muscular rigidity
parkinsonian signs and symptoms *(see also tests)*
parkinsonian speech, festinant quality in
parkinsonian tremor
parkinsonism, neuroleptic-induced
"parlay" (street name, crack)
parousiamania (birth)
paroxysmal activity
paroxysmal convulsion

paroxysmal dystonia, nocturnal
paroxysmal migraine headache
paroxysmal phenomenon
parrotlike speech pattern
"parsley" (street name, cannabis; phencyclidine)
partial agonist
partial amnesia
partial amnesic
partial cleft palate
partial complex seizure
partial cross-dressing
partial hospital patient populations
partial-hospital setting
partial laryngectomy, anterior
partial nominal aphasia
partial permanent disability
partial recruitment
partial reinforcement
partial remission
    early
    sustained
partial seizure
    complex (CPS)
    repetitive
    simple
    upper
partial sensory seizure
partial tone
partial tonic seizure
partial visual loss
partialis continua seizure, epilepsia
participle (parts of speech)
particle velocity
particular grammar
particular identity
particular task
partner relational problem *(see also* tests)
Partner Relationship Inventory (PRI)
parts of speech
    adjective
    adverb
    agenitive case
    conjoiner
parts of speech
    conjunction
    dative case
    factitive case
    gerund
    infinitive
    instrumental case
    interjection
    locative case
    nominative case
    noun
    objective case
    open
    participle
    pivot grammar
    preposition
    pronoun
    verb
"party and play" (re: MDMA combined with Viagra)
PAS (Prevocational Assessment Screen)
PASES (Performance Assessment of Syntax Elicited and Spontaneous)
PASS (Parent Awareness Skills Survey)
PASS (Perception of Ability Scale for Students)
pass-band filter
Passavant's bar/cushion/pad/ridge
passive accommodation
passive-aggressive personality disorder *(see also* tests)
passive bilingualism
passive-dependent
passive voice
passivity in anger expression
past experience
past ictal depression phase of seizure
past perfect progressive tense
past perfect tense
past progressive tense, simple
past tense, simple
past tics
"paste" (street name, crack)
pastoral care

pastoral counselor
"Pat" (street name, cannabis)
paternal behavior
paternal deprivation
pathogenic care, grossly
pathognomonic symptoms of
   schizophrenia
pathologic condition, abnormal
pathological behavior *(see also*
   tests)
pathological care
pathological character formation,
   psychoanalysis and
pathological lying
pathological process
pathological sensitivity to
   perceived interpersonal
   rejection
pathological sexual fantasy
pathological substance use
pathologist
       language
       speech
pathologist, voice
pathology
       brain
       central nervous system
       cigarette-related
       language
       manifestations of
       nasopharyngeal
       pelvic
       speech
       speech and language
       structural
pathology/audiology, speech
   (SPA) *(see also* tests)
pathomania (disease)
pathophysiological mechanism
       direct causative
       specific
pathophysiological process
pathophysiological significance of
   age at onset of schizophrenia
pathophysiology of Alzheimer's
   disease
pathway, cerebellar
pathway stimulation, sensory

"patico" (street name, crack)
patient
       abused
       agitated
       aphasic
       comatose
       combative
       disoriented
       incoherent
       lethargic
       Mot-dysphagia
       NONM-dysphagia
       Obst-dysphagia
       posttraumatic
       self-destructive
       stuporous
       unresponsive
patient acceptance of health care
Patient and Family Services (PFS)
patient compliance
patient encounter
Patient Health Questionnaire
patient populations
       clinic
       consultation/liaison
       inpatient
       outpatient
       partial hospital
       primary care
       private practice
"patient" role in factitious
   disorder
patient satisfaction
Patient Satisfaction
   Questionnaire, RAND
patient's palm test, number 3
   traced on
PATM (Progressive Achievement
   Test of Mathematics)
patronizing manner
pattern(s)
       acoustic reflex
       activity
       advanced sleep phase
       alveolar
       antisocial behavior
       attention seeking
       auditory

pattern(s)
- autosomal dominant
- behavior
- binge eating
- changing sleep-wake
- characteristic
- clinging behavior
- cognitive distortions
- compulsive substance use
- continued drinking
- cyclical symptoms
- detachment
- detachment from social relationships
- deviant behavior
- discomfort in close relationships
- disregard of others' rights
- distrust of others' motives
- disturbed sleep
- eccentric behavior
- enduring
- excessive emotionality
- excessive need for care
- failing grades
- familial
- feeling inadequate
- feminine speech
- functioning
- grandiosity
- habit
- hypersensitivity
- identified sleep and wakefulness
- impulsivity
- inflexible
- instability
- interpersonal relationship
- irregular sleep
- irregular sleep-wake
- lack of empathy
- long-term
- major depressive episode
- maladaptive
- maladaptive substance use
- mental control
- moderate drinking

pattern(s)
- mood disorder with seasonal
- motivational
- motor innervation
- need for admiration
- non-24 hour sleep-wake
- non-rapid-cycling
- occurrence of pain
- onset of pain
- parrot-like speech
- perceptual distortions
- persistent behavior
- personality
- pervasive unhappiness
- pessimistic outlook
- preoccupation with control
- preoccupation with orderliness
- preoccupation with perfectionism
- pressure
- proneness to guilt
- prototypical course
- rapid-cycling
- reading
- repetitive behavior
- response
- restricted emotional expression
- restrictive behavior
- seasonal
- self-administered substance
- self-criticism
- sleep
- social inhibition
- speech time
- spelling
- stable
- stable sleep-wake
- stereotyped behavior
- stress
- stuttering
- submissive behavior
- suspiciousness of others' motives
- symptom
- symptom response

pattern(s)
    syndromal
    syndrome
    underachievement
    unexplained absence from work
    unstable affect
    unstable self-image
    violating others' rights
    visual recognition
pattern completion test *(see also tests)*
pattern-induced epilepsy
Patterned Elicitation Syntax Screening Test (PESST)
patterning of speech, disturbance in the time
paucity of movement
paucity of speech content
paucity of verbalizations
pauses during sleep, breathing
pauses in speech
    filled
    unfilled
"paz" (street name, phencyclidine/PCP)
PB max score
PB words (phonetically balanced words)
P-BAP (Behavioral Assessment of Pain Questionnaire)
PCL (The Hare Psychopathy Checklist)
PCP/phencyclidine
PCP (Personal Communication Plan)
PCP (primary care physician)
PCP use disorder
"PCPA" (street name, phencyclidine/PCP)
PDI Employment Inventory
"P-dope" (re: 20-30% pure heroin)
PDRT (Portland Digit Recognition Test)
PDT (Phoneme Discrimination Test)
PE (pharyngoesophageal)

Peabody Developmental Motor Scales and Activity Cards
Peabody Mathematics Readiness Test
"peace" (street name, lysergic acid diethylamide/LSD; phencyclidine/PCP; MDMA)
"peace tablets" (street name, lysergic acid diethylamide/LSD)
"peace weed" (street name, phencyclidine/PCP)
peak acoustic gain
peak amplitude
peak and trough level
peak clipping
peak frequency, mean
peak-to-peak amplitude
"peanut butter" (street name, phencyclidine mixed with peanut butter)
"pearl" (street name, cocaine)
"pearls" (street name, amyl nitrite)
"pearly gates" (street name, lysergic acid diethylamide/PCP)
"pebbles" (street name, crack)
pectoral muscle
    greater
    smaller
pectoralis major, musculus
pectoralis minor, musculus
peculiar thoughts and language, peculiarities, voluntary movement
peculiarities of language
pedagogical grammar
pediatric audiology
Pediatric Early Elementary Examination
Pediatric Examination of Educational Readiness at Middle Childhood
Pediatric Extended Examination at Three (PEET)
pediatric growth chart
Pediatric Speech Intelligibility Test

"peddler" (re: drug supplier)
pedophile
pedophilic disorder (F65.4)
    exclusive type (F65.4)
    female attraction (F65.4)
    limited to incest (F65.4)
    male and female attraction (F65.4)
    male attraction (F65.4)
    nonexclusive type (F65.4)
peduncular hallucinosis
"Pee Wee" (re: $5 worth of crack)
"peep" (street name, phencyclidine/PCP)
"peepers" (street name, ecstasy/MDMA)
Peer Nomination Inventory of Depression
peer ostracism
Peer Profile
peer relationships, poor
PEET (Pediatric Extended Examination at Three)
"Peg" (street name, heroin)
pegboard tests *(see also* tests)
pejorative voices
"pellets" (street name, lysergic acid diethylamide/LSD)
pelvic pain
pelvic pathology
pelvis, vasocongestion of
penectomy
penile blood pressure
penile plethysmography
penile tumescence study, nocturnal
pentagons test, copy intersecting
pentazocine HCl
"pen yan" (street name, opium)
people
    aggression to
    "using"
peotillomania (pseudomasturbation)
PEP (Psychoeducational Profile)
"Pepsi habit" (re: drug use)
peracute mania

perceived attack on one's character
perceived interpersonal rejection, pathological sensitivity to
perceived neglect
perceived noise level (PNdB)
perceived poor performance
percentile rank
perception
    alterations in time
    auditory
    body-image
    central auditory
    color
    cross-modality
    depth
    developmental
    distance
    distorted odor
    distorted touch
    distortion of inferential
    disturbances in
    environment
    exaggerated
    external reality
    false
    gravity
    haptic
    inferential
    internal world of
    kinesthetic
    loudness
    LSD-type
    motion
    movement
    object
    physical sensation
    pitch
    proprioceptive
    self
    sensory
    size
    social
    sound
    space
    speech
    substance-induced
    tactile

perception
    taste
    time
    touch
    true
    visual
    visual sensations
    weight
perception deficit, speech
perception disorder, hallucinogen persisting
perception due to a psychotic disorder, abnormal
perception due to drug effect, abnormal
perception in schizophrenia
    distorted
    exaggerated
perception inventory
Perception of Ability Scale for Students (PASS)
Perception-Of-Relationships-Test (PORT)
perception tests *(see also* tests)
perceptive deafness
perceptive epilepsy
perceptive hearing loss
perceptual analysis
perceptual assessment
perceptual closure
perceptual consistency
perceptual defense
perceptual disorder *(see also* tests)
perceptual distortion, pattern of
perceptual disturbance
    delusional interpretation of a high level
    mixed symptom picture with
perceptual evaluation *(see also* tests)
perceptual filter
perceptual immaturity
perceptual masking
Perceptual Maze Test
perceptual-motor ability
    disturbance in
    impairment in

Perceptual-Motor Assessment for Children & Emotional/Behavior Screening Program (P-MAC/ESP)
perceptual-motor impairment
perceptual-motor match
Perceptual Organization Test
perceptual retardation
perceptual set of disturbances
perceptual skills, impaired
perceptual skills inventory *(see also* tests)
perceptual symptoms, reexperiencing
perceptually handicapped
"perfect high" (street name, heroin)
perfect negative relationship
perfect performance
perfect positive relationship
perfect progressive tense, future
perfect tense
perfection, state of
perfectionism, preoccupation with
performance
    abnormality in
    academic
    decline in
    decline in classroom
    impaired
    impaired motor
    job
    linguistic
    perceived poor
    perfect
    poor work
    public
    quality of
    school
    self-imposed high standards of
    sexual
    standards of sexual
    strict standards of
    task
performance abnormality
performance and analysis, task
performance anxiety

performance articulation
Performance Assessment of Syntax Elicited and Spontaneous (PASES)
performance characteristics, psychometric
Performance Efficiency Test
performance evaluation *(see also* tests)
performance fear
performance-intensity function
Performance Levels of a School Program Survey
performance objective, elements of
Performance Profile for the Severely and Moderately Retarded
performance report
performance scales
performance screening of articulation *(see also* tests)
performance situation, feared single
performance test *(see also* tests)
performative, lost
performative pragmatic structures
"perico" (street name, cocaine)
perimeter earmold
perinatal development
period
    apneic
    apneustic
    concrete operations
    decay
    depressive
    developmental
    drinking
    endogenous circadian
    formal operations
    ictal
    interictal
    non-REM
    preoperational thought
    refractory
    REM
    sadness

period
    sensorimotor intelligence
    sleep onset REM
period of growth
period of illness
period of learning, critical
periodic wave
periodical mania
periodicity
perioral tremor
peripheral autonomic neuropathy
peripheral dysarthria
peripheral electromyographic activity
peripheral examination, oral
peripheral field images
peripheral masking
peripheral nervous system
peripheral sensation, decreased
peripheral sensory loss
peripheral sympathomimetic effect
peripheral vascular disease
periphery
periventricular white matter
permanence, object
permanent disability, partial
permanent epilation
permanent residual impairment
permanent teeth
permanent threshold shift (PTS)
permanently damaged, feeling
permutation
"perp" (re: fake crack)
perpetrator of adult physical abuse by nonspouse or nonpartner
perpetrator of adult psychological abuse by nonspouse or nonpartner
perpetrator of adult sexual abuse by nonspouse or nonpartner
perpetrator of non-parental child abuse
perpetrator of parental child abuse
perpetrator of spousal or partner neglect
perpetuating factors
perpetuation of abuse

Psychiatric Words and Phrases

persecution, idea of
persecutory delusions
persecutory type delusions
persecutory type schizophrenia
perseverance (theory in stuttering)
perseveration, infantile
perseverative movements
perseverative response
persistence of visual image
persistent (chronic) motor or vocal tic disorder (F95.1)
persistent (chronic) motor or vocal tic disorder with motor tics only (F95.1)
persistent (chronic) motor or vocal tic disorder with vocal tics only (F95.1)
persistent depressive disorder (dysthymia) (F34.1)
persistent discomfort with gender role
persistent fear
persistent heavy drinkers
persistent inappropriate ideas
persistent inappropriate images
persistent inappropriate impulses
persistent inappropriate thoughts
persistent inappropriate urges
persistent intrusive ideas
persistent intrusive images
persistent intrusive impulses
persistent intrusive thoughts
persistent intrusive urges
persistent pain
persistent pattern of behavior
persistent sleep problems
persistent thoughts
persistent vegetative state (PVS)
persisting amnestic disorder
    alcohol-induced
    substance-induced
persisting dementia
    alcohol-induced
    substance-induced
persisting disorder
    alcohol-induced
    substance-induced

persisting perception disorder, hallucinogen
person
    dominant
    inner-directed
    other-directed
    single
    time, place and (TP&P)
personal adjustment inventory *(see also* tests)
personal assault, violent
personal care
Personal Communication Plan, The (PCP)
personal construct theory
personal counselor
Personal Experience Screening Questionnaire (PESQ)
personal gain, desire for
personal history, other circumstances of
personal history of military deployment (Z91.82)
personal history of psychological trauma, other (Z91.49)
personal history of self-harm (Z91.5)
personal history (past history) of neglect in childhood (Z62.812)
personal history (past history) of physical abuse in childhood (Z62.810)
personal history (past history) of psychological abuse in childhood (Z62.812)
personal history (past history) of sexual abuse in childhood (Z62.810)
personal history (past history) of spousal or partner neglect (Z91.412)
personal history (past history) of spousal or partner violence
    physical (Z91.410)
    sexual (Z91.410)
personal hygiene
    impaired
    minimal

personal identity, sense of
personal information
Personal Inventory of Needs
Personal Problems Checklist for
  Adolescents (PPC)
personal profile inventory
Personal Relationship Inventory
  (PRI)
Personal Resource Questionnaire
  (PRQ)
personal responsibility
personal risk factors, other
  (Z91.89)
personal satisfaction
Personal Skills Map, The
personal sound amplification
  product (PSAP)
personal space
Personal Strain Questionnaire
  (PSQ)
personal unappeal, feelings of
personal values survey
personality
  affective
  aggressive
  alexithymic
  allotropic
  alternating
  amoral
  anancastic
  antisocial (ASP)
  asocial
  asthenic
  authoritarian
  avoidant
  basic
  borderline
  coarctated
  compliant
  compulsive
  cycloid
  cyclothymic
  dependent
  depressive
  disturbed
  double
  dual
  dyssocial
personality
  eccentric
  epileptoid
  explosive
  fanatic
  histrionic
  hypomanic
  hysterical
  hysteroid
  immature
  inadequate
  introverted
  maladaptive
  masochistic
  multiple
  narcissistic
  obsessional
  obsessive-compulsive
    (OCP)
  paranoid
  passive
  passive-aggressive (PAP)
  passive-dependent (PDP)
  pathological
  premorbid
  prepsychotic
  presenting
  psychoinfantile
  psychoneurotic
  psychopathic
  sadistic
  schizoid
  schizotypal
  seclusive
  self-defeating
  shut-in
  sociopathic
  split
  stable
  syntonic
  theory
  type A
  type B
Personality Adjective Check List
  (PACL)
personality and gender, multiple
Personality Assessment Inventory
  (PAI)

personality change due to another
  medical condition
    aggressive type (F07.0)
    apathetic type (F07.0)
    combined type (F07.0)
    disinhibited type (F07.0)
    labile type (F07.0)
    other type (F07.0)
    paranoid type (F07.0)
    unspecified type (F07.0)
personality characteristics *(see also* tests)
personality disorder
  aggressive type
  antisocial (F60.2)
  apathetic type
  associated
  avoidant (F60.6)
  borderline (F60.3)
  cluster A
  cluster B
  cluster C
  combined type
  dependent (F60.7)
  dependent-passive
  depressive
  disinhibited type
  drug treatment for
  dyssocial
  emotional instability
  histrionic (F60.4)
  hyperthymic
  hypothymic
  labile type
  moral deficiency
  multiple (MPD)
  narcissistic (F60.81)
  negativistic
  obsessional
  obsessive-compulsive (F60.5)
  other specified (F60.89)
  paranoid
  passive-aggressive
  pseudosocial
  schizoid
  schizoid-schizotypal (SSPD)

personality disorder
  schizotypal
  seductive
  unspecified (F60.9)
Personality Factor Questionnaire (PFQ)
personality features
personality formation
personality functioning
personality impoverishment
Personality Inventory for Children (PIC)
personality pattern
personality psychoneurosis
personality questionnaire
Personality Rating Scale (PRS)
personality scales
personality style
  extratensive
  introintensive
personality tests *(see also* tests)
personality trait stability
personality traits
  cognitive
  interpersonal
  intrapsychic
  maladaptive
personality type
personification (figure of speech)
personnel, service
personnel profile
Personnel Reaction Blank
Personnel Selection Inventory
personnel tests *(see also* tests)
Personnel Tests for Industry
persons, loss of significant supporting
person's culture
perspective, categorical
persuasive communication
"Peruvian" (street name, cocaine)
"Peruvian flake" (street name, cocaine)
"Peruvian lady" (street name, cocaine)
pervasive and persistent maladaptive personality traits
pervasive anxiety

pervasive developmental disorder, disinhibited type of
pervasive disinhibition
pervasive disorder
pervasive distrust
pervasive impairment of development
pervasive pattern of pessimism
pervasive pattern of proneness to guilt
pervasive pattern of self-criticism
pervasive pattern of unhappiness
PESQ (Personal Experience Screening Questionnaire)
pessimism
    feelings of
    patterns of pervasive
PESST (Patterned Elicitation Syntax Screening Test)
PET (Professional Employment Test)
"Peter Pan" (street name, phencyclidine/PCP)
"peth" (street name, barbiturate)
petit mal, impulsive
petit mal (typical absence) seizure
petit mal epilepsy, impulsive
petit mal seizure, continuing
petit mal status
petit mal variant (Lennox-Gastaut) seizure
"peyote" (street term for mescaline)
    bad seed (marijuana combined with peyote)
    britton
    half moon
    hikon
    hikuli
    hyatan
    nubs
    P
    seni
    tops
PFAGH stuttering
PFS (Patient and Family Services)
"P-funk" (street name, crack and phencyclidine; heroin)
PGSR (psychogalvanic skin response)
PGSRA (psychogalvanic skin response audiometry)
phagomania (eating)
phallic overbearing
phallic phase
phallic stage psychosexual development
phalliform
phalloid
phallus
phaneromania (preoccupation with visible body parts)
phantom pain
phantom sensation
phantom speech
pharmacological aspects of drugs of abuse
pharmacological aspects of schizophrenia
pharmacological management of dementia
pharmacological provocation
pharmacological testing, intracorporeal
pharmacological treatment of dementia
pharmacological treatments
pharmacomania (drugs/medicine)
pharmacotherapy
pharyngeal constrictor
    inferior
    middle
    superior
pharyngeal flap
pharyngeal motor activity
pharyngeal raphe
pharyngeal reflex
pharyngeal speech
pharyngeal tonsil
pharyngis inferior, musculus constrictor
pharyngis medius, musculus constrictor
pharyngis superior, musculus constrictor
pharyngitis

pharyngoesophageal (PE) junction
pharyngoesophageal (PE)
  segment
pharyngopalatine arch
pharyngopalatine muscle
pharyngoplasty
pharynx (pl. pharynges)
  inferior constrictor muscle of
  middle constrictor muscle of
pharynx muscles
phase
  advance sleep-wake hours
  circadian sleep
  delayed sleep
  depressive
  developmental
  early dementia
  endogenous circadian rhythm
  excitement
  follicular
  illness
  in
  insomnia
  late luteal
  life problem
  luteal
  manic
  opposite
  out of
  pact ictal seizure
  REM sleep
  residual
  schizophrenia
  sexual response cycle
  stuttering
phase lag on EEG
phase of life problem (Z60.0)
phase of schizophrenia
  prodromal
  residual
phase of seizure, past ictal
  depression
phase of sexual response cycle
  desire
  excitement
  orgasmic
  resolution

phase of stable sleep difficulty,
  chronic
phase reversal on EEG
phase shift of sleep-wake cycle
phase spike on EEG
phasic REM activity
PHEIC (Public Health Emergency
  of International Concern)
Phelps Kindergarten Readiness
  Scale (PKRS)
phencyclidine (PCP) (street
  names)
  ace
  AD
  amoeba
  amp
  angel
  angel dust
  angel hair
  angel mist
  Angel Poke
  animal trank
  animal tranq
  animal tranquilizer
  aurora borealis
  Beam me up Scotty
  belladonna
  black acid
  black dust
  black whack
  blotter acid
  blue madman
  boat
  bohd
  bummer trip (unsettling trip
    from PCP intoxication)
  bush
  busy bee
  butt naked
  Cadillac
  cannabinol
  chips
  cigarrode cristal
  Cozmo's
  crazy coke
  Crazy Eddie
  crystal
  crystal joint

phencyclidine (street names)
- crystal T
- cycline
- cyclones
- D
- Detroit pink
- devil's dust
- dip sticks (cigarettes dipped in PCP oil)
- dipped joints (marijuana, PCP, and formaldehyde)
- dipper
- DMT
- do it Jack
- DOA
- domex (PCP and MDMA)
- donk (marijuana and PCP)
- drink
- dust
- dust blunt
- dusted parsley
- dusting (adding to PCP to marijuana)
- dust joint
- dust of angels
- dummy dust
- earth
- el diablito
- elephant
- elephant flipping (PCP and MDMA)
- elephant trank
- elephant tranquilizer
- embalming fluid
- energizer
- fake STP
- flakes
- fresh
- frios
- fry
- fry sticks
- fuel
- good
- goon
- goon dust
- gorilla biscuits
- gorilla tab
- green

phencyclidine (street names)
- green leaves
- green tea
- happy stick (marijuana & PCP combination)
- happy sticks
- HCP
- heaven and hell
- herms
- Hinkley
- hog
- horse tracks
- horse tranquilizer
- ice
- ill
- illies (marijuana dipped in PCP)
- illing (marijuana dipped in PCP)
- illy momo
- J
- jet fuel
- Jim Jones
- joy stick
- juice
- K
- kaps
- K-blast
- killer
- killer weed
- KJ
- koller joints
- kools
- krystal
- krystal joint
- KW
- LBJ
- leak (Marijuana/PCP combination)
- leaky bolla
- leaky leak
- lemon 714
- lenos
- lethal weapon
- licker
- little ones
- live ones
- log

phencyclidine (street names)
- love leaf
- loveboat (marijuana/PCP combination)
- lovelies (marijuana laced with PCP)
- lovely
- mad dog
- madman
- magic
- magic dust
- mean green
- mint leaf
- mint weed
- missile basing
- mist
- monkey dust
- monkey tranquilizer
- more
- new acid
- new magic
- niebla
- olumbo
- puffy
- O.P.P.
- octane
- oil
- orange crystal
- ozone
- P
- parachute
- parsley
- paz
- PCPA
- peace
- peace pill
- peace weed
- peanut butter
- peep
- Peter Pan
- P-funk
- Pichachu (pills with PCP and Ecstasy)
- Pig Killer
- pit
- polvo
- polvo de angel
- polvo de estrellas

phencyclidine (street names)
- poro phencyclidine
- polumbo
- puffy
- purple rain
- red devil
- rocket fuel
- scaffle
- scuffle
- sernyl
- sheets
- sherm sticks
- shermans
- sherms
- skuffle
- slum
- smoking
- snorts
- soma
- space base
- space cadet
- space dust
- spaceball
- speedboat
- spores
- squirrel
- star dust
- stardust
- stick
- STP
- super
- super joint
- super kools
- super weed
- surfer
- synthetic cocaine
- synthetic THT
- TAC
- taking a cruise
- T-buzz
- tea
- tic
- tic tac
- tish
- titch
- tragic magic
- trank
- TT1

phencyclidine (street names)
    TT2
    TT3
    uper grass
    wac
    wack
    water
    water-water
    weed
    wet
    whack
    white horizon
    white powder
    wicky
    wicky stick
    wobble weed
    wolf
    wollies
    wolly blunts
    worm
    wt sticks
    yellow fever
    yerba mala
    zombie
    zombie weed
    zoom
phencyclidine dose-related signs of withdrawal
phencyclidine-induced anxiety disorder
phencyclidine-induced disorder
phencyclidine intoxication delirium
phencyclidine intoxication with use disorder, mild (F16.129)
phencyclidine intoxication with use disorder, moderate/severe (F16.229)
phencyclidine intoxication without use disorder (F16.929)
phencyclidine-like substance
phencyclidine-related disorder
phencyclidine-related disorder, unspecified (F16.99)
phencyclidine use disorder in a controlled environment
    mild (F16.10)
        moderate/severe (F16.20)

phencyclidine use disorder with phencyclidine-induced anxiety disorder
phencyclidine use disorder with phencyclidine-induced bipolar or related disease
phencyclidine use disorder with phencyclidine-induced brief psychotic disorder
phencyclidine use disorder with phencyclidine-induced delirium
phencyclidine use disorder with phencyclidine-induced delusional disorder
phencyclidine use disorder with phencyclidine-induced depressive disorder
phencyclidine use disorder with phencyclidine-induced major or mild neurocognitive disorder
phencyclidine use disorder with phencyclidine-induced schizoaffective disorder
phencyclidine use disorder with phencyclidine-induced schizophreniform disorder
phencyclidine use disorder with phencyclidine-induced schizophrenia
phencyclidine use disorder with phencyclidine-induced schizotypal (personality) disorder
phenethylline *(see also* fenethylline)
phenobarbital, Karachi (heroin, phenobarbital & methaqualone mix)
phenomenological features, shared
phenomenological subgroups
phenomenology
phenomenon
    Bell
    clasp-knife
    dissociative
    Doppler
    freezing

phenomenon
    hesitation
    interactive
    motoric
    normal voluntary napping
    on-off
    paroxysmal
    psychic
    psychomotor
    Raynaud's
    tip-of-the-tongue
    Wever-Bray
phenothiazine-based neuroleptics
phenothiazine-based tranquilizer
pheochromocytoma
PHI (Protected Health Information)
Philadelphia Head Injury Questionnaire (PHIQ)
philopatridomania (patriotism)
philoponia (love of training)
philtrum (pl. philtra)
PHIQ (Philadelphia Head Injury Questionnaire)
phobia
    acarophobia (itching; mite or tick infestation)
    acerophobia (sourness; sharp flavors)
    achluophobia (darkness)
    acousticophobia (sounds; noise)
    acrophobia (heights)
    aelurophobia (cats)
    aerophobia (drafts; air; flying)
    agoraphobia (open spaces)
    agyiophobia (streets)
    aichmophobia (pointed objects; knife)
    ailurophobia (cats)
    alcoholophobia (alcoholism)
    algophobia (pain)
    altophobia (heights)
    amathophobia (dust)
    amaxophobia (vehicles)

phobia
    amychophobia (being scratched; scratches)
    androphobia (men, males)
    anemophobia (wind; drafts)
    anginophobia (angina pectoris attack)
    Anglophobia (England/ anything English)
    animal (e.g. spiders, snakes) (F40.218)
    anthophobia (flowers)
    anthropophobia (human companionship; people)
    antlophobia (flood)
    aphephobia (touching; being touched)
    apiphobia (bees)
    aquaphobia (water)
    arachnephobia (spiders)
    asthenophobia (being weak; weakness)
    astraphobia (thunder & lightning)
    astrapophobia (thunder & lightning)
    astrophobia (celestial space; stars)
    ataxiophobia (disorder)
    ataxophobia (disorder)
    atelophobia (imperfection)
    atephobia (ruin, personal; reckless impulse)
    aurophobia (gold)
    auroraphobia (dawn; northern lights)
    automysophobia (uncleanliness; being dirty; personal body odor)
    autophobia (self; solitude; being alone)
    bacillophobia (bacilli; germs)
    bacteriophobia (bacteria; germs)
    ballistophobia (missiles)
    barophobia (gravity)

phobia
- bathmophobia (walking)
- bathophobia (deep spaces)
- batophobia (being on tall buildings; high objects)
- batrachophobia (frogs and toads)
- belonephobia (sharp objects; pins and needles)
- bibliophobia (books)
- bogyphobia (demons and goblins)
- bromidrosiphobia (body odors; sweat)
- brontophobia (thunder; thunderstorms)
- cainophobia (novelty)
- cainotophobia (novelty)
- cancerophobia (cancer; malignancy)
- carcinophobia (cancer; malignancy)
- cardiophobia (heart disease)
- carnophobia (flesh; meat)
- cathisophobia (sitting down)
- catoptrophobia (mirrors)
- Celtophobia (Celts)
- cenophobia (open spaces; barrenness; emptiness)
- ceraunophobia (thunder and lightening)
- chaetophobia (hair)
- cheimaphobia (cold)
- cherophobia (gaiety)
- chionophobia (snow)
- cholerophobia (cholera)
- chrematophobia (wealth)
- chromatophobia (colors)
- chromophobia (colors)
- chronophobia (time)
- cibophobia (food)
- claustrophobia (confinement; enclosed space; being locked in)
- cleptophobia (loss through thievery)

phobia
- climacophobia (climbing; stairs)
- clithrophobia (being locked in)
- cnidophobia (stings)
- coitophobia (sexual intercourse)
- cometophobia (comets)
- coprophobia (excrement; feces; rectal excreta)
- counterphobia (confronting one's phobia)
- cremnophobia (precipices)
- cryophobia (ice; frost)
- crystallophobia (glass)
- cynophobia (dogs; pseudorabies)
- cypridophobia (sexual intercourse; venereal disease)
- demonophobia (demons and devils; spirits)
- demophobia (people; crowds)
- dendrophobia (trees)
- dermatopathophobia (skin disease)
- dermatophobia (skin disease)
- dermatosiophobia (skin disease)
- dextrophobia (objects on the right side of the body)
- diabetophobia (diabetes)
- dinophobia (whirlpools)
- diplopiaphobia (double vision)
- domatophobia (home)
- doraphobia (animals skins; fur; skins of animals)
- dromophobia (crossing streets)
- dysmorphophobia (deformity; becoming deformed)
- ecclesiophobia (churches)

phobia
  ecophobia (environment;
    home surroundings; home
    life)
  electrophobia (electricity)
  elurophobia (cats)
  emetophobia (vomiting)
  entomophobia (insects)
  eosophobia (dawn)
  eremiophobia (deserted
    places; solitude; being
    along; aloneness)
  eremophobia (deserted
    places; solitude; being
    alone; aloneness)
  ereuthrophobia (blushing;
    color red)
  ergasiophobia (working;
    functioning)
  ergophobia (work)
  erotophobia (physical love;
    sexual feelings)
  erythrophobia (blushing;
    color red)
  eurotophobia (female
    genitalia)
  fear of blood (F40.230)
  fear of
    injections/transfusions
    (F40.231)
  fear of injury (F40.233)
  fear of other medical care
    (F40.232)
  febriphobia (fever)
  felinophobia (cats)
  fibriphobia (fibers)
  Francophobia
    (France/anything French)
  frigophobia (cold)
  Gallophobia
    (France/anything French)
  gamophobia (marriage)
  gatophobia (cats)
  genophobia (sexual
    intercourse)
  gephyrophobia (crossing a
    bridge)

phobia
  gerascophobia (growing
    old)
  Germanophobia
    (Germany/anything
    Germanic)
  gerontophobia (the elderly;
    old people)
  geumophobia (taste;
    flavors)
  glossophobia (speaking;
    talking)
  graphophobia (writing)
  gringophobia (white
    strangers in Latin
    America)
  gymnophobia (nakedness)
  gynephobia (women)
  gynophobia (women)
  hadephobia (the
    underworld; the dead;
    hell)
  hagiophobia (sacred
    objects; saints)
  hamartophobia (sin; error)
  hamaxophobia (vehicles)
  haphephobia (being
    touched; touching)
  haphophobia (being
    touched; touching)
  haptophobia (being
    touched; touching)
  harpaxophobia (robbers)
  hedonophobia (pleasure)
  heliophobia (sun's rays;
    sunlight)
  helminthophobia (worms)
  hematophobia (blood;
    bleeding)
  hemophobia (blood;
    bleeding)
  herpetophobia (reptiles;
    amphibians)
  hierophobia (religious
    objects; sacred objects)
  hippophobia (horses)
  hodophobia (traveling)
  homichlophobia (fog)

phobia
- homilophobia (sermons)
- homophobia (homosexuality)
- hormephobia (rapid motion; shock)
- hyalophobia (glass)
- hydrophobia (choking/ gagging on liquids; water)
- hydrophobia (medical term for rabies in humans)
- hydrophobophobia (fear of rabies)
- hygrophobia (dampness; moisture; liquids esp. wine, water)
- hylephobia (forests; wood)
- hypengyophobia (responsibility)
- hypnophobia (sleep)
- hypsiphobia (heights)
- hypsophobia (heights)
- iatrophobia (going to the doctor)
- ichthyophobia (fish)
- ideophobia (ideas)
- iophobia (being poisoned; rusty objects)
- isopterophobia (termites)
- Japanophobia (Japan/ everything Japanese)
- Judaeophobia (Jews, Jewish culture)
- Judophobia (Jews, Jewish culture)
- kainophobia (newness; change; novelty)
- kakorrhaphiophobia (failure; defeat)
- katagelophobia (ridicule)
- kathisophobia (sitting down)
- kenophobia (emptiness; open spaces; barrenness; voids)
- keraunophobia (thunder and lightning)

phobia
- kinesophobia (movements; motions)
- kleptophobia (loss through thievery)
- koniophobia (dust)
- kopophobia (fatigue)
- kynophobia (pseudorabies)
- laliophobia (speaking; talking)
- lalophobia (speaking; talking)
- lepraphobia (leprosy)
- levophobia (objects on the left side of the body)
- linonophobia (string)
- logophobia (words)
- lyssophobia (rabies; insanity)
- maieusiophobia (pregnancy)
- maniaphobia (insanity)
- mastigophobia (whipping)
- mechanophobia (machinery)
- megalophobia (large objects)
- melissophobia (bees)
- meningitophobia (meningitis; brain disease)
- merinthophobia (being bound)
- metallophobia (metal objects)
- meteorophobia (weather; climate; meteors)
- microbiophobia (microbes; microorganisms; germs)
- microphobia (small objects)
- misophobia (contamination by dirt)
- molysmophobia (infection; contamination)
- monopathophobia (specific diseased body part)
- monophobia (solitude; being alone; aloneness)

phobia
- motorphobia (motor vehicles)
- musicophobia (music)
- musophobia (mice)
- mysophobia (dirt; infection; contamination; filth)
- mythophobia (myths; stating an untruth; stories)
- myxophobia (slime)
- natural environment (e.g. heights, storms) (F40.228)
- necrophobia (corpses; death)
- negrophobia (black people)
- neophobia (novelty; newness; innovation)
- nephophobia (clouds)
- noctiphobia (night; darkness)
- nomatophobia (names)
- nosophobia (illness; disease)
- nostophobia (home, returning to)
- nudophobia (unclothed; nude)
- nyctophobia (darkness; night)
- ochlophobia (crowds)
- ochophobia (vehicles)
- odontophobia (teeth)
- odynophobia (pain)
- oenopnobia (wine)
- oikophobia (home; family)
- oinophobia (wine)
- olfactophobia (odors; smells)
- ombrophobia (rain; rainstorms)
- ommatophobia (eyes)
- oneirophobia (dreams)
- onomatophobia (names; words, certain)
- ophidiophobia (snakes; reptiles)
- ophiophobia (snake venom)

phobia
- ornithophobia (birds)
- osmophobia (odors; smells)
- osphresiophobia (body odors)
- other (e.g. choking) (F40.298)
- panophobia (general anxiety; nonspecific fear)
- panphobia (general anxiety; nonspecific fear)
- pantophobia (general anxiety; nonspecific fear; fear of everything)
- paralipophobia (omission of duty; neglect of duty)
- paraphobia (sexual perversion)
- parasitophobia (parasites)
- parthenophobia (young girls)
- pathophobia (disease)
- patriophobia (hereditary disease)
- peccatiphobia (sinning)
- pediculophobia (lice)
- pediophobia (children; dolls)
- pedophobia (children; dolls)
- pellagraphobia (rough skin)
- peniaphobia (poverty)
- phagophobia (eating; swallowing)
- pharmacophobia (drugs; medicines)
- phasmophobia (ghosts)
- phengophobia (daylight)
- philosophobia (philosophers)
- phobanthropy (human companionship)
- phobophobia (phobias; being afraid; fearing)
- phonophobia (voices; sounds; noise; one's own voice)

phobia
- photalgiophobia (fear of photalgia)
- photaugiaphobia (glare of light)
- photophobia (light)
- phronemophobia (mind; thoughts; thinking)
- phthiriophobia (lice)
- phthisiophobia (tuberculosis)
- pneumatophobia (air; breathing)
- pnigophobia (choking)
- pogonophobia (beards)
- poinephobia (punishment)
- politicophobia (politicians)
- polyphobia (many things)
- ponophobia (fatigue; overwork)
- potamophobia (rivers)
- potophobia (drinking)
- proctophobia (rectal disease; rectum)
- psychophobia (mind)
- psychrophobia (cold temperatures)
- pteronophobia (feathers)
- pyrexiophobia (fever)
- pyrophobia (fire)
- radiophobia (radiation)
- rectophobia (rectal disease; rectum)
- rhabdophobia (being beaten; punishment by rod)
- rhypophobia (filth; dirt; defecation; feces)
- rupophobia (filth; dirt)
- Russophobia (Russia/anything Russian)
- Satanophobia (Satan; things satanic)
- scabiophobia (scabies)
- scatophobia (excrement; using obscene language)
- sciophobia (shadows)
- scoleciphobia (worms)

phobia
- scopophobia (being stared at)
- scotophobia (darkness)
- siderodromophobia (railways) (trains)
- siderophobia (iron; stars)
- sitiophobia (eating; food)
- sitophobia (eating; food)
- situational (e.g. elevators, airplanes) (F40.248)
- spectrophobia (seeing one's image in a mirror; phantoms)
- spermatophobia (semen, loss of)
- spermophobia (germs)
- sphecidophobia (wasps)
- stasibasiphobia (attempting to stand and/or walk)
- stasiphobia (standing still)
- stygiophobia (hell)
- symbolophobia (perceptions; symbolism)
- syphilophobia (being infected with syphilis)
- tabophobia (wasting sickness)
- tachophobia (speed)
- taeniophobia (tapeworms)
- taphephobia (being buried alive; graves)
- taphophobia (being buried alive; graves)
- tapinophobia (small things)
- taurophobia (bulls)
- teleophobia (teleology)
- telephonophobia (telephone)
- teratophobia (bearing a deformed child)
- Teutonophobia (Germany, things German)
- Teutophobia (Germany, things German)
- thaasophobia (sitting)
- thalassophobia (sea)
- thanatophobia (death)

phobia
    theatrophobia (theaters)
    theophobia (God)
    thermophobia (heat)
    thixophobia (shaking)
    tocophobia (childbirth)
    tomophobia (surgery)
    tonitrophobia (thunder)
    topophobia (places)
    toxicophobia (poison)
    toxiphobia (poison)
    toxophobia (poison)
    traumatophobia (trauma; wounds; injury)
    tremophobia (trembling)
    trichinophobia (trichinosis)
    trichopathophobia (hair abnormalities and disease)
    trichophobia (loose hair on clothing etc.)
    tridecaphobia (thirteen)
    triskaidekaphobia (thirteen)
    trypanophobia (injections)
    tuberculophobia (tuberculosis)
    tyrannophobia (morbid cruelty; tyrants)
    urophobia (passing urine)
    vaccinophobia (vaccination)
    venereophobia (venereal disease)
    vermiphobia (worms)
    xenophobia (strangers; foreigners)
    xerophobia (dry places; deserts)
    zelophobia (jealousy)
    zoophobia (animals)
phobias
    marked and excessive specific
    marked and persistent specific
    marked and unreasonable specific
    specific animal types of
phobic avoidance of situations
phobic situation
phobic stimulus
phobic trends
phon/phono
phonasthenia
phonation break
phonation
    maximum duration of
    myoelastic-aerodynamic theory of
    reverse
    ventricular
    voice disorders of
phonatory disorder
phonatory seizure
phoneme
    acute
    anterior feature English
    back
    back feature English
    compact
    consonantal feature English
    continuant feature English
    coronal feature English
    diffuse
    front
    grave
    high feature English
    lax
    lenis
    low feature English
    nasal feature English
    round feature English
    segmental
    strident feature English
    suprasegmental
    tense
    tense feature English
    vocalic feature English
    voiced feature English
Phoneme Discrimination Test (PDT)
phonemic alphabet, international
phonemic analysis
phonemic articulation error
phonemic paraphasia
phonemic regression
phonemic synthesis

phonemic transcription, broad
phonetic analysis, traditional
phonetic-analysis skills
phonetic articulation error
phonetic context
phonetic features
phonetic inventory
phonetic placement
phonetic power
phonetic skills
phonetic symbolization, visual-tactile
phonetic transcription
    close
    narrow
phonetic variations
Phonetically Balanced Kindergarten Word Lists
phonetically balanced words (PB words)
phonetician
phonetics
    acoustic
    applied
    articulatory
    auditory
    descriptive
    evolutionary
    experimental
    general
    historical
    impressionistic
    linguistic
    normative
    physiologic
phonetics of juncture
phoniatrics
phoniatrist
phonics, vocal
phonics criterion tests *(see also* tests)
phonics proficiency scales *(see also* tests)
phonics surveys *(see also* tests)
phonogram
phonological agraphia
phonological analysis *(see also* tests)
phonological conditioning
phonological disorder
phonological impairment, aphasic
Phonological Process Analysis (PPA)
phonological processes *(see also* tests)
phonological processes
    developmental
    natural
phonological rules
phonomania (voices/sounds)
phosphene
photalgiophobia
photaugiaphobia
photic epilepsy
photogenic seizure
photographic articulation tests, structured *(see also* tests)
photographic expressive language tests, structured
photomania (light)
photosensitive epilepsy *(see also* tests)
phrase
    absolute construction of
    carrier
    endocentric construction of
    exocentric construction of
    incomplete
phrase level, automatic
phrase repetition
phrase structure grammar
phronemomania (thoughts/the mind)
phthiriomania (lice)
phthiriophobia
phylogenesis
phylogeny
physical abuse
    adult, by nonspouse or nonpartner, confirmed, initial encounter (T74.11XA)
    adult, by nonspouse or nonpartner, confirmed, subsequent encounter (T74.11XD)

Psychiatric Words and Phrases

physical abuse
   adult, by nonspouse or nonpartner, suspected, initial encounter (T76.11XA)
   adult, by nonspouse or nonpartner, suspected, subsequent encounter (T76.11XD)
   childhood
physical abuse in childhood
physical abuse of adolescents
physical abuse of adults
physical abuse of children
physical activity, reduced
Physical and Architectural Features Checklist
physical attack
physical bondage (restraint)
Physical Capacities Battery - Rand
physical change, age-related
physical concomitant of anxiety
physical defect
physical environment
physical experience
physical fights, recurrent
physical harm, prevention of
physical health
physical independence
physical manifestation of pain
physical problem
physical sensations, distorted perception of
physical signs and symptoms
physical spousal or partner violence
   confirmed, initial encounter (T74.11XA)
   confirmed, subsequent encounter (T74.11XD)
   suspected, initial encounter (T76.11XA)
   suspected, subsequent encounter (T76.11XD)
physical strain
physical support
physical symptoms inventory *(see also* tests)
physical tension
physical therapy, outpatient
Physical Tolerance Profile (PTP)
physical trauma
physically endangered
physician
   family
   primary care (PCP)
physician-patient relations
physician's role
physiogenic
physiologic mechanism
physiologic phonetics
physiologic tremor
physiological dependence
   substance dependence with
   substance dependence without
physiological effect, direct
physiological factor
physiological functional variation
physiological intoxication
physiological measurements
physiological norm, deviation from
physiological process
physiological reactivity
physiological response(s), stress-related
physiological signs of withdrawal
physiological sleepiness, index of
physiological tremor
physiology of successful aging
phytocannabinoid
Piaget's cognitive development stages
"pianoing" (re: crack acquisition)
pica disorder
pica in adults (F50.4)
pica in children (F98.3)
Picha-Seron Career Analysis (PSCA)
Pick inclusion bodies, intraneuronal argentophilic
picking at bodily orifices, nonfunctional and repetitive

picking at skin, nonfunctional and repetitive
Picks disease, dementia due to
PICSYMS (picture symbols)
pictographs
pictorial completion test *(see also* tests)
pictorial reasoning test *(see also* tests)
picture from memory test, draw a
picture(s) test *(see also* tests)
    complex
    complex thematic
    thematic
picture with perceptual disturbances, mixed symptom
pidgin Sign English (PSE)
"piece" (re: 1 ounce drug quantity)
"piedras" (street name, crack)
Pierre Robin syndrome
"Pig Killer" (street name, phencyclidine/PCP)
"piggybacking" (re: injecting two drugs together)
"Pikachu" (re: pills containing PCP and ecstasy)
Pike dementia
"piles" (street name, crack)
pill-rolling tremor
pills, diet
"pimp" (street name, cocaine)
"pimp your pipe" (re: crack equipment)
Pimsleur Language Aptitude Battery
"pin" (street name, cannabis)
"ping-in-wing" (re: drug injection)
"pin gon" (street name, opium)
pin sticking sensation
Pin Test, The
"pin yen" (street name, opium)
"pink" (street name, synthetic opioid)
"pink blotters" (street name, lysergic acid diethylamide/LSD)
"pink hearts" (street name, amphetamine)
pink noise
"Pink Panther" (street name, lysergic acid diethylamide/PCP)
"Pink Panthers" (street name, ecstasy/MDMA)
"pink robots" (street name, lysergic acid diethylamide/LSD)
"pink witches" (street name, lysergic acid diethylamide/LSD)
pinna (pl. pinnae)
pinning and piercing (infibulation)
pins and needles sensation
"pipe" (re: cannabis or crack equipment; drug injection; mixed drugs)
pipe smoking, straight
"pipero" (re: crack user)
"pit" (street name, phencyclidine)
pitch
    ascending
    basal
    descending
    habitual
    natural
pitch brake
pitch discrimination
pitch perception
pitch range
pitch shift
pivot grammar (parts of speech)
pivot word
"pixies" (street name, amphetamine)
PKRS (Phelps Kindergarten Readiness Scale)
placebo medication trial
place hearing theory
placement
    alveolar consonant
    bilabial area consonant
    glottal area consonant
    labiodental area consonant

placement
    lingua-alveolar area
      consonant
    linguadental area consonant
    palatal area consonant
    phonetic
    sense of
    velar area consonant
placement exam *(see also* tests)
placement test *(see also* tests)
plan
    formulate a
    management
    meticulously detailed
    organizational
    realistic
    suicide
plan ahead, failure to
plan of action
plane
    coronal
    frontal
    horizontal
    median sagittal
    sagittal
planigraphy
planning
    disturbance in
    inventory for client and
      agency
"plant" (re: drug concealment)
plantar response, extensor
plasma homovanillic acid (HVA)
plasma HVA levels in
  schizophrenia
plasma protein metabolism
plateau masking technique
plateau method
play
    expression of traumatic
      themes through repetitive
    fantasy
    group
    imaginative
    make-believe
    rough-and-tumble
    symbolic
    verbal

play audiometry
play hunches, tendency to
play vocal range, vocal
"Playboy bunnies" (street name,
  ecstasy/MDMA)
"playboys" (street name,
  ecstasy/MDMA)
playing with hands, nonfunctional
  and repetitive
playmate, imaginary
pleasurable activities, neglect of
pleasurable activity
pleasure
    inability to experience
    lack of
    loss of
    sexual
    subjective sense of sexual
pleasure in everyday activities,
  diminished
pleasure in few activities, take
pleasure-pain principle
pleasure-seeking
plethysmography, penile
plosive consonant formation
plosive-injection method
plus juncture
plutomania (delusions of great
  wealth)
P-MAC/ESP (Perceptual-Motor
  Assessment for Children &
  Emotional/Behavior Screening
  Program)
PMEI (polymorphic epilepsy in
  infancy)
PMPQ (Professional and
  Managerial Position
  Questionnaire)
PNdB (perceived noise level)
pneumatic artificial larynx
pneumogram
pneumograph
pneumotachogram
pneumotachograph
PNS (peripheral nervous system)
p.o. (by mouth)
p.o. (probation officer)

"pocket rocket" (street name, cannabis)
"pod" (street name, cannabis)
point, alveolar
point of activity, major
point of articulation
pointing test *(see also* tests)
"poison" (street name, fentanyl; heroin)
poisoning, lead
"poke" (street name, cannabis)
polar opposites
polarities, sorting
polarity response
Police Officer Selection Test - National (POST)
Policy and Program Information Form
political activity
political values, acculturation problems with
politicomania (politics)
Politte Sentence Completion Test
Pollack-Branden Inventory: For Identification of Learning Disabilities, Dyslexia and Classroom Dysfunction
"pollutants" (street name, ecstasy/MDMA)
pollution, noise
Pollyanna-like view
"polvo" (street name, heroin; phencyclidine/PCP)
"polvo blanco" (street name, cocaine)
"polvo de angel" (street name, phencyclidine/PCP)
"polvo de estrellas" (street name, phencyclidine/PCP)
Polyfactorial Study of Personality
polyglot
polygraph
polymorphemic utterances
polymorphic epilepsy in infancy (PMEI)
polyneuropathy
polyphasic potential
polyphyria

polypoid degeneration of the true folds
polypoid vocal nodules
polysomnographic abnormalities
polysomnographic study
polysomnography
polysubstance-related disorder
polysyllabic word
polytomography
pons
"pony" (street name, crack)
poor concentration
poor form quality
poor impulse control
poor insight
poor interpersonal rapport
poor judgment
"poor man's pot" (street name, inhalant)
poor memory
poor method
poor peer relationships
poor sense of responsibility
poor work performance
"pop" (re: cocaine use)
"poppy" (street name, heroin)
population setting, general
populations, community
poriomania (wander or journey from home)
pornographomania (pornography)
pornography, paraphiliac
porphyrin metabolism
port
    nasal
    velopharyngeal
PORT (Perception-Of-Relationships-Test)
Portland Digit Recognition Test (PDRT)
Portland Problem Behavior Checklist--Revised
portmanteau word
Portuguese Speaking Test (PST)
position
    body
    cortical thumb
    final consonant

position
    initial consonant
    intervocalic consonant
    medial consonant
    medically related
    observer
    postvocalic consonant
    prevocalic consonant
    seated
    second
    sustained
    third
position/index, self
position of responsibility
positional tremor
positioning of distal limbs, abnormal
positive ability
Positive and Negative Syndrome Scale (PANSS)
positive comparison
positive correlation
positive emotion
positive emotionality
positive events, potential
positive frontal release signs
positive ion
positive reinforcer
positive relationship, perfect
positive response
positive schizophrenic symptoms
    disorganization dimension of
    psychotic dimension of
positive spikes
    fourteen-and-six Hertz
    six Hertz
positive spike-waves, six Hertz
positive symptoms of schizophrenia
positive symptoms scale assessment *(see also* tests)
positivity
positron-emission tomography (PET)
possessing agent(s)
possession, drug
possession trance state
possession trance symptom

possessive case
possessor-possession
possible effect
POST (National Police Officer Selection Test)
post stroke depression
postanalytic supervision, boundaries in
postanoxic encephalopathy
postanoxic epilepsy
postcentral gyrus
postcentral sulcus
postconcussion disorder
postconcussion headache
postconcussion neurosis
postconcussion syndrome
postconcussive amnesia
postconsonantal vowel
postcontusion brain syndrome
postdormital sleep paralysis
postencephalitic syndrome
posterior alexia
posterior cricoarytenoid muscle
posterior digastric muscle
posterior inferior, musculus serratus
posterior superior, musculus serratus
posterior vertical canal
postictal confusion
postictal depression
postictal state
post-incident care for the assaulted staff
postlingual deafness
postmortem studies of suicide victims
postoperative status
postpartum counseling and addition treatment
postpartum major depression
postponements
postpsychotic depression
postpsychotic depressive disorder
postpsychotic depressive disorder of schizophrenia
postpubertal
postpuberty

postpubescence
postpubescent
postrotary nystagmus test
postsynaptic receptor
posttermination, boundaries
posttetanic facilitation
posttetanic potentiation (PTP)
posttraumatic amnesia (PTA)
posttraumatic cerebral syndrome
posttraumatic chronic disability
posttraumatic cortical dysfunction
posttraumatic encephalopathy
posttraumatic headache
posttraumatic pain
posttraumatic seizure
posttraumatic stress disorder (children 6 YO and younger) (F42.10)
posttraumatic stress disorder (PTSD0 (F42.10)
posttraumatic stress disorder with delayed expression (F42.10)
posttraumatic stress disorder with dissociative symptoms (F42.10)
postulates, conversational
postural awareness
postural seizure
postural tremor
    anticonvulsant medication-induced
    antidepressant medication-induced
    beta-adrenergic medication-induced
    caffeine-induced
    dopaminergic medication-induced
    fine
    lithium-induced
    medication-induced (G25.1)
    methylxanthime-induced
    neuroleptic-induced
    stimulant-induced
    valproate-induced
posture
    bizarre
    body

posture
    inappropriate
    unusual sleep
posture disorganization in dyspraxic children *(see also tests)*
posturing
postvocalic consonant position
postvocalic obstruent singleton omissions
"potato" (street name, lysergic acid diethylamide)
"potato chips" (street name, crack cut with benzocaine)
potential
    acoustic evoked
    acting out
    action
    assessment of suicide
    biphasic
    brain stem auditory evoked (BAEP)
    brain stem evoked
    cerebral
    cortical evoked
    EEG
    electrical
    glossokinetic
    high tolerance
    low tolerance
    motor evoked (MEP)
    polyphasic
    resting
    sensory evoked (SEP)
    system for testing and evaluation of
    visual evoked (VEP)
potential adverse effects
potential energy
potential evaluation by others, anxiety due to
potential external awards
potential external rewards
potential for injury
potential for painful consequences, high
potential impact

Psychiatric Words and Phrases

potential impairment of immune functioning
potential inventory *(see also* tests)
potential learning disability tests *(see also* tests)
potential positive events
potential problems
potential risks for malnutrition
potential secondary gain
potential targets
potentiometer
potomania (drinking)
"potten bush" (street name, cannabis)
pounding or racing heart (a panic attack indicator)
pounding pain
poverty
    extreme (Z59.5)
    problems related to extreme (Z59.5)
poverty of content
poverty of movement
poverty of speech
poverty of speech content
POW (prisoner of war)
Powassan viral encephalitis
"powder" (street name, amphetamine; heroin)
"powder diamonds" (street name, cocaine)
power
    degrees of reading
    distribution of
    inflated
    instantaneous
    manipulative behavior to attain
    phonetic
power CROS (contralateral routing of signals)
power density, sound
power output, maximum (MPO)
"power puller" (re: crack equipment)
powerful emotion
"pox" (street name, opium)

PPA (Phonological Process Analysis)
PPC (Personal Problems Checklist for Adolescents)
PPCP (Parent Perception of Child Profile)
PPSRT (Printing Performance School Readiness Test)
"P.R." (street name, Panama Red)
practical aspects of assaultive client care
Practical Judgment Form 62 Test
Practical Maths Assessments
practical reasoning
practice
    family
    negative
    psychology
practice test
pragmatic aphasia
Pragmatic Language Test
Pragmatic Skills Test
pragmatic structures, performative
Pragmatics Profile of Early Communication Skills, The
Pragmatics Screening Test
praxis tests, sensory integration and PRE MOD II
pre-article
precentral gyrus
precentral seizure
precentral sulcus
precipitant exposure, common
precipitating factor
precipitating tremor, emotional stress
precipitation of epilepsy
precipitation of seizure
precision therapy
preconsonantal vowel
precounseling inventory, couple's
predators
predicate
    complete
    simple
predicate adjective
predicate nominative
predicate noun

predicate objective
predicate truncation
prediction from the acoustic reflex, sensitivity (SPAR)
prediction of dangerousness
Predictive Screening Test of Articulation
predisposed, situationally
predisposed panic attack(s), situationally
predisposing factor
predominant affect
predominant current defense level
predominant defense level
predominant mood disturbance
predominant symptom presentation
predominantly hyperactive-impulsive attention-deficit/hyperactivity disorder
predominantly predormital sleep paralysis
preepisode status
preexisting cognitive variables
preexisting dementia
preexisting mental disorder, exacerbated symptoms of a
preexisting tremor
preexisting underlying emotional issues
preference, consonant-vowel
preferences, paraphiliac
preferred method
preferred representational system
prefix
pregnancy
    complications of
    hysterical
    management of
    objective signs of
    psychiatric illness during
    vomiting throughout
Prekindergarten Screening Test
pre-language battery *(see also* tests)
Preliminary Diagnostic Questionnaire
prelingual deafness
prelinguistic language
premature (early) ejaculation, (lifetime, acquired, generalized, situational) (F52.4)
premature death
premaxilla
premenstrual dysphoria disorder (N94.3)
premenstrual syndrome
premolar teeth
    first
    second
premonition of seizure
premonitory sign
premorbid adjustment
premorbid history
premorbid level of functioning
premorbid state
premotor area
prenatal counseling and addition treatment
preoccupation with control
preoccupation with death
preoccupation with defect
preoccupation with details
preoccupation with lists
preoccupation with order
preoccupation with orderliness
preoccupation with organization
preoccupation with perfectionism
preoccupation with rules
preoccupation with schedules
preoperational thought period
prepalatal
preparatory set
preposition (parts of speech)
Pre-Professional Skills Test
prepsychotic
prepubertal psychopathology
preputial sensation, reduced
prerequisite skills screening test *(see also* tests)
presbyacusis
Pre-School and Primary Self-Concept Screening Test
preschool tests *(see also* tests)
Prescreening Development Questionnaire

prescribed treatment
"prescription" (street name, cannabis cigarette)
prescription drug(s) *(see also medications)*
prescription drug-related disorder
prescription-drug therapy
prescriptive grammar
presence of motivation
presentation
    atypical
    catatonic
    equivalent symptomatic
    mixed
    pain
    predominant symptom
    psychotic
    substance-induced
    subthreshold
    symptom
presenting problem
presenting psychopathology
presenting symptom
present perfect progressive tense
present perfect tense
present progressive tense, simple
present tense, simple
preservation of affect
"press" (street name, cocaine; crack)
press
    glossopharyngeal
    tongue
press limits, to
pressure
    environmental
    intraoral
    intrapleural
    intrapulmonic
    intrathoracic
    minimum audible (MAP)
    pulmonary
    time
pressure level
    saturation sound (SSPL)
    sound (SPL)
pressure level range, sound
pressure of speech
pressure pattern
pressure wave, sound
pressured behavior
presumed causality
presupposition
presyntactic devices
"pretendica" (street name, cannabis)
"pretendo" (street name, cannabis)
pretentious
prevalence of insomnia
prevalence of schizophrenia
prevention
    anxiety
    dropout prediction and stress
prevention of disclosure
prevention of extrapyramidal symptoms
prevention of physical harm
prevention of weight gain
prevention of withdrawal
preventive intervention
previous history
previously stabilizing social situations, loss of
prevocalic consonant position
prevocalic singleton
prevocalic voicing of consonants
Prevocational Assessment and Curriculum Guide, The (PACG)
Prevocational Assessment Screen (PAS)
prevocational deafness
PRI (Partner Relationship Inventory)
PRI (Personal Relationship Inventory)
priapism
pride, excessive
primary anxiety disorder
primary auditory cortex
primary autism
primary care patient populations
primary care physician (PCP)
primary care setting
primary case

primary characteristics of
    stuttering
primary degenerative dementia
primary function
primary hypersomnia
primary identity
primary insomnia
primary language
Primary Language Screen, The
    (TPLS)
Primary Measures of Music
    Audiation
primary mental disorder
primary mood disorder with
    psychotic features
primary oppositional attitude
primary palate
primary Parkinson's disease
primary process thinking
primary psychotic disorder
primary reinforcement
primary reinforcer
primary responsibility
primary seizure
Primary Self-Concept Screening
    Test
primary sex characteristics
primary sleep disorder
primary stress
primary stuttering (theory in
    stuttering)
primary support group
    problems related to
    problems with
Primary Test of Cognitive Skills
    (PTCS)
primary theory of stuttering
"primo" (street name, cannabis
    and crack)
primobolan (injectable and oral
    steroid)
"primos" (street name, cigarettes
    laced with cocaine and heroin)
principle
    binary
    organizing
    pleasure-pain
    psychophysiologic

principal clause
principal diagnosis
principal focus
principal investigation
principal objective
Printing Performance School
    Readiness Test (PPSRT)
prior diseases, dementia due to
prior history
prison
    problems related to release
        from (Z65.2)
    psychiatric
prisoner of war (POW)
private practice patient
    populations
probability curve, normal
probability learning
probability scale for suicide *(see
    also* tests)
probation officer (p.o.)
probe microphone measurements
probe tube microphone
Probes of Articulation
    Consistency - Clinical
problem(s)
    abuse and neglect
    academic
    acculturation
    adolescent identity
    adult maltreatment and
        neglect
    age-related cognitive
        decline
    alcohol
    alcoholism with cirrhosis
        and concurrent psychiatric
    cancer and concurrent
        psychiatric
    cardiovascular disease and
        concurrent psychiatric
    career change
    child maltreatment and
        neglect
    child neglect
    cocaine
    delirium and concurrent
        psychiatric

problem(s)
- disturbing
- divorce
- drug
- economic
- educational
- emotional
- environmental
- existence of a
- expressive language
- faith conversion
- gait
- gastrointestinal conditions and concurrent psychiatric
- gender identity
- health
- HIV infection and concurrent psychiatric
- housing
- identity
- impulse-control
- individuation
- kidney disease and concurrent psychiatric
- leaving parental control
- leaving school
- loss of faith
- marriage
- memory
- new career
- occasional erectile
- occasional orgasmic
- occupational
- opioid
- parent-child relational
- partner relational
- persistent sleep
- phase of life (Z60.0)
- physical
- potential
- presenting
- psychological
- psychosocial
- pulmonary disease and concurrent psychiatric
- questioning faith
- real-life
- receptive language

problem(s)
- relational
- religious or spiritual (Z65.8)
- retirement
- school change
- school discipline
- school drop-out
- school entering
- separation
- sexual arousal
- sibling relational
- spiritual
- stress-related
  - psychophysiological
- substance-related
- word-finding
- work-related

problem-based learning
problem checklist, health
Problem Experiences Checklist
problem inventory, time
problem(s) related to abuse
problem(s) related to access of medical care (Z75.3)
problem(s) related to access of other healthcare (Z75.4)
problem(s) related to adequate food (Z59.4)
problem(s) related to a general medical condition
problem(s) related to a mental condition
problem(s) related to current military deployment status (Z56.82)
problem(s) related to employment, other (Z56.9)
problem(s) related to exposure to disaster, war, or other hostilities (Z65.5)
problem(s) related to extreme poverty (Z59.5)
problem(s) related to inadequate social insurance (Z59.7)
problem(s) related to inadequate welfare support (Z59.7)

problem(s) related to interaction with the legal system
problem(s) related to lifestyle (Z72.9)
problem(s) related to living along (Z60.2)
problem(s) related to living in a residential institution (Z59.3)
problem(s) related to low income (Z59.6)
problem(s) related to multiparity (Z64.1)
problem(s) related to neglect
problem(s) related to other legal circumstances (Z64.3)
problem(s) related to primary support group
problem(s) related to psychological circumstances
    other (Z65.6)
    unspecified (Z65.9)
problem(s) related to release from prison (Z65.2)
problem(s) related to religion or spirituality (Z65.8)
problem(s) related to safe drinking water (Z59.4)
problem(s) related to sexual abuse
problem(s) related to social environment, unspecified (Z60.9)
problem(s) related to unwanted pregnancy (Z64.0)
problem scales *(see also* tests)
problem solving
    difficulties with
    visuo-spatial
problem-solving communication
Problem Solving Inventory
problem-solving negotiation
problem-solving profiles *(see also* tests)
problem-solving strategies
problem solving tests *(see also* tests)
problem(s) with access to health care services
problem(s) with acculturation (Z60.3)
problem(s) with homelessness (Z59.0)
problem(s) with inadequate housing
problem(s) with landlord (Z59.2)
problem(s) with lodger (Z59.2)
problem(s) with neighbor (Z59.2)
problem(s) with primary support group
problem(s) with sexual arousal
problem(s) with sexual desire
problem(s) with social exclusion or rejection (Z60.4)
procaine (street name: "double rock" - crack diluted with procaine)
procedures *(see also* tests)
    auditory tests and
    language tests and
    operant
    set of
procedures for the elderly *(see also* tests)
Procedures for the Phonological Analysis of Children's Language
Process for the Assessment of Effective Student Functioning, A
process of clinical evaluation
process of dementia, psychobiological
process of maxilla, alveolar
Process Skills Rating Scales (PSRS)
process thinking, primary
process words
processes *(see also* tests)
    auditory
    automatic psychological
    biological
    bizarre thought
    central auditory
    closure
    concrete thought
    decision-making

processes *(see also* tests)
   dementing
   developmental
     phonological
   disease
   egocentric thought
   empirical
   escalative
   evidence-based
   explicit
   feature contrasts
   goal-oriented
   harmony
   idiosyncratic
   mastoid
   mental
   monosyllabic
   natural phonological
   normative aging
   pathological
   pathophysiological
   phonological
   physiological
   psychosocial
   psychotic
   revision
   schizophrenic
   systematic
   therapeutic
   transition
processing
   affective experience
   auditory
   dissociative state
   disturbance in speed of information
   higher integrative language
   language
   temporal auditory
   traumatic experience
   visuo-spatial
processing assessment *(see also* tests)
processing disorder, auditory
processing issues
processing of affective experience, unconscious
processing of dissociative states and disorders, unconscious
processing of traumatic experience, unconscious
prodromal phase of schizophrenia
prodromal symptoms
prodrome, visual
prodrome of schizophrenia, prolonged
produced symptoms
   intentionally
   unintentionally
product moment
production
   constricted vocal
   electrical measurement of speech
   speech sound
   stressful word
   work skills
production of symptoms, intentional
productivity, decreased
productivity of speech, decreased
productivity of thought
productivity of thought and speech
Professional and Managerial Position Questionnaire (PMPQ)
professional burnout
professional counselor
Professional Employment Test (PET)
professional exploiters
professional gambling
professional-family relations
professional-patient relations
proficiency tests *(see also* tests)
profile(s) *(see also* tests)
   left-out sibling
   neurotic direction
   spiked
profit, manipulative behavior to gain
profound amnesia
profound hearing impairment
profound hearing loss

Prognostic Value of Imitative and
    Auditory Discrimination Tests
programmed tests *(see also* tests)
programmed therapy
programming
    articulation
    neuro-linguistic
progress, educational
progressive assimilation
progressive cerebellar tremor
progressive degenerative disease,
    inherited
progressive dementing illness
progressive deterioration,
    uniformly
progressive disability
progressive multifocal
    leukoencephalopathy
progressive palsy
progressive relaxation
progressive subcortical
    encephalopathy
progressive supranuclear palsy
progressive tense
    future perfect
    past perfect
progressive tests *(see also* tests)
progressive traumatic
    encephalopathy
progressive vowel assimilation
projection, delusional
projection tests *(see also* tests)
Projective Assessment of Aging
    Method
projective identification
projective technique
projects, field-trial
prolabium
prolongation, sound
prolongation of sounds
prolonged episode
prolonged nocturnal sleep
    episodes
prolonged prodrome of
    schizophrenia
prolonged sleep episodes
prolonged sleep latency
prominence, laryngeal

prominent anxiety
prominent deterioration
prominent grimacing
prominent hallucination
prominent irritable mood
prominent mood symptoms
prominent negative symptoms of
    schizophrenia
promiscuous sex
promiscuous sexual behavior
prompting
proneness to guilt, patterns of
    pervasive
pronoun (parts of speech)
    anaphoric
    exophoric
pronunciation
propaganda
prophylactic treatment, need for
proportions, delusional
proposed treatment
propositional speech
proprioception
proprioceptive feedback
proprioceptive perception
prosocial emotions
prosody of speech, minimal
Prosody-Voice Screening Profile
    (PVSP)
prosthesis (pl. prostheses)
prosthetic management of cleft
    palate
prosthodontist
prostitutes, services of
prostitution
Protected Health Information
    (PHI)
protection device
    canal caps hearing
    circumaural hearing
    earmuffs hearing
    earplugs hearing
    hearing (HPD)
    insert hearing
    semiaural hearing
protective "survival strategy"
"protector" identity

protein
- beta-amyloid
- Crk

protocol, test
protolanguage
prototypical case
prototypical course patterns
protoword
protrusion, tongue
protrusion lisp
proverb interpretation test
provider, health care
proviron (oral steroid)
provisional tic disorder (F95.0)
provocation
- aggression without pharmacological

provoked anxiety
provoking stimulus, emotionally
proximal renal tubular acidosis
proxy, factitious disorder by
PRQ (Personal Resource Questionnaire)
PRT (Pantomime Recognition Test)
PSAP (personal sound amplification product)
PSCA (Picha-Seron Career Analysis)
PSE (Pidgin Sign English)
pseudobinaural hearing aid
pseudobulbar palsy
pseudobulbar paralysis
"pseudocaine" (re: adulterated crack)
pseudocyesis
pseudohypacusis
pseudolaryngeal paralysis
pseudomania (factitious mental disorder)
pseudoneurological symptoms
pseudoseizure
pseudostuttering
pseudotumor cerebri
PSI Basic Skills Test for Business, Industry, and Government

psilocybin/psilocin (street names)
- boomers
- caps
- flower flipping (ecstasy mixed with mushrooms)
- God's flesh
- hippieflip (use of mushrooms and MDMA)
- hombrecitos
- las mujercitas
- little smoke
- magic mushroom
- Mexican mushroom
- mushrooms
- musk
- sacred mushroom
- sherm (psychedelic mushrooms)
- shrooms
- Silly Putty
- Simple Simon

PSQ (Personal Strain Questionnaire)
PSRS (Process Skills Rating Scales)
PST (Portuguese Speaking Test)
Psych Evaluation - Rule Eleven
Psychasthenia "7" Scale
psychedelic agents (see *psychodysleptic agents)*
psychiatric brain disorders, in vivo magnetic resonance spectroscopy in
psychiatric case history
psychiatric consequences of stroke
psychiatric consulting remote video telemedicine
psychiatric diagnosis, Robins-Guze criteria for
psychiatric diagnosis and assessment
Psychiatric Diagnostic Interview
psychiatric disorders, male-female differences
psychiatric disturbance, overall severity of

psychiatric drug
psychiatric education
psychiatric examination
psychiatric factors affecting
   medical conditions
psychiatric genetics
psychiatric illness during
   pregnancy
psychiatric inpatient
psychiatric interview
psychiatric manifestations
psychiatric nomenclature
psychiatric nurse practitioner
psychiatric nursing
psychiatric problems
    alcoholism with cirrhosis
     and concurrent
    cancer and concurrent
    cardiovascular disease and
     concurrent
    delirium and concurrent
    gastrointestinal conditions
     and concurrent
    HIV infection and
     concurrent
    kidney disease and
     concurrent
    menstrual problems and
     concurrent
    pulmonary disease and
     concurrent
    sexual disorders and
     concurrent
    sleep disorder and
     concurrent
psychiatric professional services:
    academic centers
    hospitals
    large health systems
    managed care
    pharmaceutical industry
    private practice
psychiatric setting, inpatient
psychiatric social work
psychiatric somatic therapies
Psychiatric Status Rating Scale
psychiatric syndrome
    anger and violence

psychiatric syndrome
    anxiety-related
    apathy and failure to
     rehabilitate
    dementia-related
    depression-related
    disinhibition
    gender difference
    pain, touch, and stroke
    paranoia and delusions
    sex and stroke
    speaking and understanding
psychiatric system interface
   disorder
psychiatric treatment
psychiatrist
    public
    social
Psychiatrists in Alcoholism and
   Addictions, American Academy
   of (AAPAA)
psychiatry
    academic
    addiction
    administrative
    adolescent
    adulthood
    Clunis inquiry forensic
    geriatric
    hospital-based
    military
    multidisciplinary group
    nutritional
    old age
    organized-care
    outpatient-based
    prison
    psychopharmacologic
    public
    rehabilitation
    rural
    small-city
    speech and language
     disorders in
    staff HMO-based
    urban
Psychiatry and the Law,
   American Academy of (AAPL)

psychiatry of stroke
psychic disturbance
psychic numbing
psychic phenomena
psychic seizure
psychoactive effect(s)
psychoactive substance, illicit
psychoanalysis
    boundaries in
psychoanalysis
    violation of boundaries in
psychoanalysis and character disorder
psychoanalysis and depression
psychoanalysis and neuroses
psychoanalysis and object relations
psychoanalysis and paranoid states
psychoanalysis and pathological character formation
psychoanalysis and psychopathology
psychoanalysis and psychosomatics
psychoanalysis and schizophrenia
psychoanalysis and self-psychology
psychoanalysis and sexual disorders
psychoanalysis and symptom formation
psychoanalysis and the borderline concept
psychoanalysis and the mind
psychoanalytic interpretation
psychoanalytic psychotherapies
psychoanalytic technique
psychoanalytic theorists
    Abraham, Karl
    Adler, Alfred
    Bandura, Albert
    Binet, Alfred
    Cattell, Raymond
    Erikson, Erik
    Fenichel, Otto
    Freud, Sigmund
    Hall, G. Stanley

psychoanalytic theorists
    Hartmann, Heinz
    Horney, Karen
    James, William
    Jung, Carl
    Klein, Melanie
    Kraepelin, Emil
    Lewin, Kurt
    Maslov, Abraham
    McKeen, James
    Muensterberg, Hugo
    Pavlov, Ivan
    Reich, Wilhelm
    Rogers, Carl
    Skinner, B.F.
    Wundt, Wilhelm
psychoanalytic theory
psychoanalytic therapy
psychobiology, clinical
psychobiological process of dementia
psychobiological view
psychodynamic concepts
psychodynamic conflicts
psychodynamic formulations
psychodynamic orientation
psychodynamic research orientation
psychodynamic treatments
psychodysleptic agents (dissociative drugs)
    dextromethorphan
    ketamine
    PCP
    phencyclidine
    psilocin
    psilocybin
psychodysleptic agents (hallucinogens)
    cocaine
    bufotenine (toad skin secretions)
    cannabis
    heroin
    LSD
    marijuana
    peyote

Psycho-Educational Battery *(see also* tests)
Psychoeducational Profile (PEP)
psychogalvanic skin response (PGSR)
psychogalvanic skin response audiometry (PGSRA)
psychogenic deafness
psychogenic headache
psychogenic seizure
psychoimmunology
Psycholinguistic Rating Scale *(see also* tests)
psychologic desensitization
psychological abuse
    adult, by nonspouse or nonpartner, confirmed, initial encounter (T74.31XA)
    adult, by nonspouse or nonpartner, confirmed, subsequent encounter (T74.31XD)
    adult, by nonspouse or nonpartner, suspected, initial encounter (T76.31XA)
    adult, by nonspouse or nonpartner, suspected, subsequent encounter (T76.31XD)
psychological abuse in childhood
psychological affliction, childhood
psychological changes, maladaptive
psychological development scales *(see also* tests)
psychological disorder affecting GMC
psychological distress, intense
Psychological Distress Inventory
psychological dysfunction
    manifestation of
    symptoms of
Psychological Evaluation of Children's Human Figure Drawings

psychological examination
psychological factors
    dyspareunia due to
    female orgasmic disorder due to
    female sexual arousal disorder due to
    hypoactive sexual desire disorder due to
    male erectile disorder due to
    male orgasmic disorder due to
    sexual aversion disorder due to
    sexual dysfunction due to unspecified
    vaginismus due to
psychological interventions
psychological interview
Psychological Inventory - Bipolar
psychological management of dementia
psychological mindedness
psychological models
psychological motivation
psychological needs
psychological problems
psychological process, automatic
psychological reaction
psychological refractory period
psychological related symptoms
psychological response
psychological screening *(see also* tests)
psychological signs and symptoms
psychological spousal or partner abuse
    confirmed, initial encounter (T74.31XA)
    confirmed, subsequent encounter (T74.31XD)
    suspected, initial encounter (T76.31XA)
    suspected, subsequent encounter (T76.31XD)
psychological strain
psychological stress

psychological stressor (F44.7)
psychological syndrome
psychological techniques
psychological tests *(see also* tests)
psychological trauma, other personal history of (Z91.49)
psychologically meaningful
psychologically mediated response
psychology
    adolescent
    applied
    medical
    military
    schizophrenic
psychology of deceit
psychology practice
psychometric performance characteristics
psychometric tests *(see also* tests)
psychomotor activity
psychomotor agitation
psychomotor attacks
psychomotor behavior
psychomotor changes
psychomotor development
psychomotor fit
psychomotor phenomenon (pl. phenomena)
psychomotor seizure, olfactory
psychomotor slowing
psychomotor symptom
psycho-optical reflex controls
Psychopathic Deviance "4" Scale
psychopathology
    impulsive/compulsive
    levels of
    prepubertal
    presenting
    psychoanalysis and related
psychopathology and non-Mendelian inheritance
psychopathology of gender
psychopaths
psychopathy
psychopathy checklists *(see also* tests)

psychopharmacologic psychiatry
psychopharmacological treatment
psychopharmacology
    clinical
    gender-sensitive
psychopharmacology in child psychiatry
psychophysiologic correlates
psychophysiologic principle
psychophysiological change
psychophysiological insomnia
psychophysiological problem, stress-related
psychophysiological tests *(see also* tests)
psychosensory stimulus/stimuli
psychosensory symptom
psychosexual development
    anal stage
    gender identity
    latency period
    oral stage
    phallic stage
psychosexual history
psychosexual sphere
psychosis
    brief reactive
    childhood
    chronic
    organic brain syndrome with
    symbiotic
psychosocial and environmental problem
psychosocial aspects of schizophrenia
psychosocial complications
psychosocial deprivation
psychosocial development
psychosocial event
psychosocial factor
psychosocial function
psychosocial functioning
psychosocial problem
psychosocial process
psychosocial setting
psychosocial stigma
psychosocial stress

psychosocial stressor
psychosocial treatments
psychosomatics, psychoanalysis
  and psychostimulant agents
  (e.g. ADHD medications)
    Adderall
    Adderall XR
    amphetamine
    atomoxetine
    benzedrine (amphetamine)
    Biocapton
    biphetamine
    butalbital (with caffeine)
    caffeine
    Captagon
    Concerta
    Daytrana (patch)
    Desoxyn
    Dexedrine
    dexmethylphenidate
    dextroamphetamine
    DextroStat
    Fitton
    Focalin
    Focalin XR
    lisdexamfetamine
      dimesylate
    Metadate CD
    Metadate ER
    methamphetamine
    Methylin
    methylphenidate
    modafinil
    multiple
    rational
    rational-emotive
    Ritalin
    Ritalin LA
    Ritalin SR
    Strattera (non-stimulant)
    Vyvanse
psychostimulant intoxication
psychotherapeutic agents (see also
  psychotropic agents)
psychotherapeutic measures
psychotherapeutic treatments
psychotherapies, psychoanalytic
psychotherapist

psychotherapy
  individual
  remote
psychotic denial
psychotic dimension of positive
  schizophrenic symptoms
psychotic dimension of
  schizophrenia
psychotic disorder
  abnormal perceptions due
    to a
  brief (F23)
  brief, with abnormal
    psychomotor behavior
    (F23)
  brief, with catatonia (F23)
    and (F06.1)
  brief, with marked
    stressor(s) (F23)
  brief, with postpartum
    onset (F23)
  brief, without marked
    stressor(s) (F23)
  brief, with delusions (F23)
  brief, with depression (F23)
  brief, with disorganized
    speech (F23)
  brief, with hallucinations
    (F23)
  brief, with impaired
    cognition (F23)
  brief, with manic
    symptoms (F23)
  brief, with negative
    symptoms (F23)
  primary
  shared
psychotic disorder due to another
  medical condition
  with delusions (F06.2)
  with hallucinations (F06.0)
psychotic disorder with delusions
  alcohol-induced
  amphetamine-induced
  cannabis-induced
  cocaine-induced

psychotic disorder with hallucinations
      alcohol-induced
      amphetamine-induced
      cannabis-induced
      cocaine-induced
psychotic disorganization
psychotic disorganization in
   schizophrenia
psychotic distortion
psychotic disturbance
psychotic drug
psychotic episode, recurring
psychotic episode of
   schizophrenia
psychotic factor in schizophrenia
psychotic features
      mood-congruent
      mood-incongruent
      primary mood disorder
         with
      severe bipolar I disorder
         with
      severe bipolar I disorder
         without
psychotic illness
psychotic presentation
psychotic process
psychotic state
psychotic symptom(s)
      active
      residual
psychotic symptomatology
psychotomimetic agents *(see also*
   psychodysleptic agents*)*
psychotropic agents *(see also*
   specific entries for the agents
   listed below)
      antipanic agents
      alcohol therapy agents
      antibulimic agents
      antidepressant agents
      antidipsotropic agents
      antimanic agents
      antiobsessional agents
      antipsychotic agents
      anxiolytic agents
      hallucinogenic agents

psychotropic agents
      hypnotic agents
      mood stabilizer agents
      neuroleptic agents
      non-psychotropic hypnotics
         (see also sedative &
         hypnotic agents)
      psychodysleptic agents
      psychostimulant agents
      tranquilizer agents,
         benzodiazepine-based
      tranquilizer agents,
         butyrophenone-based
      tranquilizer agents, major
         tranquilizers
      tranquilizer agents, other
         tranquilizers
      tranquilizer agents,
         phenothiazine-based
psychotropic drugs (PTD) *(see
   also* individual psychotropic
   agents)
PTA (posttraumatic amnesia)
PTCS (Primary Test of Cognitive
   Skills) *(see also* tests)
PTD (psychotropic drug)
PTP (Physical Tolerance Profile)
PTP (posttetanic potentiation)
PTS (permanent threshold shift)
PTS (posttraumatic stress)
PTSD (posttraumatic stress
   disorder) (F43.10)
      aging and
      early-age trauma and
      elder maltreatment and
      late-age trauma and
public display of emotion
public health
Public Health Emergency of
   International Concern (PHEIC)
public opinion
public performance
public psychiatrist
public psychiatry
public psychological states
public urination
puerperal convulsion
puerperal mania

"puff the dragon" (re: cannabis use)
"puffer" (re: crack user)
"puffy" (street name, phencyclidine/PCP)
pugilistica
"pulborn" (street name, heroin)
pull out
"pullers" (re: crack user)
pulmonary absorption of inhalants
pulmonary disease and concurrent psychiatric problems
pulmonary heart disease, chronic
pulmonary pressure
pulmonary valve disease, rheumatic
pulsated voice
pulsating headache
pulsating pain
pulse
    alternating
    chest
    glottal
pulsing light frequency
"pumping" (re: crack dealing)
punch-drunk encephalopathy
punishment, deserved
pupillary reaction
pupils, unreactive
"pure" (street name, heroin)
pure agraphia
pure alexia
pure aphasia
pure aphemia
pure chance
"pure ivory" (re: substance mimicking ecstasy effect)
"pure love" (street name, lysergic acid diethylamide/LSD)
pure tone air-conduction
pure tone air-conduction threshold
pure-tone audiometer
pure-tone audiometry (AC; BC)
pure tone average
pure tone bone conduction
pure tone bone-conduction threshold
pure vowel

pure wave
pure word deafness
purgation
purging disorder (50.8)
purging methods
purine metabolism
"purple" (street name, ketamine)
"purple barrels" (street name, lysergic acid diethylamide/LSD)
"purple flats" (street name, lysergic acid diethylamide/LSD)
"purple haze" (street name, lysergic acid diethylamide/LSD)
"purple hearts" (street name, amphetamine; barbiturate; LSD)
"purple ozoline" (street name, lysergic acid diethylamide/LSD)
"purple rain" (street name, phencyclidine/PCP)
"purple wave" (re: substance mimicking ecstasy effect)
purposeful behavior
purposeless agitation
purposeless motor activity
purposeless movement
purposes, educational
pursuit movement, visual
pursuits, family
purulent otitis media push back
"push" (re: drug dealing)
push back, purulent otitis media
"push shorts" (re: drug dealing)
"pusher" (re: drug dealer; re: crack equipment)
PVS (Beery Picture Vocabulary Screening Series)
PVS (persistent vegetative state)
PVSP (Prosody-Voice Screening Profile)
PVT (Beery Picture Vocabulary Test)
pyloric stenosis, congenital hypertrophic
Pyramid Scales, The

pyramidal cerebral palsy (CP)
pyramidal system
pyramidal tract
pyrexiophobia
pyrimidine metabolism
pyromania (fire) (F63.1)

"Q" (street name, barbiturate)
Q (clerical perception)
Q (clerical response)
Q (coulomb)
q (every)
QA (Quality Assessment)
Qat (methcathinone)
q.d. (every day)
q.h.s. (every night)
q.i.d. (four times a day)
QLQ (Quality of Life Questionnaire)
q.n.s (quantity not sufficient)
q.o.d. (every other day)
QPS (Quick Phonics Survey)
QPVT (Quick Picture Vocabulary Test)
q.s. (sufficient quantity)
q-set
q-sort
QSP (Quick Screen of Phonology)
qt (quiet)
QT (Quick Test)
q.2h. (every two hours)
"Qua" (street name, methaqualone)
Quaalude (methaqualone)
"quack" (street name, methaqualone)
"quad" (street name, barbiturate)
quadrangular therapy
quadrilateral, vowel
quadriplegia
qualifier
qualitative difference
qualitative impairment in communication
quality
    poor form
    sound
    subjective

quality in parkinsonian speech, festinant
quality of caring
Quality of Life Questionnaire (QLQ)
quality of life rehabilitation assessment
quality of obsessions
    inappropriate
    intrusive
quality of performance
quality of sexual functioning
quality of sleep
Quality of Well-Being Scale
quality sound
quality speech
quantified cognitive assessment (*see also* tests)
quantifier, universal
quantitative electroencephalography
quantitative variable
quantity
    absolute
    objective
    relative
    sound
    subjective
quantity not sufficient (q.n.s.)
quarrelsomeness
"quarter" (re; 1/4 ounce or $25 worth of drugs)
"quarter bag" (re: $25 worth of drugs)
"quarter bag" (street name, cocaine)
"quarter moon" (street name, hashish)
"quarter piece" (re: 1/4 ounce)
quartile
"quartz" (street name, smokable speed)
"quas" (street name, barbiturate)
quasi contract
quasipurposive movement
"Queen Ann's lace" (street name, cannabis)
querulous paranoia

Psychiatric Words and Phrases

question
  tag
  yes-no
questioning, Socratic
questioning faith problem
Questionnaire(s) *(see also* tests)
  Abbreviated Conners Teachers
  Adult Neuropsychological (ANQ)
  Adult Suicidal Ideation (ASIQ)
  alcohol use
  Anorectic Attitude
  Attributional Style
  Beck
  Behavioral Assessment of Pain
  CAGE alcohol use
  Cattell Personality Factor
  Child Neuropsychological (CNQ)
  Class Activities
  Cognitive Failures (CFQ)
  Community College Student Experiences (CCSEQ)
  Denver Prescreening Development
  Disability Screening
  Eight State
  everyday memory
  Eysenck Personality
  Functional Status (FSQ)
  Functional Time Estimation (FTEQ)
  Health Assessment
  Health Care
  Home Environment
  Home Screening
  Illness Behavior
  Inquiry Mode (IMQ)
  International Version of the Mental Status
  Intrex
  Kenny Self-Care
  Lambeth Disability Screening

Questionnaire(s) *(see also* tests)
  Leatherman Leadership (LLQ)
  Levine-Pilowsky Depression
  life quality
  McGill Pain
  McMaster Health Index
  Measure of How You Think and Make Decisions
  Menstrual Distress (MDQ)
  Mental Status
  Minnesota Importance
  Modified Health Assessment (MHAQ)
  Multidimensional Functional Assessment
  Multifactor Leadership (MLQ)
  Neuropsychological – Adult (ANQ)
  Neuropsychological – Child (CNQ)
  OARS Multidimensional Functional Assessment (OMFAQ)
  Occupational Roles (ORQ)
  Offer Parent-Adolescent
  Offer Self-Image (OSIQ)
  Offer Self-Image, for Adolescents
  Pain
  Parent-Adolescent
  Parental Acceptance-Rejection
  Patient Health
  Personal Experience Screening (PESQ)
  Personal Resource (PRQ)
  Personal Strain (PSQ)
  Personality Factor (PFQ)
  Philadelphia Head Injury (PHIQ)
  Preliminary Diagnostic
  Prescreening Development
  Professional and Managerial Position (PMPQ)

Questionnaire(s) *(see also* tests)
    Quality of Life (QLQ)
    Rand Patient Satisfaction
    Sales Personality (SPQ)
    Self-Description (SDQ)
    Sense of Coherence
    Sixteen Personality Factor (16PF)
    Speech
    Street Survival Skills
    Student Adaptation to College (SACQ)
    Substance Abuse (SAQ)
    Suicidal Ideation - Adult (ASIQ)
    Teacher Feedback
    Toronto Functional Capacity (TFCQ)
    Verbalizer-Visualization (VVQ)
    Vocational Interest (VIQ)
    Work Attitudes (WAQ)
Questionnaire of Basic Personality Supports
Quick Neurological Screening Test
Quick Picture Vocabulary Test (QPVT)
Quick Phonics Survey (QPS)
Quick-Score Achievement Test *(see also* tests)
quick screen tests *(see also* tests)
Quick Screen of Mental Development
Quick Screen of Phonology (QSP)
Quick Screener, Voc-Tech (VTQS)
"quicksilver" (street name, isobutyl nitrite)
Quick Test
Quick Word Test
quiescent
quiet (qt), wakefulness
quiet sleep
"quill" (street name, cocaine; heroin; methamphetamine)
quinolone (injectable steroid)
quotes

quotient
    achievement (AQ)
    adolescent language
    custody
    educational (EQ)
    expressive language
    grammar language
    intelligence (I.Q.)
    language test *(see also* tests)
    listening language
    memory (MQ)
    open
    positive-negative ambivalent
    reading language
    receptive language-processing
    social (SQ)
    speed
    spoken language
    verbal language
    vocabulary language
    written language

R

R or r (roentgen)
"Racehorse Charlie" (street name, cocaine; heroin)
racing thoughts
radiation
    acoustic
    visual
radiation-induced mental deterioration
radical candor
radical mastoidectomy
radicals, free
radicular low back pain
radicular pain
radiogram
radiography
radiophobia
RADS (Reynolds Adolescent Depression Scale)
rageful feelings
"ragweed" (street name, cannabis; heroin)
"railroad weed" (street name, cannabis)
"rainy day woman" (street name, cannabis)
rambling flow of thought
rambling speech
"Rambo" (street name, heroin)
Ramsay Hunt syndrome
Rand Functional Limitations Battery
Rand Patient Satisfaction Questionnaire
Rand Physical Capacities Battery
random activity
random movement
random noise
"Randy Mandies" (street name, methaqualone)
"rane" (street name, cocaine; heroin)
range
    age
    audible
    central speech
    dynamic
    frequency
    maximum frequency
    most comfortable loudness (MCLR)
    pitch
    tolerance
    T-score
range of affect, labile
range of emotion, restricted
range of emotional expression, reduced
range of feelings
range of frequencies
"Rangood" (street name, wild cannabis)
rank, percentile
rank order
"rap" (re: criminally charged; talking with someone)
rape, sadistic act of
raphe
    lingual
    median longitudinal
    palatine
    pharyngeal
rapid-alternating movement (RAM)
rapid change in activity
rapid cycling, mood disorder with
rapid-cycling course
rapid-cycling pattern
rapid eye movement (REM)
rapid eye movement latency, reduced
rapid eye movement sleep behavior disorder (G47.52)
rapid fine movements
rapid movement
rapid-onset gender dysphoria (ROGD)
Rapid Prompting Method (RPM)

rapid repetitive movements,
    impaired
rapid shifting of emotions
rapid speech
rapid tremor, small-amplitude
rapidity of analyzing information,
    disturbance in
rapidity of assimilating
    information, disturbance in
Rapidly Alternating Speech
    Perception Test (RASP)
rapidly shifting emotion
rapists
rapport, poor interpersonal
raptus of attention
rare clefts
rarefaction
rash, glue sniffer's
rashes, breast
RASP (Rapidly Alternating
    Speech Perception Test)
"raspberry" (re: crack prostitute)
"rasta weed" (street name,
    cannabis)
rate
    altered speech
    alternate motion (AMR)
    death
    decay
    fluency
    language development
    maturation
    mentation
    metabolic
    response
rate control
Rathus Assertiveness Scale
Rating Inventory for Screening
    Kindergartners (RISK)
rating scales *(see also* tests)
ratio
    characteristic sex
    equal sex
    high affectivity
    s/z
    signal to noise (S/N)
    the oral-nasal acoustic
        (TONAR)

ratio reinforcement schedule
    fixed
    variable
rational/cognitive coping
rational-emotive psychotherapy
rational psychotherapy
rationalist theory of language
"rave" (re: hallucinogenic drug
    use)
"rave energy" (street name,
    ecstasy/MDMA)
"raver" (re: rave club attendee)
"raver, candy" (re: club drug user)
"raw" (street name, crack)
raw score
Ray mania
Raynaud's phenomenon
"razed" (re: drug influence)
RBH Test of Learning Ability
    (TLA)
RBMT (Rivermead Behavioural
    Memory Test)
RCDS (Revised Children's
    Depression Scale)
RCDS (Reynolds Child
    Depression Scale)
RCPsych (Royal College of
    Psychiatrists)
RCS (Reality Check Survey)
RDI (Job Descriptive Index and
    Retirement Descriptive Index)
reactance, inductive
reaction
    angry
    catastrophic
    dangerous behavior
    doll's eye
    emotional
    escape
    idiosyncratic
    justifiable
    maladaptive
    minor stimulus
    manic
    nonpathological
    pain
    psychological
    pupillary

reaction
    stress
    toxic
reaction time, slowed
reaction time test, visual choice
reaction to death
reactive, symptomatically
reactive attachment disorder (F94.1)
    disinhibited type
    inhibited type
reactive inhibition
reactive psychosis, brief
reactive response
reactivity
    affective
    decreased
    environmental
    physiological
readiness tests *(see also* tests)
reading
    choral
    mind
reading aphasia, speech *(see also* tests)
Reading Comprehension Battery for Aphasia
reading comprehension impairment
Reading Comprehension Inventory
reading disorder
reading epilepsy
Reading/Everyday Activities in Life
reading tests *(see also* tests)
"ready rock" (street name, cocaine; crack; heroin)
real abandonment
real-life circumstances
real-life problems
realistic plan
reality
    abnormal perceptions of
    external
    external world of
    inconsistent contact with
    map of

reality ability testing
Reality Check Survey (RCS)
reality testing
    diminished
    gross impairment in
reality testing ability (Rorschach)
reanalysis, data
reanalysis strategy
reanalyzed data
rearing, child
reasonable fear
reasoning, practical
reasoning mania
reasoning skills, numerical
reasoning tests *(see also* tests)
Reasons for Living Inventory (RLI)
reassignment
    hormonal sexual
    surgical sexual
reassurance
    excessive need for
    need for
re-attribute
rebound, REM sleep
rebound REM
rebus
recalcitrant pain
recall
    auditory
    dream
    memory
recall 5 items after 5 minutes test
recall of information
recall of information test
recall test
    forward digital span
    paragraph
    reverse digit span
recalled information
recalling new information, disturbance in
receiver
    air-conduction
    bone-conduction
recent data
recent depressed mood episode
recent episode

recent hospital discharge
recent hypomanic mood episode
recent manic mood episode
recent memory test
recent mixed mood episode
recent unspecified mood episode
reception, speech (SR) *(see also tests)*
reception audiometry, speech
reception in noise, speech
reception threshold, speech (SRT)
receptive development *(see also tests)*
Receptive-Expressive Emergent Language Test (REEL)
receptive-expressive language disorder, mixed
Receptive-Expressive Observation Scale (REO)
receptive language development
receptive language disorder
receptive language problem
Receptive One Word Picture Vocabulary Test (ROWPVT)
receptor, sensory
receptor alterations, NMDA
receptor functioning
receptors
    delta
    delta opiate
    kappa
    kappa opiate
    mu
    mu opiate
    opiate
reciprocal assimilation
reciprocal social interaction
reciprocity, emotional
reckless behavior
reckless driving habits
recklessness, tendency toward
recognition, visual pattern
Recognition Memory Test
recognition test *(see also tests)*
recognition vs. recall
recollection of trauma
recompensated

"recompress" (re: cocaine processing)
reconstitute
recovery
    full interepisode
    spontaneous
recreation
recreational use of cannabis
recruitment
    complete
    incomplete
    partial
rectal bleeding, self-inflicted
rectal fissures
rectal pain
rectovaginal fistula
recurrence of a memory
recurrent brief depressive disorder
recurrent convulsion
recurrent duration
recurrent episode
recurrent episode mania
recurrent headache
recurrent laryngeal nerve paralysis
recurrent migraine headache
recurrent mood episodes
recurrent nightmares
recurrent panic attacks
recurrent physical fights
recurrent suicidal behavior
    assessment of
    case management of
    crisis management of
    treatment of
recurrent suicidal ideation
recurrent thoughts
recurring psychotic episode
recurring seizure
"recycle" (street name, lysergic acid diethylamide/LSD)
"red" (re: drug influence)
"red and blue" (street name, barbiturate)
"red bullets" (street name, barbiturate)
"red caps" (street name, crack)

"red chicken" (street name, heroin)
"red cross" (street name, cannabis)
"red devil" (street name, barbiturate; phencyclidine/PCP; MDMA/ecstasy)
"red dirt" (street name, cannabis)
"red eagle" (street name, heroin)
"red phosphorus" (street name, smokable amphetamine)
reduced attention ability
reduced body language
reduced fluency
reduced physical activity
reduced preputial sensation
reduced range of emotional expression
reduced rapid eye movement latency
reduced responsiveness
reduced screening audiometry
reduced sensation of the foreskin
reduced sleep duration
reduction
    anxiety
    cluster
    syllable
    trial of dosage
reduction of Adam's apple, surgical
reduplicated babbling
reed artificial larynx
Reed report forensic psychiatry
REEL-2 (Receptive-Expressive Emergent Language Test
reenactment, trauma-specific
re-exacerbation
reexperienced traumatic event
reexperiencing perceptual symptoms
reference
    standard
    transient ideas of
reference group
    cultural
    ethnic
    social

reference zero level
referential delusions
referential function
referential index
    shift
    switch
referential semantics
referred pain
reflected wave
reflex
    acoustic
    acoustic contralateral
    acoustic ipsilateral
    acoustic stapedial
    acousticopalpebral
    auditory
    auditory-oculogyric
    auropalpebral (APR)
    Babinski
    brain stem
    cochlear
    cochleo-orbicular
    cochleopalpebral (CPR)
    delayed
    depressed
    diminished
    doll's eye
    facial
    flexion
    gag
    intra-aural
    laryngeal
    middle ear muscle
    Moro
    Myerson
    myotatic
    orienting (OR)
    pharyngeal
    sensitivity prediction from the acoustic (SPAR)
    stapedial acoustic
    stapedius
    startle
    stretch
reflex amplitude, acoustic
reflex arc
reflex asymmetries

reflex audiometry, conditioned
    orientation (COR)
reflex changes
reflex controls, psycho-optical
reflex convulsion
reflex decay, acoustic
reflex eye movement
reflex latency, acoustic
reflex pattern, acoustic
reflex seizure
reflex threshold, acoustic
reflex time
reflexes
    exaggeration of deep
        tendon
    intact
reflexive movement
re-focus
reform, thought
reformulation
refracted wave
refractory period, psychological
reframing
    context
    six-step
    meaning
refreshing sleep attacks
refusal, treatment
refusal to treat
regard
regional dialect
regions, brain
register
    loft
    vocal
    voice
regression, phonemic
regressive assimilation
regressive behavior
regressive speech
regular determiner
"regular P" (street name, crack)
regulation
    impulse
    lack of impulse
rehabilitation
    acoupedic method of
    acoustic method of aural

rehabilitation
    bimodal aural
    bimodal method of aural
    combined aural
    grammatic method of aural
    kinesthetic method of aural
    lipreading aural
    manual method of aural
    natural method of aural
    oral-aural method of aural
    simultaneous aural
    speech
    speechreading aural
    vocal
rehabilitation assessment, quality
    of life
rehabilitation behavior
rehabilitation counselor
rehabilitation evaluation
Rehabilitation Indicators (RIs)
rehabilitation psychiatry
rehabilitation treatment
rehabilitative audiology
Reid Report
"reindeer dust" (street name,
    heroin)
reinforcement
    differential
    frequency of
    partial
    primary
    social
    verbal
reinforcement operant
    conditioning audiometry,
    tangible (TROCA)
reinforcement schedule
    continuous
    extinction
    fixed interval
    fixed ratio
    intermittent
    variable interval
    variable ratio
reinforcer
    conditioned
    delayed
    generalized

reinforcer
    negative
    positive
    primary
    secondary
    unconditioned
Reissner's membrane
Reitan Evaluation of Hemispheric Abilities and Brain Improvement Training
Reitan-Indiana Neuropsychological Test Battery for Adults
Reitan-Indiana Neuropsychological Test Battery for Children
rejecting parent
rejection
    fear of
    increased sensitivity to
    pathological sensitivity to perceived interpersonal
    perceived interpersonal
    problems with social exclusion or (Z60.4)
rejection sensitivity
re-label
relapse-prevention technique
related by marriage
related position, medically
related psychopathology
related sleep disorder
related symptoms, psychological
related problems
    abuse
    interaction with the legal system
    neglect
    social environment
relatedness
    developmentally inappropriate social
    disturbed social
    social
relation addiction
relation to age
relational concepts
relational functioning
    competent
    disrupted
    dysfunctional
    optimal
relational functioning scale *(see also* tests)
relational problem
    parent-child
    partner
    sibling
relational unit
relational utterance, mean (MRU)
relational word(s)
relations
    community-institutional
    extramarital
    family (se also tests)
    hospital-patient
    hospital-physician
    interdepartmental
    intergenerational
    interinstitutional
    interpersonal
    interprofessional
    nurse-patient
    physician-patient
    professional-family
    professional-patient
    semantic
    sibling
relations case
relations tests *(see also* tests)
relationship(s)
    addiction
    apparent
    appropriate
    causal
    chronological
    clearly demarcated
    close
    doctor-patient
    dysfunctional
    early
    effect of trauma on
    etiological
    good
    incestual

relationship(s)
    intense
    interpsychic
    intrafamilial
    lack of meaningful
    last
    long-term
    meaningful
    monogamous
    pattern of discomfort in close
    perfect negative
    perfect positive
    poor peer
    replacement
    sexual
    social
    special
    stability in
    stress-strain
    temporal
    transference
    unstable
    working
relationship distress with spouse or intimate partner (Z63.0)
Relationship Evaluation, The Mother-Child (MCRE)
relationship inventory *(see also* tests)
relationship to a deity or famous person
relative, biological
relative elective mutism
relative lack of self-destructiveness
relative quantity
relative scotoma
relative slow-wave sleep stability
relative stability of self-image
relativity, linguistic
relaxants, depolarizing muscle
relaxation
    differential
    progressive
    sense of muscular
relaxation technique training, hypnotic

release of sexual tension
release of tension
release sign
    frontal
    positive frontal
releasing consonant
relevant diagnostic criteria
reliability coefficient
    alternate forms
    comparable forms
    odd-even method
    split half
    test-retest
relief, sense of
relief of tension
religious activity
religious institution
religious mania
religious or spiritual problems (Z65.8)
religious problem
religious values, acculturation problems with expression of
reliving an event, sense of
REM (rapid eye movement)
    descent through non-REM to rebound
REM activity, phasic
REM onset sleep
REM period, sleep onset (SOREMP)
REM sleep behavior disorder
REM sleep rebound
REM stage of sleep
remarks, parenthetical
remedial intervention
remedial teaching
reminding test *(see also* tests)
remission
    early full
    early partial
    in early
    in sustained
    sustained full
    sustained partial
remissions, long-term
remitting dementia
remorse, lack of

remote memory test
remote psychotherapy
remote video psychiatric
  consulting
removed affect
remuneration
  benefit
  financial
renal disease
  chronic
  end-stage
  hypertensive
renal function
renal tubular acidosis
  distal
  proximal
renumerative
repeat tendency
repeated heavy drinkers
repeated painful experience
repeated substance self-
  administration, pattern of
Repeated Test of Sustained
  Wakefulness (RTSW)
repeated thoughts
repetition
  monosyllabic whole word
  phrase
  senseless imitative word
  sound and syllable
repetition of sounds
repetition test
  digit
  sentence
repetitious activity
repetitive behavior, patterns of
repetitive convulsion
repetitive imitative movement
repetitive lying
repetitive motor behavior
repetitive movements, impaired
  rapid
repetitive partial seizure
repetitive pattern(s) of behavior
repetitive play, expression of
  traumatic themes through
repetitive restricted behavior
repetitive speech

repetitive task
replacement, glottal
replacement relationship
representational system, preferred
representational systems
representative sample
repressed need (theory in
  stuttering)
repression, cognitive approaches
  to dreaming and
repression-sensitization scales
repressive behavior
reproductive function
reproductive hormonal
  measurement
reptilian stare
required task
research, comparative
research orientation
  behavioral
  biological
  cognitive
  family/system
  interpersonal
  psychodynamic
reserve air
reserve volume
  expiratory (ERV)
  inspiratory (IRV)
Resident and Staff Information
  Form
residential treatment
residual air
residual capacity, functional
  (FRC)
residual impairment, permanent
residual pain
residual period of illness
residual phase
residual phase of schizophrenia
residual psychotic symptom
residual schizophrenia
residual schizophrenic
residual symptoms, minimal
residual symptoms of
  schizophrenia, interepisode
residual volume (RV)

resistance
    galvanic skin
    overt compliance masking
      covert
resolution phase of sexual
  response cycle
resolving conflict skills
resonance
    facilitation of
    nasal
    vocal
    voice disorders or
resonance disorders
resonance-volley theory
resonant frequency
resonator
    subglottic
    supraglottic
resource, health
resource state
respect
respiration
    abdominal-diaphragmatic
    bronchial
    Cheyne-Stokes
    clavicular
    cortical
    diaphragmatic-abdominal
    laryngeal
    nasal
    opposition
    oral
    thoracic
respiratory capacity
respiratory disorder
respiratory frequency
respiratory infection, upper (URI)
respiratory system
respiratory tract
respiratory volume
respirometer
response(s)
    adaptive
    anxiety
    auditory brainstem (ABR)
    brain stem auditory evoked
      (BAER)
    catastrophic

response(s)
    chaining
    clasp-knife
    clerical (Q)
    color
    conditioned
    covert
    culturally sanctioned
    culturally unsanctioned
    delayed
    differential
    disorders of sexual
    emotional
    evoked (ER)
    evoked somatosensory
    exaggerated startle
    expectable
    extensor plantar
    fabulized
    false-negative
    false-positive
    frequency
    generalization
    hostile
    human movement
    latent
    long latency
    maladaptive
    mean length of (MLR)
    middle latency
    morbid
    negative
    overt
    paradigmatic
    pattern of
    perseverative
    polarity
    positive
    psychogalvanic skin
    psychological
    psychologically mediated
    reactive
    satiety
    sexual
    small detail
    space
    state
    stress

response(s)
    stress-related physiological
    syntagmatic, target
    texture
    treatment
    unconditioned
    unexpected
    vibrotactile
    vista
    visual evoked (VER)
response/anchor, integrating
response audiometry
    auditory brainstem (ABR)
    average evoked (AERA)
    brain stem evoked (BSER)
    cardiac response (CERA)
    electric (ERA)
    evoked (ERA)
    galvanic skin (GSRA)
    psychogalvanic skin
response audiometry (EDRA) test, electrodermal
response cradle, neonatal auditory
response cradle audiometry, neonatal auditory
response curve, frequency
response cycle
    desire phase of sexual
    excitement phase of sexual
    orgasmic phase of sexual
    resolution phase of sexual
    sexual
response hierarchy
response magnitude
response pattern, symptom
response rate
response scales
response set, difficulty in changing
response strength
response system
response test, visual evoked
response time
response to pain, diminished
response to speech dysfluencies, emotional
responsibility (pl. responsibilities)
    assigned

responsibility (pl. responsibilities)
    avoidance of
    generational
    greater
    homemaking
    household
    important
    increased
    individual
    interpersonal
    job
    lack of
    legal
    neglect of
    new
    noxious
    personal
    poor sense of
    position of
    primary
    sense of
    social
Responsibility and Independence Scale for Adolescents (RISA)
responsibility scales *(see also tests)*
responsiveness
    abnormal
    diminished
    emotional
    facial
    general
    mutual affective
    reduced
rest tremor
resting, wakefulness
resting energy expenditure
resting potential
resting tremor
restless behavior
restless legs syndrome (G25.81)
restlessness
    feelings of
    motor
restraint (physical bondage)
restraints
    four-point
    leather

restricted affect
restricted behavior
    repetitive
    stereotyped
restricted diet
restricted range of affect
restricted range of emotion
restricted range of emotional expression, pattern of
restriction(s)
    activity
    building
    close watch
    gown
    mandibular
    open seclusion
    shoe
    unit (UR)
restrictive behavior, patterns of
restrictive food intake disorder (F50.8)
restrictive food intake disorder, in remission (F50.8)
restrictive modifier
restructuring, cognitive
results
    field-trial
    inconsistent laboratory test
    knowledge of
"resuscitative" snores
resynthesis, binaural
retardation
    idiopathic language
    perceptual
retarded, educationally mentally (EMR)
retention
    fluid
    linguistic
    memory
    urinary
retention tests *(see also* tests)
reticence scales *(see also* tests)
reticular formation, brain stem
retino-neuropathy, toxic
retirement problem
retribution, fear of
retrieval, method of

retrieval problem, word
retrieval task, word
retroauricular
retrocochlear deafness
retrocollis
retroflex consonant formation
retroflex vowel
retrognathic
retrograde amnesia, shrinking
retrograde loss of memory
retropulsion of gait
retrospective gaps in memory
Rett disorder
return of sensation
reuptake inhibitor antidepressant medications, serotonin-specific
re-value
revenge, desire for
reverberation room
reverberation time
reversal, letter
reversal learning
reversal on EEG, phase
reversal test
    digit
    Jordan Left-Right
reverse digit span recall test
reverse discrimination or persecution, target of (perceived) (Z60.5)
reverse phonation
reverse swallowing
reversible affective disorder syndrome (SADS)
reversible amnesia
reversible memory impairment
ReVia (naltrexone)
review
    comprehensive
    empirical
    literature
    systematic
review method
review of symptoms
Review of Test Results
revision process
revulsion, sexual stimuli

reward
    token economy
    potential external
reward dependence
Reynell-Zinkin Scales: Developmental Scales for Young Handicapped
Reynolds Adolescent Depression Scale (RADS)
Reynolds Child Depression Scale (RCDS)
Rey-Ostereith Complex Figure Test
rheobase
rheumatic pulmonary valve disease
"Rhine" (street name, heroin)
rhinitis
rhinolalia aperta voice disorder
rhinolalia clausa
rhinolalia clause voice disorder
rhinophonia
rhinoplasty
rhotacised vowel
rhotacism
"rhythm" (street name, amphetamine)
rhythm
    alpha
    beta
    delta
    endogenous circadian phase
    erratic speech
    speech
    stuttered
    theta
rhythmic contraction
rhythmic movement
rhythmic slow eye movement
rhythmic tremor
rhythmical twitch/twitching
rhythmicity of tremor, steady
"rib" (street name, ecstasy/MDMA)
rib, elevator muscles of
RIBLS (Riley Inventory of Basic Learning Skills)
ridge
    rugal
    alveolar
ridicule, fear of
"riding the wave" (re: drug influence)
"rig" (re: drug injection)
right hemisphere dominance
right-left disorientation
Right-Left Orientation Test (RLO)
"righteous bush" (street name, cannabis)
"righteous weed" (street name, cannabis)
rigid attitude
rigid cerebral palsy (CP)
rigid sex roles
rigidity
    catatonic
    cognitive
    cogwheel
    "lead-pipe"
    muscle
    parkinsonian muscular
Riley Inventory of Basic Learning Skills (RIBLS)
Riley Motor Problems Inventory
Ring and Peg Tests of Behavior Development
"ringer" (re: crack use)
Rinne Hearing Conduction Test
"rippers" (street name, amphetamine)
RIs (Rehabilitation Indicators)
RISA (Responsibility and Independence Scale for Adolescents)
RISB (Rotter Incomplete Sentences Blank)
rising curve, gradual
rising curve audiogram configurations
RISK (Rating Inventory for Screening Kindergartners)
risk
    determining
    elevated

risk
- health
- significant
- specific
- suicide

risk activities, high
risk behavior, high
risk factor(s)
- other personal (Z91.89)
- significant

risk factors for mental disorders
risk factors for suicide
risk for accidents, alcohol-related
risk for depression
risk for malnutrition
risk for schizophrenia
risk for suicide
- alcohol-related
- high

risk for violence, alcohol-related
risk inventories *(see also* tests)
risk of suicide attempts
risk reduction
risk-taking
- sex-related
- sexual

risk-taking behavior, adolescent
Ritalin (methylphenidate) (street names)
- crackers (re: Talwin/Ritalin injection simulates heroin/cocaine injection effect)
- hyper drug
- hyper pill
- one and ones (re: Talwin/Ritalin injection simulating heroin/cocaine effect)
- pharming (re: doctor-shopping for prescription medication)
- poor man's heroin (re: Talwin/Ritalin injections)
- Ritz and Ts (re: Ritalin/Talwin injection simulating heroin/cocaine effect)

Ritalin (methylphenidate) (street names)
- set (re: Ritalin/Talwin injection simulating heroin/ cocaine effect)
- speedball (heroin mixed with Ritalin)
- study drug
- Ts and Rits, (re: Talwin/Ritalin injection simulating heroin/cocaine effect)
- Ts and Rs (re: Talwin/Ritalin injection simulating heroin/cocaine effect)
- vitamin R
- West Coast

ritual abuse
ritual behavior, culturally prescribed
"ritual spirit" (street name, ecstasy/MDMA)
ritualized makeup application
rituals, healing
Rivermead ADL Test
Rivermead Behavioural Memory Test (RBMT)
Rivermead Mobility Index
Rivermead Motor Assessment
Rivermead Perceptual Assessment Battery
RLO (Right-Left Orientation Test)
"roach" (re: butt of cannabis cigarette)
"roach clip" (re: cannabis equipment)
"road dope" (street name, amphetamine)
robbery
Robbins Speech Sound Discrimination and Verbal Imagery Type Tests
Robert's Apperception Test for Children
"roca" (street name, crack; ecstasy/MDMA)

Psychiatric Words and Phrases

"roche" (street name, Rophynol)
Rochester method
"rock attack" (street name, crack)
"rock house" (street name, crack house)
"rock star" (re: crack prostitute)
"rocket" (street name, cannabis cigarette)
"rocket caps" (re: crack containers)
"rocket fuel" (re: drug injection)
"rocket fuel" (street name, phencyclidine/PCP)
"Rockette" (re: female crack user)
rocking, nonfunctional and repetitive
"rocks of hell" (street name, crack)
"Rocky III" (street name, crack)
Roeder Manipulative Aptitude Test
roentgen (R,r)
roentgenogram
roentgenography
ROGD (rapid-onset gender dysphoria)
Rogers Criminal Responsibility Scale
Rogers Personal Adjustment Inventory
Rohypnol (tranquilizer used to facilitate sexual assault)
Rohypnol (flunitrazepam) (street names)
    circles (S-H-A)
    forget me drug (S-H-A)
    forget pill (S-H-A)
    forget-me pill (S-H-A)
    getting roached (re: using Rohypnol)
    La rocha (S-H-A)
    lunch money drug (S-H-A)
    Mexican valium (S-H-A)
    pingus (S-H-A)
    R-2 (S-H-A)
    Reynolds (S-H-A)
    rib (S-H-A)
    roach-2 (S-H-A)

Rohypnol (flunitrazepam) (street names)
    roachas dos (S-H-A)
    roaches (S-H-A)
    roachies (S-H-A)
    robutal (S-H-A)
    roche (S-H-A)
    roofies (S-H-A)
    rope (S-H-A)
    rophies (S-H-A)
    rophy (S-H-A)
    ropies (S-H-A)
    roples (S-H-A)
    row-shay (S-H-A)
    ruffies (S-H-A)
    ruffles (S-H-A)
rohypnoled (date raped)
"roid range" (re: steroid use)
Rolando, fissure of
role(s)
    adultomorphic behavior
    contributing
    cross-sex
    important
    intangible benefits of the "sick"
    interpersonal
    minimal
    persistent discomfort with gender
    physician's
    significant
    social
    social stereotypical gender
    victim
role ambiguity
role boundary
role disorder, false
role function
role insufficiency
role obligations, major
role of giving, transgenerational
role overload
role-play activity
roles questionnaire
"roller" (re: drug injection)
"rollers" (re: police)

"rolling" (street name, methylenedioxy-methamphetamine; MDMA)
"Rolls Royce" (street name, ecstasy/MDMA)
romantic fantasy
Romberg sign
"roofies" (street name, Rophynol)
room
    dead (no-echo chamber)
    reverberation
"rooster" (street name, crack)
"root" (street name, cannabis)
root of the tongue
root word
roots of addiction, biological
"roples" (street name, Rophynol)
Rorschach Inkblot Test
"Rosa" (street name, amphetamine)
"Rose Marie" (street name, cannabis)
"roses" (street name, amphetamine)
Ross Information Processing Assessment
Ross Test of Higher Cognitive Processes
Roswell-Chall Auditory Blending Test
Roswell-Chall Diagnostic Reading Test of Word Analysis Skills:
Rotation test
rote memory
Rothwell-Miller Interest Blank
Rotter Incomplete Sentences Blank
rotunda, fenestra
rough-and-tumble play
rough hoarseness
round feature English phoneme
round window
rounded vowel
rounding, lip
routine
    family
    hospital

routine skills, negotiating
routing of signals
    bilateral contralateral (BICROS)
    contralateral (CROS)
    focal contralateral (FOCALCROS)
    front (FROS)
    hearing aid contralateral (CROS)
    ipsilateral (IROS)
    ipsilateral frontal (IFROS)
roving eye movement
roving ocular movement
ROWPVT (Receptive One Word Picture Vocabulary Test)
"rox" (street name, crack)
"Roxanne" (street name, cocaine; crack)
"royal blues" (street name, lysergic acid diethylamide/LSD)
Royal College of Psychiatrists (RCPsych)
"Roz" (street name, crack)
R-PDQ (Revised Denver Prescreening Development Questionnaire)
RPM (Rapid Prompting Method)
RSCCD (Rating Scale of Communication in Cognitive Decline)
RTSW (Repeated Test of Sustained Wakefulness)
rubral tremor
"ruderalis" (street name, cannabis)
"ruffles" (street name, Rophynol)
ruga (pl. rugae)
rule(s)
    as a general
    base
    McNaughton
    phonological
    preoccupation with
    semantic
    sequencing
    serious violation of

rule(s)
    syntactic
    Tarasoff
rule bending
Rule Eleven Psych Evaluation
rule in a diagnosis
rule of thumb
rule out a diagnosis
rules skills, negotiating
rumination, morbid
rumination disorder (F98.2)
ruminative, introspective and
run, cocaine
runaway from home
"runners" (re: drug dealers)
"running" (street name, methylenedioxy-methamphetamine/MDMA)
running speech
ruptures, gastric
rural psychiatry
"rush snappers" (street name, isobutyl nitrite)
Russell Version Wechsler Memory Scale
"Russian drug" (street name, "krocodil" for synthetic desomorphine)
"Russian sickles" (street name, lysergic acid diethylamide/LSD)
Russian spring-summer viral encephalitis
Russiomania
Rust Inventory of Schizotypal Cognitions
rustle, nasal

S

S (schizophrenia)
S (spatial aptitude)
S (systems)
SA (self-analysis)
SA (sensory awareness)
SA (social acquiescence)
SA (social age)
SA (suicide attempt)
sabotage
saboteur
sac, alveolar
saccadic eye movements
saccule
"sack" (street name, heroin)
SACL (Sales Attitude Check List)
SACQ (Student Adaptation to College Questionnaire)
"sacrament" (street name, lysergic acid diethylamide/LSD)
"sacred mushroom" (street name, psilocybin)
SAD (seasonal affective disorder)
SAD (Self-Assessment Depression) scale
SAD (separation anxiety disorder)
SAD (social avoidance and distress)
sad, feeling suddenly
sad mood
SADAG (South African Depression and Anxiety Group, The)
SADD (Standardized Assessment of Depressive Disorders)
saddle curve audiogram configurations
sadism, sexual
sadism and masochism (S&M)
sadist
sadistic act of rape
sadistic behavior
sadistic mutilation
sadistic personality
SADL (simulated activities of daily living)
sadness
    feelings of
    intense, due to bereavement
    intense, due to financial ruin
    intense, due to significant loss from natural disaster
    intense, due to significant loss from serious disability
    intense, due to significant loss from serious medical illness
    periods of
sadomasochism (SM, S/M)
sadomasochistic relationship
SADS (Schedule for Affective Disorders and Schizophrenia)
SADS (seasonal affective disorder syndrome)
SADS (Shipman's Anxiety Depressive Scale)
SADS-C (Schedule for Affective Disorders and Schizophrenia–Change)
SADS-L (Schedule for Affective Disorders and Schizophrenia–Lifelong)
SAE (Standard American English)
"safe" situation
Safran Student's Interest Inventory
SAGES-P (Screening Assessment for Gifted Elementary Students–Primary)
sagittal orientation
sagittal plane, median
SAI (Student Adjustment Inventory)
SAL test (sensorineural acuity level) *(see also* tests)
salaam convulsion

Salamon-Conte Life Satisfaction in the Elderly Scale (LSES)
Sales Attitude Check List (SACL)
Sales Personality Questionnaire (SPQ)
Sales Style Diagnostic Test
salience
Salience Inventory (SI)
saliva smearing
salpingopharyngeal muscle
salpingopharyngeus, musculus
"salt" (street name, heroin)
"salt and pepper" (street name, cannabis)
SALT-P (Slosson Articulation Language Test with Phonology)
"sam" (re: federal narcotics agent)
SAM (sex arousal mechanism)
same period of illness
same-sex marriage
same-sex orientation
sample
    language
    representative
"sancocho" (re: to steal)
sanctioned behavior, culturally
sanctioned response, culturally
sanctions
    imposition of legal
    imposition of social
S&M (sadism and masochism)
"sandwich" (re: heroin in between layers of cocaine)
SANS (Scale for the Assessment of Negative Symptoms)
"Santa Marta" (street name, cannabis)
SAPS (Scale for the Assessment of Positive Symptoms)
SAQ (Substance Abuse Questionnaire)
SAQ-Adult Probation
SAS (School Assessment Survey)
"sasfras" (street name, cannabis)
SASSI (Substance Abuse Subtle Screening Inventory)
SAT (speech awareness threshold) *(see also* tests)

SATA (Scholastic Abilities Test for Adults)
satanic worship
"satan's secret" (street name, inhalant)
"satch" (re: drug smuggling)
"satch cotton" (re: drug injection)
satiation
satiety response
    satisfaction
        job
        patient
        personal
satisfaction tests *(see also* tests)
satisfaction with life
"sativa" (street name, cannabis)
saturation, oxyhemoglobin
saturation output
saturation sound pressure level (SSPL)
saturation sound pressure level 90, high-frequency average
satyromania
saucer curve audiogram configurations
saw-tooth noise
SBAI (Social Behavior Assessment Inventory)
"scaffle" (street name, phencyclidine/PCP)
scaffolded language-learning environment
"scag" (street name, heroin)
scala (pl. scalae)
scala media
scala tympani
scala vestibuli
SCALE (Scaled Curriculum Achievement Levels Test)
SCALE (Scales of Creativity and Learning Environment)
scale(s) *(see also* tests)
    content
    developmental *(see also* tests)
    Generalized Anxiety Disorder
    Impact of Event-Revised

repression-sensitization
Self-Rating Anxiety (SAS)
Self-Rating Depression (SDS)
repression-sensitization
    sensory
Scale for the Assessment of Negative Symptoms (SANS)
Scale for the Assessment of Positive Symptoms (SAPS)
Scale of Social Development
    scale score(s)
        full
        GAF
scale norms, adaptive
Scaled Curriculum Achievement Levels Test (SCALE)
scalene muscle
    anterior
    middle
    posterior
scalenus anterior, musculus
scalenus medius, musculus
scalenus posterior, musculus
Scales for Early Communication Skills for Hearing-Impaired Children (SECS)
Scales of Functional Independence
Scales of Independent Behavior
Scales of Psychological Development
Scales of Self-Regard for Preschool Children
Scales of Social Adaptation
scalp, "itchlike" sensation of the
SCAN-TRON Reading Test
scanning, eye
scanning communication board
Scanning Instrument for the Identification of Potential Learning
scanning quality speech, cerebellar
scanning speech
scanning type speech, cerebellar
scanning visage
scapgoated subsystem

scar tissue formation
"scat" (street name, heroin)
"scate" (street name, heroin)
scatophobia
scatter, intratest
Schaie-Thurstone Adult Mental Abilities Test
schedule
    abnormal sleep-wake
    continuous reinforcement
    extinction reinforcement
    fixed interval reinforcement
    fixed ratio reinforcement
    intermittent reinforcement
    reinforcement
    variable interval reinforcement
    variable ratio reinforcement
Schedule for Affective Disorders & Schizophrenia (SADS)
Schedule for Affective Disorders & Schizophrenia–Change (SADS-C)
Schedule for Affective Disorders & Schizophrenia–Lifetime (SADS-L)
Schedule of Growing Skills, The
Schedule of Recent Experience
schedules, preoccupation with
Scheibe deafness
schema (pl. schemata)
schizoaffective disorder
    bipolar type (F25.0)
    bipolar type, unspecified (F25.0)
    bipolar type, with abnormal psychomotor behavior (F25.0)
    bipolar type, with catatonia (F25.0) and (F06.1)
    bipolar type, with delusions (F25.0)
    bipolar type, with depression (F25.0)
    bipolar type, with disorganized speech (F25.0)

schizoaffective disorder
   bipolar type, with
     hallucinations (F25.0)
   bipolar type, with impaired
     cognition (F25.0)
   bipolar type, with manic
     symptoms (F25.0)
   bipolar type, with negative
     symptoms (F25.0)
   depressive type (F25.1)
   depressive type,
     unspecified (F25.1)
   depressive type, with
     abnormal psychomotor
     behavior (F25.1)
   depressive type, with
     catatonia (F25.1) and
     (F06.1)
   depressive type, with
     delusions (F25.1)
   depressive type, with
     depression (F25.1)
   depressive type, with
     disorganized speech
     (F25.1)
   depressive type, with
     hallucinations (F25.1)
   depressive type, with
     impaired cognition
     (F25.1)
   depressive type, with manic
     symptoms (F25.1)
   depressive type, with
     negative symptoms
     (F25.1)
schizoaffective episode
schizoid features *(see also* tests)
schizoid personality disorder
   (F60.1)
schizophasia, glossomanic
   (subtype)
schizophrenia (F20.9)
     abnormal frontotemporal
       interactions in
     abnormal psychomotor
       behavior with (F20.9)
     active phase of
     acute exacerbation of

schizophrenia
   alternative dimensional
     descriptors for
   behavioral disorganization
     in
   behavioral genetics of
   biology of
   categorization in
   characteristic sign of
   characteristic symptoms of
   communication disorder in
   continuous (F20.9)
   corticolimbic alterations in
   delusions with (F20.9)
   depression with (F20.9)
   disorder of
   disorganized behavior in
   disorganized factor in
   disorganized speech with
     (F20.9)
   dissolution of cerebral
     cortical mechanisms in
   distorted communication in
   distorted inferential
     thinking in
   distorted language in
   distorted perception in
   early onset of
   early sign of
   epidemiology of
   erotomanic-type
   exaggerated
     communication in
   exaggerated inferential
     thinking in
   exaggerated language in
   exaggerated perception in
   excitotoxicity in
   executive speech
     dysfunction in
   familial transmission of
   first sign of
   fragmentary delusions in
   fragmentary hallucinations
     in
   gender differences in
   grandiose type
   hallucinations with (F20.9)

schizophrenia
    impaired cognition with
      (F20.9)
    increased risk for
    insights from neuroimaging
      into
    interepisode residual
      symptoms of
    jealous type
    language disorder in
    language impairments in
    late onset of
    linguistic disorganization in
    manic symptoms with
      (F20.9)
    mimics of
    mixed type
    mood symptoms in
    negative factor in
    neuroleptic treatment of
      childhood
    neuroleptics as treatment
      for
    pathognomonic symptoms
      of
    pathophysiological
      significance of age at
      onset of
    pathophysiology of
    persecutory type
    pharmacological aspects of
    plasma HVA levels in
    positive symptoms of
    postmortem studies in
    postpsychotic depressive
      disorder of
    prevalence of
    prodromal phase of
    prolonged prodrome of
    prominent negative
      symptoms of
    psychoanalysis and
    psychosocial aspects of
    psychotic dimension of
    psychotic disorganization
      in
    psychotic episode of
    psychotic factor in

schizophrenia
    residual phase of
    semantic memory in
    semantic processing in
    somatic type
    speech disorder in
    subchronic
    syntactic processing in
    thought disorder in
    3-factor dimensional model
      of
    undifferential type
    unspecified (F20.9)
    water balance in
Schizophrenia "8" Scale
schizophrenia spectrum and other
    psychotic disorders
    other specified (F28)
    unspecified (F29)
schizophrenia with catatonia
    (F20.9) and (F06.1)
schizophrenia with negative
    symptoms (F20.9)
schizophrenic affect
    residual
    short-lived
schizophrenic disturbance of
    speech and language
schizophrenic process
schizophrenic psychology
schizophrenic speech and
    language disorder
    neuropsychology of
    pathology of
schizophrenic symptoms
    disorganization dimension
      of positive
    psychotic dimension of
      positive
schizophrenic thought disorder,
    Descartes' "cogito" as
schizophrenic thought disorder
    linguistic analysis of
    psychology of
    psychopathology of
schizophreniform disorder
    (F20.81)
      abnormal psychomotor

schizophreniform disorder
  behavior with (F20.81)
  delusions with (F20.81)
  depression with (F20.81)
  disorganized speech with
    (F20.81)
  hallucinations with
    (F20.81)
  impaired cognition with
    (F20.81)
  manic symptoms with
    (F20.81)
  negative symptoms with
    (F20.81)
schizophreniform disorder with
  good prognostic features
  (F20.81)
schizophreniform disorder
  without good prognostic
  features (F20.81)
schizotypal personality disorder
  (F21)
"schmeck" (street name, cocaine)
Schmidt syndrome
Schneider's list of first-rank
  symptoms
Scholastic Abilities Test for
  Adults (SATA)
School Administrator Assessment
  Survey
School and College Ability Tests
School Apperception Method
School Assessment Survey (SAS)
School Attitudes Survey
school aversion
school battery *(see also* tests)
School Climate Inventory
school counselor
school discipline problem
school drop-out
school dysfunction
school entering problems *(see
  also* tests)
school environment, inadequate
School Environment Preference
  Survey
school functioning impairment
  (see also tests)

School Handicap Condition Scale
  (SEH)
School Interest Inventory
School language
School Library/Media Skills Test
school performance *(see also*
  tests)
School Situation Survey (SSS)
school skills inventory, basic *(see
  also* tests)
School Social Skills Rating Scale
  (S3 Rating Scale)
school truancy
school work, neglect of
school/work activities,
  interference with
"schoolboy" (street name,
  cocaine; codeine/
  methylmorphine-opioid)
"Schoolcraft" (street name, crack)
Schubert General Ability Battery
Schutz Measures, The
Schwabach Test
schwannoma
science
  cognitive
  communication
  hearing
  speech
  speech and hearing
science of aging
scientific grammar
scintillating scotoma,
  homogenous
"scissors" (street name, cannabis)
SCL-90-R (Symptom Checklist-
  90-Revised)
sclerosing panencephalitis,
  subacute
sclerosis
  amyotrophic lateral (ALS;
    Lou Gehrig's disease)
  multiple
  tuberous
sclerotic area
sclerotome area
scoleciphobia

scopolamine (street names)
    homicide (heroin cut with scopolamine and strychnine)
    spice (heroin cut with scopolamine and strychnine)
"score" (re: purchase OF drugs)
score
    Apgar
    Children's Coma
    finger-tapping
    Full Scale
    GAF scale
    high
    PB max
    raw
    standard
    test
score discrimination
"scorpion" (street name, cocaine)
scotoma (pl. scotomata)
    absolute
    bilateral
    cecocentral
    central
    dense
    fortification
    homogenous scintillating
    mental
    negative
    paracentral
    relative
    scintillating
"Scott" (street name, heroin)
Scott Mental Alertness Test
"Scottie" (street name, cocaine)
"Scotty" (street name, cocaine; crack cocaine; crack influence)
SCRA (Society for Community Research and Action)
"scramble" (street name, crack)
"scratch" (re: currency)
SCREEN (Screening Children for Related Early Educational Needs)
screen
    blood drug
    heavy metal
    THC elevation
    urine drug
screen for drugs test, blood
screen out irrelevant stimuli
Screening and Referral Form for Children with Suspected Learning and Behavioral Disabilities, Basic
screening articulation test
Screening Assessment for Gifted Elementary Students—Primary
screening audiometry, reduced
screening batteries *(see also* tests)
Screening Children for Related Early Educational Needs (SCREEN)
Screening Deep Test of Articulation
screening evaluation
screening exam, neuropsychological *(see also* tests)
screening instruments
screening inventories
screening profiles
screening tests *(see also* tests)
scribblemania
scribomania
"scruples" (street name, crack)
scrupulous
scrutiny, fear of
SCT-B (Short Category Test - Booklet Format)
"scuffle" (street name, phencyclidine/PCP)
SD (speech discrimination)
SD (standard deviation)
SD, sd (stimulus drive)
SD, S-D (suicide-depression)
S-D Proneness Checklist
SDD (specific developmental disorder) *(see also* tests)
SDL (Serial Digit Learning Test)
SDL task, ninc-digit (SD9)

SDQII (Self-Description
   Questionnaire II)
SDS (speech discrimination
   score) *(see also* tests)
SDT (speech detectability
   threshold)
SDT (speech detection threshold)
(S/E) subsequent encounter
SEA (Survey of Employee
   Access)
search
   transderivational
   word
Search and Attention Test -
   Visual (VSAT)
searching for words
searing pain
Seashore Measures of Musical
   Talents
seasonal headache
seasonal migraine headache
seasonal pattern
seasonal pattern, mood disorder
   with
seasonal-related psychosocial
   stressors
seated position
seclusion
   office
   locked
second, cycles per (CPS)
second deciduous molar teeth
second episode
"second messenger" system
second messengers, lithium's
   action on
second premolar teeth
secondary articulation
secondary autism
secondary characteristics of
   stuttering
secondary gain, potential
secondary palate
secondary reinforcer
secondary sex characteristics
secondary stress
secondary stuttering
secondary verb

secretion, cortisol
secretive manner
SECS (Scales for Early
   Communication Skills for
   Hearing-Impaired
secure video connections
sedative/hypnotic agents (non-
   psychotic)
   Alurate
   aprobarbital
   butabarbital
   Butisol
   divalproex sodium
   Duralith
   Epitol
   Epival
   Imovane
   Lotusate
   Mysoline
   Nembutal
   pentobarbital
   primidone
   secobarbital
   Seconal
   talbutal
   zopiclone
Sedative-Hypnotic-Anxiolytic (S-
   H-A)
sedative/hypnotic use
sedative-induced anxiety disorder
sedative-induced disorders
sedative intoxication delirium
sedative intoxication with use
   disorder
       mild (F13.129)
       moderate/severe (F13.229)
sedative intoxication without use
   disorder (F13.929)
sedative-related disorder
sedative-related disorder,
   unspecified (F13.99)
sedative-type withdrawal
sedative use disorder
       mild (F13.10)
       moderate/severe (F13.20)
sedative use disorder with
   sedative-induced anxiety
   disorder

sedative use disorder with
  sedative-induced bipolar or
  related disease
sedative use disorder with
  sedative-induced brief psychotic
  disorder
sedative use disorder with
  sedative-induced delirium
sedative use disorder with
  sedative-induced delusional
  disorder
sedative use disorder with
  sedative-induced depressive
  disorder
sedative use disorder with
  sedative-induced
  schizoaffective disorder
sedative use disorder with
  sedative-induced schizophrenia
sedative use disorder with
  sedative-induced
  schizophreniform disorder
sedative use disorder with
  sedative-induced schizotypal
  (personality) disorder
sedative-use lifestyle
sedative withdrawal with
  perceptual disturbance
  (F13.232)
sedative withdrawal without
  perceptual disturbance
  (F13.239)
seductive tendency
seductiveness
SEE (Seeing Essential English)
SEE (Signing Exact English)
SEED Development Profile
"seeds" (street name, cannabis)
seekers, care
seeking, novelty
Seeking of Noetic Goals Test, The
"seggy" (street name, barbiturate)
segment, pharyngoesophageal
  (PE)
segmental analysis
segmental phoneme
SEH (severe emotional handicap)
SEI (Self-Esteem Index, The)

seizure
  absence
  acute
  akinetic
  alcohol as cause of
  alcohol withdrawal
  alcohol-related
  aphasic
  apneic
  asteric
  asymptomatic
  atonic absence
  atypical absence
  audiogenic
  auditory
  benign neonatal familial
  bilateral myoclonic
  cardiovascular
  centrencephalic
  cephalic
  cerebellar fits
  cerebral
  cessation of
  clonic
  clonic-tonic-clonic
  complex partial (CPS)
  continuing petit mal
  conversion
  convulsive
  cryptogenic
  diencephalic
  drug-induced
  drug-withdrawal
  emotion as cause of
  epilepsia partialis continua
  epileptic
  fatigue as cause of
  generalized tonic-clonic
    (GTC)
  grand mal (tonic-clonic)
  history of
  hysterical
  iatrogenic
  ictal confusional
  jacksonian
  Lennox-Gastaut (petit mal
    variant)
  major motor

seizure
   myoclonic
   new-onset
   olfactory psychomotor
   partial complex
   partial sensory
   partial tonic
   past ictal depression phase
     of
   petit mal (typical absence)
   petit mal variant (Lennox-
     Gastaut)
   phonatory
   photogenic
   post-traumatic
   postural
   precentral
   precipitation of
   premonition of
   primary
   psychic
   psychogenic
   psychomotor
   recurring
   reflex
   repetitive partial
   sensory-evoked
   simple partial
   situation-related
   sleep-related
   sleep-waking cycle and
     occurrence of
   somatosensory
   subclinical
   symptomatic
   tonic
   tonic-clonic (grand mal)
   traumatic
   typical
   typical absence (petit mal)
   uncinate
   unilateral
   vertiginous
   visual
   withdrawal
seizure type of symptom

selection
   hearing aid
   treatment
selection battery
selection communication board,
   direct
selection of sounds, errors of
selective attachments
selective auditory agnosia *(see
   also* tests)
selective focusing on
   environmental stimuli
selective listening, auditory
selective mutism
selective mutism (F94.0)
Selective Reminding Test
self
   aniled sense of
   effect of trauma on
   experience of the
   perception of
   sense of
self-absorbed tendencies
self-administered penectomy
self-administration of drugs,
   frequency of
self-assertion
Self-assessment test *(see also*
   tests)
self-biting
   nonfunctional and
     repetitive
   severe
self-care, fear of
self-care activity
self-care dysfunction
self-care skills *(see also* tests)
self-castration
self-centered attitude
self-centeredness
self-compassion, lack of
self-concept scales *(see also* tests)
self-confidence, low
self-consciousness
Self-Consciousness Scale, The
self-criticism, patterns of
   pervasive
self-damaging behavior

self-damaging impulsivity
self-deprecating thoughts
self-derogatory concepts
self-derogatory content
self-derogatory themes
Self-Description Questionnaire (SDQ)
self-destructiveness, relative lack of
self-discipline
self-disclosure *(see also* tests)
self-disgust, feelings of
self-dramatization
self-dramatizing behavior
self-esteem
    denigrated
    lack of
    low
    negative
self-evaluation *(see also* tests)
self-harm, personal history of (Z91.5)
self-help skills, age-appropriate *(see also* tests)
self-hypnosis training, cognitive
self-image
    relative stability of
    splitting of
    unstable
self-importance, sense of
self-imposed high standards of performance
self-individuation
self-induced alopecia
self-induced hair loss
self-induced injury
self-inflicted bodily injury
self-inflicted gunshot wound
self-inflicted rectal bleeding
self-initiated activity
self-injury, motivation for
self-loathing
self-observation *(see also* tests)
self position/index
self-propagation
self-psychology, psychoanalysis and
Self-Rating Anxiety Scale (SAS)
Self-Rating Depression Scale (SDS)
self-regulatory capacity
self-report measure of social adjustment *(see also* tests)
self-report personalities inventories *(see also* tests)
self-responsibility, lack of
self-role concept
self-stimulation behavior
self-stimulatory behaviors in sensory deficit individuals
self-stimulatory behaviors in the young, developmentary appropriate *(see also* tests)
self-sufficiency, economic
self-sufficient, need to be
self-support, minimum
"self-talk"
self-treatment, hormonal
self-worth, feelings of low
selfishness
semantic constraints
semantic differential
semantic feature
semantic implication
semantic interference
semantic memory
semantic relations
semantic rule
semantic theory of stuttering
semantics
    behavioral
    extension
    general *(see also* tests)
    generative
    intention
    referential
semantics of autism
semen loss, excessive
semiaural hearing protection device
semiautomatic action
semi-autonomous systems concept of brain function
semicircular canal(s)
scmiology
semipurposeful behavior

semistarvation
semitone
semi-vowel consonant formation
Semon law
Semon-Rosenbach law
"sen" (street name, cannabis)
Senf Comrey Ratings of Extra
    Educational Needs
"seni" (street name, mescaline)
senile chorea
senile dementia, Alzheimer type
    (SDAT)
senile mania
senile osteoporosis
senile tremor
Senior Apperception Technique
sensation
    altered
    buzzing
    creeping-crawling
    decreased peripheral
    deep
    diminished
    distorted perception of
      physical
    distorted perception of
      visual
    drug-induced floating
    dysesthetic
    ejaculatory inevitability
    electric shock
    facial
    fear
    fetal movement
    fine tactile
    flying
    impaired hearing
    insect infestation
    "itchlike" scalp
    lack of control
    light touch
    loss of pain
    loss of touch
    numbing
    orgasmic
    out-of-body
    out-of-mind
    pain
sensation
    phantom
    pins and needles
    pins sticking
    reduced preputial
    reduced foreskin
    return of
    slowed time
    smell
    sound-produced color
    superficial
    tactile
    taste
    temperature
    tingling
    touch
    vibration/vibratory
    wakefulness
    well-being
sensation level (SL)
sensation of numbness (a panic
    attack indicator)
sensation of shortness of breath
    (SOB) (a panic attack indicator)
sensation of smothering (a panic
    attack indicator)
sensation of tingling (a panic
    attack indicator)
sensation unit (SU)
sense
    aniled
    common
    rejection
    time
sense of
    arousal
    being out of control
    being overwhelmed
    detachment
    difficulty concentrating,
      subjective
    emptiness
    entitlement
    foreshortened future
    frustration
    humor
    muscular relaxation
    numbing

sense of
    other people's boundaries, little
    personal identity
    placement
    relief
    reliving an event
    responsibility, poor
    self, aniled
    self-importance
    sexual pleasure
    tension, increasing
    time
Sense of Coherence Questionnaire
senseless imitative word repetition
sensitivity
    contrast
    rejection
sensitivity group
sensitivity prediction from the acoustic reflex (SPAR)
sensitivity reaction of adolescence
Sensitivity reaction of childhood
sensitivity to perceived interpersonal rejection, pathological
sensitivity to rejection, increased
sensitivity training group (T-group)
sensor operation
sensorial epilepsy
sensorimotor act
sensorimotor arc
sensorimotor intelligence period
sensorimotor system
sensorineural acuity level masking technique
sensorineural acuity level technique
sensorineural deafness
sensorium, clear
sensory acuity
sensory anesthesia
sensory aphasia, transcortical
sensory ataxia
sensory aura
sensory-based

sensory bondage (blindfolding)
sensory cortex
sensory deficit individuals, self-stimulatory behaviors in
sensory deficit, central
sensory discrimination, oral
sensory dissociation, syndrome of
sensory disturbance, global assessment of
sensory-evoked potential (SEP)
sensory-evoked seizure
sensory function, intact
sensory functioning, voluntary
sensory impairment
Sensory Integration and Praxis Tests (SIPT)
sensory level
sensory loss
    central
    cortical
    dense
    dissociated
    level of
    peripheral
    stocking-glove
sensory modalities, loss of
sensory modality
    auditory
    gustatory
    olfactory
    tactile
    visual
sensory/motor behavior
sensory nerve
sensory paralysis, laryngeal
sensory pathway stimulation
sensory perception
sensory receptor
sensory scale
sensory seizure, partial
sensory shock
sensory stimulation
sensory stimulus
sensory symptoms
sensory testing, level of demarcation in
sensory threshold
sensory type of symptom

sentence
    complex
    compound
    compound-complex
    constituent
    declarative
    derivation of a
    derived
    embedded
    exclamatory
    imperative
    interrogative
    kernel
    matrix
    simple
sentence classification
sentence closure task
Sentence Closure Test
sentence completion blank
sentence constituents
sentence derivation
sentence structure, evaluating *(see also* tests)
sentence test
    need a
    write a
sentence types
sentimental value
SEP (somatosensory evoked potential) brain test
separation
    binaural
    family
    fear of
    marital
separation anxiety disorder (F93.0)
separation anxiety of infancy and childhood
separation-individuation phase
separation of ideas from feelings
separation problem
separator state
septal area
septum
    alveolar
    deviated
    nasal

sequela (SQ)
sequence
    memory
    syllable
    ungrammatical
    word *(see also* tests)
    work
sequence memory
sequence of sounds and memory
Sequenced Inventory of Communication Development - Adapted (A-SICD)
sequencing, auditory
sequencing rule of syntax *(see also* tests)
sequencing rules
Sequential Assessment of Mathematics Inventories: Standardized Inventory
Sequential Inventory of Language Development (SILD)
sequential multiple analysis (SMA)
SER (somatosensory evoked response) brain test
serial content speech *(see also* tests)
Serial Digit Learning Test (SDL)
serial killers
serial learning
serial list learning
serial observation
serial sevens (7's) test
serial sexual killers
serial threes (3's) test
seriatim speech
seriation skills
series of numbers
serious assaultive acts
serious illness
serious impairment in communication
serious impairment in judgment
serious impairment of functioning
serious suicide act
serious traumatic stress
serious violation of rules

"sernyl" (street name,
  phencyclidine/PCP)
serotonin-specific reuptake
  inhibitor (SSRI) antidepressant
  medications
serotonin syndrome
serous otitis media (SOM)
"Serpico 21" (street name,
  cocaine)
serratus anterior muscle
serratus anterior, musculus (Latin)
serratus posterior inferior,
  musculus (Latin)
serratus posterior inferior muscle
serratus posterior superior,
  musculus (Latin)
serratus posterior superior muscle
serum calcium level
"server" (re: crack dealer)
service(s)
    armed
    community mental health
    general hospital
      consultation/liaison
    health care
    hospital
      consultation/liaison
    medical
    problems with access to
      health care
    psychiatric emergency
      (PES)
    social and rehabilitation
      (RS)
    vocational rehabilitation
      (VRS)
service agency, social
service personnel
services of prostitutes
servomechanism
"sess" (street name, cannabis)
sessile vocal nodules
session
    fixed-ended
    open-ended
SET (support, empathy, truth)
  therapy
"set" (re: drug-buying place)

set
    criteria
    data
    difficulty in changing
      response
    preparatory
    single criteria
set of disturbances
    affective
    attentional
    behavioral
set of disturbances
    cognitive
    linguistic
    perceptual
set of procedures
set system, symbol
setter, fire (FS)
setting
    clinical
    community
    cultural
    educational
    fire
    general population
    group
    home
    inpatient psychiatric
    institutional
    novel
    outpatient
    partial-hospital
    psychosocial
    social
"Seven-up" (street name, cocaine;
  crack)
severe anxiety
severe aphasia
severe ataxia
severe bipolar I disorder with
  psychotic features
severe bipolar I disorder without
  psychotic features
severe dementia
severe depression
severe diffuse brain dysfunction
severe disability
severe emotional handicap (SEH)

severe environmental deprivation
severe headache
severe hearing impairment, moderately
severe hearing loss, moderately
severe intoxication
severe life stress
severe memory impairment
severe mental illness
severe myoclonic epilepsy in infancy (SMEI)
severe self-biting
severe stress in children
severe substance use disorder
severity of headache pain
severity of psychiatric disturbance
severity rating scales for speech and language impairments *(see also* tests)
"sewer" (re: drug injection)
sex
 anal
 assigned
 biological
 forced
 indeterminate
 promiscuous
 trading
 unprotected
 "wrong"
sex acts, criminal
sex addiction
sex characteristics
 primary
 secondary
sex chromosomes
sex counseling (Z70.9)
sex drive
sex for drugs
sex headache
sex ratio
 characteristic
 equal
sex-reassignment, hormonal
sex-reassignment surgery
sex-related risk-taking
sex-role behavior, stereotypic
sexomnia

sexual abstinence
sexual abuse
 adult, by nonspouse or nonpartner, confirmed, initial encounter (T74.21XA)
 adult, by nonspouse or nonpartner, confirmed, subsequent encounter (T74.21XD)
 adult, by nonspouse or nonpartner, suspected, initial encounter (T76.21XA)
 adult, by nonspouse or nonpartner, suspected, subsequent encounter (T76.21XD)
 childhood
 problems related to
sexual abuse as major childhood stressor
sexual abuse in childhood
sexual abuse of a child
sexual abuse of an adult
sexual activity, masochistic
sexual and gender identity disorder
sexual arousal
 oxygen-deprived
 problems with
sexual arousal disorder
 acquired type female
 female
 generalized type female
 lifelong type female
 situational type female
sexual arousal disorder due to combined factors, female
sexual arousal disorder due to psychological factors, female
sexual arousal problems
sexual assault, drug facilitated (DFSA)
sexual aversion, occasional
sexual aversion disorder
 acquired type
 generalized type

sexual aversion disorder
    lifelong type
    situational type
sexual aversion disorder due to combined factors
sexual aversion disorder due to psychological factors
sexual behavior
    cultural-related standards of
    inappropriate
    intense
    masochistic
    promiscuous
    unusual
    voyeuristic
sexual boundary violations
sexual coercion
sexual contact, genital
sexual desire
    absent
    deficient
    disturbance in
    hyperactive
    hypoactive
    loss of
    low
    problems with
sexual desire disorder
    acquired type hypoactive
    generalized type hypoactive
    hypoactive
    lifelong type hypoactive
    situational type hypoactive
sexual desire disorder due to combined factors, hypoactive
sexual desire disorder due to psychological factors, hypoactive
sexual development
sexual deviance disorder
sexual disorders
    drug treatment for
    psychoanalysis and
sexual dysfunction
    acquired
    alcohol-induced

sexual dysfunction
    amphetamine-induced
    cocaine-induced
    generalized
    life-long
    other specified (F52.8)
    situational
    unspecified (F52.9)
sexual dysfunction due to combined factors
sexual dysfunction due to GMC
sexual dysfunction due to psychological factors
sexual dysfunction due to a substance
sexual dysfunction with impaired arousal
sexual dysfunction with impaired desire
sexual dysfunction with impaired orgasm
sexual dysfunction with sexual pain
sexual encounters
    frequency of
    indiscriminate
    types of
sexual excitement, adequate
sexual experience, fantasied
sexual expression, excessive need for
sexual fantasy
    female object of
    intense
    masochistic
    nonpathological
    pathological
sexual fears
sexual function, adequate
sexual functioning, quality of
sexual identity, adolescent
sexual identity disorder
sexual indifference
sexual interaction
sexual intercourse, pain during
sexual interest
    diminished
    low

sexual masochism (F65.51)
sexual masochism in a controlled
  environment (F65.51)
sexual masochism in full
  remission (F65.51)
sexual masochism with
  asphyxiophylia (F65.51)
sexual maturity
sexual misconduct in the helping
  professions
sexual opportunity
sexual orientation
sexual pain, sexual dysfunction
  with
sexual pain disorder
sexual performance
sexual physiology
sexual pleasure, subjective sense
  of
sexual reassignment
    hormonal
    surgical
sexual relationships
sexual response, disorders of
sexual response cycle
    desire phase of
    excitement phase of
    orgasmic phase of
    resolution phase of
sexual risk-taking
sexual sadism disorder (F65.52)
sexual spousal or partner violence
    confirmed, initial encounter
      (T74.21XA)
    confirmed, subsequent
      encounter (T74.21XD)
    suspected, initial encounter
      (T76.21XA)
    suspected, subsequent
      encounter (T76.21XD)
sexual stimulation
sexual stimuli revulsion
sexual symptoms, somatization
sexual tension, release of
sexual urges
    intense
    masochistic
    voyeuristic

sexual values
sexually addictive behavior
sexually arousing behavior
sexually arousing fantasies,
  voyeuristic
sexually seductive behavior
sexually transmitted disease
  (STD)
"sezz" (street name, cannabis)
S-H-A (Sedative-Hypnotic-
  Anxiolytic)
shading, emotional
shadow, object
shadow curve
shadow effect, head
shadowing masking technique
shadowing method
"shake" (street name, cannabis)
"shaker/baker/water" (re: cocaine
  use)
shaking (a panic attack indicator)
shaking palsy
shaking tremor
shaking voice
shallow expression of emotion(s)
shamanism
shame, feelings of
shamed, fear of being
shape
    body
    syllable
shared delusional belief (folie a
  deux)
shared mechanism
shared phenomenological features
shared psychotic disorder
shared understanding
shared values
sharing drug paraphernalia
sharp pain
sharply falling curve audiogram
  configurations
"sharps" (re: razor blades;
  needles)
"she" (street name, cocaine)
"sheet rocking" (street name,
  crack and lysergic acid
  diethylamide/LSD)

"sheets" (street name, phencyclidine/PCP)
shell earmold
Sheltered Care Environment Scale
"shermans" (street name, phencyclidine/PCP)
"sherms" (street name, crack; phencyclidine/PCP)
shift
    Doppler
    gradual topic
    method threshold
    paradigmatic
    permanent threshold (PTS)
    pitch
    temporary threshold (TTS)
    voice
shift ability
shift in mood
shift masking technique, threshold
shift referential index
shift work
shift work type dyssomnia
shifting of emotions
shifting sleep-wake cycle
shimmer, amplitude
Shipley Institute of Living Scale
Shipman Anxiety Depressive Scale
SHM (simple harmonic motion)
"shmeck/schmeek" (street name, heroin)
shock
    auditory
    cultural
    electrical
    neurogenic
    psychic
    sensory
    spinal
shock exhibitionism
shock syndrome
    neurogenic
    psychogenic
shock therapy
Shock treatment
shoe restrictions

"shoot/shoot up" (re: drug injection)
"shoot the breeze" (street name, nitrous oxide)
"shooting gallery" (re: drug-using place)
shooting pain
short cycle(s)
Short Employment Tests
Short Imaginal Processes Inventory (SIPI)
Short Increment Sensitivity Index (SISI)
short-lived schizophrenic affect
short orientation-memory-concentration test (OMC)
short sleep duration
short sleep latency
Short-Term Auditory Retrieval and Storage Test (STARS)
Short Test for Use With Cerebral Palsy Children
Shortened Edinburgh Reading Tests, The
"shot" (re: drug injection)
"shot down" (re: drug influence)
shoulders, stooped
shower collar
shrinking retrograde amnesia
shrinking retrograde amnesic
"shrooms" (street name, psilocybin/psilocin)
Shubo-kyofu (F42)
shuffling gait
shuffling steps
shunting
shy behavior
    culturally appropriate
    developmentally appropriate
shyness
SI (Salience Inventory)
SI (self-inflicted)
SI (social introversion)
SI (structure of intellect)
(S/I) suspected/initial episode
SIB (self-injurious behavior)
sibilant consonant formation

sibling jealousy
sibling lifestyle
sibling profile
sibling relational problem
  (Z64.891)
sibling relations
sibship
"sick" role, intangible benefits of
  the
sickness, sleeping
Sickness Impact Profile Test
"Siddi" (street name, cannabis)
side effect
       extrapyramidal medication
       medication
side effects of treatment
siderodromomania
SIFTER (Screening Instrument
  for Targeting Educational Risk)
sign
       arithmetic
       autonomic
       autonomic hyperactivity
       Babinski
       brain stem
       cerebellar
       cerebral
       Claude hyperkinesis
       focal neurologic
       focal nonextrapyramidal
        neurologic
       frontal release
       increased autonomic
       neurological soft
       Omega (+ or - for suicide)
       operational
       pathognomonic
       positive frontal release
       premonitory
       psychological
       root
       sheet
       soft neurological
       withdrawal
       vital (VS)
sign language
sign marker
sign systems

sign words
signal
       acoustic
       speech
       therapeutic error (TES)
signal anxiety
signal detection
signal speech
signal-to-noise ratio (S/N)
signals
       bilateral contralateral
        routing of (BICROS)
       contralateral routing of
        (CROS)
       focal contralateral routing
        of (FOCALCROS)
       front routing of (FROS)
       hearing aid contralateral
        routing of (CROS)
       ipsilateral routing of
        (IROS)
signed English
significance of age at onset of
  schizophrenia,
  pathophysiological
significant deterioration
significant distress, clinically
significant insomnia
significant risk
significant risk factor
significant role
significant subjective distress
significant supporting persons,
  loss of
significant underachievement,
  pattern of
significantly subaverage
Signing Exact English (SEE)
signs and symptoms
       bodily
       constellation of
       parkinsonian
       physical
       psychological
       withdrawal
signs of affective expression
signs of alcohol intoxication
signs of compulsive substance use

signs of depression
signs of pregnancy
signs of schizophrenia
signs of substance tolerance or
    withdrawal
signs of withdrawal
    anchor
    phencyclidine dose-related
    physiological
SIL (speech interference level)
silent blocking in speech
silent speech blocking
silliness, childlike
"Silly Putty" (street name,
    psilocybin/psilocin)
similar shared features
similarities mental status test
similarities test, understanding of
similarity disorders of aphasia
simile (figure of speech)
Similes Test
simple aphasia
simple deteriorative disorder
simple future progressive tense
simple future tense
simple hallucination
simple harmonic motion (SHM)
simple motor tics
simple partial seizure
simple past progressive tense
simple past tense
simple predicate
simple present progressive tense
simple present tense
simple schizophrenia
simple sentence
"Simple Simon" (street name,
    psilocybin/psilocin)
simple sound source
simple subject
simple syllabic
simple tense
simple tone
simple vocal tics
simple wave
simple word
simplex virus meningitis, herpes
simplification

simultaneous auditory feedback
simultaneous aural rehabilitation
simultaneous method sine wave
simultaneous nerve impulse
sine wave, simultaneous method
singer's formant frequency
singer's nodes
Single and Double Simultaneous
    Stimulation Test
single criteria set
single episode mania
single hypomanic episode
single major depression episode
single manic episode
single parent
single performance situation,
    feared
single person
singleton, prevocalic
singleton omissions, postvocalic
    obstruent
sinistral
sinistrality
"sinse" (street name, cannabis)
sinus of the ventricle
sinusoidal wave
SIOP (Society for Industrial and
    Organizational Psychology)
SIPI (Short Imaginal Processes
    Inventory)
SIPT (Sensory Integration and
    Praxis Tests)
SIRS (Structured Interview of
    Reported Symptoms)
SIs (Status Indicators)
SIS (Stress Impact Scale)
SISI (Short Increment Sensitivity
    Index)
sissyish behavior
site of pain, anatomical
sitomania
SIT (Slosson Intelligence Test
sitting balance
situation(s)
    avoiding speech
    cluster of
    conflictual
    dreaded

situation(s)
    educational
    emotion-laden
    family
    feared
    feared single performance
    loss of previously
      stabilizing social
    low-activity
    low-stimulation
    My Vocational
    one-to-one
    performance
    phobic
    phobic avoidance of
    "safe"
    social
situation-related epilepsy
situation-related seizure
Situation Survey - School (SSS)
situational sexual dysfunction
situational stressor, specific
situational type dyspareunia
situational type female orgasmic disorder
situational type female sexual arousal disorder
situational type hypoactive sexual desire disorder
situational type male erectile disorder
situational type male orgasmic disorder
situational type sexual aversion disorder
situational type vaginismus
situationally appropriate atmosphere
situationally bound (cued) panic attack(s)
situationally optimistic atmosphere
situationally predisposed panic attack(s)
Siuvo Intelligent Psychological Assessment Platform
SIV (Survey of Interpersonal Values)

SIW (self-inflicted wound)
six Hertz positive spikes
six Hertz positive spike-waves
six-step reframing
Sixteen Personality Factor Questionnaire (16PF)
sixth cycle noise hum
"sixth sense," belief in
sixty-cycle hum noise
"sixty-two" (re: drug injection)
size
    body
    chunk
size perception
"skee" (street name, opium)
"skeeger/skeezer" (re: crack user)
skeleton earmold
"sketching" (re: drug withdrawal)
"skid" (street name, heroin)
"skied" (re: drug influence)
skill(s) *(see also* tests)
    activities of daily living (ADLs)
    age-appropriate self-help
    assertiveness
    assessment of
    attentional
    auditory
    basic
    calculation
    communication
    comprehension
    conceptual
    cross-dressing
    decision making
    decoding
    deterioration of social
    ego-coping
    encoding
    individual
    intellectual
    interpersonal
    leisure
    linguistic
    mathematical
    memory
    minimum acceptable
    negotiating goals

skill(s) *(see also* tests)
    negotiating routines
    negotiating rules
    numerical reasoning
    organizational
    perceptual
    perceptual-motor
    phonetic
    phonetic-analysis
    problem-solving
    resolving conflict
    self-care
    seriation
    social
    socialization
    stress adaptability
    verbally mediated
    visual-perceptual
    word attack
    wordfinding
skill areas
skill competencies *(see also* tests)
skill domains, adaptive
Skill Indicators (SKIs)
skill training
    occupational
    social
SKILLSCOPE for Managers
skills disorder, motor
skin, picking at
skin infection
"skin popping" (re: drug injection)
skin resistance, galvanic
skin response audiometry
    galvanic (GSRA)
    psychogalvanic
skin response, psychogalvanic
skipping
SKIs (Skill Indicators)
Sklar Aphasia Scale
"skuffle" (street name, phencyclidine/PCP)
skull asymmetry
skull bone(s)
    ethmoid
    frontal
    inferior maxillary

skull bone(s)
    inferior nasal concha
    inferior turbinated
    lacrimal
    malar
    mandible
    maxilla
    medial nasal concha
    medial turbinated
    nasal
    occipital
    palatine
    parietal
    sphenoid
    sphenoidal nasal conchae
    superior maxillary
    superior nasal concha
    superior turbinated
    supreme nasal concha
    temporal
    turbinate
    vomer
    zygomatic
"skunk" (street name, cannabis)
SL (sensation level)
SL (sublingual)
"slab" (street name, crack)
"slam" (re: drug injection)
"slanging" (re: drug dealing)
sleep
    active
    alcohol-induced nighttime
    arousal from
    breathing pauses during
    choking during
    circadian phase of
    confusional arousals from
    consolidated
    daytime
    decreased
    decreased need for
    deep
    depth of
    difficulty maintaining
    disorder of initiating and maintaining (DIMS)
    disordered
    disrupted

sleep
- disturbed
- dreamless
- easily disturbed
- forced
- fragmented nighttime
- gasping during
- impaired ventilation during
- inability to
- increased
- increased arousal from
- indeterminate
- insufficient nocturnal
- lack of excessive
- negative conditioning for
- non-REM
- nonrestorative
- onset of
- overconcern with
- paradoxical
- quality of
- quiet
- REM onset
- REM stage of
- slow-wave
- stage 1-4 NREM
- stage of REM
- stage W (wakefulness)
- timing of
- transitional
- undisturbed nocturnal
- unintended
- unrefreshing
- very deep
- very light

sleep abnormalities
sleep and wakefulness
- mixed
- obstructive
- pattern of

sleep apnea, central
sleep apnea hypopnea, obstructive
sleep apnea syndrome
- adult obstructive
- central
- obstructive

sleep architecture
sleep arousal
sleep attacks
- refreshing
- sudden
- uncontrollable

sleep behavior disorder, REM
sleep complaint
sleep continuity
- better
- specific
- worse

sleep continuity disturbance(s)
sleep cycle
sleep deprivation
sleep difficulty, chronic phase of
- stable

sleep disorder
- alcohol-induced
- amphetamine-induced
- breathing-related
- caffeine-induced
- circadian rhythm
- cocaine-induced
- gender differences in
- insomnia type
- insomnia type caffeine-induced
- insomnia type substance-induced
- medical/psychiatric
- parasomnia type
- parasomnia type substance-induced
- primary
- related

sleep disorder due to epilepsy, parasomnia type
sleep disorder due to GMC
sleep disorder insomnia
sleep disruption, increased
sleep disturbance
- breathing-related
- chronic

"sleep drunkenness"
sleep duration
- nocturnal
- normal
- reduced
- short

sleep efficiency, good
sleep episodes
    daytime
    prolonged
    prolonged nocturnal
    unintentional daytime
sleep hygiene, inadequate
sleep latency
    mean
    prolonged
    short
sleep loss, mild
sleep-onset episode
sleep-onset insomnia
sleep-onset REM period (SOREMP)
sleep organization, disrupt
sleep paralysis
    postdormital
    predormital
sleep pattern(s)
    disturbed
    irregular
sleep phase, delayed
sleep phase pattern, advanced
sleep phase syndrome
    advanced
    delayed
sleep phase type dyssomnia, delayed
sleep postures, unusual
sleep problems, persistent
sleep rebound, REM
sleep-related epilepsy
sleep-related hallucination
sleep-related hypoventilation
    comorbid (G47.36)
    idiopathic G47.34)
sleep-related seizures
sleep-related sexual behavior (sexomnia)
sleep spindle on EEG
sleep spindles
sleep stability, relative slow-wave
sleep stage(s)
sleep state misperception
sleep tendency

sleep-terror episodes, frequency of
sleep-terror event, amnesia for
sleep-wake abnormality
sleep-wake cycle, phase shift of
sleep-wake disorders
sleep-wake hours, phase-advance
sleep-wake pattern
    changing
    irregular
    non-24 hour
    stable
sleep-wake schedule, abnormal
sleep-wake syndrome, non-24-hour
sleep-wake system
sleep-wake timing mechanisms, endogenous abnormalities in
sleep-wake transition
sleep-wakefulness cycle
sleep-waking cycle
sleep-waking cycle and occurrence of seizure
"sleeper" (street name, barbiturate; heroin; sleeping pills)
sleeper, long
sleepiness
    daytime
    excessive
    index of physiological
    physiological
sleeping, difficulty
sleeping sickness
sleeplessness
sleeptalking
sleepwalking behavior
"sleet" (street name, crack)
SLES (Speech and Language Evaluation Scale)
"slick superspeed" (street name, methcathinone)
slight defect
slight hearing impairment
slight impairment of functioning
"slime" (street name, heroin)
"slip off the track"
slit fricative consonant formation

Psychiatric Words and Phrases

slope curve audiogram configurations, ski
Slosson Articulation Language Test with Phonology (SALT-P)
Slosson Children's Version Family Environment Scale
Slosson Drawing Coordination Test
Slosson Intelligence Test for Children and Adults
Slosson Oral Reading Test (SORT)
Slosson Test of Reading Readiness (STRR)
slow-acting viral encephalitis
slow eye movement, rhythmic
slow-frequency (delta) EEG activity
slow rate of language development
slow release drug (SR)
slow speech
slow-wave activity
slow-wave sleep
slow-wave sleep stability
slowed reaction time
slowed time, sensation of
slowing, psychomotor
slowing activity
slowness
slurred speech
slurring
small-amplitude rapid tremor
small-city psychiatry
small detail responses
small shuffling steps
smearing, saliva
"smears" (street name, lysergic acid diethylamide/LSD)
SMEI (severe myoclonic epilepsy in infancy)
smell sensation
Smith-Johnson Nonverbal Performance Scale
"smoke" (street name, crack or heroin and crack)
"smoke Canada" (street name, cannabis)
"smoke-out" (re: drug influence)
"smoking" (street name, phencyclidine/PCP)
smoking
    marijuana
    straight pipe
smoking cessation
"smoking gun" (street name, heroin and cocaine)
S/N (signal to noise ratio)
"snap" (street name, amphetamine)
"sniff" (re: cocaine use)
"sniff" (street name, inhalant; methcathinone)
sniff method of esophageal speech
sniffing
sniffing death, sudden
"snop" (street name, cannabis)
snores, "resuscitative"
snoring, loud
"snort" (re: cocaine use; inhalant use)
snort, nasal
"snorts" (street name, phencyclidine/PCP)
"snot" (re: amphetamine use)
"snot balls" (street name, burned rubber cement)
"snow" (street name, amphetamine; heroin)
"snow pallets" (street name, amphetamine)
"snow seals" (street name, cocaine and amphetamine)
"snow soke" (street name, crack)
"Snow White" (street name, cocaine)
"snowball" (street name, cocaine and heroin)
"snowcones" (street name, cocaine)
"soaper" (street name, methaqualone)
sobriety
    long-term
    "white knuckling"
    Youth Enjoying (YES)

sociability
social activities, interference with
social adjustment guides *(see also* tests)
social adjustment measure, modified self-report measure of
social alienation
Social and Occupational Functioning Assessment Scale (SOFAS)
social anxiety, excessive
social anxiety disorder (F40.10)
social apprehensiveness
social attachment(s)
social babbling
Social Behavior Assessment Inventory (SBAI)
Social Behaviour Assessment Schedule
social class
Social Climate Scale (SCS)
social (pragmatic) communication disorder (F80.89)
social communication impairments
social competence
social conformity
social desirability
social detachment
Social Development Scale
social disability
social distance
social dominance
social drinking
social dysfunction
Social-Emotional Dimension Scale
social environment
social exclusion or rejection, problems with (Z60.4)
social facilitation
social functioning
    anxiety-induced impaired
    frustration-induced impaired
    impairment in
    level of
    marked distress in

social gambling
social gesture speech
social hierarchy
social history (SH; S.H.)
social identification
social immaturity
social inappropriateness
social ineptness
social inhibition, pattern of
social insecurity
social integration
Social Intelligence Test
Social Interaction Scale
social interaction
    impaired
    impairment in reciprocal
Social Introversion "0" Scale
social isolation
social learning theory
social maturity scales *(see also* tests)
social media addiction
social perception
social phobia (e.g. public speaking) (F40.10)
social phobia experience
social phobic-like behavior
social psychiatrist
social reference group
social reinforcement
social relatedness
    developmentally inappropriate
    disturbance in
    disturbed
    marked disturbances in
social relationship
social responsibility
Social Reticence Scale
social role
social sanctions, imposition of
social service agency
social setting
social situation(s)
social situations, loss of previously stabilizing
social skills, deterioration of

Social Skills Rating System (SSRS)
social skill training
social status
social stereotypical behavior
social stereotypical gender role(s)
social stimulation
social stress
social support
social tension
social values
social work, psychiatric
societal norms
    age-appropriate
    demands of
    functioning in
    levels of
    majority
    marginal member of
    traditional
    violation of age-appropriate
Society for Community Research and Action (SCRA)
Society for Industrial and Organizational Psychology (SIOP)
Society for Personality and Social Psychology (SPSP)
Society for Psychotherapy Research (SPR)
Society for Research in Child Development (SRCD)
Society for the Teaching of Psychology (STP)
"society high" (street name, cocaine)
Society of Teachers of Family Medicine (STFM)
sociocultural background
Socioemotional Development, Test of Early
socioenvironmental status
socioenvironmental therapy
sociolinguistics
sociology, medical
"soda" (street name, injectable cocaine)

SOFAS (Social and Occupational Functioning Assessment Scale)
soft neurological signs
soft palate, elevator muscle of
soft palate cleft
soft signs, neurological
soft whisper
"softballs" (street name, barbiturate)
soldiers in combat, trauma effects on
"soles" (street name, hashish)
solitariness
solitary activities
SOM (serous otitis media)
"soma" (street name, phencyclidine/PCP)
Somatic "3" Scale
somatic complaints
somatic focus
Somatic Inkblot Series
somatic symptom and related disorders (F45.1)
    other specified (F45.8)
    unspecified (F45.9)
somatic symptom disorder (F45.1)
somatic symptom disorder with predominant pain (F45.1)
somatic symptoms
somatic therapies, psychiatric
somatic treatment for depression
somatic treatments
somatic type delusions
somatic type schizophrenia
somatization, tendency to
somatization gastrointestinal symptom
somatization pain symptoms
somatization pseudoneurological symptoms
somatization sexual symptoms
somatoform disorders, gender differences in
somatoform interface disorder
somatosensory response, evoked
somatosensory seizure
somesthetic
somesthetic area

somesthetic dysarthria
SOMPA (System of multicultural assessment)
sonant consonant formation
sone
sonogram
sonority
"sopers" (street name, barbiturate)
"sopes" (street name, methaqualone)
sophomania
Sopor (methaqualone)
SOREMP (sleep onset REM period)
sorting polarities
SORT (Slosson Oral Reading Test)
"soul loss"
sound(s)
    air-blade
    attention to
    consonantal
    developmentally expected speech
    discrimination of
    distorted perception of
    embedded
    errors of ordering of
    errors of selection of
    fricative
    gross
    non-nasal
    nonspeech
    nonsyllabic speech
    Ohio Tests of Articulation and Perception of (OTAPS)
    prolongation of
    repetition of
    speech
sound analysis
sound and memory, sequence of
sound and syllable repetition *(see also* tests)
sound and symbol, association of
sound blending
sound development, speech
sound discrimination, speech
sound discrimination test *(see also* tests)
sound field
sound flow, speech
sound intensity
sound level, overall
sound level meter
sound localization
sound power density
sound pressure level (SPL)
sound pressure level, saturation (SSPL)
sound pressure level 90, high-frequency average saturation
sound pressure level range
sound pressure wave
sound production, speech
sound-produced sensation of color
sound prolongation
sound quality sound quantity
sound source, simple
sound spectrogram
sound spectrograph
sound spectrum
sound-symbol association
sound wave
source of information
sources, collateral
Southern California Motor Accuracy Test
Southern California Postrotary Nystagmus Test
Southern California Sensory Integration Tests
SP (scale of psychosis)
S/P (status post)
SP (systolic pressure)
SPA (speech pathology/audiology)
space
    alveolar
    personal
"space base" (street name, cigar laced with phencyclidine and crack)
"space cadet" (street name, crack dipped in phencyclidine/PCP)

"space dust" (street name, crack dipped in phencyclidine/PCP)
space perception
space responses
"space ship" (re: crack equipment)
spacial balance
Spadafore Diagnostic Reading Test
span
 auditory memory
 auditory retention
 comprehension
 digit
 language-structured auditory retention
 life
 memory
Spanish Computerized Adaptive Placement Exam, A (S-CAPE)
SPAR (sensitivity prediction from the acoustic reflex)
"spark it up" (re: cannabis use)
"sparkle plenty" (street name, amphetamine)
"sparklers" (street name, amphetamine)
sparsity of verbalizations
SPAR Spelling and Reading Tests
spasm
 hemifacial
 laryngeal-pharyngeal
spasmodic convulsion
spasmodic croup
spasmodic laryngitis
spastic cerebral palsy (CP)
spastic dysarthria
spastic dysphonia
spastic paralysis
spastic state
spasticity
spatial agraphia
spatial behavior
spatial disorganization
spatial disorientation
spatial neglect, unilateral
spatial orientation

speak
 consistent failure to
 unwillingness to
speaker's nodes
speaking, choral
speaking capacity
special caution
special "K" (street name, ketamine)
"special la coke" (street name, ketamine)
special relationship
specialized language assessment *(see also* tests)
specific, culture
specific age features
Specific Aptitude Test Battery
specific competencies
specific culture, age and gender features
specific culture features
specific developmental disorder (SDD)
specific diagnosis (provisional)
specific employment skill competencies
specific gender features
Specific Language Disability test
specific learning disorder
specific learning disorder with impairment in mathematics memorization of arithmetic facts (F81.2)
specific learning disorder with impairment in mathematics with accurate or fluent calculations (F81.2)
specific learning disorder with impairment in mathematics with accurate math reasoning (F81.2)
specific learning disorder with impairment in mathematics with number sense (F81.2)
specific learning disorder with impairment in reading with reading rate (F81.0)

specific learning disorder with
    impairment in reading with
    reading fluency (F81.0)
specific learning disorder with
    impairment in reading with
    reading comprehension (F81.0)
specific learning disorder with
    impairment in reading with
    word reading accuracy (F81.0)
specific learning disorder with
    impairment in written
    expression with spelling
    accuracy (F81.81)
specific learning disorder with
    impairment in written
    expression with grammar and
    punctuation accuracy (F81.81)
specific learning disorder with
    impairment in written
    expression with clarity (F81.81)
specific learning disorder with
    impairment in written
    expression with organization of
    written expression (F81.81)
specific phobia
        animal type
        marked and excessive
        marked and persistent
        marked and unreasonable
specific risk
specific situational stressor
specific sleep continuity
specific treatment
specified neurodevelopmental
    disorder (F88)
specified tic disorder, other
    (F95.8)
SPECS (System to Plan Early
    Childhood Services)
SPECT scan
spectin, brain
spectrogram (or spectrograph),
    sound
spectrum (pl. spectra or
    spectrums)
        acoustic
        band
        schizophrenia (SS)

spectrum
    sound
    tonal
SPECT scan
speech
    accelerated
    agrammatic
    alaryngeal
    alteration in rate of
    altering the rate of
    aphasic
    arrest of
    articulate
    atoxic
    audible blocking in
    automatic
    breathing method of
        esophageal
    buccal
    cerebellar scanning quality
    cerebellar scanning type
    circumlocution of
    cold-running
    compressed
    confabulation of
    connected
    cued
    dactyl
    deaf
    decreased fluency of
    decreased productivity of
    delayed
    deviant
    digressive
    disorganized
    displaced
    disturbance in
    disturbance in the normal
        fluency of
    disturbance in the time
        patterning of
    dysrhythmic
    echo
    egocentric
    emotive
    erratic rhythm of
    esophageal
    excessively impressionistic

speech
    executive
    festinant quality in
      parkinsonian
    filled pauses in
    filtered
    flaccid
    fluency of
    fluent aphasic
    fluent paraphasic
    halting
    high-stimulus
    hyperkinetic
    hypokinetic
    impaired
    impediment of
    impoverished
    impressionistic
    incoherent
    incomprehensible
    infantile
    inhalation method of
      esophageal
    injection method of
      esophageal
    inner
    internal
    irrelevant
    labored
    limited
    loss of
    loud
    manic
    metaphorical
    methods of esophageal
    mimic
    minimal prosody of
    monosyllabic
    narrative
    nonelaborative
    nonfluent aphasic
    nonpropositional
    nonsensical
    overabstract
    overconcrete
    over-elaborate
    paraphasic
    pattern in

speech
    phantom
    pharyngeal
    poverty of
    pressure of
    productivity of
    productivity of thought and
    propositional
    rambling
    rapid
    regressive
    repetitive
    repressed
    rhythm of
    running
    scanning
    serial content
    seriatim
    silent blocking in
    slow
    slurred
    sniff method of esophageal
    social gesture
    spontaneous
    staccato
    stereotyped
    subvocal
    suction method of
      esophageal
    swallow method of
      esophageal
    tangential
    telegraphic
    thickened
    tolerance threshold for
    tremulous
    unfilled pauses in
    unintelligible
    unvoiced
    vague
    visible
speech acts
speech and hearing science
speech and language behavior
speech and language
    characteristics of cleft palate
speech and language clinician

speech and language disorder, schizophrenic
speech and language disorders in psychiatry
Speech and Language Evaluation Scale (SLES)
speech and language pathologist
speech and language pathology
speech and language tests *(see also* tests)
speech apraxia
speech articulation
speech articulation test
speech aspects
speech assessment, disorganized
speech audiometer, limited range
speech audiometry, limited range
speech awareness audiometry
speech awareness threshold (SAT)
speech blocking
    audible
    silent
speech center
speech community, dialect
speech conservation
speech content
    paucity of
    poverty of
speech correction
speech correctionist
speech defect
speech derailment
speech detectability threshold (SDT)
speech detection threshold (SDT)
speech development, late
speech difficulty(ies)
speech discrimination (SD)
speech discrimination audiometry
Speech Discrimination in Noise
speech discrimination test
speech disorder
speech distortion
speech dysfluencies
    avoidance of
    emotional response to

Speech-Ease Screening Inventory (K-1)
speech education
speech frequency
speech impairment
speech impediment
Speech Improvement Cards
speech in schizophrenia, disorganized
speech innateness theory
speech intelligibility test
speech interference level (SIL)
Speech-Language & Audiology Canada
speech/language behavior *(see also* tests)
speech/language pathology
speech mannerism(s)
speech mechanism
speech-motor deficit
speech-motor function
speech noise
speech or language, difficulties in
speech pathologist
speech pathology/audiology (SPA)
speech pattern
    feminine
    parrotlike
speech perception
speech perception deficit
speech perception test *(see also* tests)
speech production, electrical measurement of
Speech Questionnaire
speech range, central
speech-reading aphasia
speech-reading aural rehabilitation
speech reception (SR)
speech reception audiometry
speech reception in noise
speech reception threshold (SRT)
speech rehabilitation
speech rhythm, erratic
speech science
speech situations, avoiding

speech sound
    developmentally expected
    nonsyllabic
    standard
    syllabic
speech sound development
speech sound discrimination test
speech-sound disorder (F80.0)
speech sound flow
Speech Sound Memory Test
speech sound production
speech tests *(see also* tests)
speech therapist
speech therapy
speech time patterns
speech training units
Speech With Alternating Masking Index (SWAMI)
"speed" (methamphetamine) (street names)
    biker coffee (coffee mixed with methamphetamine)
    red phosphorus (smokable speed)
    sketching (re: coming down from a speed-induced high)
    superlab (re: clandestine labs producing 10 pounds of methamphetamine in 24 hours)
    tweaking (re: drug-induced paranoia; peaking on speed)
"speed boat" (street name, cannabis, phencyclidine, and crack)
"speed for lovers" (street name, methylenedioxy-methamphetamine/MDMA)
"speed freak" (re: methamphetamine user)
speed of information processing, disturbance in
speed quotient
speed "runs"
"speedball" (street name, amphetamine; heroin and cocaine)

spell a word backwards test
spell backwards test
spelling tests *(see also* tests)
SPELT (Structured Photographic Expressive Language Test)
sphecidophobia
sphenoid bone
sphenoid skull bone
sphenoidal nasal conchae skull bones
sphenoidal turbinated bones
sphere, psychosexual
SPI (ACT Study Power Assessment and Inventory)
SPI (self-perception inventory
SPI (Shipley Personal Inventory)
"Spice/K2" (street name, designer drug; synthetic cannabinoids; hallucinogen)
"spider blue" (street name, heroin)
"spike" (re: needle; drug injection)
spike, diphasic
spike on EEG, phase
spike-waves
    negative
    six Hertz positive
spiked profile
spikes
    fourteen-and-six Hertz positive
    negative
    six Hertz positive
spina bifida
spinal accessory (cranial nerve XI)
spinal accessory nerve
spinal shock
spindle on EEG, sleep
spindles, sleep
spiral effect
spirant consonant formation
spirits, controlling external
spiritual aspects of the body
spiritual counselor
spiritual function
spiritual possession, experience of

spiritual problem
Spiritual Well-Being Scale (SWBS)
spirituality, religion or, problems with (Z65.8)
spirometer
SPL (sound pressure level)
"splash" (street name, amphetamine)
"spliff" (street name, cannabis cigarette)
"splim" (street name, cannabis)
"split" (street name, half and half)
split half reliability coefficient
split word
splitting of image of others
splitting of self-image
"splivins" (street name, amphetamine)
Spondee Threshold Test
spondee word
spontaneity
    lack of
    loss of
spontaneous convulsion
spontaneous imitation
spontaneous recovery
spontaneous speech
"spoon" (re: heroin injection; 1/16 ounce of heroin)
"spores" (street name, phencyclidine/PCP)
"sporting" (re: cocaine use)
spot, figurative blind (scotoma)
spousal abuse
spousal or partner abuse
    psychological, confirmed, initial encounter (T74.31XA)
    psychological, confirmed, subsequent encounter (T74.31XD)
    psychological, suspected, initial encounter (T76.31XA)
    psychological, suspected, subsequent encounter (T76.31XD)
spousal or partner neglect confirmed
    initial encounter (T74.01XA)
    subsequent encounter (T74.01XD)
spousal or partner neglect suspected
    initial encounter (T76.01XA)
    subsequent encounter (T76.01XD)
spousal or partner violence
    physical, confirmed, initial encounter (T74.11XA)
    physical, confirmed, subsequent encounter (T74.11XD)
    physical, suspected, initial encounter (T76.11XA)
    physical, suspected, subsequent encounter (T76.11XD)
    sexual, confirmed, initial encounter (T74.21XA)
    sexual, confirmed, subsequent encounter (T74.21XD)
    sexual, suspected, subsequent encounter (T76.21XD)
    sexual, suspected, initial encounter (T76.21XA)
SPQ (Sales Personality Questionnaire)
SPR (Society for Psychotherapy Research)
Spravata (esketamine)
"spray" (street name, inhalant)
spring-summer viral encephalitis, Russian
"sprung" (re: drug user)
SPSP (Society for Personality and Social Psychology)
(SQ) sequela
squandermania
square brackets

"square mackerel" (street name, cannabis)
"square time Bob" (street name, crack)
squatting
"squirrel" (re: cocaine, cannabis and PCP use)
SR (slow release)
SR (speech reception)
SRA Achievement Series
SRA Nonverbal Form
SRA Pictorial Reasoning Test
SRA Verbal Form
SRCD (Society for Research in Child Development)
"SRP" (street name, designer drug: psychedelic)
SRT (speech reception threshold)
(S/S) suspected/subsequent episode
SSA (ACT Study Skills Assessment and Inventory)
SSI (ACT Study Skills Assessment and Inventory)
SSPL (saturation sound pressure level)
SSPL 90
    HF average
    high-frequency average
SSPL output HF average
SSRS (Social Skills Rating System)
SSS (School Situation Survey)
SST (Slingerland Screening Tests)
SST for Identifying Children with Specific Language Disability
St. Louis viral encephalitis
stabbing pain
stability
    personality trait
    relative slow-wave sleep
stability in relationships
stability of self-image
stability of vocational functioning
stabilization
stabilizing social situations
stable pattern

stable sleep difficulty, chronic phase of
stable sleep-wake pattern
staccato speech
"stack" (street name, cannabis)
"stacking" (re: taking prescription steroids)
stacking anchors
Staff Burnout Scale for Health Professionals
staff HMO-based psychiatry
stage
    cognitive development (Period I-IV)
    dementia
    developmental
    Piaget's cognitive development
    sleep
    stuttering
stage 1-4 NREM sleep
stage I of non-REM (drowsiness)
stage II of non-REM (light sleep)
stage III of non-REM (deep sleep)
stage IV of non-REM (very deep sleep)
stage fright
stage of anesthesia, first
stage of REM sleep
stage W (wakefulness) sleep
stage whisper
staggering gait
STAI (State-Trait Anxiety Inventory)
STAIC (State-Trait Anxiety Inventory for Children)
stalker
stance
    approach-avoidance
    norm-assertive
standard earmold
standard language
standard of living
Standard Progressive Matrices
standard reference
standard score
standard speech sound
Standard Timing Model, The

standard word
Standard Written English Test
standardized cognitive assessment
  technique(s)
Standardized Test of Computer
  Literacy (STCL)
standards of performance, self-
  imposed high
standards of performance, strict
standards of sexual behavior,
  cultural-related
standards of sexual performance
standing balance
standing trial
standing wave
Stanford Achievement Test
Stanford-Binet Intelligence Scale:
  Form L-M
Stanford Diagnostic Mathematics
  Test
Stanford Early School
  Achievement Test
Stanford Hypnotic Clinical Scale
  for Children
Stanford Profile Scales of
  Hypnotic Susceptibility,
  Revised
stanine
Stanton Survey
stapedectomy
stapedial acoustic reflex
stapedial reflex, acoustic
stapedius reflex
stapes (pl. stapes)
stapes mobilization
"star" (street name,
  methcathinone)
STAR Profile (Student Talent and
  Risk Profile)
"star-spangled powder" (street
  name, cocaine)
"stardust" (street name, cocaine;
  phencyclidine)
stare, reptilian
staring eyes
staring face
staring facial expression

START (Screening Test for the
  Assignment of Remedial
  Treatment)
startle reflex
startle response
startle technique
startling stimulus
STAS (State-Trait Anger Scale)
"stash" (re: drug storage)
"stash areas" (re: drug storage)
stasiphobia
"stat" (street name,
  methcathinone)
stat or STAT (immediately)
STAT (Suprathreshold Adaptation
  Test)
state
   acute confusional (ACS)
   affective and paranoid
   agitated
   alert awake
   alertness
   alpha
   altered
   amnesic
   amnestic
   anxiety (AS)
   anxiety-tension (ATS)
   apprehensive
   borderline
   break
   catatonic
   central excitatory
   clouded
   confusional
   consciousness
   constitutional psychopathic
   (CPS)
   convulsive
   crepuscular
   current
   delirium-like
   dependent memory
   depressive
   disequilibrium
   dissociative
   dream
   dreamy

state
- ego
- emotional
- epileptic confusional (ECS)
- epileptic fugue
- euthymic
- feeling
- fugue
- fully wakefulness
- hallucinatory
- heightened attention
- heightened awareness
- hyperdopaminergic
- hypnagogic
- hypnoid
- hypnopompic
- hypnotic
- hysterical
- hysterical coma-like
- hysterical fugue
- identity
- lacunar
- locked in
- marked heavy drinking (GGT)
- mental
- mind
- mixed-mood
- moribund
- multiple ego
- negative mood
- neurotic
- nonresponsive
- obsessional
- oneiroid
- organic psychotic
- panic
- paranoid
- parasomniac conscious
- perfection
- persistent vegetative (PVS)
- phobic
- possession trance
- postictal
- premorbid
- psychotic
- rapid eye movement
- resource

state
- schizophrenic residual (SRS)
- separator
- sleep
- spastic
- subacute confusional (SCS)
- subjectively experienced feeling
- substance-induced
- tension
- toxic-confusional
- trance
- transient mental
- twilight
- unresponsive
- vegetative
- vulnerability to life's stressors
- wakeful
- withdrawal

state licensing board
state mental hospital (SMH)
state response
state test, city and
State-Trait Anger Expression Inventory (STAXI)
State-Trait Anger Scale (STASI)
State-Trait Anxiety Index
State-Trait Anxiety Inventory (STAI)
State-Trait Anxiety Inventory for Children (STAIC)
stated desire
statements, "I"
static acoustic impedance
static dementia
static encephalopathy State-Trait
static tremor
stationary focus
statistical deviation
statistical information
statistical lives
status
- absence
- altered mental
- ambulatory
- clinical

status
    confident
    current cognitive
    deterioration of
    disordered mental
    grand mal
    hostage
    immigrant
    petit mal
    postoperative
    preepisode
    social
    Social Adaptation (SAS)
    socioenvironmental
    symptomatic
    temporal lobe
status aura
status dysgraphicus
status epilepsy
status epilepticus organic psychotic
status epilepticus
    convulsive
    nonconvulsive
status examination
status index
Status Indicators (Sis)
status inventory
status post (S/P)
status questionnaire
status scale
status schedule
status value
STAXI (State-Trait Anger Expression Inventory)
stay on task
STCL (Standardized Test of Computer Literacy)
STD (sexually transmitted disease)
steady pain
steady rhythmicity of tremor
stealing, solitary
stealing an anchor
steep curve audiogram configurations
steep drop curve
"steerer" (re: drug dealing)

Stein Sentence Completion test
Stekel, Wilhelm (1868-1940)
"stem" (re: crack equipment)
"stems" (street name, cannabis)
Stenger Test
stenosis (pl. stenoses)
    carotid artery
    congenital hypertrophic pyloric
    urethral
"step on" (re: dilute drugs)
STEPS (Screening Test for Educational Prerequisite Skills)
steps, small shuffling
steps in therapy, branching
Steps Up Developmental Screening Program
stereognosis, oral
stereotyped activity
stereotyped behavior, patterns of
stereotyped body movements
stereotyped interests
stereotyped motor movement, nonrhythmic
stereotyped motor vocalization, nonrhythmic
stereotyped movements, intentional
stereotyped restricted behavior
stereotyped speech
stereotyped stress
stereotypical behavior, social
stereotypical gender roles, social
stereotypical movements
stereotypic behavior
stereotypic motor movement
stereotypic movement disorder (F98.4)
stereotypic movement disorder associated with a known genetic condition (F98.4)
stereotypic movement disorder associated with a known medical condition (F98.4)
stereotypic movement disorder associated with a neurodevelopmental disorder (F98.4)

stereotypic movement disorder associated with an environmental factor (F98.4)
stereotypic movement disorder with self-injurious behavior (F98.4)
stereotypic movement disorder without self-injurious behavior (F98.4)
stereotypic sex-role behavior
stereotypy/habit disorder
sternoclavicular muscle
sternoclavicularis, musculus
sternocleidomastoid muscle
sternocleidomastoideus, musculus
sternohyoid muscle
sternohyoideus, musculus
sternothyroid muscle
sternothyroideus, musculus
steroid hormones
steroids
    abolic
    anabolic
    anadrol
    anatrofin
    anavar
    bolasterone
    deca-duabolin
    delatestryl
    dep-testosterone
    dianabol
    dihydrolone
    durabolin
    dymethzine
    enoltestovis
    equipose
    finajet/finaject
    maxibolin
    methatrol
    methyltestosterone
    parabolin
    primbolin
    primobolan
    proviron
    quinolone
    sustanon 250
    synthetically prepared

steroids
    testosterone-produced hormone
    therobolin
    trophobolene
steroids (street names)
    Arnolds
    Georgia home boy
    GHB
    gym candy
    juice
    pumpers
    roid rage
    stackers
    stacking
STFM (Society of Teachers of Family Medicine)
STG (short-term goals)
S3 Rating Scale (School Social Skills Rating Scale)
"stick" (street name, cannabis; phencyclidine/PCP)
sticking sensation, pins
stigma, psychosocial
stigma of mental illness, unwarranted
stigmatism
stimulant effect
stimulant-induced anxiety disorder
stimulant-induced disorder
stimulant-induced obsessive-compulsive and related disorders
stimulant-induced postural tremor
stimulant intoxication (see specific stimulant)
stimulant-related disorders
stimulant use disorder with stimulant-induced anxiety disorder with use disorder
stimulant use disorder with other stimulant-induced obsessive-compulsive and related disorders
stimulants (drugs, street names)
    A
    aimies

stimulants (drugs, street names)
- amp
- amped
- amped-out
- back dex
- bain
- bathtub crank
- batu
- beans
- bennie
- bennies
- benz
- benzidine
- biker coffee
- black
- black and white
- black beauties
- black beauty
- black birds
- black bombers
- black cadillacs
- black mollies
- blue boy
- blue meth
- blue mollies
- bolt
- bombido
- bombita (Spanish)
- bottles
- brain ticklers
- brown
- brownies
- cartwheels
- chalk
- chicken powder
- chocolate
- Christina
- Christmas tree
- clear
- coasts to coasts
- co-pilot
- CR
- crank
- crink
- cris
- crisscriss
- Cristina (Spanish)
- Cristy

stimulants (drugs, street names)
- croak
- cross tops
- crossies
- crossroads
- crypto
- crystal
- crystal meth
- desocsins
- desogtion
- dexies
- diet pills
- disco pellets
- dominoes
- double cross
- dropping
- eye openers
- fast
- fire
- geeter
- geigo
- glass
- go-fast
- granulated orange
- hanyak
- head drugs
- hearts
- hironpon
- horse heads
- hot ice
- hugs and kisses
- ice
- inbetweens
- jam
- jam cecil
- jelly baby
- jelly bean
- jolly bean
- jugs
- kaksonjae
- L.A.
- L.A. glass
- L.A. ice
- leapers
- lemon drop
- lid poppers
- lid proppers
- lightning

stimulants (drugs, street names)
- lithium scabs
- little bomb
- M-cat
- meth
- meth head
- meth monster
- methlies quik
- Mexican crack
- Mexican speedballs
- miaow
- minibennie
- Nazimeth
- nugget
- oranges
- peaches
- peanut butter
- pep pills
- pink
- pink hearts
- pixies
- poppers
- powder
- purple hearts
- quartz
- quill
- red
- red phosphorus
- rhythm
- rippers
- road dope
- robin's egg
- rock
- Rosa (Spanish)
- roses
- Shabu
- snot
- snow pallets
- snow seals
- soap
- soap dope
- sparkle plenty
- sparklers
- speed
- speed freak
- speedball
- speedballing
- speedies

stimulants (drugs, street names)
- splash
- splivins
- star
- stove top
- sunshine
- super ice
- super lab
- super X
- sweets
- The C
- thrusters
- tic
- Tina
- TR-6s
- truck driver
- twisters
- uppers
- uppies
- wake ups
- water
- West Coast
- West Coast turnarounds
- wet
- white
- white cross
- whites
- work
- X
- Ya Ba
- yellow barn
- yellow powder

stimulating experience

stimulation
- angry reaction to minor
- auditory
- environmental
- epileptogenic
- erotic
- external
- genital
- insufficient
- lack of
- linguistic
- manual
- noncoital
- oral
- psychosensory

stimulation
    screen out irrelevant
    sensory
    sensory pathway
    sexual
    social
    subliminal
    synesthetic
    tactile
    tactile genital
    visual
stimulation fatigue
stimuli revulsion, sexual
stimulus (pl. stimuli)
    alerting
    appropriate
    auditory
    conditioned
    emotional
    emotionally provoking
    environmental
    epileptogenic
    external
    musical
    neutral
    novel
    noxious
    outside
    painful
    paraphiliac
    phobic
    psychosensory
    sensory
    startling
    tactile
    terrifying
    thermal
    threshold of
    triggering
    unconditioned
    visual
stimulus generalization
Stimulus Recognition Test
stimulus-response
stimulus substitution
stinging pain
"stink weed" (street name, cannabis)
stirrup
stocking-glove anesthesia
stocking-glove sensory loss
stoma (pl. stomas or stomata)
stoma blast
stoma button
stomata
Stone and Neale Daily Coping Assessment
"stoned" (re: drug influence)
"stones" (street name, crack)
stooped shoulders
stop
    glottal
        ubiquitous glottal
stop-and-think technique
stop consonant formation
"stoppers" (street name, barbiturate)
stopping of fricatives
storage, auditory
stormed defense
Story Articulation Test
story-like dream sequence
"STP" (2,5-dimethyloxy-4-methylamphetamine)
"STP" (Serenity-Tranquility-Peace) (street drug name)
"STP" (street name, pseudo-phencyclidine)
STP (Society for the Teaching of Psychology)
straight pipe smoking
strain
    interpersonal
    psychological
    vocational
strains, Alpha-wave
strategy (pl. strategies)
    bibliotherapeutic
    conflict-resolution
    coping
    data reanalysis
    gambling
    problem-solving
    protective survival
Strauss syndrome

"straw" (street name, cannabis
   cigarette)
"strawberries" (street name,
   barbiturate)
"strawberry" (re: crack prostitute)
stream
   breath
   coherent thought
   mental activity
   misdirected urinary
stream of consciousness
Street Survival Skills
   Questionnaire
street-drug culture
strength
   antagonistic muscle
   fatigue
   response
stress
   biology of
   Coping With
   family
   fatigue
   iambic
   medical
   nonpathological reactions
      to
   primary
   psychological
   psychosocial
   secondary
   serious traumatic
   severe life
   social
   stereotyped
   tertiary
   trochaic
   Understanding and
      Managing
   war-related
   wax weak
   weak
stress adaptability skills
Stress Audit
stress disorder, acute (F43.0)
Stress Evaluation Inventory
Stress Impact Scale (SIS)
stress in children, severe

stress patterns
stress precipitating tremor
stress prevention
stress-related disturbance
stress-related paranoid ideation
stress-related physiological
   responses
stress-related psychophysiological
   problem
stress response
Stress Response Scale
stress-strain relationship(s)
stressful life experiences
stressful word production
stressor(s)
   childhood
   external
   extreme
   handling of
   identifiable
   initial
   intermediate
   internal
   major
   maladaptive reaction to a
   natural disasters as a major
   psychological
   psychosocial
   seasonal-related
      psychosocial
   sexual abuse as a major
   situational
   terminal
   violence as a major
   vulnerability to life's
stretch reflex
stria, acoustic
striatal hypometabolism
striatocerebral tremor
strict standards of performance
stricture, vaginal
stridency deletion
strident feature English phoneme
strident lisp
stridor
stridulous laryngitis
stroboscope

stroke (CVA)
    brain stem
    glottal
    lacunar
    psychiatric consequences of
    psychiatry of
strong emotion
Strong-Campbell Interest Inventory
strongly held idea
Stroop Color and Word Test
STRR (Slosson Test of Reading Readiness)
structural abnormality
Structural Analysis of Social Behavior
structural atrophy
structural brain abnormalities
structural brain imaging
structural linguistics
structural pathology
structural rule morpheme
structure
    abnormal brain
    base
    deep
    external
    grammatical
    group
    hierarchical
    intermediate
    lack of
    language
    organizational
    performative pragmatic
    pragmatic
    surface
    syllable
    underlying
    Wachs Analysis of Cognitive
structure grammar, phrase
Structure of Intellect Learning Abilities Test
structure word
structured hallucination
Structured Interview of Reported Symptoms (SIRS)
Structured Photographic Articulation Test (SPAT)
Structured Photographic Expressive Language Test
Structured Sentence Completion Test
structured task(s)
struggle behavior, anticipatory and (theory in stuttering)
"strung out" (re: drug addiction)
strychnine (street names)
    back breakers (LSD and strychnine)
    homicide (heroin cut with scopolamine or strychnine)
    red rock opium (heroin, barbital, strychnine, and caffeine)
    red rum (heroin, barbital, strychnine, and caffeine)
    red stuff (heroin, barbital, strychnine, and caffeine)
    spike (heroin cut with scopolamine or strychnine)
stubbornness
Student Adaptation to College Questionnaire (SACQ)
Student Adjustment Inventory (SAI)
student dropouts
student evaluations *(see also* tests)
Student Talent and Risk Profile (STAR Profile)
study (pl. studies)
    community
    double-bind
    epidemiological
    hospital-based
    nerve conduction
    nocturnal penile tumescence
    polysomnographic
    systematic
    time and motion
study case
study design

study of values
"stuff" (street name, heroin)
"stumbler" (street name, barbiturate)
stupor mania
stuporous patient
stuttered rhythm
stuttering
    adaptation effect of
    cognitive
    consistency effect of
    coping
    exteriorized
    extratensive coping
    extratensive personality
    fixation in
    hysterical
    implicit
    incipient
    interiorized
    laryngeal
    laterality theory of
    learning theory of
    PFAGH
    phases of
    primary
    primary characteristics of
    secondary
    secondary characteristics of
    stages of
    theory in anticipatory and struggle behavior
    theory in approach-avoidance
    theory in breakdown
    theory in cerebral dominance and handedness
    theory in communication failure
    theory in conditioned disintegration
    theory in cybernetic
    theory in diagnosogenic
    theory in dysphemia and biochemical
    theory in instrumental avoidance act
    theory in neurotic
    theory in operant behavior
stuttering
    theory in perseverance
    theory in primary
    theory in repressed need
    transitional
stuttering gait
stuttering pattern
style(s)
    cognitive
    coping
    deception
    extratensive coping
    extratensive personality
    introtensive
    introtensive personality
    introtensive problem-solving
style inventories *(see also* tests)
Style of Leadership and Management
Style of Leadership Survey
Style of Management Inventory
styloglossus, musculus
styloglossus muscle
stylohyoideus, musculus
stylohyoid muscle
stylopharyngeal muscle
stylopharyngeus, musculus
SU (sensation unit)
subacute sclerosing panencephalitis
subarachnoid hemorrhage
subaverage academic functioning
subaverage intellectual functioning
subaverage motor coordination
subchronic schizophrenia
subclavian muscle
subclavius, musculus
subclinical seizure
subcortical aphasia
subcortical brain involvement
subcortical dementia
subcortical encephalopathy
subcortical motor aphasia
subcortical white matter
subcultural language
subculture norms

subdural hemorrhage
subglottic laryngitis
subglottic resonator(s)
subgroups, phenomenological
subject
    complete (parts of speech)
    simple (parts of speech)
subjective case (parts of speech)
subjective drive
subjective doubles, syndrome of
subjective experience
subjective fear
subjective feelings
subjective quality
subjective quantity
subjective sensation of fetal movement
subjective sensation of wakefulness
subjective sense of difficulty concentrating
subjective sense of sexual pleasure
subjective symptoms of impairment
subjectively experienced feeling state
subjectivity
    out of control
    overwhelmed
subjunctive mood (parts of speech)
subliminal behavior
subliminal stimulation
sublingual drug (SL)
submania
submissive behavior
submodalities, critical
submucous cleft palate
suboccipital headache
subordinate clause (parts of speech)
Suboxone (buprenorphine/naloxone)
subsequent amnesia
subsequent development
subsequent encounter (S/E)
subsonic

substance
    amphetamine-like
    anxiolytic
    character of a
    high-dose use of
    illicit psychoactive
    mood-altering
    phencyclidine-like
    psychoactive
    sexual dysfunction due to a
substance abuse
substance abuse counselor
Substance Abuse Problem Checklist
Substance Abuse Questionnaire
Substance Abuse Subtle Screening Inventory (SASSI)
substance abuser, anxious
substance dependence
substance dependence with physiological dependence
substance dependence without physiological dependence
substance group
substance-induced anxiety disorder due to:
    alcohol
    amphetamines/stimulants
    caffeine
    cannabis
    cocaine
    hallucinogens
    inhalants
    opioids
    phencyclidine (PCP)
    sedatives/hypnotics/anxiolytics
    unknown/other substances
substance-induced bipolar disorder due to:
    alcohol
    amphetamines/stimulants
    cocaine
    hallucinogens
    phencyclidine (PCP)
    sedatives/hypnotics/anxiolytics
    unknown/other substances

substance-induced condition
    anxiety disorder as a
    bipolar disorder as a
    delirium as a
    depressive disorder as a
    intoxication as a
    neurocognitive disorder as a
    obsessive-compulsive disorder as a
    psychotic disorder as a
    sexual dysfunction as a
    sleep disorder as a
    withdrawal as a
substance-induced delirium due to:
    alcohol
    amphetamines/stimulants
    cannabis
    cocaine
    hallucinogens
    opioids
    phencyclidine (PCP)
    sedatives/hypnotics/anxiolytics
    unknown/other substances
substance-induced dementia
substance-induced depressive disorder due to:
    alcohol
    amphetamines/stimulants
    cocaine
    hallucinogens
    inhalants
    opioids
    phencyclidine (PCP)
    sedatives/hypnotics/anxiolytics
    unknown/other substances
substance-induced disorders
substance-induced dystonia
substance-induced mental disorder
substance-induced persisting amnestic disorder
substance-induced persisting dementia
substance-induced persisting disorder
substance-induced presentations
substance-induced neurocognitive disorder due to:
    alcohol (major NCD amnestic)
    alcohol (major NCD non-amnestic)
    alcohol (mild)
    inhalants (major or mild NCD)
    sedatives/hypnotics/anxiolytics (major or mild NCD)
    unknown/other substances (major or mild NCD)
substance-induced obsessive-compulsive disorder due to:
    amphetamines/stimulants
    cocaine
    unknown/other substances
substance-induced psychotic disorder due to:
    alcohol
    amphetamines/stimulants
    cannabis
    cocaine
    hallucinogens
    phencyclidine (PCP)
    sedatives/hypnotics/anxiolytics
substance-induced psychotic disorder due to:
    unknown/other substances
substance-induced sexual dysfunction due to:
    alcohol
    amphetamines/stimulants
    cocaine
    opioids
    sedatives/hypnotics/anxiolytics
    unknown/other substances
substance-induced sleep disorder
    insomnia type
    parasomnia type

substance-induced sleep disorder
  due to:
    alcohol
    amphetamines/stimulants
    caffeine
    cannabis
    cocaine
    opioids
    sedatives/hypnotics/
      anxiolytics
    tobacco
    unknown/other substances
substance-induced state
substance intoxication
    other/unknown with mild
      use disorder (F19.129)
    other/unknown with
      moderate/severe use
      disorder (F19.229)
substance intoxication delirium
substance/medication-induced
  anxiety disorder with
  intoxication
substance/medication-induced
  anxiety disorder with
  withdrawal
substance/medication-induced
  bipolar/related disorder during
  intoxication
substance/medication-induced
  bipolar/related disorders during
  withdrawal
substance/medication-induced
  brief psychotic disorder during
  intoxication
substance/medication-induced
  brief psychotic disorder during
  withdrawal
substance/medication-induced
  delirium
substance/medication-induced
  delusional disorder during
  intoxication
substance/medication-induced
  delusional disorder during
  withdrawal
substance/medication-induced
  depressive disorder during
  intoxication
substance/medication-induced
  depressive disorder during
  withdrawal
substance/medication-induced
  disorders
substance/medication-induced
  major/mild neurocognitive
  disorder
substance/medication-induced
  obsessive-compulsive disorder
  during intoxication
substance/medication-induced
  obsessive-compulsive disorder
  during withdrawal
substance/medication-induced
  psychotic disorder
substance/medication-induced
  schizoaffective disorder during
  intoxication
substance/medication-induced
  schizoaffective disorder during
  withdrawal
substance/medication-induced
  schizophrenia during
  intoxication
substance/medication-induced
  schizophrenia during
  withdrawal
substance/medication-induced
  schizophreniform disorder
  during intoxication
substance/medication-induced
  schizophreniform disorder
  during withdrawal
substance/medication-induced
  schizotypal (personality)
  disorder during intoxication
substance/medication-induced
  schizotypal (personality)
  disorder during withdrawal
substance/medication-induced
  sexual dysfunction during
  intoxication

substance/medication-induced sexual dysfunction during medication use
substance/medication-induced sexual dysfunction during withdrawal
substance/medication-induced sleep disorder during intoxication
substance/medication-induced sleep disorder during withdrawal
substance-related and addiction disorders
substance-related causes
substance-related disorder (other/unknown/unspecified) (F19.99)
substance-related problems
substance-seeking behavior
substance self-administration
substance tolerance or withdrawal, signs of
substance use
    compulsive
    escalating pattern of
    maladaptive pattern of
    pathological
    pattern of compulsive
    signs of compulsive
substance use disorder (F19.239)
substance use disorder (other/unknown)
    mild (F19.10)
    moderate/severe (F19.20)
substance use disorder (other/unknown)
    with other substance-induced anxiety disorder
    with other substance-induced bipolar disease
    with other substance-induced brief psychotic disorder
    with other substance-induced delusional disorder
substance use disorder (other/unknown)
    with other substance-induced depressive disorder
    with other substance-induced major/mild neurocognitive disorder
    with other substance-induced obsessive-compulsive disorder
    with other substance-induced schizoaffective disorder
    with other substance-induced schizotypal (personality) disorder
    with other substance-induced schizophreniform disorder
    with other substance-induced schizophrenia
substance-using friends
substance withdrawal
    alcohol (no perceptual disturbance) with moderate/severe comorbid presence (F10.232)
    amphetamines/stimulants with m/s comorbid presence (F15.23)
    caffeine with m/s comorbid presence (F15.93)
    cannabis with m/s comorbid presence (F12.288)
    cocaine with m/s comorbid presence (F14.23)
    opioids with m/s comorbid presence (F11.23)
    other/unknown with m/s comorbid presence (F19.239)
    sedatives/hypnotics/anxiolytics with m/s comorbid presence, with m/s perceptual disturbance (F13.232)

substance withdrawal
    sedatives/hypnotics/
      anxiolytics with m/s
      comorbid presence, with
      no perceptual disturbance
      (F13.239)
    tobacco with a m/s
      comorbid presence
      (F17.203)
substance withdrawal delirium
substance withdrawal tremor
substandard language
substantive universals
substitute object
substituted-phenylethylamine structure
substituting behavior
substitution, stimulus
substitution analysis
substitution articulation
substitution test
substitutional lisp
subsystem
    depreciated
    individuals
    parents
    scapegoated
    siblings
    spouses
subsystem boundaries
subthreshold presentations
subtotal cleft palate
subtotal laryngectomy
subvocal speech
successive approximation
Sucher-Allred Reading Placement Inventory
sucking behavior
sucking technique, high-amplitude (HAS)
suction method of esophageal speech
Sudafed (pseudoephedrine) (street terms)
    robotripping (re: under the influence of pseudoephedrine and DXM dextromethorphan)

Sudafed (pseudoephedrine) (street terms)
    skittle-ing (re: under the influence of pseudoephedrine and DXM dextromethorphan)
sudden drop curve audiogram configurations
sudden fear
sudden loss of vision
sudden-onset headache
sudden sleep "attack"
sudden-sniffing-death
suffering death
suffix, tainting
"sugar" (street name, cocaine; heroin; lysergic acid diethylamide/LSD)
"sugar block" (street name, crack)
"sugar lumps" (street name, lysergic acid diethylamide/LSD)
"sugar weed" (street name, cannabis)
suggestible
suggestion hypnosis
suicidal behavior, recurrent
    assessment of
    case management of
    consequences of
    crisis management of
suicidal gestures
suicidal ideation, recurrent
Suicidal Ideation Questionnaire - Adult (ASIQ)
suicidal patients
    assessment of
    case management of
    crisis management of
    treatment of
suicidal potential
suicidal thinking, consequences of
suicidality, repetitious
suicide
    adolescent
    alcohol-related risk for
    completed
    death from

Psychiatric Words and Phrases

suicide
    high risk for
    risk factors for
suicide act, serious
suicide attempt, failed
suicide by cop
Suicide Intervention Response Inventory
suicide motivation
suicide plan
suicide potential, assessment of
Suicide Probability Scale
suicide risk factor
suicide threats
suicide victims, postmortem studies of
sulcus (pl. sulci)
    callosal
    central
    frontal
    inferior frontal
    inferior temporal
    lateral
    lateral occipital
    median lingual
    middle frontal
    postcentral
    precentral
    superior frontal
    superior temporal
    temporal
    terminal
summation, binaural
"sunshine" (street name, lysergic acid diethylamide/LSD)
"super" (street name, phencyclidine/PCP)
"super acid" (street name, ketamine)
"super C" (street name, ketamine)
"super grass" (street name, phencyclidine/PCP)
"super ice" (street name, smokable methamphetamine)
"super joint" (street name, phencyclidine/PCP)
"super kools" (street name, phencyclidine/PCP)
"super weed" (street name, phencyclidine/PCP)
superego control
superficial affect
superficial charm
superficial pain
superficial sensation
superficiality, tendency toward
"supergrass" (street name, cannabis)
superior
    musculus constrictor pharyngis
    musculus serratus posterior
superior constrictor muscle of pharynx
superior frontal sulcus
superior laryngotomy
superior linguae, musculus longitudinalis
superior longitudinal muscle of tongue
superior manner
superior maxillary bone
superior meatus, nasi
superior nasal concha
superior pharyngeal constrictor
superior temporal sulcus
superior to others, feeling
superior turbinate bone
superimposed delirium
superlative comparative
supernumerary teeth
superoxides
superciliousness
supervision, need for
Supervisory Practices Inventory
Supervisory Profile Record
supplemental air
simpleton
supplies, drug
support
    child
    empirical
    excessive need for
    fear of loss of
    informational
    instrumental

support
    lack of
    limited
    need for
    physical
    social
support for the assaulted staff
support group
    primary
    problems with primary
supporting bone, alveolar
supporting persons, loss of significant
suppression, bone marrow
suppression test, dexamethasone
suppurative otitis media, chronic
supra nuclear gaze palsy
supraglottic resonator(s)
suprahyoid extrinsic muscles
supramarginal gyrus
supranuclear palsy, progressive
suprasegmental analysis
suprasegmental phoneme
supraversion of teeth
supreme nasal concha
supreme turbinated bone
surd
surface structure
"surfer" (street name, phencyclidine/PCP)
surgical reduction of Adam's apple
surgical sex-reassignment
surgical sexual reassignment
survey *(see also* tests)
survival, nerve cell
survival strategy, protective
survivor of child abuse, adult
survivor of neglect, adult
survivors of death
suspected disease
suspected/initial episode (S/I)
suspected/subsequent episode (S/S)
suspension laryngoscopy
suspicious ideation
suspiciousness of others
suspiciousness of others motives

sustained belief
sustained blowing, maximum duration of
sustained fatigue
sustained full remission
sustained manner
sustained partial remission
sustained position
sustained remission
Sustained Wakefulness, Repeated Test of (RTSW)
sustention/intention tremor
Sveriges Psykologförbund (Swedish Psychological Association)
swallow method of esophageal speech
swallowing
    deviant
    difficulty
    infantile
    reverse
    visceral
swallowing automatism
swallowing dysfunction
swallowing habit, normal
SWAMI (Speech With Alternating Masking Index)
swaying, body
swaying gait
SWBS (Spiritual Well-Being Scale)
sweat gland activity
sweating (a panic attack indicator)
sweep check test audiometry
"Sweet Jesus" (street name, heroin)
"Sweet Lucy" (street name, cannabis)
"sweet stuff" (street name, cocaine; heroin)
"sweets" (street name, amphetamine)
"swell up" (street name, crack)
swelling, external genitalia
swing
    decreased arm
    mood

swing phase control
Swinging Story Test
swish
switch referential index
sycophant
Sydenham's chorea
syllabic aphonia
syllabic speech sound
syllabication
syllabics
    complex
    simple
syllabification
syllable
    closed
    consonant-vowel
    consonant-vowel-
      consonant
    nonsense
    open
    vowel-consonant
syllable deletion
    unstressed
    weak
syllable duplication
syllable reduction
syllable repetition, sound and
syllable sequence
syllable shape
syllable structure
syllables, paired
Sylvius, fissure of
symbiotic attachment
symbol, Wing's
symbol set system
symbol test, digit
symbolic play
Symbolic Play Test
symbolic thinking
symbolization
symbols
    association of sounds and
    letter
    mathematical
    numerical
symmetromania
sympathetic dysfunction
sympathetic vibration

sympathic mimetic addiction
sympathomimetic addiction
sympathomimetic effect,
    peripheral
symptom(s)
    active psychotic
    active-phase
    anchor
    anxiety
    attention-deficit
    auditory
    avoidance
    baseline
    behavioral dysfunction
    biological dysfunction
    bodily signs and
    brain stem
    catatonic
    constellation of
    constellation of signs and
    conversion
    cyclical pattern of
    deficit
    delusional
    depressive
    disorganized schizophrenic
    dissociative
    emotional
    equivalent
    evaluation of
    extrapyramidal
    fatigue
    feigned
    gastrointestinal
    impairment
    insomnia
    intentionally produced
    manic
    mental disorder type of
    minimal residual
    mixed type of
    mood
    motor
    motor type of
    movement
    objective impairment
    pain
    painful

symptom(s)
- parkinsonian signs and
- perceptual disturbances
- physical signs and
- preexisting
- presenting
- prodromal
- prominent mood
- pseudoneurological
- psychological
- psychological dysfunction
- psychological related
- psychological signs and
- psychomotor
- psychosensory
- psychotic
- reexperiencing perceptual
- residual
- residual psychotic
- review of
- schizophrenia type of
- seizure type of
- sensory
- sensory type of
- sexual
- somatic
- somatization gastrointestinal
- somatization pain
- somatization pseudoneurological
- somatization sexual
- subjective impairment
- trance
- unintentionally produced
- visual

Symptom Checklist-90 (SCL-90)
symptom criteria, full
symptom diary
symptom formation, psychoanalysis and
Symptom History (SH)
symptom in schizophrenia
- depressive
- mood

symptom inventories *(see also tests)*
symptom pattern(s)

symptom presentation, predominant
symptom ratings, daily
symptom relief through hypnosis
symptom response pattern
symptomatic epilepsy
symptomatic presentation, equivalent
symptomatic seizure
symptomatic status
symptomatic therapy
symptomatic treatment
symptomatically reactive
symptomatology
- mood
- psychotic

synapse (pl. synapses)
synaptic
synchronic linguistics
syncope
syncretic thoughts
syncretism
syndromal pattern
syndrome(s)
- absence
- acute organic brain
- adult obstructive sleep apnea
- advanced sleep phase
- amnestic-confabulatory
- androgen insensitivity
- antidepressant discontinuation, initial encounter (T43.205A)
- antidepressant discontinuation, sequela (T43.205D)
- antidepressant discontinuation, subsequent encounter (T43.205S)
- approximate answers
- Asperger's
- attenuated psychosis (F28)
- Avellis
- behavioral
- brain death
- brain stem
- Brissaud

syndrome(s)
    Brissaud-Marie
    callosal disconnection
    cannabinoid hyperemesis
      (CHS)
    Capgras
    cat cry (cri du chat)
    central alveolar
      hypoventilation
    central sleep apnea
    cerebellar
    characteristic
    characteristic withdrawal
    chromosome 21-trisomy
    Collet-Sicard
    contralateral neglect
    Costen
    cri-du-chat
    culturally bound
    culture-bound (CBS)
    de Lange
    Dejerine
    delayed sleep phase
    delusional misidentification
    Dravet
    epileptic
    evolution of the
    fetal alcohol
    fragile X
    Franceschetti's
    frontal lobe
    Gerstmann
    headache
    hepatorenal
    Hunt's
    intoxication
    isolation
    Jackson
    lacunar
    Landau-Kleffner
    Lennox-Gastaut (petit mal
      variant)
    Lesch-Nyhan
    Marfan
    migrainous
    Mobius
    narcolepsy cataplexy
    neglect

syndrome(s)
    neonatal abstinence,
      antidepressant
      discontinuation
    neurobehavioral
    neuroleptic malignant
    neuroleptic malignant
      (G21.0)
    nocturnal drinking
    nocturnal eating
    non-24-hour sleep-wake
    obstructive sleep apnea
    pain
    Pierre Robin
    post concussion
    posttraumatic cerebral
    premenstrual
    psychological
    Ramsay Hunt
    restless legs (G25.81)
    reversible affective
      disorder (SADS)
    Schmidt
    sensory dissociation
    serotonin
    Strauss
    Tapia
    tardive Tourette
    temporomandibular joint
    time zone change
    Usher's
    Vernet
syndrome aphasia, callosal
    disconnection
syndrome of subjective doubles
syndrome of intermetamorphosis
syndrome pattern
Syndrome Scale - Positive and
    Negative (PANSS)
syndrome with psychosis, organic
    brain
synecdoche (figure of speech)
synesthesia
synesthetic stimulation
synkinesis
synkinetic motor movement
synonym
syntactic aphasia

syntactic rule
syntagmatic response
syntagmatic word
syntax tests *(see also* tests)
synthesis
    aculturated into a
    auditory
    autonomic nervous
    categorical
    circadian
    classification
    coding
    endocrine
    five-axis
    focus of delusional
    genitourinary
    haptic
    ICD-10-CM
    IDEA
    integumentary
    lead
    legal
    Medicare
    motor
    multiaxial
    nervous
    nigrostriatal
    peripheral nervous (PNS)
    peripheral vascular
    phonemic
    preferred representational
    pyramidal
    respiratory
    response
    "second messenger"
    sensorimotor
    sleep-wake
    symbol set
    sympathetic nervous
synthesis tests *(see also* tests)
synthetic cannabis/marijuana
  (street names)
    Black Mamba
    Joker
    Kronic
    K2
    Kush
    Spice

"synthetic cocaine" (street name, phencyclidine/PCP)
synthetic method
"synthetic morphine" (desomorphine, street name: "krocodil")
synthetic opioid
Synthetic Sentence Identification Test
"synthetic THT" (street name, phencyclidine/PCP)
synthetically prepared steroids
syphilitic meningitis
system(s)
    academic instruction measurement
    categorical
    hearing aid
    man-machine
    neurotransmitter
    representational
    sign
System for Testing and Evaluation of Potential
System of Phonetic Symbolization – Visual/Tactile
System to Plan Early Childhood Services (SPECS)
systematic method
systematic process
systematic review
systematic study
systematized amnesia
systems interface disorders, psychiatric
Szondi Test
s/z ratio

T

"T" (street name, cannabis; cocaine)
T (transformation)
taboo
tabophobia
"tabs" (street name, lysergic acid diethylamide/LSD)
tabular index
tabulation, allophone
tachistoscope
tachylalia
tachyphemia
TACL-R (Tests for Auditory Comprehension of Language-R)
tact operant
tactile alexia
tactile anomia
tactile feedback
Tactile Form Recognition Test (TFRT)
tactile genital stimulation
tactile hallucinations, transient
tactile illusions, transient
tactile information with motor activity, disturbance in integrating
tactile kinesthetic perception
tactile perception
tactile sensation, fine
tactile sensory modality
tactile stimulation
tactile stimulus
tag question(s)
Taijin kyofusho (F42)
tail, velar
"tail lights" (street name, lysergic acid diethylamide/LSD)
"taima" (street name, cannabis)
tainting suffix
take pleasure in few activities
"taking a cruise" (street name, phencyclidine/PC)
taking control
"Takkouri" (street name, cannabis)
talent, exaggerated
talk
    baby
    parallel
talk therapy
Talwin (pentazocine) (Street Names)
    crackers (re: Talwin/Ritalin simultaneous injections for heroin/cocaine effect)
    one and ones (re: Talwin/Ritalin injections for heroin/cocaine effect)
    pharming (re: doctor-shopping for prescription medication)
    poor man's heroin (re: Talwin/Ritalin injections)
    Ritz and Ts (re: Ritalin/Talwin injections)
    set (re: Ritalin/Talwin injections)
    Ts and Rits, (re: Talwin/Ritalin injections)
    Ts and Rs (re: Talwin/Ritalin injections)
Talwin Nx (pentazocine/naloxone)
tangential speech
tangible reinforcement operant conditioning audiometry (TROCA)
tangles
    Alzheimer
    neurofibrillary
"Tango and Cash" (street name, fentanyl)
tantrums, temper
TAP (Trainer's Assessment of Proficiency)
TAP-D (Test of Articulation Performance-Diagnostic)

tape-editing
taphophobia
Tapia syndrome
tapinophobia
TAP-S (Test of Articulation
    Performance-Screen)
"tar" (street name, heroin; opium)
Tarasoff Decision
Tarasoff Rule
TARC Assessment System
tardive akathisia (G25.71)
tardive dyskinesia (G24.91)
tardive dyskinesia, neuroleptic-
    induced
tardive dystonia (G24.09)
tardive orobuccal dyskinesia
tardive Tourette syndrome
target, potential
target of (perceived) reverse
    discrimination or persecution
    (Z60.5)
target response
TAS (Test of Attitude toward
    School)
task
    added purpose
    complex multistep
    dichotic listening
    instrumental
    manipulatory
    necessary
    nine-digit SDL (SD9)
    particular
    repetitive
    required
    sentence closure
    structured
    three-step
    visual-motor
    word retrieval
task analysis
Task Assessment Scales
task completion
Task-Oriented Assessment
task performance
"taste" (re: drug dealing)
"taste" (street name, heroin)
taste, distorted perception of

taste sensation
taste threshold
TAT (Thematic Apperception
    Test)
TAT (Thematic Aptitude Test)
tautologous
TAWF (Test of Adolescent/Adult
    Word Finding)
"taxing" (re: crack-house entrance
    fee; drug dealing)
Taylor-Johnson Temperament
    Analysis
Tay-Sachs disease
TBI (traumatic brain injury) *(see
    also* tests)
TBS (Transition Behavior Scale)
"T-buzz" (street name,
    phencyclidine/PCP)
TCMP (Thematic Content
    Modification Program)
TCSM (Test of Cognitive Style in
    Mathematics)
TD (threshold of discomfort)
TDD (telephone device for the
    deaf)
TDE (thiamine deficiency
    encephalopathy)
"tea" (street name,
    phencyclidine/PCP)
"tea party" (re: cannabis use)
Teacher Evaluation Scale (TES)
    (see also tests)
Teacher Feedback Questionnaire
Teacher Occupational
    Competency Test: Child Care
    and Guidance
Teacher Occupational
    Competency Test: Mechanical
    Technology
Teacher Opinion Inventory
Teacher's School Readiness
    Inventory (TSRI)
Teacher Stress Inventory
teaching
    diagnostic
    remedial
teaching alphabet, initial

Teaching Style Inventory *(see also* tests)
"teardrops" (re: crack containers)
tearfulness, breakthrough
tears, esophageal
"tecate" (street name, heroin)
"tecatos" (re: Hispanic heroin addicts)
technique
    ascending
    bounce (stuttering)
    cognitive-behavioral
    communicative
    compensatory
    descending
    head turn
    high-amplitude sucking (HAS)
    Hood
    Hood masking
    kinesthetic
    plateau masking technique, projective
    psychoanalytic
    psychological
    relapse-prevention
    shadowing masking
    standardized cognitive assessment
    startle
    stop-and-think
    theoretical
    threshold shift masking
    sensorineural acuity level masking
technique audiometry
    ascending
    descending
technological detection of deceit
technologies, brain imaging
TEEM (Test for Examining Expressive Morphology)
teen vaping
"teenage" (re: 1/16 gram of methamphetamine)
"teeth" (street name, cocaine; crack)
teeth (sing. tooth)
    axioversion of
    bicuspid
    buccoversion of
    canine
    central incisor
    closed bite malposition of
    cross-bite malposition of
    cuspid
    deciduous
    distoclusion of
    eye
    facioversion of
    first deciduous molar
    first premolar
    incisor
    infraversion of
    jumbling of
    labioversion of
    lateral incisor
    linguoversion of
    mesioclusion of
    mesioversion of
    molar
    "moth-eaten"
    neutroclusion of
    open bite malposition of
    overbite malposition of
    overjet of
    permanent
    premolar
    second deciduous molar
    second premolar
    supernumerary
    supraversion of
    torsiversion of
    transversion of
    underbite malposition of
    wisdom
teeth malocclusion
teeth malpositions
TEL (Test of Economic Literacy)
TELD (Test of Early Language Development) *(see also* tests)
tele-psychiatrist
tele-psychiatry, effective
telecoil

telegraphic speech
telegraphic utterance
telehealth treatment
telemedicine psychiatric
  consulting
teleophobia
telepathy, belief in
telephone device for the deaf
  (TDD)
telephone hearing theory
telephone volley theory
telescoped words
television-induced epilepsy
Tell-Me-A-Story (TEMAS)
TEMAS (Tell-Me-A-Story)
temper dyscontrol
temper tantrums
Temperament and Values
  Inventory
Temperament Assessment Battery
  for Children
temperature
    body
      core body
temperature measurement, core
  body
temperature sensation
Temple University Short Syntax
  Inventory (TUSSI)
temporal association
temporal auditory processing
temporal bones
temporal characteristics of pain
temporal gyri
temporal headache
temporal lobe
temporal lobe status
temporal organization
temporal orientation
temporal relationship
temporal skull bones
temporal sulci
temporal sulcus
    inferior
    superior
temporary epilation
temporary habit
temporary threshold shift (TTS)

temporomandibular joint (TMJ)
temporomandibular joint
  syndrome
temptation, failure to resist
tendency (pl. tendencies)
    acting-out
    destructive
    excitement-seeking
    familial
    impulsive
    insightless
    introversive
    repeat
    seductive
    self-absorbed
    sleep
    tough-minded
tendency for dependence
tendency to externalize blame
tendency to overreact
tendency to play hunches
tendency to somatization
tendency toward amelioration
tendency toward boredom
tendency toward impulsivity
tendency toward recklessness
tendency toward superficiality
tense
    feeling
    future perfect
    future perfect progressive
    past perfect
    past perfect progressive
    perfect
    present perfect
    present perfect progressive
    progressive
    simple
    simple future
    simple future progressive
    simple past
    simple past progressive
    simple present
    simple present progressive
tense feature English phoneme
tense phoneme
tense vowel
"tension" (street name, crack)

tension
   combat
   feeling of
   increased muscle
   increasing sense of
   inner
   marked
   muscular
   physical
   release of
   release of sexual
   relief of
   sense of
   sexual
   social
tension migraine headache
tension-type headache
tension-vascular headache
tensor muscle of soft palate
tensor palati, musculus
tensor veli palatini, musculus
TERA-D/HH (Test of Early Reading Ability--Deaf or Hard of Hearing)
terminal
   axon
   clause
terminal achievement behavior
terminal behavior
terminal insomnia
terminal juncture
terminal lag
terminal string
terminal sulcus
terminal tremor
termination time, voice (VTT)
terrifying experience
terrifying stimulus
territoriality
terrorist attack
tertiary stress
TES (Teacher Evaluation Scale)
TES (Therapeutic error signal)
test (general descriptive terms)
   ability
   audiometric
   audiometry
   behavioral hearing

test (general descriptive terms)
   calculations
   complex thematic pictures
   confrontation naming
   continuous performance task or test
   copy geometric designs
   copy intersecting pentagons
   count backwards from 100
   criterion-referenced
   day of month
   deep articulation
   dexamethasone suppression
   diagnostic
   diagnostic articulation
   digit repetition
   digit reversal
   digit span
   digit symbol
   draw a clock face
   draw a house
   draw a picture from memory
   drug screening
   electrodermal response (EDRA)
   forward digital span recall
   fund of information
   immediate memory
   immittance
   ink blot
   intelligence
   language
   letter cancellation
   liver function
   logical memory
   memory for digits
   mini mental status
   misplaced objects
   month of year
   multi-item
   name the date
   naming common objects
   need a sentence
   neuropsychologic battery of
   neuropsychological
   neuropsychometric

test (general descriptive terms)
    nonverbal
    norm-referenced
    number 3 traced on
      patient's palm
    paragraph recall
    performance
    personality
    proverb interpretation
    psychological
    psychometric
    psychophysiological
    recall 5 items after 5
      minutes
    recall of information
    recent memory
    remote memory
    reverse digit span recall
    rotation
    serial threes (3's)
    short orientation-memory-
      concentration (OMC)
    similarities mental status
    16PF
    spell a word backwards
    spell backwards
    sweep check
    thematic picture
    three-stage command
    tyramine challenge
    understanding of
      similarities
    urine for drug screen
    visual choice reaction time
    visual evoked response
    visual field
    visual threat
    wall chart vision
    word association
    word retrieval
    write a sentence
test protocol
test results
    inconsistent laboratory
    interpretation of
    review of
test-retest reliability coefficient
test scores, full

testing
    cortical
    diminished reality
    gross impairment in reality
    immittance
    intracorporeal
      pharmacological
    level of demarcation in
      sensory
    neurophysiological
    psychometric
testing ability, reality (Rorschach)
testing program
testosterone drug addiction
testosterone-produced hormone
    steroids
tests (Eponymous and Other
  Proper Names)
    (select list of *tests* is
      arranged in these
      categories: *Achievement;
      Behavior Assessment;
      Developmental;
      Education-related;
      English / Language;
      Intelligence and General
      Aptitude; Neuropsycho-
      logical; Other (e.g.
      Career / General Health /
      Leadership); Personality;
      and Speech and Hearing)*
tests, *Achievement*
    Adult Basic Learning
      Examination
    Basic Achievement Skills
      Individual Screener
    Bracken Basic Concept
      Scale
    Canadian Comprehensive
      Assessment Program
      (Achievement Series)
    Collis-Romberg
      Mathematical Problem
      Solving Profiles
    Diagnostic Achievement
      Battery (DAB)
    Gifted and Talented
      Screening

tests, *Achievement*
    Group Achievement Identification Measure
    Group Inventory for Finding Creative Talent
    Measures of Musical Abilities
    Quick-Score Achievement Test
    Riley Inventory of Basic Learning Skills (RIBLS)
    Scaled Curriculum Achievement Levels Test)
    Screening Assessment for Gifted Elementary Students--Primary (SAGES-P)
    Seashore Measures of Musical Talents
    Sequential Assessment of Mathematics Inventories
    Skill Indicators (SKIs)
    Student Talent and Risk Profile (STAR Profile)

tests, *Behavior Assessment*
    Activity Pattern Indicators (APIs)
    Adaptive Behavior Evaluation Scale (ABES)
    Adaptive Behavior Inventory
    ADL Index
    Adolescent Alienation Index
    Adolescent Drinking Index (ADI)
    Adolescent-Family Inventory of Life Events and Changes
    AMD Adaptive Behavior Scale
    Attributional Style Questionnaire
    Balthazar Scales for Adaptive Behavior I (Scales of Functional Independence)

tests, *Behavior Assessment*
    Balthazar Scales for Adaptive Behavior II (Scales of Social Adaptation)
    Barthel ADL Index
    Behavior Disorders Identification Scale (BDIS)
    Behavior Evaluation Scale (BES)
    Behavior Rating Profile (BRP)
    Behavioral Assessment of Pain Questionnaire (BAPQ)
    Behavioral Deviancy Profile
    Behavioral Observation Scale for Autism
    Blessed Behavior Scale
    Burks' Behavior Rating Scale
    CAGE Alcohol Use Questionnaire
    Child and Adolescent Adjustment Profile
    Child Behavior Rating Scale
    Children's Academic Intrinsic Motivation Inventory
    Children's Adaptive Behavior Scale
    Children's Version/Family Environmental Scale
    Cognitive Behavior Rating Scales
    Communication Sensitivity Inventory
    Community-Oriented Programs Environment Scale (COPES)
    Cooper-Farran Behavioral Rating Scales (CFBRS)
    Correctional Institutions Environment Scale

tests, *Behavior Assessment*
    Couple's Pre-Counseling Inventory
    Devereux Adolescent Behavior Rating Scale
    Devereux Child Behavior Rating Scale
    Diversity Awareness Profile (DAP)
    Drug Use Index
    Emotional and Behavior Problem Scale (EBPS)
    Emotional/Behavior Screening Program (ESP)
    Emotions Profile Index
    Family Adaptability and Cohesion Evaluation Scales
    Family Environment Scale (FES)
    Family Inventory of Life Events and Changes
    Family Satisfaction Scale
    Frenchay Activities Index
    Gordon Personal Profile Inventory
    Group Styles Inventory (GSI)
    Hahnemann Elementary School Behavior Rating Scale
    Hahnemann High School Behavior Rating Scale
    Home Environment Questionnaire
    Home Observation for Measurement of the Environment
    Home Screening Questionnaire
    Hutchins Behavior Inventory (HBI)
    Illness Behavior Questionnaire
    Inferred Self-Concept Scale
    Interpersonal Style Inventory

tests, *Behavior Assessment*
    Inventory of Individually Perceived Group Cohesiveness
    Katz ADL Index
    Kenny ADL Index
    Life Satisfaction Index (LSI)
    Life Styles Inventory (LSI)
    Marital Communication Scale
    Michigan Screening Profile of Parenting
    Millon Behavioral Health Inventory (MBHI)
    Motivational Patterns Inventory
    Motivation and Decision-Making Inventory on Leadership
    Multiphasic Environmental Assessment Procedure
    Neonatal Behavioral Assessment Scale , The (NBAS)
    Neonatal Behavioral Assessment Scale, The (NBAS)
    Northwick Park Index of Independence in ADLs
    Nottingham Extended ADL Index
    Parent Perception of Child Profile (PPCP)
    Personal Experience Screening Questionnaire (PESQ)
    Personal Relationship Inventory (PRI)
    Profile of Adaptation to Life
    Rivermead ADL
    Rivermead Behavioural Memory (RBMT)
    Scales of Independent Behavior
    Self-Esteem Questionnaire

tests, *Behavior Assessment*
   Self-Perception Profile for Children
   Social Behavior Assessment Inventory (SBAI)
   Social Behaviour Assessment Schedule
   Street Survival Skills Questionnaire
   Temperament Assessment Battery for Children
   Thurstone Temperament Schedule
   Time Problems Inventory
   Transition Behavior Scale (TBS)
   Vineland Adaptive Behavior Scales
   Walker-McConnell Scale of Social Competence and School Adjustment
   Weller-Strawser Scales of Adaptive Behavior for the Learning Disabled
   Work Environment Scale (WES)

tests, *Developmental*
   Adapted Sequenced Inventory of Communication Development (A-SICD)
   AGS Early Screening Profiles
   Assessment for Children & Emotional/Behavior Screening
   Barber Scales of Self-Regard for Preschool Children
   Basic Screening and Referral Form for Children with Suspected Learning and Behavioral Disabilities
   Basic Skills Assessment Program

tests, *Developmental*
   Battelle Developmental Inventory
   Beery Picture Vocabulary Screening (PVS)
   Beery Picture Vocabulary Test (PVT)
   Behaviour Assessment Battery
   Birth to Three Assessment and Intervention System
   Birth to Three Developmental Scale
   BRIGANCE Diagnostic Inventory of Early Development
   BRIGANCE K & 1 Screen for Kindergarten and First Grade Children
   Bristol Language Development Scales (BLADES)
   Cain-Levine Social Competency Scale
   Canadian Comprehensive Assessment Program (Developing Series)
   Caregiver's School Readiness Inventory (CSRI)
   Child Care Inventory
   Children's Inventory of Self-Esteem (CISE)
   CID Preschool Performance Scale
   Clark Picture Phonetic Inventory
   Communication Abilities Diagnostic Screen
   Communication Screen, The (A Pre-school Speech-Language Screening Tool)
   Communicative Evaluation Chart from Infancy to Five Years

tests, *Developmental*
    Comprehensive Developmental Evaluation Chart
    Conners Hyperkinesis Index (Parent Form)
    Conners Hyperkinesis Index (Teacher Form)
    Cooperation Preschool Inventory
    Daberon Screening for School Readiness
    Denver Prescreening Development Questionnaire (DPDQ)
    Developmental Assessment of Learning (AGS Edition)
    Developmental Indicators for Assessment of Learning
    Developmental Sentence Scoring (DOS)
    Diagnostic Skills Battery
    Differential Ability Scales
    Early Child Development Inventory
    Early Coping Inventory
    Early Development Scale for Preschool Children
    Early Language Milestone Scale
    Early School Assessment (ESA)
    Early Screening Inventory
    Early Screening Profiles
    Early Years Easy Screen (EYES)
    Edinburgh Functional Communication Profile (EFCP)
    Environmental Pre-Language Battery,
    Erhardt Developmental Prehension Assessment (EDPA)

tests, *Developmental*
    Erhardt Developmental Vision Assessment (EDVA)
    Family Adaptability and Cohesion Evaluation Scales (FACES)
    Family Relationship Inventory
    Florida Kindergarten Screening Battery, The
    Fuld Object-Memory Evaluation
    Functional Assessment Inventory
    Gesell Child Development Age Scale, The (GCDAS)
    Howell Prekindergarten Screening Test
    Infant/Toddler Environment Rating Scale (ITERS)
    Instructional Environment Scale The (TIES)
    Inventory for Counseling and Development
    Inventory of Natural Language, Basic
    Joseph Pre-School and Primary Self-Concept Screening Test
    Kaufman Development Scale
    Kaufman Infant and Preschool Scale
    Kent Infant Development Scale
    Learning Disability Evaluation Scale (LDES)
    Learning Inventory of Kindergarten Experiences (LIKE)
    Lincoln-Oseretsky Motor Development Scale
    Measurement of Language Development
    Measures of Psychosocial Development (MPD)

Psychiatric Words and Phrases

tests, *Developmental*
- Memory Assessment Scales (MAS)
- Michigan Picture Inventory
- Miller Assessment for Preschoolers
- Minnesota Infant Development Inventory
- Minnesota Preschool Scales
- Missouri Kindergarten Inventory of Developmental Skills
- Mother/Infant Communication Screening (MICS)
- Mother-Child Relationship Evaluation, The (MCRE)
- Motor Steadiness Battery
- Mullen Scales of Early Learning
- Need for Cognition Scale
- Oral-Motor/Feeding Rating Scale
- Parent as a Teacher Inventory (PAAT)
- Parent Opinion Inventory
- Perceptual-Motor Assessment for Children (P-MAC)
- Phelps Kindergarten Readiness Scale (PKRS)
- Pimsleur Language Aptitude Battery
- Pragmatics Profile of Early Communication Skills, The
- Prereading Expectancy Screening Scale
- Preschool Development Inventory
- Preschool Language Assessment Instrument (PLAI)
- Preschool Language Screening Test
- Preschool Screening Test

tests, *Developmental*
- Preschool Speech and Language Screening Test
- Quick Screening of Mental Development, A
- Rand Functional Limitations Battery
- Rand Physical Capacities Battery
- Rating Inventory for Screening Kindergartners (RISK)
- Recognition Memory
- Reynell-Zinkin (Developmental) Scales
- Rey-Ostereith Complex Figure
- Right-Left Orientation (RLO)
- Rivermead Motor Assessment
- S.E.E.D. Developmental Profiles
- Scale of Social Development
- School Readiness Screening Test
- Screening Kit of Language Development (SKOLD)
- Sequenced Inventory of Communication Development
- Speech-Ease Screening Inventory (K-1)
- System for Testing and Evaluation of Potential
- Temperament Assessment Battery for Children
- WHO Handicap Scales
- Wide Range Assessment of Memory and Learning

tests, *Education-Related*
- Academic Instruction Measurement System, A
- ACT Evaluation/Survey Service, The (ESS)

tests, *Education-Related*
    ACT Study Power Assessment and Inventory (SPA; SPI)
    ACT Study Skills Assessment and Inventory (SSA; SSI)
    ADD-H: Comprehensive Teacher's Rating Scale (ACTeRS)
    Analytic Learning Disability Assessment
    Ann Arbor Learning Inventory and Remediation Program
    Assessment and Placement Services for Community Colleges
    Assessment in Mathematics
    Attitudes Toward Mainstreaming Scale (ATMS)
    Autism Screening Instrument for Educational Planning
    Basic Reading Inventory (BRI)
    Basic School Skills Inventory Diagnostic Screen
    Burns/Roe Informal Reading Inventory: Preprimer to Twelfth Grade
    Canadian Comprehensive Assessment Program (School Attitude Measure)
    Canfield Instructional Styles Inventory
    Career Assessment Inventories (For the Learning Disabled)
    Child Assessment Schedule
    Class Activities Questionnaire
    Classroom Environment Index

tests, *Education-Related*
    Classroom Environment Scale
    College Major Interest Inventory (CMII)
    Colorado Educational Interest Inventory
    Community College Student Experiences Questionnaire (CCSEQ)
    Conners Parent Rating Scale (CPRS)
    Conners Teacher Rating Scale (CTRS-28, CTRS-39)
    Content Mastery Examinations for Educators (CMEE)
    Diagnostic Assessments of Reading (DAR)
    Diagnostic Mathematics Profiles
    DMI Mathematics Systems Instructional Objectives Inventory
    Enhanced ACT Assessment
    Environmental Language Inventory (ELI)
    Evaluating Educational Programs for Intellectually Gifted Students
    Evaluation and Development Program, Instructional
    Gifted Evaluation Scale, (GES)
    Gifted Program Evaluation Survey, The
    Graduate and Managerial Assessment
    Indicators for the Assessment of Learning
    Instructional Leadership Inventory
    Learning and Study Strategies Inventory (LASSI)

tests, *Education-Related*
   Learning Style Profile
     (LSP)
   Practical Math
     Assessments
   Prevocational Assessment
     and Curriculum Guide,
     The (PACG)
   Prevocational Assessment
     Screen (PAS)
   Process for Assessment of
     Effective Student
     Functioning, A
   Psychoeducational Profile
     (PEP)
   School Administrator
     Assessment Survey
   School Assessment Survey
     (SAS)
   School Climate Inventory
   School Handicap Condition
     Scale (SEH)
   School Interest Inventory
   School Social Skills Rating
     Scale (S3 Rating scale)
   Screening Assessment for
     Gifted Elementary
     Students, Primary Grade
   Screening Children for
     Related Early Educational
     Needs (SCREEN)
   Screening Instrument for
     Targeting Educational
     Risk (S.I.F.T.E.R.)
   Screening Test for
     Educational Prerequisite
     Skills (STEPS)
   Screening Test of
     Academic Readiness
   Sequential Assessment of
     Mathematics Inventories
   Steps Up Developmental
     Screening Program
   Student Adaptation to
     College Questionnaire
     (SACQ)
   Student Adjustment
     Inventory (SAI)

tests, *Education-Related*
   Teacher Evaluation Scale
     (TES)
   Teacher Evaluation Scale
     (TES)
   Teacher Feedback
     Questionnaire
   Teacher Opinion Inventory
   Teacher Stress Inventory
   Teacher's School
     Readiness Inventory
     (TSRI)
   Teaching Style Inventory
   Test Anxiety Profile
   Time Use Analyzer
   TLC-Learning Preference
     Inventory
   Woodcock-Johnson
     Psycho-Educational
     Battery (WJ)
tests, *English and Language*
   Adolescent Language
     Screening Test
   Analytical Reading
     Inventory
   Basic School Skills
     Inventory Screen
   Bilingual Syntax Measure
     (BSM)
   Botel Reading Inventory
   Bzoch-League Receptive-
     Expressive Emergent
     Language Scale, The
   CAP Assessment of
     Writing
   Coarticulation Assessment
     in Meaningful Language
     (CAML)
   Compton Speech and
     Language Screening
     Evaluation
   Diagnostic Reading Scales
   Dos Amigos Verbal
     Language Scales
   English/Spanish Del Rio
     Language Screening Test
   Evaluating Acquired Skills
     in Communication

tests, *English and Language*
- Evaluating Communicative Competence (Pragmatic Program)
- Functional Communication Profile
- Functional Limitation Profile
- Gillingham-Childs Phonics Proficiency Scales
- Illinois Children's Language Assessment Test
- Interpersonal Language Skills and Assessment (ILSA)
- Inventory of Language Abilities
- Iowa's Severity Rating Scales for Speech and Language Impairments
- Johnston Informal Reading Inventory (JIRI)
- Language Assessment (Oral) Scales (LAS-O)
- Language Assessment (Reading and Writing) Scales (LA-R/W)
- Language Assessment Remediation and Screening Procedure
- Language Sampling, Analysis, and Training
- Learning Styles Inventory
- Michigan English Language Assessment Battery
- Mill Hill Vocabulary Scale
- Multilevel Informal Language Inventory
- New Sucher-Allred Reading Placement Inventory, The
- Oral Language Evaluation
- Oral Language Sentence Imitation Diagnostic Inventory (OLSIDI)

tests, *English and Language*
- Patterned Elicitation Syntax Screening Test (PESST)
- Performance Assessment of Syntax Elicited and Spontaneous (PASES)
- Primary Language Screen, The (TPLS)
- Proficiency Assessment Report (PAR)
- Prosody-Voice Screening Profile (PVSP)
- Quick Phonics Survey (QPS)
- Quick Word Test
- Reading Comprehension Inventory
- Receptive One Word Picture Vocabulary (ROWPVT)
- Receptive-Expressive Emergent Language Scale (REEL)
- Screening Test of Adolescent Language
- Slingerland Screening Tests for Identifying Children with Specific Language Disability
- Smith-Johnson Nonverbal Performance Scale
- Speech and Language Evaluation Scale (SLES)
- Temple University Short Syntax Inventory (TUSSI)
- Verbal Language Development Scale
- Vocabulary Comprehension Scale
- Woodcock Language Proficiency Battery (WLPB)
- Written Language Assessment

tests, *Intelligence and General Aptitude*
- Aptitude Interest Measurement
- Basic Concept Inventory
- Brief Cognitive Rating Scale (BCRS)
- California Critical Thinking Dispositions Inventory
- Cognitive Skills Assessment Battery
- College Basic Academic Subjects Examination
- College-Level Examination Program General Examination (CLEP)
- Decision Making Inventory
- Gifted Evaluation Scale
- Inventory of Perceptual Skills (IPS)
- Khatena-Torrance Creative Perception Inventory
- Kolbe Cognitive Index (KCI)
- Leiter Adult Intelligence Scale
- Measure of How You Think and Make Decisions, A (Inquiry Mode Questionnaire)
- Musical Aptitude Profile
- Pediatric Early Elementary Examination
- Pediatric Examination of Educational Readiness at Middle Childhood
- Perception of Ability Scale for Students (PASS)
- Pragmatics Screening Test
- Problem Solving Inventory
- Process Skills Rating Scales (PSRS)
- Roeder Manipulative Aptitude
- Roswell-Chall Analysis Skills

tests, *Intelligence and General Aptitude*
- Scales of Creativity and Learning Environment
- Short Imaginal Processes Inventory (SIPI)
- Slingerland College-Level Screening for the Identification of Language Learning Strengths and Weaknesses
- Stanford-Binet Intelligence Scale
- Wechsler Intelligence Scale for Children (WISC)

tests, *Neuropsychological*
- Acceptance of Disability Scale (AD scale)
- Ackerman-Schoendorf Scales for Parent Evaluation of Custody (ASPECT)
- Adjustment Inventory, The (Adult Form)
- Adolescent Alienation Index
- Adolescent Diagnostic Interview (ADI)
- Adolescent Drinking Index (ADI)
- Adult Neuropsychological Questionnaire (ANQ)
- Adult Suicidal Ideation Questionnaire (ASIQ)
- Affects Balance Scale
- Alcohol Assessment and Treatment Profile
- Alzheimer's Disease Assessment Scale (ADAS)
- Anxiety Scales for Children and Adults (ASCA)
- Aphasia Clinical Battery
- Aphasia Language Performance Scales (ALPS)
- Appraisal of Language Disturbances (ALD)

tests, *Neuropsychological*
- Apraxia Battery for Adults (ABA)
- Arizona Battery for Communication Disorders of Dementia, The (ABCD)
- Assessment Link Between Phonology and Articulation
- Assessment of Chemical Health Inventory
- Assessment of Conceptual Organization (ACO)
- Assessment of Core Goals (ACG)
- Assessment of Intelligibility of Dysarthric Speech
- Assessment of Suicide Potential
- Attention Deficit Disorder Behavior Rating Scales (ADDBRS)
- Attention Deficit Disorders Evaluation Scale (ADDES)
- Autistic Behavior Composite Checklist and Profile
- Barthel ADL Index
- Bay Area Functional Performance Evaluation
- Beck Hopelessness Scale (BHS)
- Bedside Evaluation and Screening Test of Aphasia
- Behavioral Assessment of Pain Questionnaire (BAP)
- Bell Object Relations-Reality Testing Inventory
- Bem Sex-Role Inventory
- Bexley-Maudsley Automated Psychological Screening
- Biographical Inventory
- Bipolar Psychological Inventory

tests, *Neuropsychological*
- Blessed Dementia Rating Scales
- Bloom Analogies Test
- Boston Assessment of Severe Aphasia (BASA)
- Boston Diagnostic Aphasia Examination (BDAE)
- Brief Drinker Profile
- Brief Life History Inventory (BLHI)
- Brief Symptom Inventory
- California Life Goals Evaluation Schedules
- California Marriage Readiness Evaluation (CMRE)
- Canadian Neurological Scale
- Caregiver Strain Index
- Cattell Scales
- Center for Epidemiological Studies Depression Scale
- Checklist for Child Abuse Evaluation, (CCAE)
- Checklist of Adaptive Living Skills (CALS)
- Child "At Risk" for Drug Abuse Rating Scale, The (DARS)
- Child Abuse Potential Inventory
- Child Anxiety Scale
- Child Neuropsychological Questionnaire (CNQ)
- Children's Depression Inventory
- Children's Depression Scale
- Children's Hypnotic Susceptibility Scale
- Children's Manifest Anxiety Scale (CMAS)
- Clifton Assessment Procedures for the Elderly
- Clinical Dementia Rating Scale (CDR)

tests, *Neuropsychological*
    Clinical Evaluation of
      Language Functions
      (CLEF)
    Clinical Rating Scale
      (CRS)
    Clinical Scales (MMPI)
    Clinical Support System
      Battery
    Cognitive Control Battery
    Cognitive Diagnostic
      Battery
    Comprehensive
      Assessment of Symptoms
      and History (CASH)
    Comprehensive Drinker
      Profile
    Comprehensive Level of
      Consciousness Scale
      (CLCS)
    Conflict Management
      Appraisal (CMA)
    Conflict Tactics Scale
    Conners Hyperkinesis
      Index (Parent Form)
    Conners Hyperkinesis
      Index (Teacher Form)
    Content Scales (MMPI)
    Coopersmith Self-Esteem
      Inventories
    Coping Resources
      Inventory (CRI)
    Cornell Scale for
      Depression and Dementia
      (CSDD)
    Culture Shock Inventory
    Culture-Free Self-Esteem
      Inventories for Children
      and Adults
    Defense Functioning Scale
      (DFS)
    Defense Mechanism
      Inventory (DMI)
    Dementia Behavior
      Disturbance Scale (DBD)
    Dementia Mood
      Assessment Scale
      (DMAS)

tests, *Neuropsychological*
    Dementia Rating Scale
    Depression "2" Scale
    Developmental Assessment
      of Life Experiences
      (D.A.L.E. System)
    Diagnostic Screening
      Batteries (Adolescent,
      Adult, and Child)
    Disability Factor (General)
      Scales
    Dissociative Experiences
      Scale (DES)
    Driver Risk Inventory
      (DRI)
    Drug Use Index
    Dyslexia Screening Survey,
      The
    Eating Disorder Inventory
      (EDI)
    Edinburgh Rehabilitation
      Status Scale
    Edinburgh-2 Coma Scale
    Emotions Profile Index
    Endler Multidimensional
      Anxiety Scales (EMAS)
    Evaluation and Screening
      Test of Aphasia, Bedside
    Evaluation of Children's
      Human Figure Drawings
    Evaluation of Hemispheric
      Abilities and Brain
      Function
    Examining for Aphasia
    Follow-up Drinker Profile
    Folstein Mini-Mental
      Status Examination
    Frenchay Aphasia
      Screening Test (FAST)
    Frenchay Dysarthria
      Assessment
    Functional Assessment
      Inventory
    Functional Independence
      Measure (FIM)
    Functional Needs
      Assessment (FNA)

tests, *Neuropsychological*
    Functional Status Questionnaire (FSQ)
    Functional Time Estimation Questionnaire (FTEQ)
    Geriatric Depression Scale
    Glasgow Coma Scale (GCS)
    Global Assessment of Relational Functioning Scale (GARF)
    Golombok Rust Inventory of Marital State, The (GRIMS)
    Grief Experience Inventory (GEI)
    Halstead-Russell Neuropsychological Evaluation S system (HRNES)
    Halstead-Wepman Aphasia Screening Test
    Hamilton Rating Scale for Depression
    Hilson Adolescent Profile
    Hospital Anxiety and Depression Scale
    Hypnotic Induction Profile (HIP)
    Impact Message Inventory (IMI)
    Impact of Event Scale
    Index of Well Being (IWB)
    Integrated Assessment System (IAS)
    Inventory of Personal Needs
    IPAT Anxiety Scale
    IPAT Depression Scale
    Jette Functional Status Index
    Katz ADL Index
    Keegan Type Indicator
    Kenny ADL Index
    Kenny Self-Care Questionnaire

tests, *Neuropsychological*
    Kolbe Cognitive Index (KCI)
    Lambeth Disability Screening Questionnaire
    Leeds Scales for the Self-Assessment of Anxiety and Depression
    Leiter Recidivism Scale
    Levine-Pilowsky Depression Questionnaire
    Life Event Scale: Adolescents
    Life Event Scale: Children
    Life Satisfaction Index (LSI)
    Luria-Nebraska Neuropsychological Battery
    Mania "9" Scale
    Marital Satisfaction Inventory
    Marriage Adjustment Inventory (MAI)
    Masculinity-Femininity "5" Scale
    McGill Pain Questionnaire
    Menstrual Distress Questionnaire (MDQ)
    Mental Status Intrex Questionnaire
    Millon Adolescent Clinical Inventory (MACI)
    Mini Inventory of Right Brain Injury (MIRBI)
    Miskimins Self-Goal-Other Discrepancy Scale
    Multidimensional Self-Concept Scale (MSCS)
    Murphy-Meisgeier Type Indicator for Children (MMTIC)
    Neurobehavioral Cognitive Status Examination
    Neurobehavioral Rating Scale
    Neuropsychological Screening Exam

tests, *Neuropsychological*
    Neuropsychological Status Examination
    NIH Stroke Scale
    North American Depression Inventories for Children and Adults
    Northwick Park Index of Independence in ADLs
    Nottingham Extended ADL Index
    Nottingham Ten-Point ADL Scale
    Number three (3) traced on patient's palm test
    OARS Multidimensional Functional Assessment Questionnaire (OMFAQ)
    Obsessive-Compulsive Personality Disorder Inventory, Subscale-2
    Offer Parent-Adolescent Questionnaire, The
    Offer Self-Image Questionnaire (OSIQ)
    Offer Self-Image Questionnaire for Adolescents
    Ordinal Scales of Psychological Development
    Orzeck Aphasia Evaluation
    Paranoia "6" Scale
    Parent Attachment Structured Interview
    Parent-Adolescent Communication Scale
    Parental Acceptance-Rejection Questionnaire
    Parenting Stress Index
    Partner Relationship Inventory (PRI)
    Peer Nomination Inventory of Depression
    Peer Profile
    Personal Experience Screening Questionnaire (PESQ)

tests, *Neuropsychological*
    Personal Resource Questionnaire (PRQ)
    Personal Strain Questionnaire (PSQ)
    Philadelphia Head Injury Questionnaire (PHIQ)
    Physical Tolerance Profile (PTP)
    Pollack-Branden Inventory (For Identification of Learning Disabilities, Dyslexia and Classroom Dysfunction
    Positive and Negative Syndrome Scale (PANSS)
    Preliminary Diagnostic Questionnaire
    Projective Assessment of Aging Method
    Psychasthenia "7" Scale
    Psychiatric Diagnostic Interview
    Psychiatric Status Rating Scales
    Psycholinguistic Rating Scale
    Psychological Distress Inventory
    Psychopathic Deviance "4" Scale
    Quality of Life Questionnaire (QLQ)
    Quality of Well-Being Scale
    Questionnaire on Resources and Stress for Families with Chronically Ill or Handicapped Members
    Quick Neurological Screening Test
    Rathus Assertiveness Scale
    Rating Scale of Communication in Cognitive Decline (RSCCD)

tests, *Neuropsychological*
- Reading Comprehension Battery for Aphasia
- Receptive-Expressive Observation Scale (REO)
- Rehabilitation Indicators (RIs)
- Reitan-Indiana Neuropsychological Test Battery for Children
- Responsibility and Independence Scale for Adolescents (RISA)
- Reynolds Adolescent Depression Scale (RADS)
- Reynolds Child Depression Scale (RCDS)
- Riley Motor Problems Inventory
- Rivermead Mobility Index
- Rogers Criminal Responsibility Scale
- Rorschach Inkblot Test
- Rule Eleven Psych Evaluation
- Russell Version Wechsler Memory Scale
- Rust Inventory of Schizotypal Cognitions
- Salamon-Conte Life Satisfaction in the Elderly Scale (LSES)
- Salience Inventory (SI)
- Scale for the Assessment of Negative Symptoms (SANS)
- Scale for the Assessment of Positive Symptoms (SAPS)
- Schizophrenia "8" Scale
- Screening Procedure for Emotional Disturbance (Draw A Person) (DAP:SPED)
- Screening Test for Developmental Apraxia of Speech
- Self-Consciousness Scale

tests, *Neuropsychological*
- Self-Description Questionnaire (SDQ)
- Self-Esteem Index (SEI)
- Sense of Coherence Questionnaire
- Sheltered Care Environment Scale
- Short Increment Sensitivity Index (SISI)
- Sickness Impact Profile Test
- Sklar Aphasia Scale
- Social and Occupational Functioning Assessment Scale (SOFAS)
- Social Interaction Scale
- Social Introversion "0" Scale
- Social Reticence Scale
- Somatic "3" Scale
- Social-Emotional Dimension Scale
- Spiritual Well-Being Scale (SWBS)
- Stanford Hypnotic Clinical Scale for Children
- Stanford Profile Scales of Hypnotic Susceptibility
- State-Trait Anger Expression Inventory
- Stone and Neale Daily Coping Assessment
- Stress Evaluation Inventory
- Stress Impact Scale (SIS)
- Stress Response Scale
- Structured Interview of Reported Symptoms (SIRS)
- Substance Abuse Questionnaire (SAQ)
- Substance Abuse Subtle Screening Inventory (SASSI)
- Suicidal Ideation Questionnaire
- Suicide Intervention Response Inventory

tests, *Neuropsychological*
   Suicide Probability Scale
   Task Assessment Scales
   Temperament and Values
     Inventory
   Test Anxiety Scale
   Test for Examining
     Expressive Morphology
     (TEEM)
   Time Perception Inventory
   Toronto Functional
     Capacity Questionnaire
     (TFCQ)
   Trait Evaluation Index
   Trites Neuropsychological
     Test Battery
   Values Scale, The
   Wakefield Self-Assessment
     Depression Inventory
   Ways of Coping Scale
   Wechsler Memory Scale
   Wechsler Scales
   Western Aphasia Batter,
     The (WAB)
   Yale-Brown Obsessive-
     Compulsive Scale
     (YBOCS)
   Zung Self-Rating
     Depression Scale
tests, *Other (e.g. career / general health / leadership)*
   Adult Career Concerns
     Inventory (ACCI)
   Armed Services Vocational
     Aptitude Battery
   Assessing Specific
     Employment Skill
     Competencies
   Assessment of Career
     Decision Making
     (ACDM)
   Campbell Leadership Index
   Career Assessment
     Inventories (For the
     Learning Disabled)
   Career Assessment
     Inventory

tests, *Other*
   Career Beliefs Inventory
     (CBI)
   Career Decision Scale
   Career Development
     Inventory
   Description of Body Scale
   Differential Aptitude Tests
     for Personnel and Career
     Assessment
   Employability Inventory,
     The
   Employee Attitude
     Inventory
   Employee Effectiveness
     Profile
   Employee Reliability
     Inventory (ERI)
   Evaluating the Participant's
     Employability Skills
   Executive Profile Survey
   Health Assessment
     Questionnaire (HAQ)
   Health Care Questionnaire
   Hogan Personnel Selection
     Series
   Index of Well-Being (IWB)
   Job Descriptive Index (JDI)
   Job Seeking Skills
     Assessment
   Leadership Ability
     Evaluation
   Leadership Practices
     Inventory (LPI)
   Leadership Skills Inventory
   Leatherman Leadership
     Questionnaire (LLQ)
   Management Development
     Profile
   Management Readiness
     Profile
   Management Styles
     Inventory
   Manager Profile Record
   Manager Style Appraisal
   Maslach Burnout Inventory
     (MBI)

tests, *Other*
- McMaster Health Index Questionnaire
- Military Environment Inventory
- Minnesota Clerical Assessment Battery
- Modified Health Assessment Questionnaire (MHAQ)
- Multifactor Leadership Questionnaire (MLQ)
- Nottingham Health Profile
- Occupational Environment Scales
- Occupational Roles Questionnaire (ORQ)
- Occupational Stress Indicator (OSI)
- Organizational Climate Index, The
- Organizational Culture Inventory (OCI)
- Personnel Selection Inventory
- Prevocational Assessment Screen (PAS)
- Professional and Managerial Position Questionnaire
- Program for Assessing Youth Employment Skills
- Retirement Descriptive Index (RDI)
- Staff Burnout Scale for Health Professionals
- Styles of Management Inventory
- Supervisory Practices Inventory
- Supervisory Profile Record
- United States Employment Service Interest Inventory
- Vocational Interest Inventory and Exploration S Survey

tests, *Other*
- Voc-Tech Quick Screener (VTQS)
- Wahler Physical Symptoms Inventory
- Work Attitudes Questionnaire (WAQ)
- Work Interest Index

tests, *Personality*
- Adolescent Multiphasic Personality Inventory
- Adult Personality Inventory (API)
- Basic Personality Inventory (BPI)
- Cattell Personality Factor Questionnaire
- Comrey Personality Scales
- Hogan Personality Inventory
- Inwald Personality Inventory (IPI)
- Maudsley Personality Inventory
- Millon Adolescent Personality Inventory
- Minnesota Multiphasic Personality Inventory (MMPI)
- Minnesota Multiphasic Personality Inventory (Adolescent) (MMPI-A)
- NEO Personality Inventory (NEO-PI)
- Personality Assessment Inventory (PAI)
- Personality Inventory for Children
- Sales Personality Questionnaire (SPQ)
- Sixteen Personality Factor Questionnaire (16PF)
- Western Personality
- Western Personality Inventory

tests, *Speech and Hearing*
- Advanced Measures of Music Audiation

tests, *Speech and Hearing*
   Arizona Articulation
     Proficiency Scale
   Assessment of
     Phonological Processes,
     The (APP)
   Central Institute for the
     Deaf Preschool
     Performance Scale
   Compton-Hutton
     Phonological Assessment
   Deep Test of Articulation
     Screening
   Elicited Articulatory
     System Evaluation
   Flowers Auditory
     Screening Test (FAST)
   Goldman-Fristoe-
     Woodcock Auditory
     Skills Battery
   Haws Screening Test for
     Functional Articulation
     Disorders
   Predictive Screening Test
     of Articulation
   Primary Measures of Music
     Audiation
   Prosody-Voice Screening
     Profile (PVSP)
   Quick Screen of Phonology
     (QSP)
   Rapidly Alternating Speech
     Perception (RASP)
   Rey Auditory Verbal
     Learning
   Rinne Hearing Conduction
   Robbins Speech Sound
     Discrimination and
     Verbal Imagery Type
   Roswell-Chall Auditory
     Blending
   Scales for Early
     Communication Skills for
     Hearing-Impaired
     Children (SECS)
   Screening Speech
     Articulation Test

tests, *Speech and Hearing*
   Screening Test for
     Auditory Comprehension
     of Language
   Screening Test for
     Auditory Perception
   Screening Test for
     Auditory Processing
     Disorders, A
   Screening Test for
     Identifying Central
     Auditory Disorders
     (SCAN)
   Speech Questionnaire
   Speech with Alternating
     Masking Index (SWAMI)
tetanic convulsion
tetism
tetrahydrocannabinol (THC)
tetrahydrocannabinolic acid
   (THCA)
tetrahydrol-soquinoline (THIQ)
Teutonomania
Teutophobia
"Tex-mex" (street name,
   cannabis)
"Texas pot" (street name,
   cannabis)
Texas Research Society on
   Alcoholism (TRSA)
"Texas tea" (street name,
   cannabis)
text
   nonobtrusive
   obtrusive
   pragmatic
textual operant
texture responses
TFCQ (Toronto Functional
   Capacity Questionnaire)
TFRT (Tactile Form Recognition
   Test)
thalamic epilepsy
thalassomania
thanatomania
THC (tetrahydrocannabinol)
THC elevation screen

THCA (tetrahydrocannabinolic
    acid)
the "blahs"
the oral-nasal acoustic ratio
    (TONAR)
theatricality
theatrophobia
Thematic Apperception Test
    (TAT)
Thematic Aptitude Test (TAT)
Thematic Content Modification
    Program (TCMP)
thematic paralogia
thematic paraphasia
thematic pictures test, complex
thematic role
themes
    grandiose
    self-derogatory
theomania
theophylline
theoretical linguistics
theoretical techniques
theory (pl. theories)
    aggressive behavior
    biolinguistic
    biolinguistic language
    decision
    double bind
    empiricist
    etiology
    frequency hearing
    freudian
    game
    hearing
    information
    innateness
    jungian
    language
    language empiricist
    language innateness
    language learning
    language mixture
    language nativist
    language rationalist
    learning
    mixture
    nativist

theory (pl. theories)
    personal construct
    place
    place hearing
    psychoanalytic
    resonance-volley
    speech innateness
    telephone (volley)
    telephone hearing
    traveling wave hearing
    violence
    volley
    volley hearing
theory in stuttering
    anticipatory and struggle
      behavior
    approach-avoidance
    breakdown
    cerebral dominance and
      handedness
    communication failure
    conditioned disintegration
    cybernetic
    diagnosogenic
    dysphemia and biochemical
    instrumental avoidance act
    laterality
    learning
    neurotic
    operant behavior
    perseverance
    primary stuttering
    repressed need
    semantic
theory of language, rationalist
Theory of Pain, Gate
theory of phonation, myoelastic-
    aerodynamic
theotromania
therapeutic action of lithium
therapeutic approaches for
    deceitfulness
therapeutic drug holiday
therapeutic error signal (TES)
therapeutic modality
therapeutic processes
therapeutic trial

therapist
    language
    music
    occupational
    physical
    speech
    voice
therapy (pl. therapies)
    adjuvant
    adolescent group
    adult group
    agonist
    behavioral
    biological
    branching steps in
    child group
    cognitive
    cognitive-behavioral
    color
    contextual
    deliberate
    diagnostic (DX)
    EMDR
    light
    myofunctional
    nondirective
    operant
    orthomolecular
    outpatient physical
    pharmacological
    precision
    programmed
    psychiatric somatic
    socioenvironmental
    speech
    symptomatic
    talk
    tongue thrust
therapy-induced mood disorder, electroconvulsive
thermal noise
thermal stimulus
therobolin (injectable steroid)
theta activity, EEG
theta index
theta rhythm
theta wave

thiamine deficiency encephalopathy (TDE)
thickened speech
"thing" (street name, cocaine; heroin; drug of choice)
thinking
    avoid
    circular
    combinative
    delusional
    difficulty
    disorganized
    distortion of inferential
    exaggeration of inferential
    futuristic
    impoverishment in
    inferential
    odd
    primary process
    suicidal
    symbolic
thinking ability, impaired
Thinking About My School
thinking and paganism, magical
Thinking Creatively in Action and Motion
"Thinking Good" Profile
thinking in schizophrenia
    distorted inferential
    exaggerated inferential
thinness, drive for
THIQ (tetrahydrol-soquinoline)
third octave filter
third position
thirst drive
"thirst monsters" (re: crack users)
"thirteen" (street name, cannabis)
thoracic respiration
thoracis, musculus iliocostalis
thorax (pl. thoraces)
thorax, iliocostal muscle of
"thoroughbred" (re: drug dealer)
thought(s)
    alien
    blasphemous
    coherent stream of
    compulsive
    considered

thought(s)
    delusional
    diminution of
    distressing
    disturbing
    fluency of
    impoverished
    intrusive
    obsessional
    persistent
    persistent inappropriate
    persistent intrusive
    productivity of
    racing
    rambling flow of
    recurrent
    repeated
    self-deprecating
    syncretic
    unacceptable
    wide circles of
thought and speech, productivity of
thought blockade
thought content
thought period, preoperational
thought processes
    bizarre
    concrete
    egocentric
thought reform
thoughts of death
threat, suicide
threat of death
threat test, visual
threatened, feeling constantly
threatening voices
3DBCT (Three-Dimensional Block Construction Test)
Three-Dimensional Block Construction Test (3DBCT)
3-factor dimensional model of schizophrenia
Three Minute Reasoning Test
3-R's Test, The
three-stage command test
three-step task

threshold
    absolute
    acoustic reflex
    audibility
    auditory
    detectability
    detection
    differential
    discomfort
    equivalent speech reception
    false
    intelligibility
    intelligible
    noise detection (NDT)
    pain
    pure tone air-conduction
    pure tone bone-conduction
    sensory
    speech awareness (SAT)
    speech detectability (SDT)
    speech detection (SDT)
    speech reception (SRT)
    taste
    tickle
    vibrotactile
threshold for speech, tolerance
threshold hearing level
threshold level, hearing (HTL)
threshold of discomfort
threshold of feeling
threshold of stimulus
threshold shift
    permanent (PTS)
    temporary (TTS)
threshold shift masking technique
threshold shift method
throat, frog in the
throat clearing
throbbing headache
throbbing pain
"thrust" (street name, isobutyl nitrite)
thrust, tongue
thrust therapy, tongue
"thrusters" (street name, amphetamine)
"thumb" (street name, cannabis)

thumb
    cerebral
    rule of
thumb position, cortical
Thurstone Temperament Schedule
thyroarytenoideus, musculus
thyroarytenoid muscle
thyroepiglottic muscle
thyroepiglotticus, musculus
thyrohyoideus, musculus
thyrohyoid muscle
thyroid cartilage
thyroid cartilage shaving
thyrotoxicosis
"tic" (street name, phencyclidine in powder form)
tic(s)
    articulatory
    complex motor
    complex vocal
    current
    facial
    motor
    past
    simple motor
    simple vocal
    vocal
    body
tic disorder
    chronic motor
    chronic vocal
    transient
    unspecified (F95.9)
"tic tac" (street name, phencyclidine/PCP)
tick-borne viral encephalitis
"ticket" (street name, lysergic acid diethylamide/LSD)
tickle threshold
ticlike behavior
tidal air
tidal volume
"tie" (re: drug injection)
TIES (The Instructional Environment Scale)
timbre
timbromania

time
    reaction
    reflex
    response
    reverberation
    sense of
    slowed reaction
    voice onset (VOT)
    voice termination (VTT)
time and motion studies
Time Compressed Speech Test
time management
time of evaluation
Time of Your Life, The
time-out (TO)
time patterning of speech (see also tests)
time patterns
time perception, alterations in
Time Perception Inventory
time preceding evaluation
time pressure
Time Problems Inventory
time sense
Time Use Analyzer
time zone change syndrome
times three, alert and oriented (A+Ox3)
timing mechanisms, endogenous abnormalities in sleep-wake
timing of sleep
TIN (Tone in Noise)
"tin" (re: cannabis container)
tin ear
tingling sensation
Tinker Toy Test
tinnitus (cocaine-related)
tip-of-the-tongue phenomenon
tiredness, chronic
"tish" (street name, phencyclidine/PCP)
"tissue" (street name, crack)
tissue, connective
tissue damage, chronic
"titch" (street name, phencyclidine/PCP)
TLA (RBH Test of Learning Ability)

TLC (Test of Language
    Competence)
TLC (total lung capacity)
TLC-C (Test of Language
    Competence for Children)
TLC Learning Preference
    Inventory
TMH (trainable mentally
    handicapped)
TMJ (temporomandibular joint)
TMJ Scale
TMR Performance Profile for the
    Severely and Moderately
    Retarded
"TNT" (street name, fentanyl;
    heroin)
TO (time out)
to-and-fro tremor
tobacco
    cigarette
    roll-your-own
    smokeless
tobacco products
tobacco-related disorder,
    unspecified (F17.209)
tobacco use disorder
    mild (Z72.0)
    moderate/severer (F17.200)
tobacco withdrawal with a
    comorbid moderate/severe
    tobacco use disorder (F17.203)
TOEFL Test of Written English
toilet training
    delayed
    lax
"toilet water" (street name,
    inhalant)
"toke" (re: cannabis use; cocaine
    use)
"toke up" (re: cannabis use)
token economy reward
token reward
Token Test for Aphasia
Token Test for Children
Token Test for Receptive
    Disturbances in Aphasia
TOLD (Tests of Language
    Development)

TOLD-I (Test of Language
    Development-Intermediate)
TOLD-P (Test of Language
    Development-Primary)
tolerance level of discomfort
tolerance of drug
tolerance or withdrawal, signs of
    substance
tolerance potential
    high
    low
tolerance range
tolerance threshold for speech
tomboy behavior
tomboyishness
tomomania
tomophobia
tonal spectrum
TONAR (the oral-nasal acoustic
    ratio)
"toncho" (re: octane booster
    which is inhaled)
tone
    complex
    difference
    emotional
    glottal
    inhibitory
    modal
    normal muscle
    partial
    pure
    simple
    warble
tone air-conduction, pure
tone air-conduction threshold,
    pure
tone audiometer
    brief (BTA)
    pure
tone average, pure
tone bone-conduction threshold,
    pure
tone control
tone deafness, low
tone decay
Tone Decay Test
tone focus, voice

Tone in Noise (TIN)
tone of feelings
tone of voice
tongue
    apex of
    bifid
    blade of the
    body of the
    dorsum of
    extrinsic muscles of the
    fasciculations of
    forked
    hypertonic
    inferior longitudinal muscle of
    intrinsic muscles of the
    muscles of the
    root of the
    superior longitudinal muscle of
    transverse muscle of
    vermiform movement of
    vertical muscle of
tongue clucking
tongue dysfunction
tongue habits
tongue height
tongue press
tongue protrusion
tongue thrust
tongue thrust therapy
tongue-tie
tongue tremor
TONI (Test of Nonverbal Intelligence)
tonic block (in stuttering)
tonic/clonic convulsion
tonic-clonic movement
tonic-clonic seizure, generalized (GTC)
tonic seizure, partial
tonometer
tonsil
    palatine
    pharyngeal
tonsillectomy
tonsillectomy and adenoidectomy (T&A)

tool, educational
"tooles" (street name, barbiturate)
"tools" (re: equipment for injecting drugs)
"toot" (re: cocaine use)
"tooties" (street name, barbiturate)
"Tootsie Roll" (street name, heroin)
"top gun" (street name, crack)
"top surgery" (euphemism for double mastectomies)
"topi" (street name, mescaline)
topic shift
    abrupt
    gradual
TOPL (Test of Pragmatic Language)
topographical agnosia
topography
"tops" (street name, mescaline)
"torch" (street name, cannabis)
"torch cooking" (re: cocaine use)
"torch up" (re: cannabis use)
Toronto Functional Capacity Questionnaire (TFCQ)
"torpedo" (street name, crack and cannabis)
torque
torsional wave
torsiversion of teeth
torticollis
torture
TOSF (Test of Oral Structures and Functions)
"toss up" (re: crack prostitute)
total cleft palate
total communication
total laryngectomy
total lung capacity
total period of illness
"totally spent" (re: methylene-dioxy-methamphetamine/MDMA hangover)
touch, loss of
touch perception

touch sensation
    light
    loss of
touched, distorted perception of being
"toucher" (re: crack user)
tough-minded tendency
Tourette disorder (F95.2)
Tourette syndrome
    neuroleptic treatment of
    childhood
    tardive
"tout" (street name, opium)
toxic action of lithium
toxic amblyopia
toxic-confusional state
toxic deafness
toxic effect of drug
toxic effects
    acute
    alcohol
    chronic
    cocaine
    hallucinogens
    narcotics
    other substances
toxic hepatitis
toxic hypoxia
toxic injury
toxic levels
toxic lithium tremor
toxic masculinity
toxic nystagmus
toxic reaction
toxic retino-neuropathy
toxic substances
toxicity
    current drug
    drug
    lithium
toxicological analysis
toxicomania
toxin-provoked amnesia
"toxy" (street name, opium)
TPLS (The Primary Language Screen)
TPS (Test of Pragmatic Skills)

"TR-6s" (street name, amphetamine)
trachea (pl. tracheae)
tracheobronchial tree
tracheoesophageal fistula, Blom-Singer
tracheotomy
tracing, I (interrupted tracing)
"track" (re: drug injection)
"tracks" (re: drug injection)
tract
    extrapyramidal
    nasal
    pyramidal
    respiratory
    vocal
trading sex
traditional feminine identity
traditional grammar
traditional masculine identity
traditional phonetic analysis
traditional society
traditional traits of femininity
traditional traits of masculinity
trafficking survivors
trafficking victims
"tragic magic" (street name, crack dipped in phencyclidine/PCP)
tragus (pl. tragi)
trailing images
"trails" (re: lysergic acid diethylamide (LSD) use)
trainer
    desk-type auditory
    frequency-modulation auditory
    hard-wire auditory
    loop-induction auditory
Trainer's Assessment of Proficiency (TAP)
training
    auditory
    autogenic
    clinical
    cognitive self-hypnosis
    cultural
    delayed toilet
    ear

training
  hypnotic relaxation
    technique
  lax toilet
  occupational skill
  social skill
  visual
  vocational
training discrimination
training units
  auditory
  speech
trait(s)
  cognitive personality
  dominant
  ego-syntonic
  interpersonal personality
  intrapsychic personality
  personality
  pervasive and persistent
    maladaptive personality
Trait Evaluation Index
trait stability, personality
trance
  amnesia after
  dissociative
  hysterical
  involuntary state of
  possession
trance disorder, dissociative
trance identification, deep
trance state, possession
trance symptom, possession
trancelike behavior
"trank" (street name,
  phencyclidine/PCP)
"tranq" (street name, barbiturate)
tranquilizer agents (major)
  acepromazine
  acetophenazine maleate
  butaperazine
  butyrophenone
  chlorpromazine
  clozapine
  Clozaril
  Etrafon
  Fluanxol
  flupenthixol

tranquilizer agents (major)
  fluphenazine decanoate
  Haldol
  haloperidol
  Largactil
  Loxapac
  loxapine
  Loxitane
  Mellaril
  mesoridazine
  methtrimeprazine
  Modecate
  Navane
  nozinan
  olanzepine
  Orap
  Permitil
  perphenazine
  phenothiazine
  pimozide
  Piportil
  pipotiazine palmitate
  prochlorperazine
  Prolixin
  promazine
  quetiapine
  Risperdal
  risperidone
  Serentil
  Stelazine
  sulpiride
  thioridizine
  thiothixene
  Thixol
  Thorazine
  trifluoperazine
  Trilafon
tranquilizer agents (minor/other)
  alprazolam
  aminophenylpyridone
  amphenidone
  Anx
  Anxanil
  Anzenet
  ataractics
  Atarax
  Ativan
  azacyclonol

tranquilizer agents (minor/other)
    benzodiazepines
    Centrax
    chlordiazepoxide
    clorazepate
    Dalmane
    diazepam
    flunitrazepam
    flurazepam
    halazepam
    hydroxyzine
    Librium
    lorazepam
    medazepam
    meprobamate
    nitrazepam
    oxazepam
    Paxipam
    prazepam
    prochlorperazine
    promazine
    Serax
    spiperone
    Tranxene
    trifluperidol
    Valium
    Xanax
transcortical aphasia
transcortical apraxia
transcortical mixed aphasia
transcortical motor aphasia
transcortical sensory aphasia
transcription
    broad
    broad phonemic
    close
    close phonetic
    narrow
    narrow phonetic
    phonemic
    phonetic
transderivational search
transducer
transducing
transfer, intersensory
transference
transference feelings
transference relationship
transferred meaning
transformational grammar, generative
Transformational Leadership Development Program
transformer
transgender
transgender orientation
transgenerational role of giving
transient amnesic
transient auditory hallucinations
transient auditory illusions
transient distortion
transient hallucinatory experience
transient ideas of reference
transient ideation
transient image
transient ischemic attack (TIA)
transient mental states
transient receptor potential ankyrin 1 (TRPA1)
transient receptor potential vanilloid 1 (TRPV1)
transient tactile hallucinations
transient tactile illusions
transient tic disorder
transient vibration
transient visual hallucinations
transient visual illusions
transillumination
transistor
transition
    life-cycle
    normal
    sleep-wake
Transition Behavior Scale (TBS)
transition process
transitional change
transitional sleep
transitional stuttering
transitory mania
translating
transmissible agent(s)
transmission of ideas by language
transmission of schizophrenia, familial
transmitted disease, sexually (STD)

transpeople
transsexual voice
transverse arytenoid muscle
transverse muscle of tongue
transverse orientation
transverse temporal gyri
transverse wave
transversion of teeth
transversus, musculus arytenoideus
transversus linguae, musculus
transvestic disorder (F65.1)
transvestic disorder with autogynephilia (F65.1)
transvestic disorder with fetishism (F65.1)
transvestic fetishism
transvestic phenomena
transvestic subculture
"trap" (re: drug concealment)
trauma
    acoustic
    aftermath of
    brain
    cerebral
    closed head
    craniocerebral
    extreme
    head
    occult head
    original
    physical
    recollection of
    reexperiencing the
trauma and PTSD, early-age
trauma- and stress-related disorder
    other specified (F43.8)
    unspecified (F43.9)
trauma deafness, acoustic
trauma effects on soldiers in combat
trauma-induced delirium
trauma in women, vulnerability to
trauma-specific reenactment
Trauma Symptom Checklist for Children Ages 8-15
traumatic anesthesia

traumatic brain injury (TBI)
    dementia due to
    diffuse, with loss of consciousness, of unspecified duration, sequela with behavioral disturbance (S06.2X9S) and (F02.81)
    diffuse, with loss of consciousness of unspecified duration, sequela without behavioral disturbance (S06.2X9S) and (F02.80)
traumatic cataracts
traumatic dementia
traumatic encephalopathy, progressive
traumatic epilepsy
    early
    late
traumatic event, reexperienced
traumatic experience, unconscious processing of
traumatic headache
traumatic injury
traumatic loss
traumatic seizure
traumatic stress, serious

traumatic themes through repetitive play, expression of
"travel agent" (street name, LSD supplier)
traveling wave hearing theory
"trays" (re: drug containers)
treat, refusal to
treatment
    active
    adequate
    antidepressant
    appropriate
    change in
    cognitive-behavioral
    communication/cognition
    complications of
    course of

treatment
    daily
    diet
    educational
    exercise
    expense of
    factors that interfere with
    family
    focus of
    institution of
    medical
    need for
    need for prophylactic
    neuroleptic *(see also* tests)
    noncompliance with
    nutrition
    pharmacological
    pharmacotherapeutic
    postpartum counseling and addition
    prenatal counseling and addition
    prescribed
    proposed
    psychodynamic *(see also* tests)
    psychopharmacological
    psychosocial
    psychotherapeutic *(see also* tests)
    rehabilitation
    residential
    side effects of
    somatic
    specific
    symptomatic
    ultrasound
treatment for depression, somatic
treatment for personality disorders, drug
treatment for schizophrenia, neuroleptics as
treatment for sexual disorders, drug
treatment for the elderly, drug
treatment frequency
treatment of childhood autism, neuroleptic
treatment of childhood conduct disorders, neuroleptic
treatment of childhood schizophrenia, neuroleptic
treatment of childhood Tourette's syndrome, neuroleptic
treatment of dementia, pharmacological
treatment of recurrent suicidal behavior
treatment program
treatment refusal
treatment response
treatment selection
tree, tracheobronchial
tree diagram, branching
trees, decision
trembling (panic attack specifier)
trembling voice
tremor
    action
    anticonvulsant medication-induced postural
    antidepressant medication-induced postural
    benign essential
    beta-adrenergic medication-induced postural
    caffeine-induced postural
    cerebral outflow
    coarse
    counting-money
    cps (cycle per second)
    dopaminergic medication-induced postural
    dystonic
    emotional stress precipitating
    end point
    essential
    essential cerebellar
    essential cerebral
    facial
    factors to increase
    familial
    fine postural
    flapping

tremor
    hand
    head and neck
    hepatic encephalophy
    heredofamilial
    hysterical
    increased hand
    intentional
    kinetic
    lip
    lithium-induced postural
    medication-induced postural
    medication-induced postural (G25.1)
    metabolic
    methylxanthime-induced postural
    neuroleptic medication-induced postural
    neuroleptic-induced Parkinson
    neuroleptic-induced postural
    non-neuroleptic-induced
    no-no
    nonparkinsonian
    nonpharmacologically induced
    nontoxic lithium
    oscillating
    parkinsonian
    perioral
    physiologic
    physiological
    pill-rolling
    positional
    postural
    preexisting
    progressive cerebellar
    rest
    resting
    rhythmic
    rubral
    senile
    shaking
    small-amplitude rapid
    static

tremor
    stimulant-induced postural
    striatocerebral
    substance withdrawal
    sustention/intention
    terminal
    to-and-fro
    tongue
    toxic lithium
    valproate-induced postural
    vocal
    voice
    volitional
    writing
    yes-yes
tremor from cerebellar disease
tremulous cerebral palsy (CP)
tremulous movement
tremulous speech
trends
    anxiety
    phobic
trial
    placebo medication
    standing
    therapeutic
trial of dosage reduction
trials, field
triangular wave
trichomania
trichophagia
trichorrhexomania
trichotillomania (hair-pulling) disorder (F63.3)
trichotillomania-induced alopecia
tricuspid valve disease
tricyclic antidepressant
tricyclic antidepressants for mood disorders
tridecaphobia
trigeminal (cranial nerve V)
trigeminal neuralgia
trigger an obsession
triggering mechanism
triggering stimulus
trill consonant formation
trim of the adenoid, lateral

"trip" (re: lysergic acid diethylamide/LSD use)
"trip" (street name, alpha-ethyltyptamine; lysergic acid diethylamide/LSD)
triphthong
"trippier" (re: more intoxicating)
trismus
tristimania
Trites Neuropsychological Test Battery
TROCA (tangible reinforcement of operant conditioning audiometry)
trochaic stress
trochlear (cranial nerve IV)
tromomania
"troop" (street name, crack)
trophobolene (re: injectable steroid)
troubling experience
trough curve audiogram configurations
trough level, peak
Troxyca ER (oxycodone/naltrexone)
TRPA1 (transient receptor potential ankyrin 1)
TRPV1 (transient receptor potential vanilloid 1)
TRSA (Texas Research Society on Alcoholism)
truancy, school
"truck drivers" (street name, amphetamine)
true amnesia
true belief
true folds, polypoid degenerative of the
true language
true perception
true vertigo
true vocal folds
truncation, predicate
truth disclosure
T-score range
TSRI (Teacher's School Readiness Inventory)
"TT 1" (street name, phencyclidine/PCP)
"TT 2" (street name, phencyclidine/PCP)
"TT 3" (street name, phencyclidine/PCP)
TTMAD (Testing-Teaching Module of Auditory Discrimination)
TTO (Test of Temporal Orientation)
tube
    auditory
    eustachian
    tympanotomy
    ventilation
tube microphone, probe
tubercle, acoustic
tuberosa, chorditis
tuberous sclerosis
tubular acidosis
    distal renal
    proximal renal
tubular vision
"tuie" (street name, barbiturate)
tumescence, penile
tumescence study, nocturnal penile
tumor
    brain
    brain stem
    dementia due to brain
    eighth nerve
tunnel vision
turbinate bone
    medial
    superior
    supreme
turbinated skull bone
    inferior
    medial
    superior
"turbo" (street name, crack and cannabis)
turbulence, nasal
"turf" (re: drug-buying place)
"turkey" (street name, amphetamine; cocaine)

Turkomania
turmoil, emotional
turn technique, head
"turnabout" (street name, amphetamine)
"turned on" (re: introduced to drugs; drug influence)
TUSSI (Temple University Short Syntax Inventory)
"tutti-frutti" (street name, flavored cocaine)
twang, nasal
"tweak" (street name, methamphetamine-like substance)
"tweak mission" (re: crack acquisition)
"tweaker" (re: crack user; methamphetamine user; methcathinone)
"tweaking" (re: drug-induced paranoia; amphetamine use)
Twelve Step Program
"twenty" (re: $20 rock of crack)
"twenty-five" (street name, lysergic acid diethylamide/LSD)
21-trisomy syndrome, chromosome
TWF (Test of Word Finding)
TWFD (Test of Word Finding in Discourse)
twilight state
twin language
twirling of objects, nonfunctional and repetitive
"twist" (street name, cannabis cigarette)
twist, octave
"twistum" (street name, cannabis cigarette)
twitch/twitching
    facial
    focal
    involuntary
    muscle
    rhythmical
"two for nine" (re: two $5 vials of crack for $9)
two-tones voice
tympani, scala
tympanogram classification (Feldman model)
tympanogram classification (Jerger model)
tympanophonia
tympanoplasty
tympanostomy
tympanotomy tube
type
    blood-injection-injury
    catatonic
    disinhibited
    inhibited
    natural environment
    other
    sentence
    sexual encounters
    situational
    with poor insight
type of symptom
    mixed
    motor
    seizure
    sensory
type of speech, cerebellar scanning
typical absence seizure
typical age
typical seizure
typomania
tyramine challenge test
tyrannical decision making

U

"U-4" (street name, synthetic opioid)
U-47700 (designer drug; synthetic opioid)
ubiquitous glottal stop
UCL (uncomfortable loudness level)
"ugly" body parts
ulcer
    contact
    psychogenic duodenal
    psychogenic gastric
    psychogenic peptic
"ultimate" (street name, crack)
ultrasonic frequency
ultrasound treatment
umbo
unable to control
unable to function
unacceptable actions
unacceptable feelings
unacceptable thoughts
unaided augmentative communication
unavailability or inaccessibility of health care facilities (Z75.3)
unavailability or inaccessibility of other helping agencies (Z75.3)
unawareness of environment, complete
unbecoming
unbiased information
uncinate convulsion
uncinate seizure
"uncle" (re: Federal agents)
"Uncle Milty" (street name, barbiturate)
uncomfortable loudness level (UCL)
uncomplicated bereavement (Z63.4)
unconditioned reinforcer
unconditioned response
unconditioned stimulus
unconscious, collective
unconscious concern
unconscious conflict
unconscious homosexuality
unconscious process
unconscious processing of affective experience
unconscious processing of dissociative states and disorders
unconscious processing of traumatic experience
unconscious rage
unconsciousness conversion
uncontrollable action
uncontrollable sleep attacks
uncoordinated gait
uncoupling, nasal
uncued behavior
under control
    behavior is
    emotions are
underbite malposition of teeth
undercontrol
    behavioral
    emotional
underextension
underlip
underlying emotional issues, preexisting
underlying structure
undermasking
underproductive speech
undersocialized conduct disorder
    aggressive type
    unaggressive type
undersocialized reaction
    aggressive type
    unaggressive type
undersocialized runaway reaction
undersocialized socialized disturbance
    aggressive type
    unaggressive type

understanding
    shared
    speech
    word (WU)
Understanding and Managing
    Stress (see also tests)
understanding of similarities test
understatement (figure of speech)
understatement, environmental
understimulating environment,
    academically
understimulation, environmental
undescended testicle
undetermined origin (UO)
undifferential type schizophrenia
undifferentiated schizophrenia
undisturbed nocturnal sleep
undoing (defense mechanism)
undue social anxiety
unemployment
unethical behavior
unexpected behavior
unexpected death
unexpected (uncued) panic attacks
unexpected response
unexplained absence from work,
    pattern of
unexplained pain
unfilled pauses in speech
ungiving parent
unhappiness, patterns of pervasive
uniformly progressive
    deterioration
unilateral abductor paralysis
unilateral adductor paralysis
unilateral cleft lip
unilateral cleft palate
unilateral focus
unilateral headache
unilateral migraine headache
unilateral neglect
unilateral organic neglect
unilateral paralysis
unilateral seizure
unilateral spatial neglect
unilateral visual neglect
unimodal
unintelligible speech

unintended consequences
unintended effect
unintended sleep
unintentional daytime sleep
    episodes
unintentionally produced
    symptoms
uninterrupted period of illness
unipolar depression, gender
    differences in
unisensory
unit(s)
    addictive disease (ADU)
    auditory training
    family
    intensive care (ICU)
    intensive treatment (ITU)
    life change (LCU)
    loudness
    maximum security
    psychiatric intensive
        (PICU)
    relational
    sensation (SU)
    speech training
unit clerk (UC)
unit meter, volume (VU meter)
unit restriction (UR)
United States Employment
    Service Interest Inventory
    (USES)
United States Pharmacopeia
    (USP)
United States Public Health
    Service (USPHS)
universal grammar
universal quantifier
universality
universals
    formal
    language
    substantive
universals theory, linguistic
unjustified doubts of loyalty
unjustified doubts of
    trustworthiness
unkempt appearance
unkempt manner

"unkie" (street name, morphine)
unknown substance-induced
    mood disorder
unlawful behavior
unmet dependency needs
unmet needs
unmitigated echolalia
unpleasant hallucination
unpredictable agitation
unpredictable mood changes
unproductive mania
unprotected sex
unpublished data sets
unpurposeful behavior
unreactive pupils
unreasonable belief
unreasonable demand
unreasonable fear
unreasonable idea
unrefreshing sleep
unresolved conflict
unresponsive patient
unresponsive state
unrounded vowel
unsanctioned response, culturally
unspecified bipolar I disorder
unspecified psychological factors
unspecified type delusions
unspecified type dyssomnia
unspecified type personality
    disorder
unstable affect, pattern of
unstable attachments
unstable personality disorder
unstable relationship
unstable self-image, pattern of
unsteadiness (a panic attack
    indicator)
unsteady gait
unstressed syllable deletion
unstressed vowel
untreated episode
untriggered agitation
unusual case
unusual manner
unusual sexual behavior
unusual sleep postures
unvoiced speech

unwanted child
unwanted pregnancy
unwarranted idea
unwillingness to speak
"up against the stem" (re:
    cannabis addiction)
"up in the clouds"
upbringing away from parents
    (Z62.89)
upper bound
upper limit of age at onset
upper partial
upper respiratory infection (URI)
"uppies" (street name,
    amphetamine)
"ups and downs" (street name,
    barbiturate)
upset
        emotionally
        excessively
        mental
upward masking
UR (unit restriction)
uranoplasty
uranoschisis
urban psychiatry
uremic convulsion
urethral stenosis
urges
        intense sexual
        masochistic sexual
        persistent inappropriate
        persistent intrusive
        sexual
URI (upper respiratory infection)
urinary incontinence
urinary retention
urinary stream, misdirected
urinary symptoms with other
    specified elimination disorder
    (N39.498)
urinary symptoms with unspeci-
    fied elimination disorder (R32)
urination
        during
        pain public
urine drug screen
urine for drug screen test

usage doctrine
use
    drug
    language
use disorder
    alcohol
    amphetamine
    anxiolytic
    cannabis
    cocaine
    hallucinogen
    hypnotic
    inhalant
    nicotine
    opioid
    other or unknown
    PCP (phencyclidine)
    psychoactive substance
    sedative
    substance
use index, drug
use of aliases
used drug-injecting equipment
users, injection drug
USES (United States Employment Service)
U-shaped curve audiogram configurations
Usher's syndrome
"using" people
USP (United States Pharmacopeia)
usual activities, decreased interest in
Utah Test of Language Development (UTLD)
uteromania
utility
    clinical
    expected (EU)
UTLD (Utah Test of Language Development)
"utopiates" (street name, LSD; hallucinogens)
utricle
utterance
    holophrastic
    mean length of (MLU)
utterance
    mean relational (MRU)
    polymorphemic
    telegraphic
uvula (pl. uvulae)
uvulae, musculus
uvular muscle
"uzi" (re: crack equipment)

V

"V" (Valium)
V, Conversion (MMPI)
VA domiciliary
VABS (Vineland Adaptive Behavior Scales)
vacuous affect
vaginal lubrication
vaginal stricture
vaginismus
    acquired type
    generalized type
    lifelong type
    situational type
vaginismus due to combined factors
vaginismus due to psychological factors
vague speech
vagus (cranial nerve X)
vagus nerve
validating variables
validity
    descriptive
    discriminate
    factorial
valproate-induced postural tremor
valproic acid for mood disorders
value
    educational
    high
    idealized
    monetary
    nontrivial
    personal
    prognostic
    sentimental
value judgment
Value of Imitative and Auditory Discrimination Tests, Prognostic
values
    sharing of
    social
Values Scale, The
values survey of personal traits *(see also* tests)
values survey of work habits *(see also* tests)
valve, velopharyngeal
valve disease
    rheumatic pulmonary
    tricuspid
vape
vape cartridge
vape juice
vape oil
vape pen
vapers
vaping
vaping, teen
vapors, method of inhaling intoxicating
variable interval reinforcement schedule
variable ratio reinforcement schedule
variables
    preexisting cognitive
    validating
variant seizure, petit mal
variation(s)
    free
    linguistic
    phonetic
    physiological functional
VASC (Verbal-Auditory Screen for Children) test
vascular dementia
vascular disease, peripheral
vascular headache
vascular system, peripheral
vascular-type headache
vasculogenic loss of erectile functioning
vasocongestion of pelvis
vasomotor headache

(VAT)Vocational Apperception Test)
VC (vital capacity)
V-C (vowel-consonant)
VCDQ (Verbal Comprehension Deviation Quotient)
VD (venereal disease)
VDRS (Verdun Depression Rating Scale)
VE (vocational evaluation) *(see also* tests)
vegetative state, persistent (PVS)
vela (sing. velum)
velar area consonant placement
velar assimilation
velar insufficiency
velar tail
velarized consonant
velars, backing to
veli palatine
    musculus levator
    musculus tensor
velocity, particle
velopharyngeal closure
velopharyngeal competence
velopharyngeal incompetence
velopharyngeal insufficiency
velopharyngeal port
velopharyngeal valve
velum (pl. vela)
vented earmold
ventilation, impaired
ventilation during sleep, impaired
ventilation tube
ventilatory control
ventral cochlear nucleus
ventricle, sinus of the
ventricular dysphonia
ventricular fold
ventricular function
ventricular phonation
ventriculus laryngis
VEP (visual evoked potential)
VEP brain test
VER (visual evoked response)
VER brain test

verb (parts of speech)
    auxiliary
    helping
    linking
    modal
    modal auxiliary
    secondary
verbal aphasia
verbal apraxia
verbal auditory agnosia
Verbal Auditory Screen for Children test (VASC)
verbal behavior
verbal communication
Verbal Comprehension Deviation Quotient (VCDQ)
verbal comprehension factor (V factor)
verbal expression
verbal fluency
verbal imagery test *(see also* tests)
Verbal Intelligence quotient (VIQ)
Verbal I.Q. Score
Verbal Language Development Scale (VLDS)
verbal language quotient
verbal learning
verbal learning test *(see also* tests)
verbal mediation
verbal memory
verbal, numerical, and reasoning (V,N,R)
verbal operant
verbal paraphasia
verbal paraphrasis
Verbal Perceptual Speed
verbal play
verbal reinforcement
verbal scale (VS)
Verbal Scale Scores
verbal technique
verbal tests *(see also* tests)
verbal visual agnosia
verbalization of feelings
verbalizations
    paucity of
    sparsity of

Verbalizer-Visualization Questionnaire (VVQ)
verbally mediated function
verbally mediated skills
verbatim
verbigeration
verbomania
verborum, delirium
verbotonal method
verbous
verb phrase
Verdun Depression Rating Scale (VDRS)
veridical dream
vermicular movements
vermiform movement of tongue
vermillion border
vernacular
Vernet syndrome
vertebrobasilar insufficiency
vertical canal
    anterior
    posterior
vertical-gaze palsy
vertical muscle of tongue
vertical nystagmus
vertical-gaze palsy
verticalis linguae, musculus
vertiginous seizure
vertigo
    labyrinthine
    true
very deep sleep
very light sleep
vestibular canal
vestibular folds
vestibular function, caloric stimulation test for
vestibular hydrops
vestibular membrane
vestibular migraine headache
vestibular movement
vestibular window
vestibule
vestibuli
    fenestra
    scala
vestibulocochlear nerve

Veterans Administration (VA, V Adm.)
Veterans Hospital (VH)
veterinary steroid
    abolic
    dianabol
    equipose
    finajet/finaject
    parabolin
    winstrol V
VEWA (Vocational Evaluation and Work Adjustment)
V factor (verb comprehension factor)
VFDT (Visual Form Discrimination Test)
VH (Veterans Hospital)
VI (visual imagery)
VIB (Vocational Interest Blank)
vibrant consonant
vibration
    forced
    free
    glottal
    sympathetic
    symptomatic
    transient
vibration meter
vibration sensation
vibrato
vibrator, bone-conduction
vibratory cycle
vibrometer
vibrotactile aids
vibrotactile hearing aid
vibrotactile response
vibrotactile threshold
VIBS (vocabulary, information, block design similarities)
VIC (Values Inventory for Children)
vicarious trial and error (VTE)
vice-like pain
vicious cycle
victim
    condition of
    intended
    rape

Psychiatric Words and Phrases

victim abuse
victim of adult physical abuse by nonspouse or nonpartner
victim of adult psychological abuse by nonspouse or nonpartner
victim of adult sexual abuse by nonspouse or nonpartner
victim of child neglect
victim of crime (Z65.4)
victim of non-parental child abuse
victim of parental child abuse
victim of spousal or partner neglect
victim of spousal or partner violence
victim of terrorism or torture (Z65.4)
victim role
victim's condition
VIESA (Vocational Interest, Experience, and Skill Assessment)
view
    intropunitive
    Pollyanna-like
    psychobiological
vigilance
Vineland Adaptive Behavior Scales (VABS)
violation of age-appropriate societal norms
violation of rules, serious
violation of the rights of others, pattern of
violations
    nonsexual boundary
    sexual boundary
violations in psychoanalysis, boundary
violence
    alcohol-related risk for
    alleviating
    domestic (D-V)
    drug-related
    family
    management of
    medical management of

violence
    multidisciplinary management of
    spouse or partner
    theories of
    workplace
violence as major childhood stressor
violence in aggressive behavior alleviating
violent acts
violent agitation
violent behavior
violent death
violent outbursts
violent personal assault
"viper's weed" (street name, cannabis)
VIQ (Verbal Intelligence Quotient)
VIQ (Vocational Interest Questionnaire) *(see also* tests)
viral encephalitis
    arthropod-borne
    Australian X
    biundulant
    California
    Central European
    Czechoslovakian
    diphasic meningoencephalitis
    eastern equine
    Far Eastern
    Ilheus
    Japanese B
    Langat
    louping ill
    mosquito-borne
    Murray Valley
    other
    Powassan
    Russian spring-summer
    slow-acting
    St. Louis
    tick-borne
    western equine
viral encephalopathy
viral meningitis

Virgin Mary visions
virgules
virtual consult program
virtual program training in mental health
virtual therapy sessions
VIS (vocational interest schedule)
VISA (Vocational Interest and Sophistication Assessment)
visage, scanning
viscera (sing. viscus)
visceral disorder
visceral nervous system
visceral swallowing
visible speech
Visible Speech, Bell's
vision
    altered
    blurred
    blurring of
    darkening of
    double
    entopic
    foveal
    hemifield of
    impaired
    loss of
    sudden loss of
    tubular
    tunnel
    Virgin Mary
vision assessment *(see also* tests)
vision disparity
vision test, wall chart
visit
    trial home
    weekend
vista responses
visual agnosia
    apperceptive
    associative
    verbal
visual area
Visual-Auditory Screening Test for Children (VASC)
visual aura
Visual Aural Digit Span test (VADS)
visual blurring
visual center
visual choice reaction time test
visual cue
visual discrimination
visual disorders
visual disturbance
visual epilepsy
visual evoked potential (VEP)
visual evoked response (VER)
visual evoked response test
visual field construction
visual field cut
visual field defects
visual field disturbance
visual field exam
visual field test
visual figure-ground discrimination
Visual Form Discrimination Test (VFDT)
visual form of Wernicke aphasia
visual functioning test *(see also* tests)
visual hallucination
    formed
    transient
    unformed
visual hearing
visual illusions, transient
visual image, persistence of
visual impairment
visual information with motor activity, disturbance in integrating
visual letter dysgnosia
visual listening
visual loss
    complete
    hysterical
    partial
visual memory test *(see also* tests)
visual method
visual-motor coordination
visual-motor integration test *(see also* tests)
visual-motor tasks
visual neglect, unilateral

Visual Neglect Test
visual obstruction
visual organization test *(see also* tests)
Visual Pattern Completion Test
visual pattern recognition
visual perception
visual perception test *(see also* tests)
visual prodrome
visual pursuit movement
visual radiation
Visual Reinforcement Audiometry
visual retention test *(see also* tests)
Visual Search and Attention Test (VSAT)
visual seizure
visual sensations, distorted perception of
visual sensory modality
visual-spatial acalculia
visual-spatial distortion
visual-spatial memory
visual stimulation
visual stimulus
visual symptoms
Visual-Tactile System of Phonetic Symbolization
visual threat test
visual training
visual verbal agnosia
visualized
visuo-spatial disorders
visuo-spatial disorientation
visuo-spatial problem solving
visuo-spatial processing
vital capacity (VT)
vital energy
vitamin B12 deficiency
vitamin deficiencies, dementia due to
vitamin deficiency
"vitamin K" (street name, designer drug; ketamine; dissociative hallucinogen)
"vitamin Q" (street name, depressant)
"vitamin R" (street name, Ritalin; stimulant)
vivid dream image
vivid dream recall
Vivitrol (naltrexone)
VLDS (Verbal Language Development Scale)
VMGT (Visual-Motor Gestalt Test)
VMI (Visual-Motor Integration
VMIT (Visual-Motor Integration Test)
VMS (Visual Memory Score)
VMS (visual memory span)
VMST (Visual-Motor Sequencing Test)
V,N,R (verbal, numerical, reasoning)
vocabulary, core
Vocabulary Comprehension Scale
vocabulary placement test *(see also* tests)
vocabulary scale *(see also* tests)
vocabulary screening test *(see also* tests)
vocabulary test *(see also* tests)
vocal abuse
vocal attack
vocal bands
vocal behavior, abusive
vocal constriction
vocal cords
vocal efficiency
vocal effort
vocal fatigue
vocal focus
vocal fold approximation
vocal fold paralysis
vocal folds
    bowed
    false
    true
vocal fry
vocal mode
vocal muscle

vocal nodules
    polypoid
    sessile
vocal organs
vocal phonics
vocal pitch abnormality
vocal play
vocal production, constricted
vocal range
vocal register
vocal rehabilitation
vocal resonance
vocal tic disorder
    chronic
    chronic motor or
vocal tics
    complex
    simple
vocal tract
vocal tremor
vocalic feature English phoneme
vocalic glide
vocalis, musculus
vocalization, nonrhythmic stereotyped motor
Vocational Apperception Test (VAT) *(see also* tests)
vocational environment
vocational evaluation (VE) *(see also* tests)
Vocational Evaluation and Work Adjustment (VEWA)
vocational functioning, stability of
vocational guidance
Vocational Interest and Sophistication Assessment (VISA)
Vocational Interest Blank (VIB)
Vocational Interest Inventory and Exploration Survey
Vocational Interest Questionnaire (VIQ)
vocational interest schedule (VIS)
vocational interests test *(see also* tests)
Vocational Learning Styles (LSV2)
Vocational Opinion Index (VOI)
Vocational Planning Inventory (VPI)
Vocational Preference Inventory (VPI)
vocational rehabilitation (VR)
vocational rehabilitation and education (VR&E)
Vocational Rehabilitation Services (VRS)
vocational situations
vocational strain
vocational test *(see also* tests)
vocational training
Voc-Tech Quick Screener (VTQS)
"vodka acid" (street name, lysergic acid diethylamide/LSD)
VOI (Vocational Opinion Index)
voice(s)
    active
    adolescent
    altered
    chest
    dysphoric
    esophageal
    eunuchoid
    falsetto
    gravel
    guttural
    hearing God's
    inspiratory
    light
    muffled
    mutation
    passive
    pejorative
    pulsated
    shaking
    shaky
    threatening
    tone of
    transsexual
    trembling
    two-tones
voice audiometry
    live
    monitored live

voice clinician
"voice commenting"
voice disorder
    cul de sac
    denasality
    hypernasality
    hyperrhinolalia
    hyperrhinophonia
    mixed nasality
    rhinolalia aperta
    rhinolalia clause
voice disorder of assimilated nasality
voice disorder of phonation *(see also* tests)
voice disorder of resonance
voice fatigue
voice hostility
voice instructions
voice murmuring
voice onset time (VOT)
voice pathologist
voice register
voice shift
voice termination time (VTT)
voice therapist
voice tone focus
voice tremor
voiced consonant
voiced feature English phoneme
voiceless consonant
voicing, consonant
voicing of consonants, prevocalic
volition, hedonic
volitional drinking
volitional movement
volitional oral movement
volitional tremor
volley hearing theory
volley theory
volt
volume
    air
    expiratory reserve (ERV)
    inspiratory reserve (IRV)
    lung
    residual (RV)
    respiratory

volume control
    automatic (AVC)
    manual
volume depletion, metabolic
volume unit meter (VU meter)
voluntary hysterical overbreathing
voluntary motor functioning
voluntary movement peculiarities
voluntary muscle movement
voluntary napping phenomenon, normal
voluntary overbreathing, hysterical
voluntary sensory functioning
vomer skull bone
vomiting throughout pregnancy
"voodoo death"
VOT (Hooper Visual Organization Test, The)
VOT (voice onset time)
vowel
    back
    cardinal
    central
    close
    front
    high
    indefinite
    interconsonantal
    lax
    light
    low
    mid
    narrow
    neutral
    obscure
    open
    postconsonantal
    pure
    retroflex
    rhotacised
    rounded
    tense
    unrounded
    unstressed
vowel assimilation, progressive
vowel-consonant syllable
vowel neutralization

vowel quadrilateral
vowelization *(see also* tests)
vowels
    cardinal
    nasalization of
voyeuristic activity
voyeuristic behavior
voyeuristic disorder (F65.3)
voyeuristic sexual behavior
voyeuristic sexually arousing fantasy
VPI (Vocational Planning Inventory)
VPI (Vocational Preference Inventory)
VR (vocational rehabilitation)
VR&E (vocational rehabilitation)
VR&E (vocational rehabilitation and education)
VRS (Vocational Rehabilitation Services)
VS (verbal scale) *(see also* tests)
VS (vital signs)
VSAT (Visual Search and Attention Test)
VSMS (Vineland Social Maturity Scale)
V_T (tidal volume)
VTE (vicarious trial and error)
VTQS (Voc-Tech Quick Screener) *(see also* tests)
VTT (vocal termination time)
vulgar language
vulnerability
    genetic
    narcissistic
vulnerability to life's stressors
vulnerability to psychosis, inherent
vulnerability to trauma in women
Vulpé Assessment Battery
VU meter (volume unit meter)
VVQ (Verbalizer-Visualization Questionnaire)
Vygotsky Concept Formation Test

W-1/W-2 Auditory Tests
W-22 Auditory Test
WAB (Western Aphasia Battery)
"wac" (street name, phencyclidine or cannabis)
Wachs Analysis of Cognitive Structures
"wack" (street name, phencyclidine/PCP)
"wacky weed" (street name, cannabis)
waddling gait
"wafers" (street name, club drug; ecstasy/MDMA; stimulant)
"waffle dust" (street name, club drug; re: combined MDMA and amphetamine; timulant)
"wagon wheels" (street name, methaqualone)
Wahler Physical Symptoms Inventory *(see also* tests)
WAIS (Wechsler Adult Intelligence Scale)
WAIS Block Design Test
Wakefield Self-Assessment Depression Inventory *(see also* tests)
wakeful state
wakefulness
    identifiable pattern of sleep and
    intermittent
    repeated sustained sleep and
    state of full
    subjective sensation of
wakefulness epochs
wakefulness quiet
wakefulness resting
waking EEG

waking frequency, dominant
Walker-McConnell Scale of Social Competence and School Adjustment
wall, alveolar
wall chart vision test
wandering associated with a mental disorder (Z91.83)
WAQ (Work Attitudes Questionnaire)
war, prisoner of (POW)
war-related complex adaptation
war-related lack of self-compassion
war-related moral injury
war-related stress
war-related traumatic loss
warble tone
warm-wire anemometer
warn, duty to
washing, brain
wastage, air
"wasted" (re: drug influence; murdered)
"water" (street name, methamphetamine; phencyclidine/PCP)
water, body
water balance in schizophrenia
water deprivation
water intoxication
waterfall curve audiogram configurations
watershed area
watt
"wave" (street name, crack)
wave
    alpha
    aperiodic
    beta
    complex
    cosine
    damped
    delta
    diffracted
    electromagnetic
    incident
    Jewett

wave
    longitudinal
    negative spike
    nonperiodic
    notched
    periodic
    pure
    reflected
    refracted
    simple
    sine
    sinusoidal
    slow
    sound
    sound pressure
    standing
    theta
    torsional
    transverse
    triangular
wave activity, brain
wave filter
wave hearing theory, traveling
wave of excitation
wave on EEG, beta
wave strains, alpha
waveform distortion
wavelength
waves, six Hertz positive spike
waveshape
waving, nonfunctional and repetitive hand
wax weak stress
Ways of Coping Scale
weak parent
weak syllable deletion
weakness, localized
weakness of an extremity
wearing-off effect of drugs
web, laryngeal
webbing
Weber Test
Wechsler Adult Intelligence Scale (WAIS)
Wechsler Intelligence Scale for Children (WISC)
Wechsler Memory Scale (WMS)
Wechsler Scales

"wedding bells" (street name, lysergic acid diethylamide/LSD)
"wedge" (street name, lysergic acid diethylamide/LSD)
"weed" (street name, phencyclidine/PCP)
"weed tea" (street name, cannabis)
weekend headache
weight, body
weight-control program
weight fluctuations
weight gain, prevention of
weight loss, method of
weight-loss aids
weight perception
"weightless" (re: crack influence)
Weiss Comprehensive Articulation Test
Weiss Intelligibility Test
Welch Allyn AudioScope
well-being, exaggerated feeling of
well-being
    feeling of
    sensation of
well-being index *(see also* tests)
well-being scale *(see also* tests)
well-formed outcome
Weller-Strawser Scales of Adaptive Behavior for the Learning
Welsh Figure Preference Test
Wernicke aphasia, visual form of
Wernicke area 22, 39, 40
Wernicke-Korsakoff encephalopathy
WES (Work Environment Scale)
Wesman Personnel Classification Test
Western Aphasia Battery (WAB)
western equine viral encephalitis
Western Personality Inventory *(see also* tests)
Western Personnel Tests *(see also* tests)
wet hoarseness
Wever-Bray phenomenon

"whack" (street name, phencyclidine and heroin)
"wheat" (street name, cannabis)
"when-shee" (street name, opium)
whipping
whisper
    buccal
    forced
    soft
    stage
whispering, involuntary
"white" (street name, amphetamine)
"white ball" (street name, crack)
"white boy" (street name, heroin)
"white cloud" (street name, crack smoke)
"white cross" (street name, amphetamine; methamphetamine)
"white diamonds" (street name, ecstasy/MDMA; stimulant)
"white dove" (street name, ecstasy/MDMA; stimulant)
"white dragon" (street name, cocaine; heroin)
"white dust" (street name, lysergic acid diethylamide/LSD)
"white ghost" (street name, crack)
"white girl" (street name, cocaine; heroin)
"white-haired lady" (street name, cannabis)
"white horizon" (street name, phencyclidine/PCP)
"white horse" (street name, cocaine)
"white junk" (street name, heroin)
"white knuckling" sobriety
"white lady" (street name, cocaine; heroin)
"white lightning" (street name, LSD; hallucinogen)
white matter
    long spinal
    periventricular
    subcortical
white matter (of CNS)
white matter diseases
"white mosquito" (street name, cocaine)
white noise
"white nothing" (street name, ecstasy/MDMA; stimulant)
"white nurse" (street name, heroin)
"white Owsley's" (street name, lysergic acid diethylamide/LSD)
"white powder" (street name, cocaine; phencyclidine/PCP)
"White Russian" (street name, cannabis)
"white stick" (street name, crack cocaine)
"white stuff" (street name, heroin; opioid)
"white sugar" (street name, crack)
"white tiger" (street name, synthetic cannabis)
"white tornado" (street name, crack)
"whiteout" (street name, isobutyl nitrite)
"whiz bang" (street name, cocaine and heroin)
WHO (World Health Organization)
WHO–DAS (WHO Disability Assessment Schedule)
whole word repetition, monosyllabic
wide-band noise
wide-based gait
wide circles of thoughts
Wide Range Achievement Test (WRAT) *(see also* tests)
Wide Range Assessment of Memory and Learning
wide range audiometer
wide-set eyes
widowhood
"wild cat" (street name, methcathinone and cocaine)
Willis paracusis

window
    cochlear
    oval
    round
    vestibular
"window glass" (street name, lysergic acid diethylamide/LSD)
windpipe
wing-beating tremor
Wing's symbol
"wings" (street name, cocaine; heroin)
winstrol (oral steroid)
winstrol V (veterinary steroid)
wired on cocaine
WISC (Wechsler Intelligence Scale for Children)
WISC-R Split-Half Short Form
wisdom teeth
wish, intense
wishes
    cross-gender
    disturbing
"witch" (street name, cocaine; heroin)
"witch hazel" (street name, heroin)
withdrawal
    alcohol, with no perceptual disturbance (F10.239)
    alcohol, with perceptual disturbance (F10.232)
    amphetamine (F15.23)
    anxiolytic-type with perceptual disturbance (F13.232)
    anxiolytic-type with no perceptual disturbance (F13.239)
    caffeine (F15.93)
    cannabis (F12.288)
    cocaine (F14.23)
    hypnotic-type with no perceptual disturbance (F13.239)
    hypnotic-type with perceptual disturbance (F13.232)
    nicotine/tobacco (F17.203)
    opioid (F11.23)
    sedative-type with no perceptual disturbance (F13.239)
    sedative-type with perceptual disturbance (F13.232)
    stimulants, other (F15.23)
    substance, other or unknown (F19.239)
withdrawal criteria, equivalent
withdrawal delirium
    alcohol
    anxiolytic
    hypnotic
    sedative
    substance
withdrawal disorder, caffeine
withdrawal from social affairs
withdrawal insomnia
withdrawal movement(s)
withdrawal seizure, alcohol
withdrawal signs and symptoms
withdrawal state(s)
withdrawal symptom, sedative hypnotic
withdrawal syndrome, characteristic
withdrawal tremor, substance
WJ (Woodcock-Johnson Psycho-Educational Battery)
WJ-R ACH (Tests of Achievement)
WJ-R COG (Tests of Cognitive Abilities)
WLB (Woodcock Language Proficiency Battery)
WMI (Work Motivation Inventory)
WMS (Wechsler Memory Scale)
"wobble weed" (street name, phencyclidine)

"wolf" (street name, phencyclidine/PCP)
Wolfe Microcomputer User Aptitude Test
"wollie" (street name, crack and cannabis)
women, vulnerability to trauma in
women's counselor
Wonderlic Personnel Test, The
Woodcock Language Proficiency Battery (WLPB)
Woodcock Language Proficiency Battery—English Form
Woodcock Reading Mastery Tests (WRMT)
Woodcock-Johnson Psycho-Educational Battery (WJ)
word(s)
    ambiguous
    base
    broken
    class
    clipped
    complex
    compound
    content
    contentive
    feared
    form
    function
    heterogeneous
    homogenous
    inappropriate
    interstitial
    Jonah
    lexical
    monosyllabic
    nonsense
    nonsensical
    open
    paradigmatic
    PB (phonetically balanced)
    pivot
    polysyllabic
    portmanteau
    process
    relational
    root

word(s)
    searching for
    sign
    simple
    split
    spondee
    standard
    structure
    syntagmatic
    telescoped
word analysis test *(see also* tests)
word approximation
Word Association Test
word calling
word classes
word configuration
word count
word deafness, pure
word discrimination score
word-finding ability, disturbance in
word-finding difficulty
word-finding problem
word-finding skills
word finding tests
word lists
word method, key
Word Processing Test
Word Processor Assessment Battery
word production, stressful
word reading test *(see also* tests)
word recognition skills *(see also* tests)
Word Recognition Test
word repetition, senseless imitative
word retrieval problem
word retrieval task
Word Search
word sequence
word spelling test *(see also* tests)
work, neglect of school-
Work Attitudes Questionnaire (WAQ)
work disability
work dysfunction
Work Environment Scale (WES)

work group
Work Interest Index
Work Motivation Inventory (WMI)
work-related problem
Work Skills Series Production (WSS)
work values *(see also* tests)
"working" (re: crack dealing)
"working half" (re: crack weights)
working relationship
workplace violence
"works" (re: equipment for injecting drugs)
World Health Organization (WHO)
World Health Organization - Disability Assessment Schedule (WHO–DAS)
world of reality, external
World Psychiatric Association (WPA)
"worm" (street name, phencyclidine/PCP)
worries, hyperresponsible
worry
 constant
 excessive
 focus of
 uncontrolled
worse sleep continuity
worth, inflated
wound, self-inflicted gunshot
WPA (World Psychiatric Association)
WRAT (Wide Range Achievement Test)
"wrecking crew" (street name, crack)
write a sentence test
writer's cramp
writing, assessment of
writing ability
writing skills
writing, thinking, and reading skills *(see also* tests)
writing tremor
written English *(see also* tests)

written expression, disorder of
Written Language Assessment
written spelling test *(see also* tests)
WRMT (Woodcock Reading Mastery Tests)
"wrong" sex
wryneck
WSS (Work Skills Series) production

x (times)
"X" (street name, amphetamine; cannabis; methylendioxy-methamphetamine)
X-bar theory
xenomania
xenophobia
xerophobia
"X-ing" MDMA (re: ecstasy/methylendioxymethamphetamine use)
X-linkage
X-linked dominance
X syndrome, fragile
"XTC" (street name, ecstasy/methylenedioxy-methamphetamine)

Y

Y-cord hearing aid
"yahoo/yeaho" (street name, crack)
"Yale" (street name, crack)
Yale-Brown Obsessive-Compulsive Scale (YBOCS)
yawn-sign approach
YBOCS (Yale-Brown Obsessive-Compulsive Scale)
year test, month of
"yeh" (street name, cannabis)
"yellow" (street name, lysergic acid diethylamide/LSD; barbiturate)
"yellow bam" (street name, methamphetamine)
"yellow dimples" (street name, lysergic acid diethylamide/LSD)
"yellow fever" (street name, phencyclidine/PCP)
"yellow submarine" (street name, cannabis; LSD)
"yen pop" (street name, cannabis)
"Yen Shee Suey" (street name, opium wine)
"yen sleep" (re: lysergic acid diethylamide/LSD use)
"yerba" (street name, cannabis)
"yerba mala" (street name, phencyclidine and cannabis)
YES (Youth Enjoying Sobriety)
yes-no question
yes-yes tremor
"yesca" (street name, cannabis)
"yesco" (street name, cannabis)
"yeyo" (street name, cocaine)
"yimyom" (street name, crack)
yoke, alveolar

young, developmentary appropriate self-stimulatory behaviors in the
youth counselor
youth employment skills *(see also* tests)
Youth Enjoying Sobriety (YES)
youth ministry, determining needs in

Z

"Z" (re: 1 ounce of heroin)
"Zacatecas purple" (street name, cannabis)
"zambi" (street name, cannabis)
"zen" (street name, lysergic acid diethylamide/LSD)
"zero" (street name, opium)
zero, audiometric
zero amplitude
zero cerebral
zero hearing level
zero level, reference
zero morpheme (0)
"zig zag man" (re: cannabis equipment)
"zig zag man" (street name, lysergic acid diethylamide/LSD; cannabis)
"zip" (street name, cocaine)
"zol" (street name, cannabis cigarette)
"zombie" (re: drug user)
"zombie" (street name, phencyclidine/PCP)
"zombie weed" (street name, phencyclidine/PCP)
zone, time
"zooie" (re: cannabis equipment)
"zoom" (street name, phencyclidine/PCP; cannabis and phencyclidine)
zoomania
"zoomers" (re: dealers in fake crack)
zoster meningitis, herpes
Zubsolv (buprenorphine/naloxone)
Zung Self-Rating Depression Scale
zygomatic bones

APPENDIX

MUSCLES OF LARYNX, PALATE, PHARYNX, RESPIRATION, TONGUE

(Note: The Latin singular form "musculus" with its modifiers is used when a single muscle or a single pair of muscles is described. In a few instances multiple pairs of muscles are described. In these instances the plural form "musculi" with its modifiers is used.)

I LARYNX MUSCLES

Extrinsic Muscles (Suprahyoid)

a) digastric muscle, anterior (musculus digastricus anterior) (1 pair)
b) digastric muscle, posterior (musculus digastricus posterior) (1 pair)
c) geniohyoid muscle (musculus geniohyoideus) (1 pair)
d) mylohyoid muscle (musculus mylohyoideus)
e) stylohyoid muscle (musculus stylohyoideus) (1 pair)

Extrinsic Muscles (Infrahyoid)

a) omohyoid muscle, anterior (musculus omohyoideus anterior) (1 pair)
b) omohyoid muscle, posterior (musculus omohyoideus posterior) (1 pair)
c) sternohyoid muscle (musculus sternohyoideus) (1 pair)
d) sternothyroid muscle (musculus sternothyroideus) (1 pair)
e) thyrohyoid muscle (musculus thyrohyoideus) (1 pair)

Intrinsic Muscles

a) aryepiglottic muscle (musculus aryepiglotticus)
b) arytenoid muscle, oblique (musculus arytenoideus obliquus)
c) arytenoid muscle, transverse (musculus arytenoideus transversus)
d) cricoarytenoid muscle, lateral (musculus cricoarytenoideus lateralis)
e) cricoarytenoid muscle, posterior (musculus cricoarytenoideus posterior)
f) cricothyroid muscle (musculus cricothyroideus)
g) thyroarytenoid muscle (musculus thyroarytenoideus)
h) thyroepiglottic muscle (musculus thyroepiglotticus)
i) vocal muscle (musculus vocalis)

II PALATE MUSCLES

a) elevator muscle of soft palate (musculus levator veli palatini)
b) glossopalatine or palatoglossus muscle (musculus palatoglossus)
c) pharyngopalatine or palatopharyngeus muscle (musculus palatopharyngeus)
d) tensor muscle of the soft palate (musculus tensor palati or musculus tensor veli palatini)
e) uvula muscle or muscle of the uvula (musculus uvulae)

III PHARYNX MUSCLES

a) constrictor muscle of pharynx, inferior (musculus constrictor pharyngis inferior)
b) constrictor muscle of pharynx, middle (musculus constrictor pharyngis medius)
c) constrictor muscle of pharynx, superior (musculus constrictor pharyngis superior)
d) salpingopharyngeal or salpingopharyngeus muscle (musculus salpingopharyngeus)
e) stylopharyngeal or stylopharyngeus muscle (musculus stylopharyngeus)

IV MUSCLES OF RESPIRATION

The Diaphragm (the musculomembranous partition between the abdominal and thoracic cavities; principal muscle of inhalation, also aids in expiration)

Inhalation (Quiet) Muscles

a) elevator muscles of ribs (musculi levatores costarum) (12 pairs)
b) intercostal muscles, external (musculi intercostales externi) (11 pairs)
c) scalene muscle, anterior (musculus scalenus anterior) (1 pair)
d) scalene muscle, middle (musculus scalenus medius) (1 pair)
e) scalene muscle, posterior (musculus scalenus posterior) (1 pair)

Inhalation (Forced) Muscles

a) latissimus dorsi muscle (musculus latissimus dorsi) (1 pair)
b) pectoral muscle, greater (musculus pectoralis major) (1 pair)
c) pectoral muscle, smaller (musculus pectoralis minor) (1 pair)
d) serratus muscle, anterior (musculus serratus anterior) (1 pair)
e) serratus muscle, posterior inferior (musculus serratus posterior inferior) (1 pair)
f) serratus muscle, posterior superior (musculus serratus posterior superior) (1 pair)

g) sternoclavicular muscle (musculus sternoclavicularis) (variable)
h) sternocleidomastoid muscle (musculus sternocleido-mastoideus) (1 pair)
i) subclavian or subclavius muscle (musculus subclavius) (1 pair)

Exhalation Muscles

a) iliocostal muscle of loins or lumbar iliocostal muscle (musculus iliocostalis lumborum)
b) iliocostal muscle of thorax (musculus iliocostalis thoracis or musculus iliocostalis dorsi)
c) intercostal muscles, internal (musculi intercostales interni) (11 pairs)
d) oblique muscle of abdomen, external (musculus obliquus externus abdominis) (1 pair)
e) oblique muscle of abdomen, internal (musculus obliquus internus abdominis) (1 pair)
f) quadrate muscle of loins or lumbar quadrate muscle (musculus quadratus lumborum) (1 pair)
g) rectus muscle of the abdomen (musculus rectus abdominis) (1 pair)
h) serratus muscle, inferior posterior (musculus serratus posterior inferior) (1 pair)
i) subcostal muscle (musculus subcostalis) (1 pair)
j) transverse muscle of the abdomen (musculus transversus abdominis) (1 pair)
k) transverse muscle of the thorax (musculus transversus thoracis) (1 pair)

V   MUSCLES OF THE TONGUE

Extrinsic Muscles

a) genioglossal or genioglossus muscle (musculus genioglossus)
b) hyoglossal or hyoglossus muscle (musculus hyoglossus)
c) palatoglossus muscle (musculus palatoglossus)
d) styloglossus muscle (musculus styloglossus)

Intrinsic Muscles

a) longitudinal muscle of tongue, inferior (musculus longitudinalis inferior linguae)
b) longitudinal muscle of tongue, superior (musculus longitudinalis superior linguae)
c) transverse muscle of tongue (musculus transversus linguae)
d) vertical muscle of tongue (musculus verticalis linguae)

About the Authors

Mary Ann D'Onofrio earned and maintained credentials as a certified medical transcriptionist (CMT) and accredited record technician (ART) in the course of her 41 years of work in the health information field, until her retirement in 2013. As a graduate of the University of Michigan, with a master's degree in information/library science (AMLS), she remains committed to research. In 2018 Mary Ann received the Albert Nelson Marquis Lifetime Achievement Award as a biographee who has achieved career longevity and has demonstrated unwavering excellence in her chosen field. Her many years working in psychiatric clinic, hospital and physician office settings have provided her with a wide knowledge of psychiatric medical terminology and coding practices. During her career she was an active member of the American Association of Medical Transcriptionists (AAMT, now AHDI), from which she received the Distinguished Member Award in 1984. Her regular columns for the AAMT Journal, including "What's Your MT Quotient" and "Scope," appeared for six years. She has been a contributing author to Health Professions Institute's *Perspectives* magazine. Her first joint venture with her daughter Elizabeth was as editor of the AAMT "Annotated Bibliography." They collaborated again on *Psychiatric Words and Phrases* (Health Professions Institute, 1990) as well as the book's Second Edition (HPI, 1998). Mary Ann lives in Lexington, Kentucky. Her interests include photography, political analysis and watching the thoroughbreds race at Keeneland.

About the Authors

Elizabeth D'Onofrio joined the field of medical transcription in 1988, with a specialty in psychiatry/psychology. She and Mary Ann operated a medical transcription business together for over 25 years. A graduate of the University of Arizona, Elizabeth is a former member of the Health Professions Institute staff and has also been a contributing author to its *Perspectives* magazine. Today Elizabeth is the owner/publisher of Little Pebble Press, as well as an author of fiction and nonfiction.

other books from
Little Pebble Press:

12 Days of Christmas Coloring Book
Saints Cathedral Windows Coloring Books
Color Me Comic Book with Paper Dolls
O Antiphons Coloring Book
Distant Eyes
Sword Striker
At the Ball
Charm of the Gloaming
The Crystals of Yukitake
Casey the Crocodoodle
Living Happy: Insights from a Blind Kitty
Healing Memory: Transforming the Mind with the Holy Spirit

find them at:
www.littlepebblepress.com